Brief Contents

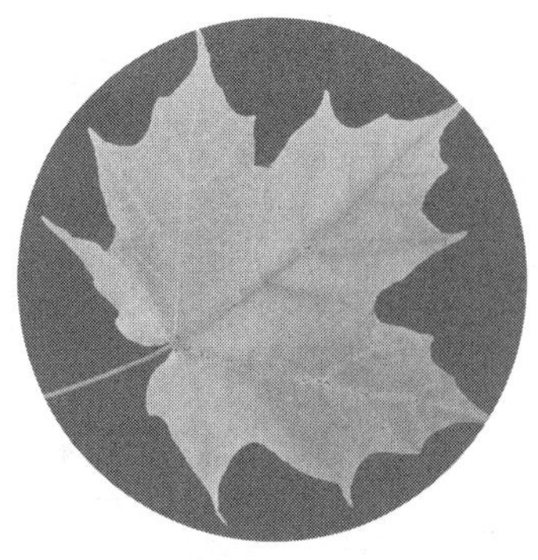

Contents

Preface

Throughout our many combined years of teaching consumer health courses, our students expressed an increasing interest in the exploration of topics related to alternative health practices. Unfortunately, we came to find that there are few consumer health texts available that explore the topic of alternative health practices and methods of healing in addition to coverage of the core topics. It became evident that a new approach was needed, and from that need this text was conceived. We wrote this text, *Complementary and Alternative Medicine for Health Professionals: A Holistic Approach to Consumer Health*, to aid our students and readers in learning more about these practices, so they might become more savvy health consumers.

Today, being a health consumer encompasses more than being knowledgeable about traditional medicine and health practices; it also includes the necessity to be knowledgeable about the expanding field of complementary and alternative medicine here in the United States.

We realized that health professionals could not learn much about these alternative modalities within one or two chapters, as was the norm in other consumer health texts. Therefore, our outline for this book provided for many chapters that would include the major alternative medicine systems and healing modalities, including Ayurvedic medicine, traditional Chinese medicine, naturopathic medicine, homeopathic remedies, chiropractic, massage, reflexology, herbals or botanicals, and essential oils.

Our vision for the consumer health portion of the text was to make the information fun to learn and applicable to students' lives. We have gone to great lengths to provide accurate and meaningful information on a vast array of practices, as well as information on how to evaluate treatments and quackery, and to leave the consumer to explore more and make their own conclusions. The mission was to increase the reader's knowledge base, not to make up their mind for them. We all make better choices related to our own personal healthcare practices when we are informed consumers.

This text includes many valuable features, including:

- *Lesson Objectives:* Each chapter opens with a short list of lesson objectives. We could have written many more, but only wanted to touch on a few main points related to the specific chapter. The lesson objectives are written as broad-based learning objectives rather than specific for each heading and paragraph content.
- *Content:* We open the text with a chapter that introduces the purpose of learning about health consumerism and the costs involved. Often we strive for good health by purchasing agents or services that we believe will make us healthier. This includes traditional or orthodox practices (seeing a medical doctor, joining a fitness facility, purchasing exercise equipment) as well as alternative medicine practices (seeing a chiropractor, getting a massage, or buying some herbal preparations). If we purchase health-related resources, we need to become knowledgeable health consumers. We also need to engage in positive health practices for the right reasons, not necessarily to avoid becoming ill but to enhance our lives.

We included a chapter on scientific method (Chapter 2) so that readers can learn more about the characteristics of research design, the types of research, and where to find valid health information. We all should decide whether a health product or practice meets certain scientific criteria, and if it doesn't, we need to consider the reasons why not. We then can make an intelligent health purchase. We can also use this knowledge when we read or listen to advertising blogs. The chapter on advertising (Chapter 3) helps us to consider the tricks involved.

The cost of health care in the United States is spiraling ever-higher. Chapter 4 outlines the reasons for rising healthcare costs, the expenditures, and ways to control costs. Healthcare programs in the United States and the healthcare delivery system are complex. We have tried to sort out the reasons for this in Chapter 5.

The reason for inserting the integrative medicine and alternative medicine chapters in the middle third of the text comes from the way that Dr. Synovitz sets up her semester classes. She finds teaching the course is more fun by starting with traditional consumer health information, following with a few weeks of alternative medicine information, and then following with more traditional consumer health information.

The chapter on integrative medicine (Chapter 6) introduces the reader to the meaning of integrative medicine and integrative medicine clinics. Early pioneers who have promoted integrative medicine and alternative healing modalities are highlighted. Chapter 7 gives the historical foundations of holistic healing and the reasons people seek alternative forms of medical care. Key historical healing modalities, events, and professionals that have impacted present-day healing methods are identified.

Each of the chapters on the alternative medical systems (Chapters 8–13) describe the historical foundations, what each system is, the main principles or beliefs, the diagnostic techniques, the therapies, and related scientific studies. Chapter 14 on mind–body interventions includes six forms of meditation, the meditation positions, and techniques. The chapter also includes a history of yoga and how it works, and offers results of clinical studies. Also included in the same chapter is information about therapeutic hypnosis and how it is used; the Alexander technique and benefits; and the origins of biofeedback, how it works, and its effectiveness. Chapter 15 on energy therapies contains historical information and how each is used as a healing modality. Topics include tai chi ch'uan, qi gong, Reiki, therapeutic touch, and pulsed fields.

Following the alternative medicine chapters is a chapter on frauds and quackery (Chapter 16). We all need to realize that quacks operate out of both orthodox and alternative medicine healing fields.

Because we believe that students (readers) need to learn medical self-care, we wrote Chapter 17 to show how they can become responsible health consumers in and out of the home. Chapter 18 is devoted to showing students their rights as consumers. There are many agencies that can help us when we feel we have been a victim of fraud, and this chapter identifies several. The last chapter gives an in-depth look at health insurance in the United States, including the newly legislated Patient Protection and Affordable Care Act. Available health insurance options are described and forms of life insurance are differentiated. Finally, an appendix explains how to find available health resources.

- *Case Studies and "In the News" Features:* Each chapter contains one or two case studies and "In the News" features so that readers can apply chapter concepts in a more personal way. Case studies are presented as scenarios intended to evoke analytical thinking skills. Application of concepts presented are made easier because of the ways in which scenarios are presented. The "In the News" feature is also intended to engage the reader in an active learning process because it relates to the chapter topics. We offer questions concerning the news feature that encourage analytical thinking and make the situation or problem personally relevant.
- *Review Questions:* Many review questions can be found at the end of each chapter. These are intended to help the reader conceptualize and reflect on main points.
- *Suggestions for Class Activities:* As in any college course, we believe that students learn better when they are actively engaged in the classroom. Therefore, suggestions for classroom activities are included at the end of most chapters. This gives all students an opportunity to present in the classroom, work in a group, or engage in an activity. A classroom activity may also involve bringing in a practitioner who explains his or her practice and who then engages the class in a particular activity.
- *References:* Rather than compiling one large reference list for the entire text, each chapter has its own reference list. Some chapters have as few as 15 references and some have over 80. We have relied on Internet references as well as journal articles and books. In this modern day, we have many tools for compiling and writing books, and we have attempted to use as many types of them as possible.
- *Ancillaries:* Supportive materials that will be available for instructors include PowerPoint lecture outlines corresponding to each chapter, a test bank, a semester syllabus, and lesson plans. A student companion website is also available and can be accessed at go.jblearning.com/synovitz using the code bound into this book.

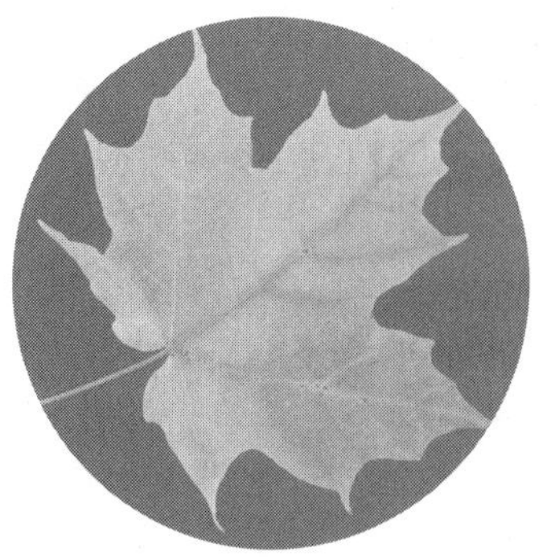

Acknowledgments

Dr. Synovitz: We could not have completed this project without the help and support of many others. First, I would like to thank my co-author, Dr. Larson, for working with me as we moved through this book writing journey. He was most cooperative and a diligent writer. I would like to thank my husband, Robert; my sons, Blake and Jared; my stepchildren, Steve, Ronald, Cathy, and Mark; and all my friends for their words of encouragement throughout the two and a half years it took to write this text. My department head, Dr. Eddie Hebert, and my department colleagues were especially supportive. I thank them for their motivating words and actions. My three graduate assistants, Katie Keen, Renee Autry, and Elizabeth Pardy were truly helpful in creating glossaries, taking photos for use in this text, and helping me create new PowerPoint lectures and edit the existing ones.

Dr. Larson: I would like to thank Dr. Synovitz for her tireless work in completing the manuscript. She is a true professional and a valued colleague. I thank my teaching colleagues at Gustavus Adolphus College for their support along the way. And, finally, my wife Kathy, for her support and love throughout the process of completing the text.

Both Authors: We would also like to thank the following reviewers for their valuable feedback:

William C. Andress, DrPH
La Sierra University
Department of Health and Exercise Science
Riverside, California

Martha Dallmeyer, PhD
Bradley University
Department of Family and Consumer Sciences
Peoria, Illinois

Ari Fisher, MA
Louisiana State University
Department of Kinesiology
Baton Rouge, Louisiana

Debra C. Harris, PhD, MST
University of Wisconsin: Oshkosh
Department of Human Kinetics and Health
Oshkosh, Wisconsin

Joseph Hudak, PhD
Ohio University Eastern
Department of Health Science
Clairsville, Ohio

Dr. Garry Ladd
Southwestern Illinois College
Department of Health and Exercise Science
Belleville, Illinois

Dr. Kirsten Lupinski
Assistant Professor, Health and Physical Education
Albany State University
Albany, Georgia

Audrey McCrary-Quarles, MSA, CHES, PhD
Assistant Professor, Health Education
South Carolina State University
Orangeburg, South Carolina

Linda Pina, PhD, RN
California University of Pennsylvania
Department of Nursing
California, Pennsylvania

Barbara Wright, MS
Virginia Western Community College
Department of Health and Physical Education
Roanoke, Virginia

We would like to thank several individuals for their help and/or permission to share materials: We thank Southeastern Louisiana University's Public Information office for use of a stock photo (Matthew in Chapter 1) and Jacob Barger, a student and Southeastern employee, for posing as John in Chapter 1. We thank Dr. Andrew Weil and Dr. Bernie Siegel for their personal correspondence and permission to use their photos in Chapter 6. Subdosha descriptions in Chapter 8 were originally published in Terra Rafael's book, *Ayurveda for the Childbearing Years* (2009). We thank her for permission to reprint them in our text. We thank Ken Chow, Dipl. OM, DNM, CBP, an acupuncturist from Baton Rouge, Louisiana, for sharing photos used in Chapter 9 depicting him conducting acupuncture and cupping. We thank Subhuti Dharmananda, PhD, Founder and Director of the Institute for Traditional Medicine in Portland, Oregon, for his review of Chapter 9 and also for allowing us to use, in that chapter, his Fifteen Most Commonly Used Herbals information. The Bach Centre in Oxon, England, was invaluable for providing and sharing information about *Bach® Original Flower Remedies*. In particular, we would like to thank Stefan Ball of the Bach Visitor & Education Centre, who was our contact. Stefan reviewed the chapter section on *Bach® Original Flower Remedies* and made several suggestions for revision. Dr. Pam Doughty wrote the initial draft of Chapter 19, and we thank her for that support.

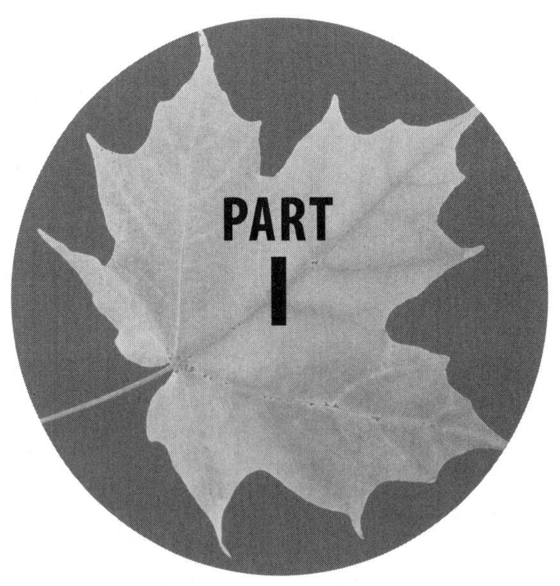

Understanding the Basics

Introduction to Consumer Health: Orthodox and Complementary and Alternative Medicine (CAM)

LEARNING OBJECTIVES

As a result of reading this chapter, students will:

1. Explain why it is important to become a responsible health consumer.
2. Describe what it means to be healthy.
3. Assess how a person in today's world could integrate traditional health practices with alternative therapies.
4. Compare and contrast similarities and differences between traditional medicine and CAM.

Note: Throughout this text, our use of the word healthcare will refer to a system that offers, provides, or delivers health care to individuals. Our use of the phrase, health care, will refer to care given to a patient by medical or health professionals.

WHAT IS THE PURPOSE OF LEARNING ABOUT HEALTH CONSUMERISM AND CAM?

This chapter is intended to get you motivated to become a better health consumer and to learn initial information regarding complementary and alternative medicine (CAM). All of us "consume" health by buying products or services to treat illnesses or to prevent disease or disorders. Those products and services encompass traditional therapies, such as prescription drugs, vitamins, minerals, pain medications, and other over the counter (OTC) drugs, and may include complementary and alternative therapies such as herbal supplements, massage therapy, and acupuncture.

As a health consumer, we join fitness centers or clubs where we "work out" or play golf or tennis. We use walking, running, or bicycle trails. So that youth can have a safe place to skateboard, many cities are building skateboard tracks within their city parks or other sites. To do many of these activities, we need to buy proper clothing: tennis or running shoes and outfits, swimsuits, and so forth. As a result of our fitness-seeking lifestyle we spend a lot of money, and we need to learn to spend wisely. We can only do that if we are knowledgeable about the services we are purchasing.

Why do we buy health products or engage in fitness activities? Why do we believe it's important to make better food choices when we go to the grocery store? Why do many people look for, and select, organic foods? It seems that we are chasing after good health.

HOW COSTLY IS CHASING AFTER GOOD HEALTH?

People want to be healthy because they perceive that healthy people feel and look better, and they appear more youthful. Because of this, individuals of every race and culture seek ways to become healthier and, in so doing, they collectively spend billions of dollars. It is wonderful that people want to become healthier, but the health care that is needed requires financing. Part of the funding for health care comes from private and governmentally funded insurance programs. For very poor countries, publicly financed development assistance is available in the form of financial resources and improved effectiveness of resources. As an example, spending on health care by health-related worldwide agencies, governmental (e.g., World Health Organization [WHO], United Nations Children's Fund [UNICEF]) and nongovernmental (e.g., Bill and Melinda Gates Foundation), has increased from $5 billion in 1990 to $21.8 billion in 2007. In 2007, $10 billion of that amount was spent by the United States.[1] Per capita, the United States spends approximately $6,714, an amount reported to be much more than two dozen other developed countries.[2]

As can be seen, we value our health and we spend great amounts of money to achieve healthier lifestyles and to seek medical treatment when needed. It is important, therefore, to gain an understanding of the meaning of health and disease/illness conditions.

WHAT IS THE MEANING OF HEALTH AND DISEASE/ILLNESS?

Disease and Illness

A disease can be either a mental or physical condition. An example of a mental disease is depression, which is treatable with certain medications and/or counseling. A physical disease generally is caused by a germ (pathogen) that could be bacterial, viral, fungal, and so forth. Depending on the type of pathogen, usually a medical doctor will order medicinal treatment. Not all physical diseases, however, are caused by pathogens. They may have a genetic (inherited) cause or may be caused by an autoimmune response, such as occurs with arthritis or gout. Even if people have a disease condition (whether mental or physical), they may not always feel unwell or uncomfortable. When people have the flu or a cold, they usually consider themselves ill. The perception of feeling the symptoms of a disease is considered an illness.

To illustrate further, examine the following case study.

Health

What is the meaning of "health"? It appears to be an elusive quality that we seem to cherish, but have difficulty maintaining. In our current world, most health professionals view health in a holistic manner, an approach to health care that aims at treating the whole person, both body and mind, rather than focusing solely on a specific set of symptoms. It encompasses the physical, mental, emotional, social, sexual, and spiritual domains. The 2000 Joint Committee on Health Education Terminology[3] has presented several definitions of health.

- A state of complete physical, mental, and social well-being, and not merely the absence of disease and infirmity (WHO definition of health).
- A quality of life involving dynamic interaction and independence among the individual's physical well-being, his (sic) mental and emotional reactions, and the social complex in which he (sic) exists.
- An integrated method of functioning that is oriented toward maximizing the potential of which the individual is capable. It requires that the individual maintain a continuum of balance and purposeful direction with the environment where he (sic) is functioning.

Because it allows for individual differences regarding levels of health, the latter health definition has great potential for more accurately assessing health status. It speaks to the potential that people have for achieving their personal, maximal level of good health. The following case study explains this health definition more clearly.

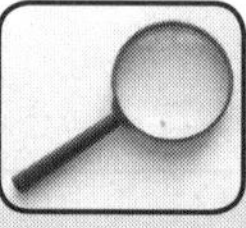

Case Study

Judy is a 19-year-old college student who has been having unprotected sexual intercourse with her boyfriend, Tom. Unknown to her, Tom has been having unprotected sexual intercourse with another college female who has chlamydia, a bacterial sexually transmitted disease (STD). Tom is having some penile discharge but it is not causing him much discomfort, so he ignores it and continues to have sex with both Judy and the other woman. Judy is one of the 80 to 90% of women who do not show immediate symptoms of chlamydia (e.g., vaginal irritation and redness, swollen labia, vaginal discharge). A couple of months after contracting the STD, Judy began to get an elevated temperature, low pelvic pain, and a discharge. When that occurred, Judy experienced symptoms of the disease and felt ill. At this point, we could say that Judy has the subjective state of illness. An illness is a description of the physical or mental condition of a person who shows symptoms of disease or sickness; an unhealthy state.[3] This event caused Judy to go to a doctor for testing and diagnosis, at which point Judy learned she had the disease called chlamydia.

All of us will experience being ill and having a disease at some point in our lives. We will turn to our traditional doctors for diagnosis and treatment; we may seek an alternative practitioner for care; or we may attempt self-care. The reason that we do this is to feel healthy.

Questions:

1. What is good health?
2. Why don't all people experience the same level of health?
3. Do we all seek health for the same reasons? If not, what are those reasons?

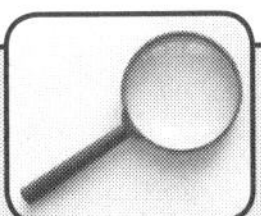

Case Study

Let's contrast the health behaviors of two males, each age 22 years. John has a chronic disease diagnosed as muscular dystrophy, which causes progressive weakness and degeneration of the skeletal muscles that control movement. His disease has progressed to the point that he is now confined to a wheelchair. Please refer to a photo of John in **FIGURE 1.1**.

Matthew is a 22-year-old college baseball player. He is handsome, lean, muscular, and has no known disease condition. Please see the photo of Matthew in **FIGURE 1.2**.

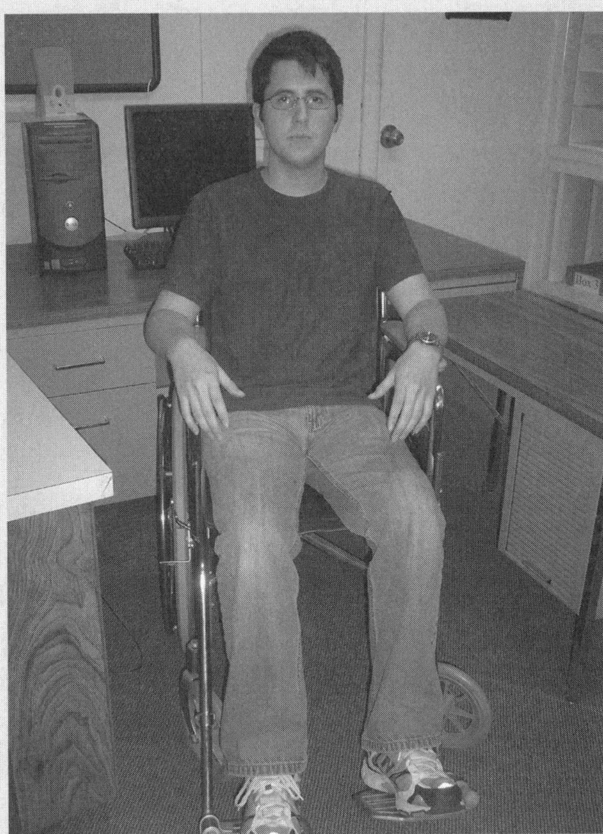

FIGURE 1.1 John.

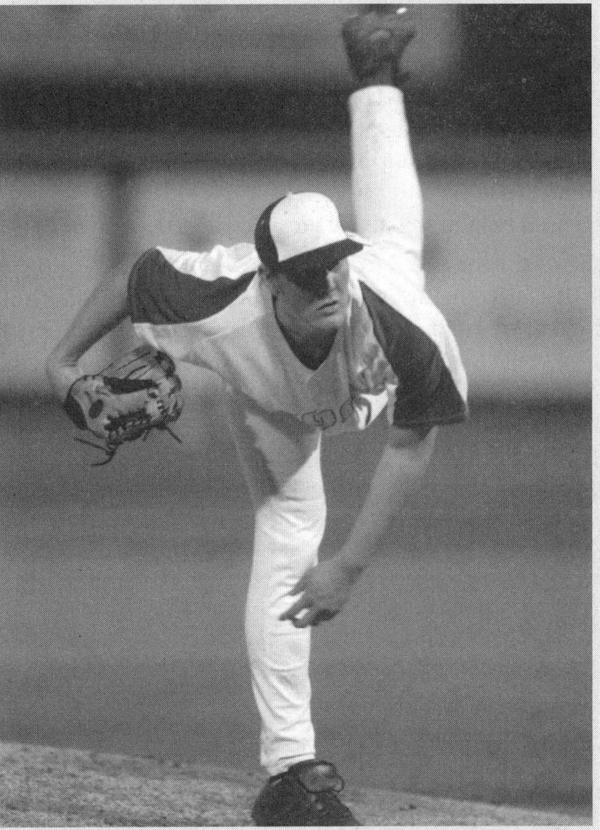

FIGURE 1.2 Matthew.

Based on the descriptions provided thus far, which of the two would you say is healthier?

Now let's learn more about each young man. John, who has muscular dystrophy, maximizes his health potential because he follows physicians' medical orders, attends physical therapy sessions, eats a diet appropriate for his health condition, and follows a prescribed exercise regimen. John spends time tutoring at-risk youth at the local high school, has a great sense of humor, and his peers love to be around him.

Matthew, the college athlete, has a less healthy lifestyle and engages in risky health behaviors. He takes steroids, does not eat a healthy diet, drinks heavily on the weekends, drives while drunk, does not use a seatbelt, and practices unsafe sexual practices. He has very few friends because he has an explosive personality and is very egocentric. Based on this description, who do you believe is healthier?

If all individuals could strive to maximize their potential for being healthy, we would see a definite decrease in morbidity (diseases) and mortality (deaths). This case study scenario has demonstrated that a person could have the physical appearance of high quality health but, in actuality, be very unhealthy.

Illness-Avoiding Behaviors and Health-Enhancing Behaviors

Health practices can be considered as illness-avoiding or health-enhancing behaviors. Individuals may practice healthy behaviors because they want to avoid getting sick or they may practice healthy behaviors because they want to enhance their health. People who practice health-enhancing behaviors do not live in fear that if they don't practice good health, they will acquire some illness or die. Rather, they practice healthy behaviors because they like the way it makes them feel, function, and look. Health-enhancing behaviors are those that should be practiced over a lifetime. As depicted in **BOX 1.1**, several major differences exist between illness avoiding and health-enhancing behaviors.

As presented in Box 1.1, one of the illness-avoiding behaviors is setting short-term health-related goals, which is discussed next in the application of concepts section.

Informed Consumer: Application of Concepts

You are in your junior year of college and the month is January. You and several of your friends are planning a spring break trip to Cancun, Mexico. It has been a stressful year because you have had to take many upper-level science courses (organic chemistry, biology, and physics) and you have been working 20 hours per week. You have been overeating and not exercising like you used to do. Because of this, you have gained 15 pounds and perceive yourself as being fat. You want to begin a diet and exercise plan so that you will lose weight in order to look "buff" or sexy.

1. What short-term goals should you set?
2. What long-term goals should you set?

You begin your training in January in preparation for the April trip. Lo and behold, the goal is met: you lose weight, acquire some level of muscle mass, and look "leaner" and "sexier."

Questions for Discussion:

1. Do you feel better about yourself?
2. What will be your health habits from now on?
3. If your behavior was only practiced to look good for spring break, once it is over, what is the chance that you will continue to eat nutritiously and keep exercising?

We can conclude that people may practice healthy behaviors because they love how it makes them feel or they may practice healthy behaviors because they have a greater fear of becoming ill. The result is that many individuals seek help in achieving a higher level of wellness. For this, they may turn to either orthodox (traditional) medicine or alternative means.

Box 1.1
Illness-Avoidance Behaviors vs. Health-Enhancing Behaviors

ILLNESS-AVOIDING BEHAVIORS	HEALTH-ENHANCING BEHAVIORS
Avoiding illness is highest priority	High health is highest priority Enjoy healthy behaviors
Motivated by return to health or alleviation of symptoms	Motivated by feeling good, better, best
Minimal goal	Maximal goal
Desire immediate or short-term results	Desire long-term results
Need measurable results	More nebulous results are okay
Time-limited activity	Ongoing activity
Medical-centered motivation	Ego-centric motivation
Authority dominated	Internal control
Fear as motivator	Accomplishment as motivator
External checks mandatory	Few external checks
External rewards	Internal rewards
Specific behaviors	Diffuse behaviors
Reactive (to symptoms or threat of symptoms)	Proactive (don't need that negative force)

WHAT ARE ORTHODOX AND COMPLEMENTARY AND ALTERNATIVE MEDICINE PRACTICES?

Orthodox Medicine

Orthodox medicine is also known as traditional medicine. Orthodox physicians may be either allopathic or osteopathic doctors. An allopathic physician is a medical doctor (MD). An osteopathic physician is a DO. Both have similar academic training and clinical experiences. These are the physicians that have been the mainstream of our traditional medical care. Other examples of orthodox practitioners are nurses, dentists, social workers, registered dietitians, and health educators. Later chapters of this text include information on how one can find a medical physician and the costs associated with diagnostics and treatment.

Complementary and Alternative Medicine (CAM)

CAM includes a myriad of approaches to health care provided by a variety of practitioners. As defined by the National Center for Complementary and Alternative Medicine (NCCAM) at the National Institutes of Health, CAM is "a group of diverse medical and health care systems, practices, and products that are not presently considered to be part of conventional medicine."[4, p1] The NCCAM was established for the purpose of scientifically testing and assessing CAM therapies for safety and efficacy. Those therapies used to complement traditional medical therapies (e.g., use of aromatherapy after surgery) are identified as complementary;

Box 1.2

Orthodox Medicine and CAM: Similarities and Differences

- Both orthodox medicine and alternative health care embrace holistic health concepts.
- Alternative practices are generally viewed as unorthodox from the standpoint of scientific medicine as currently taught in medical schools.
- Alternative health care is more emphatic about the role of the individual in maintaining his or her own health.
- Practitioners of orthodox medicine all must fulfill certain kinds and amounts of training, education, and licensing.
- Orthodox practitioners tend to treat symptoms of a disease or some other sick or unhealthy state.
- Alternative health care providers embrace a wide variety of possible practices and emphasize the body's natural self-restoration properties.

those used as a replacement for traditional medical practices (e.g., use of a special diet to treat cancer rather than surgery or chemotherapy) are known as alternative.

A major difference between traditional and alternative modalities is that CAM practices accentuate the role of the individual in maintaining his or her health.[5,6] Alternative health care practitioners also embrace a wide variety of possible practices that emphasize the body's natural self-restoration properties. Please see **BOX 1.2**, which depicts similarities and differences between traditional and alternative practices.

The NCCAM has divided CAM therapies into five categories[4]: (1) alternative medical systems (homeopathic medicine, naturopathic medicine, traditional Chinese medicine, and Ayurvedic medicine), (2) mind–body interventions (meditation, prayer, mental healing, art, music, or dance), (3) biologically-based therapies (dietary supplements, herbal medicine), (4) manipulative and body-based therapies (chiropractic, osteopathic, massage), and (5) energy therapies (qi gong, Reiki, therapeutic touch, pulsed fields, and magnetic fields). Acupuncture, acupressure, and Tai chi ch'uan are practices used in traditional Chinese medicine. Other examples of CAM therapies include prayer utilized for healing, faith healing, Alexander technique, reflexology, yoga, hypnosis, biofeedback, and deep breathing exercises. Chapters devoted to more in-depth discussion of alternative therapies are included in this text.

WHY DO PEOPLE SEEK ALTERNATIVE HEALTH CARE?

Three major reasons[7,8] have been identified to explain the increased use of alternative health care:

1. Dissatisfaction with conventional treatment as expensive, impersonal, and ineffective
2. Feeling empowered to make one's own health care decisions
3. Compatibility with users' own values and spiritual beliefs regarding the nature of their illness

One persuasive appeal of CAM is the association of CAM with nature.[6] Many of the CAM practices comprise natural rather than artificial therapies and supplements. Terms such as "pure" versus "synthetic" comprise the language. Organic rather than processed foods are bought and consumed. As a result, stores that sell herbal supplements and organic food supplies have proliferated into the thousands and can be found in most cities (e.g., Whole Foods stores). The result is that a nationwide government study, co-funded by NCCAM, found that in 2007, $34 billion[4] was spent to seek "natural" means to good health. About two-thirds of that money was spent on self-care.

Thus far in this chapter, we have discussed the meaning of health and illness and provided an introduction to orthodox and CAM helping practices. We, the consumers, have to make decisions about the type of health care we want to

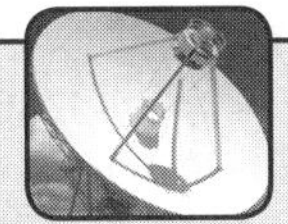

In the News

A June 9, 2010, news article from MSNBC news described the increased use of pesticides as a contributing factor to the increase in ADHD in children.[9] In fact, children who showed high markers of pesticide residue in their systems had a 93% greater likelihood of ADHD symptoms. The compound commonly found in pesticides is organophosphates, which are known to disrupt the neurological systems of insects. This is a purposeful objective in order to aid in insect control. Even children who live in cities have high markers for this pesticide because the exposure comes from the air we breath and the foods we consume. Some of those foods that may contain pesticides are blueberries, strawberries, and celery. All should be washed with cold water before eating. This is a reason that people are drawn to buying foods that are 100% organically grown.

use and the types of products we want to buy. Let's now explore what being a consumer of health means.

WHAT DOES IT MEAN TO BE A HEALTH CONSUMER?

Americans like "stuff." We like to have as much as possible, right? Stereos, iPods, video gaming systems, computers, clothing, cars, houses, boats . . . we like our stuff, and every time we buy something, we are acting as a consumer. We seek out a product, we purchase that product, we use that product, and, when it is gone or stops working, we throw the product away and replace that product. In other words, we consume the product. Our nation's economy is built on this function, called a material economy, and the economy relies on individuals to keep buying things to keep it healthy.

Because we are consumers of goods and services, including health services, we need to make wise and intelligent decisions when spending our money to buy "good health." A major goal in *Healthy People 2020*[10], reads, "Improve the health literacy of the population." Three objectives related to that goal are:

1. Increase the proportion of persons who report their health care provider always gave them easy-to-understand instructions about what to do to take care of their illness or health condition.
2. Increase the proportion of persons who report their health care provider always asked them to describe how they will follow the instructions.
3. Increase the proportion of persons who report their health care providers' office always offered help in filling out a form.

Cornacchia et al.[11] describe consumer health as follows:

> It deals with the decisions individuals make in regard to the purchase and use of the available health products and services that will have a direct effect on their health. It involves the economic, or monetary, aspects of health over which individuals have control. Consumer health includes self-motivated or self-initiated actions, which may include the purchase of a bottle of aspirin tablets or a dentifrice or the selection of a physician, dentist or nursing home. It is not what health departments or others do to control disease through clinics or information. However, a consumer's decision to use such services or information is consumer health.

The health consumer is the one who buys or otherwise acquires, consumes, or makes and then uses services or products intended to promote health. Prior to 1960, there was no history related to protecting the consumer from fraudulent or dangerous products. In 1962, President John F. Kennedy was so concerned about consumer rights that he made it a focus during a speech.[12] At that time, President Kennedy outlined four basic rights; later they were expanded to six basic rights. **BOX 1.3** shows the six basic consumer rights.

Box 1.3
Consumer Bill of Rights

President John F. Kennedy first conceptualized the Consumer Bill of Rights in 1962. This was professional regulation to serve the public interest. The following are the six basic consumer rights:

- *The right to safety:* To be protected against the marketing of goods that are hazardous to health or to life
- *The right to be informed:* To be protected against fraudulent, deceitful, or grossly misleading information, advertising, labeling, or other practices, and to be given the facts needed to make informed choices
- *The right to choose:* To be assured, wherever possible, access to a variety of products and services at competitive prices; in those industries in which competition is not workable and government regulation is substituted, an assurance of satisfactory quality and service at fair prices
- *The right to be heard:* To be assured that consumer interests will receive full and sympathetic consideration in the formulation of government policy, and fair and expeditious treatment in its administrative tribunal
- *The right to education:* To have access to programs and information that help consumers make better marketplace decisions
- *The right to redress:* To work with established mechanisms to have problems corrected and to receive compensation for poor service or for products that do not function properly

Source: John F. Kennedy Presidential Library and Museum. Special message to Congress on protecting consumer interest, 15 March 1962. Digital Identifier JFKPOF-037-028. Available at: http://www.jfklibrary.org/Asset-Viewer/Archives/JFKPOF-037-028.aspx. Accessed August 24, 2011.

WHAT IS CONSUMER ADVOCACY?

Consumer advocacy reached new levels in 1965 when Ralph Nader[13] published *Unsafe at Any Speed*, a book detailing the manufacturing flaws in the auto industry. Since that time, Nader has been a leading advocate for consumer health and safety. His followers, called Nader's Raiders, have been conducting research and providing advocacy for more than 40 years, spurring the creation and eventual passage into law of a wide range of consumer policy.

We health consumers need to take responsibility for the choices we make. A term for that is *caveat emptor*, which is a warning that means "let the buyer beware." The concept of *caveat emptor* came from the Romans and then became part of English law, the Statute of Frauds, which was enacted by the English Parliament in 1677. It held that a victim of his own mistakes had little or no recourse in the courts. Today, *caveat emptor* is a principle of commerce stating that if no warranty is provided, then a customer buys at his or her own risk. All 50 states in the United States have incorporated this into their laws, and consequentially, it is very difficult to prosecute fraud.

A term that places responsibility on the *seller* is *caveat vendor*. This is a Latin term meaning "let the seller beware." The term implies that it is the seller's responsibility rather than the purchaser's to ensure that the goods or services offered for sale are able to deliver their intended purpose. Again, without a warranty, it is very difficult to get one's money returned for defective products or to prove fraud. Fraud is a deceitful, tricky, or willful act committed to gain an unfair or dishonest advantage or to make a profit (make money off someone else).

Part of the 2010 national budget included $561 million to strengthen the integrity of Medicare and Medicaid with an emphasis on reducing health care fraud.[14] To protect the U.S. consumer, the U.S. Department of Health and Human Services Agency for Healthcare Research and Quality provides information about getting safer medical care, preventing errors, and getting quality medical care. Several states also have agencies and/or departments that focus on consumer protection. For example, the state of Maryland has an Office of Consumer Protection. Many consumer protection organizations focus on energy and environmental advocacy. An example of their efforts to protect people's health is establishing the Climate Action Plan, which focuses on reducing greenhouse gas emissions by 80% by the year 2050.[15]

CONCLUSION

In sum, information in this chapter was intended to provide an introduction to concepts regarding the meaning of health, traditional or orthodox medicine, CAM therapies, and consumer health. To improve and maintain our health, we need to make intelligent decisions and become savvy health consumers.

Suggestions for Class Activities

Select one of the following and present your findings in class.

1. Survey a group of friends to learn whether they have been ripped off when they purchased or used health products or services. Include the action taken and the results. Provide evidence relating it to the *caveat emptor/caveat vendor* concepts.
2. Find a magazine that contains unreliable nutrition information or promotes faddism. Analyze your findings by relating them to health consumer concepts learned in this chapter. Prepare a poster of cutouts from the magazine.
3. Compare and contrast high carbohydrate, low fat, and low protein diets with high protein, high fat, and low carbohydrate diets, or compare and contrast other questionable diet plans.
4. Compare and contrast two weight control plans (e.g., Nutrisystem, Weight Watchers, Atkins) to obtain information about procedures used for weight reduction, drugs used, food product prices, costs of service, and related matters. Include your opinions and conclusions.

Review Questions

1. What is the meaning of health and disease?
2. How much is spent annually on health care in the United States?
3. What do the terms "orthodox medicine" and "CAM" mean?
4. How do orthodox medicine and alternative medicine differ?
5. Why do people seek alternative care?
6. Why is it important to become an intelligent health consumer?
7. What are the meanings of *caveat emptor* and *caveat vendor*?
8. What are the six basic consumers' rights?

Key Terms

acupressure The application of pressure or localized massage to specific sites on the body to control symptoms such as pain or nausea.

acupuncture A traditional Chinese medicine treatment that uses stainless steel needles at specific points in the body to increase the flow of life energy known as Qi or Chi.

Alexander technique A technique for positioning and moving the body that is believed to reduce tension and discomfort.

allopathic medicine The traditional or conventional system of medicine that uses drugs, surgery, or radiation to prevent or treat diseases.

alternative medicine A system of practices not considered to be standard treatments. Examples are chiropractic medicine, Ayurvedic medicine, and traditional Chinese medicine.

Ayurvedic medicine (Ayurveda) A traditional system of medicine of India. The word Ayurveda is a Sanskrit word that means *Science of Life* or *Sciences of Lifespan*.

biofeedback A technique used to train people to control their own involuntary body processes such as heart rate, respirations, and even brain waves. It requires watching a monitor of some sort in order to change the rate using mental control.

consumer A person who buys and uses goods. In this text, it means the person who buys and uses health-related goods.

fraud A deceitful, tricky, or willful act committed to gain an unfair or dishonest advantage or to make a profit (make money off someone else).

holistic health Refers to the physical, emotional, spiritual, social, and mental domains of health. All should be seen as making up the whole person.

homeopathic medicine Medicines prepared by extreme dilution. The fundamental concept of homeopathic is that "like cures like." Substances in the preparations are thought to stimulate the body's own healing response.

muscular dystrophy A genetic disease group that is characterized by progressive weakness and degeneration of the skeletal muscles that control movement.

naturopathic medicine A system of medical practices that relies on more natural healing methods (herbs, massage, exercise). It encompasses a belief in the body's ability to heal itself.

References

1. Ravishankar N, Gubbins P, Cooley RJ, et al. Financing of global health: tracking development assistance for health from 1990 to 2007. *Lancet*. 2009;373(9681):2113–2124.
2. Reinhardt U. Why does U.S. health care cost so much? (Part I). *New York Times*. November 14, 2008. Found online at: http://economix.blogs.nytimes.com/2008/11/14/why-does-us-health-care-cost-so-much-part-i/. Accessed August 10, 2010.
3. Report of the 2000 Joint Committee on Health Education and Promotion Terminology. *Am J Health Educ*. 2001;32(2):89–104.
4. National Center for Complementary and Alternative Medicine. *Get the facts: what is complementary and alternative medicine?* NCCAM Publication No. D156. 2002. Available at: http://nccam.nih.gov/health/whatiscam/. Accessed October 16, 2010.
5. Ernst E, Pittler M, Stevinson C, White A. (Eds.) *Desktop guide to complementary and alternative medicine: an evidence-based approach*. St. Louis: Elsevier Health Sciences; 2001.
6. Kaptchuk T, Eisenberg D. The persuasive appeal of alternative medicine. *Ann Int Med*. 1998;129(12):1061–1065.
7. Astin J. Why patients use alternative medicine. *JAMA*. 1998;279(19):1548–1553.
8. Cauffield J. The psychosocial aspects of complementary and alternative medicine. *Pharmacotherapy*. 2000;11:1289–1294.
9. Isaacs T, MSNBC News. Increased usages of pesticides a contributing factor to the increase in ADHD. May 24, 2010. Available at: http:/www.allergiesandalternativemedicine.com/news-briefs.html. Accessed August 15, 2010.
10. HealthyPeople.gov. Healthy People 2020. Health Communication and Health Information Technology Objectives. Available online at: www.healthypeople.gov/2020/topicsobjectives2020/objectiveslist.aspx?topicId = 18. Accessed July 20, 2011.
11. Cornacchia H, London W, Baratz R, Kroger M. *Consumer health: a guide to intelligent decisions*. 8th ed., New York: McGraw-Hill; 2007.
12. Wikipedia. *Consumer bill of rights*. Available at: http://en.wikipedia.org/wiki/Consumer_Bill_of_Rights. Accessed February 21, 2010.
13. Nader R. *Unsafe at any speed: the designed-in dangers of the American automobile*. New York: Grossman; 1965.
14. U.S. Department of Health and Human Services, Agency for Healthcare Research and Quality. *Getting safer care. February 2004*. Available at: http://www.ahrq.gov/consumer/safety.html. Accessed February 22, 2010.
15. Office of Consumer Protection, Montgomery County Government. Available at: http://www.montgomerycountymd.gov/consumer. Accessed February 22, 2010.

Scientific Method

LEARNING OBJECTIVES

As a result of reading this chapter, students will:

1. Explain how to seek the truth about health products, especially when hearing conflicting information.
2. Describe six characteristics of scientific testing.
3. Analyze the importance of learning about valid and reliable scientific testing and research practices and their application when attempting to select a health-related product or therapy.
4. Assess the impact of television infomercials or fitness magazine ads on people who want to lose weight or gain muscle mass.

WHAT ARE THE CHARACTERISTICS OF SCIENTIFIC TESTING?

How many times in our lifetime do we hear someone tell us about a "proven" remedy for some condition or disorder that we may have. For example, it may have been expressed similar to this, "I heard that cherry juice will cure gout." How do we learn whether cherry juice will really cure gout? We need to know if the statement is fact or hearsay. While studying information for personal health consumerism, whether it is part of mainstream medicine or complementary and alternative therapies, individuals should learn how to assess whether a treatment modality has been scientifically tested. After reviewing the research results, one could say whether the treatment is legitimate. Research involves scientific testing of a theory or idea, and the research procedures to be used should be based on several characteristics.

Characteristics of Scientific Testing

The first characteristic of scientific testing is that the research should be self-correcting.[1,2] In other words, if the results of a research study are later found to be false, the research should be conducted again so that the conclusions or results may be modified. When conducting research, the truth is not found in one experiment or study; it often requires many studies to find the truth. An example of how attitudes change based on scientific study is the belief about acupuncture, a traditional Chinese medicine treatment. For years, western medical and health professionals believed that acupuncture was quackery. Granted, there are still those who do, but the National Center for Complementary and Alternative Medicine (NCCAM) has conducted several studies demonstrating the effectiveness of acupuncture in treating pain (i.e., low back pain, headaches, osteoarthritis) as well as providing other benefits.[3] See **BOX 2.1**. Many studies are needed to find the truth, and that is what sound research does.

Second, the study requires objectivity.[1,2] The findings must not be biased by the researcher's personal beliefs, perceptions, values, or emotions. When planning the study, the

> **Box 2.1**
>
> **U.S. Medical Physicians Becoming Certified in Acupuncture**
>
> Rather than declaring acupuncture a bogus treatment modality, numerous medical physicians here in the United States are now becoming certified in acupuncture techniques. Many now view acupuncture as a valuable medical treatment.

researchers must develop rules and procedures for the research (such as formulating specific hypotheses or research questions and setting significance levels). If the research involves a pen and paper or Internet survey, the coding procedure and statistical analyses should be planned in advance. Quantitative research methods are those in which a value, score, or scale is used. Objectivity is met fairly easily because the researcher is working with numbers.

Problems with objectivity come when researchers have not specified methods that measure qualitative research. For instance, if researchers were to measure the degree to which individuals liked or disliked television advertisements for medicines or acupuncture to cure addictions, they could record the number of times (quantitative research) the subjects changed the channel. However, if they attempted to base the level at which individuals liked or disliked television advertisements by the looks on subjects' faces (qualitative research), the results would more than likely be biased.

A third characteristic is that the findings must be made public.[1,2] Most researchers attempt to publish their findings in peer-reviewed professional journals. Certainly, findings may be made public by mass media (television, Internet, radio), but peer review is essential.

A fourth characteristic is that the experiments must be reproducible by other scientists at later times.[1,2] This requires other scientists to replicate the same research process using the same research design and methodology.

A fifth characteristic is that the experiment must be empirical,[1,2] a word derived from the Greek word for experience or observation.[4] If the research is experimental, the scientist may manipulate a variable and then observe the results. Qualitative research may entail observing without manipulating any variables. An example of the latter is Jane Goodall's studies of chimpanzees (see **FIGURE 2.1**) from the 1960s to the 1990s, when she observed and recorded them in their native environment, the Gombe Stream National Park, located in Tanzania in southeastern Africa.[5] Jane Goodall watched and observed but did not try to interact with the chimpanzees in any way. In other words, she did not manipulate the variables (the chimpanzees) and bias her research.

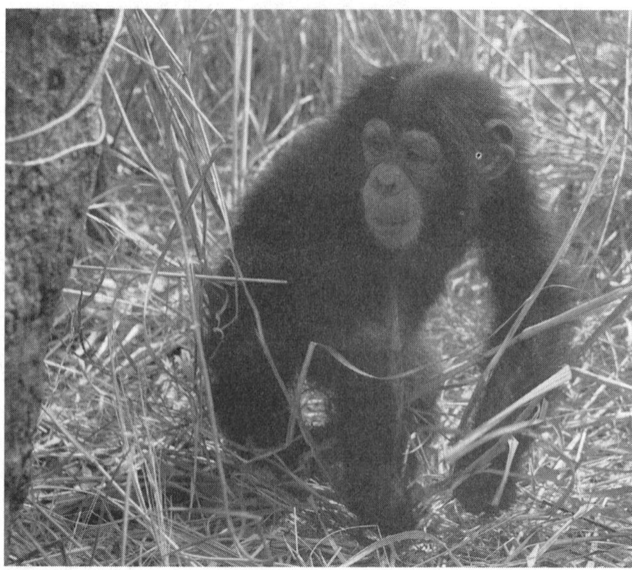

FIGURE 2.1 Chimpanzee.

A sixth characteristic is that science should be predictive.[1,2] Such predictions are demonstrated in scientific theories that arise as a result of research studies. The predictions allow for further research that tests the theories. At times, such theories are found not to be true, and more research and theories are subsequently conducted and planned.

It is true that scientific testing takes much time and money just to prove that a product or treatment will work.

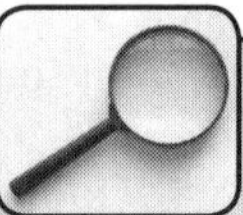

Case Study

Abbey is a college student in her senior year. Her major is health education, and she believes it is important to practice healthy behaviors, but she has had many rigorous courses over the past 2 years and has been working 30 hours per week. As a result, Abbey has not had time to exercise, and she has not eaten very nutritiously. Abbey perceives that she is overweight and out of shape. One day she is watching a 20-minute infomercial on television promoting a fat-burning product. She is impressed about the before and after results of three individuals who recounted their experience using this "wonder" drug and how their lives had changed due to all the weight they had lost. Even though the product is very expensive, Abbey is seriously considering buying it.

Questions:

1. How can Abbey learn whether the product has been scientifically tested?
2. What steps are taken to conduct scientific testing of drugs and products?
3. Do you believe that a drug will be the answer to Abbey's problems? Why or why not?

To identify effective health or medical treatments, however, the research must require exemplary scientific testing characteristics, and the researchers have to plan an appropriate research design depending on what is to be tested.

The next section will give you a brief overview of what is involved in scientific testing, starting with information about research design.

WHAT ARE THE TYPES OF RESEARCH DESIGNS?

Research design is divided into two main categories: experimental and quasi-experimental.[6] If it is experimental, the subjects are randomly selected or assigned into either a treatment or a control group. If it is quasi-experimental, comparison groups are not randomly selected, and many factors may cloud (or confound) the findings. Confounding factors (variables) may relate to both the cause and effect or outcome. For example, it could be that a statistical analysis shows that ice cream sales and heat stroke are highly positively correlated (related). A researcher could determine that eating ice cream causes heat stroke. The confounding factor, of course, is the summer season. More people eat ice cream in the summer and the summer weather is a factor in causing heat stroke. A research study may be valuable, but confounding factors need to be accounted for.

Studies are conducted in a variety of ways, ranging from pen and paper survey studies to laboratory experiments.[1,2,6] Studies may involve researching historical facts from archived materials. They may involve analyzing data from large populations over a span of years. They may involve conducting case studies on a limited number of individuals. Please refer to **BOX 2.2** for types of research study designs. No matter the type of study design, however, the researcher must abide by scientific research characteristics.

Finally, numerous types of data may be collected. Blood or other body fluids may be drawn and examined in laboratory experiments. Morbidity and mortality statistics and historical data may be sought from local, state, or national databases. Surveys may be used to collect demographic, knowledge, attitude, and behavioral information (via telephone, personal interview, or paper and pencil). As described, the researchers must carefully select the type of research design most appropriate for the particular study and determine the type of data to be collected. We, as health consumers, should become knowledgeable about the steps taken when conducting scientific research so we can determine if a health product or service is one that we should purchase. The steps in scientific research are summarized in the following section.

Box 2.2
Research Study Designs

- *Case studies:* Observation of people
- *Laboratory experiments:* Controlled environment
- *Epidemiological studies:* Analyze data from various population groups
- *Controlled clinical trials:* May involve a number of people using an experimental group and a control group

WHAT ARE THE STEPS IN SCIENTIFIC RESEARCH?

Depending on the type of research study, the scientific process may be somewhat different, but the steps listed here are very appropriate for health professionals. A needs assessment[7] may be one of the first steps completed so that a researcher can identify health or health behavioral problems existing in a community, county, or state. It is beneficial if the researcher can use findings from fairly current needs assessments because it saves a great deal of time. Usually, several health and health behavioral problems are identified within needs assessments; therefore, the researcher determines which health problems will be researched. For example, a county (parish) needs assessment may reveal high rates of diabetes, heart disease, hypertension (high blood pressure), lung cancer, sexually transmitted diseases, tobacco use, and teen pregnancy. The researcher cannot investigate all these problems at one time, but needs to select one or two for further investigation. Depending on the purpose, researchers can conduct their research in many ways. The researcher might develop an educational program that would be tested for effectiveness or the researcher might investigate the reasons (variables) related to the health problem (e.g., relationship of tobacco use to lung cancer).

A literature review is important because the researcher can identify studies that could be replicated or used as a guide. The literature review may include researching library databases such as ERIC (educational studies), Medline (medical studies), Sociofile (sociology database), or PsychInfo (psychology-behavioral database). Most of the journal articles found in the databases will be research-based. A review of dissertations or theses written during the past few years may also be accessed. The researcher could conduct Internet searches from sources such as PubMed and NCCAM Web sites.

Now it is time for the researcher to plan the research study. First, the researcher will develop the hypotheses or research questions; of which there might be four or more. These questions are the basis of the study. Next, the researcher will plan the research design and methodology and set the statistical level of significance. The researcher has to determine if this type of research requires being 95 percent confident about the results or whether the results should be 99 percent certain. Once the research questions,

> **Box 2.3**
> **Steps in Scientific Research**
>
> 1. Identify a problem.
> 2. Review existing research based on the problem.
> 3. Develop either hypotheses or research questions.
> 4. Plan the research design and methodology (complete with the type of statistics to be used and the statistical level of evaluation).
> 5. Collect and analyze the data.
> 6. Describe the results of each hypothesis or research question.
> 7. Publicize the results in peer-reviewed journals.
> 8. Other researchers may replicate the study.

design and methodology are set, it's time to collect the data, which comprises many forms: bodily liquids, body measurements, oral communication, pen and paper tests, and others. The researcher may conduct blood draws to analyze blood content levels of certain substances (e.g., glucose, lipids, hormones) before and after exercise performance. If the researcher has planned an educational program, a pre and post pen and paper test may be given to assess gains in knowledge and changes in attitudes and behaviors. No matter what the data is composed of, the statistical results are carefully recorded and analyzed.

Once the statistical work has been completed, the researcher will write the results in a formal manuscript. The manuscript is then sent to professional journals for publication and presented at professional conferences and/or seminars. It is important for the findings to be peer reviewed because it is a means to validate the study design, methodology, and results.[1,2] The steps in scientific research are summarized for you in **BOX 2.3**.

COULD YOU APPLY WHAT YOU HAVE LEARNED?

You are taking a basic research class at the undergraduate or graduate level and you have been asked to conduct a study. Your professor has told you that the study has to be a survey to assess knowledge, attitudes, and behaviors about a health topic. Because you are interested in learning more about herbal supplements, you decide that will become your health topic.

Preliminary Information

Your professor has suggested that you use college students to collect data from because they are available and would reduce time and expenses.

Of benefit to you, a health needs assessment was conducted at your university and it revealed several health problems: a large percentage of college students were overweight, did not regularly exercise, felt stressed out, were not eating nutritiously, and were not sleeping well.

Your Task

Using the needs assessment results and the steps in conducting research, describe how you would set up this study. You need to determine what you want to learn about herbal supplement use.

Step 1: Use one or more of the problems identified from the college needs assessment.

Step 2: Identify two or more databases you would use to learn about related studies.

Step 3: Formulate three research questions.

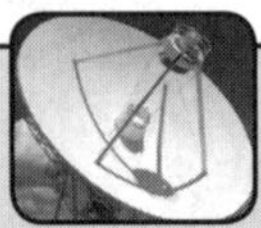

In the News

A news article published on June 15, 2010, described a study wherein smokers with higher levels of vitamin B6 and an essential amino acid were found to have less risk of developing lung cancer than those lacking the nutrients. This was a study of nearly 400,000 participants that included current and former smokers in 10 European countries.

Questions:

1. If people read this account, how might they interpret the results?
2. What might smokers do as a result of reading about this study?

Further information was also presented in this news article. The researchers did not conclude that consuming more of the nutrients would reduce the risk of getting lung cancer, and they did promote the message that it was important for smokers to give up the habit.

We as health consumers need to research information about health and medical treatments, but we must be careful not to misinterpret what we read and hear. Furthermore, most of us do not have time to find information about every medicine and treatment that we use in our everyday lives. It becomes problematic and confusing when we are unsure if a medical or health product or therapy really works. So how can we more easily obtain help?

Step 4: Plan your research design.

- What would be the best way to collect your data?
- How many participants do you want to include in your study?
- Could you do a study to investigate if herbal supplement use is related to one or more health problems identified from the college needs assessment?
- Can you think of any confounding factors that would bias your research?

When the steps in scientific research are followed, although it seems to be a slow and precise process, we can usually trust that the findings are the truth. Researchers have to be careful, however, when interpreting and publishing research results because people can become confused about the meaning of those results. See In the News for a published account of a recent research study.

HEALTH CONSUMERS: CAN WE TRUST WHAT WE READ AND HEAR ABOUT HEALTH AND MEDICAL TREATMENTS?

These days, we health consumers are bombarded with mega amounts of information. This often causes uncertainty when attempting to make a rational decision about what product, medicine, treatment, and/or therapy we should buy and use. We cannot always trust what we read and hear. Because there are many problems with health information (as listed in **BOX 2.4**), health consumers need to be able to find accurate sources.

WHERE CAN WE FIND VALID, RELIABLE, AND EVIDENCE-BASED HEALTH INFORMATION?

We should have faith in a claim if the source demonstrates that the treatment, product, or medicine is the result of evidence-based research. This is research that has been planned and executed using the techniques previously discussed in this chapter. If that has occurred, we can be assured that the health or medical product has been scientifically tested. A red flag should go up, however, when we hear or read promises from some source touting untested or unusual remedies for chronic or incurable diseases.

Box 2.4
Problems with Health Information

- Sources not reliable
- Nonprofessionals or pretend scientists promoting products
- Some medical professionals promoting products for their own financial gain
- Media hype on certain products—unwarranted

A health product or medical treatment should be tested to determine if it is scientifically sound. Testing will include assessing if the health product or medical treatment is valid and reliable. Validity is the extent to which the test predicts the outcome it is supposed to predict, and a test is said to be reliable if it yields consistent results.[2,6] For example, a procedure to use stents in carotid arteries has recently been tested and approved to lessen the probability that a person will experience a stroke. The researchers would have posed a research question such as, "Will carotid artery stents lessen the probability of stroke?" The ensuing research demonstrated that the stents did lessen the probability of stroke. Moreover, after a longer period in time, it became evident across a wide population at risk for stroke that the stents were effective. The researchers could make the claim that this treatment was indeed valid and reliable.

If there is a question about the validity of health information, there are several ways to investigate.

1. Check for verification of the product or drug, such as a peer-reviewed article or report.
2. Investigate safety research on products and side effects of medicines/drugs.
3. Don't rely on the results of one study. Remember that several studies are often required.
4. If you read a report, investigate the origin of the report. Find out if it was from a peer-reviewed study or medical institution. If not, be wary.
5. Ask your doctor.
6. Read reliable magazines and newsletters, such as the following:
    - *FDA Consumer*
    - *Consumer Reports on Health*
    - *Tufts University Diet and Nutrition Letter*
7. Obtain information from reputable sources, including
    - Governmental agencies such as the Food and Drug Administration (FDA)
    - American Medical Association
    - Volunteer agencies (e.g., American Cancer Society, American Heart Association)
    - Foundations (e.g., Arthritis Foundation)
    - U.S. Department of Health and Human Services (Office of Public Health and Sciences)
    - Trusted consumer health publications and Web sites.[8]

There are some trustworthy Internet sites. A few of these are listed for you in **BOX 2.5**.

CONCLUSION

This chapter was intended to raise your awareness of the importance of scientific research and its application in your life

Box 2.5

Trustworthy Internet Sources

Medlineplus: http://medlineplus.gov

National Institutes of Health's Senior Health: http://nihseniorhealth.gov

National Cancer Institute: http:// www.cancer.gov

CAMline: http://www.camline.ca

Consumer Health Complete Ebsco: http://www3.dbu.edu/library/documents/Consumer- Ebsco.pdf (gives directions on how to conduct your search)

Harvard Health Publications: http://www.health.harvard.edu/

National Institutes of Health Center for Complementary and Alternative Medicine (NCCAM): http://nccam.nih.gov

as a health consumer. We need to be cautious about what we read and hear, especially on the Internet and in television infomercials. To be optimal health consumers, we need to learn the important steps of scientific research, and we need to learn how to find valid and reliable information.

Suggestions for Class Activities

Select one of the two.

1. Find a Web site that deals with health issues or the sale of health products and evaluate it for reliability and scientific soundness. Web site evaluation forms are available. Here are two links to aid you in finding a tool:

   http://www.sph.emory.edu/WELLNESS/instrument.html

   http://www.hon.ch/HealthEvaluationTool/

2. Exercise.

   a) Analyze four types of exercise equipment using the Exercise Equipment Rating form provided in **TABLE 2.1**. In order to do the analysis, research necessary articles for information regarding the

Table 2.1

Exercise Equipment Rating Form

Note: The pieces of equipment listed below are heavily advertised and many are used in fitness gyms. On a scale of 1 to 5, with 5 being the highest and best number, please rate each item's effect according to fitness level, strength, muscle endurance, and cardiorespiratory endurance. Also rate how each would affect specific body parts. Research the average cost of each. Place your number in the appropriate box and total your points. The items listed below are only samples. You may use them or find different items.

F = fitness level, S = strength, ME = muscle endurance, CRE = cardiorespiratory endurance

Scale:	1	2	3	4	5
	Poor	Fair	Average	Good	Excellent

	BENEFITS				BODY PARTS AFFECTED					COST	TOTAL POINTS
Equipment	F	S	ME	CRE	Arm	Leg	Shoulder	Back	Core		
Shake weight											
Inversion table											
Exercise bike											
Elliptical machine											
Treadmill											
Fitness balls											
Ab circle pro											

Discussion Questions

1. After quantifying each of the types of exercise equipment that you chose, were you surprised at your findings? Why?
2. What advice would you offer your friends or family if they were thinking about purchasing a piece of equipment that has been heavily advertised?

particular piece of equipment. Provide a reference list.

b) Answer the two discussion questions found on the form.

Review Questions

1. How are facts determined?
2. What are the characteristics of scientific testing?
3. What are the types of research design?
4. What steps are involved in conducting scientific research?
5. What are confounding factors?
6. What is the meaning of "validity" and "reliability"?
7. To what extent should people believe what they read and hear about health matters?
8. Where can valid, reliable, and/or evidence-based information be found?

Key Terms

acupuncture A traditional Chinese medicine treatment that uses stainless steel needles at specific points in the body to increase the flow of life energy known as Qi or Chi.

biased research Errors in research during the selection of subjects, the measurements used, or the treatment process (intervention).

consumer A person who buys and uses goods. In this text, it means the person who buys and uses health-related goods.

demographic A single vital or social statistic of a human population, such as the number of births or deaths.

empirical A word derived from the Greek word for experience or observation.

experimental Subjects are randomly selected or assigned into a treatment or control group.

hypnosis The induction of a person into a state of consciousness in which he or she is responsive to a suggestion/s by a therapist.

hypothesis A research statement or proposal that the subsequent study will find truthful or not.

morbidity Refers to illness or disease.

mortality Refers to deaths.

NCCAM (National Center for Complementary and Alternative Medicine) A center in the National Institutes of Health that conducts research to prove the effectiveness of complementary and alternative therapies.

needs assessment Investigation to determine health needs. May investigate at the community, county, state, or national level.

objectivity in research Findings must not be biased by personal beliefs, perceptions, biases, values, or emotions of the researcher.

peer review Peers review the study usually when it is submitted for publication. It is a means to validate the study design, methodology, and results.

predictive approach The researcher makes a guess or prediction about the research problem based on the probability that the prediction is accurate. The study tests the prediction using specialized statistical techniques.

qualitative research Research that seeks to provide understanding of human experience, perceptions, motivations, intentions, and behaviors. It requires observation and personal interaction with subjects rather than the use of a survey instrument.

quasi-experimental Comparison groups in a study are not randomly selected, and many things may cloud (or confound) the findings.

reliability The consistency of a measurement, or the degree to which an instrument measures the same way each time it is used under the same condition with the same subjects. It refers to the repeatability of a measurement.

reputable Considered to be respectable or acceptable.

research design A design that may be experimental or quasi-experimental.

research questions Rather than a statement or statements found in hypotheses, research questions are formulated. The study tests each research question for truth or not.

self-correcting research If results of a previous research study are later found to be false, the research should be conducted again so that the conclusions or results may be modified.

significance levels The levels set before a research study is begun. If the level is not met for a particular hypothesis or research question studied, the research is said to be non-significant and is rejected.

validity The strength of conclusions, inferences, or propositions. Validity is the extent to which the test predicts the outcome it is supposed to predict.

References

1. RM Institute. *The research methods knowledge base*. 2006. Available at: http://www.researchmethods.org/rm-knowledge.htm. Accessed November 2, 2009.
2. Patten M. *Understanding research methods: an overview of the essentials.* 7th ed. Glendale, CA: Pyrczak; 2009.
3. National Institutes of Health, National Center for Complementary and Alternative Medicine. *Acupuncture*. Available at: http://nccam.nih.gov/health/acupuncture/. Accessed June 3, 2009.

4. alphaDictionary.com. *Empirical*. Available at: http://www.alphadictionary.com/goodword/word/empirical. Accessed February 28, 2009.
5. The Jane Goodall Institute. *Study corner—biography*. Available at: http://www.janegoodall.org/study-corner-biography/. Accessed July 1, 2010.
6. Berg K, Latin R. *Essentials of research methods in health, physical education, exercise science, and recreation*. 3rd ed. Philadelphia: Lippincott Williams & Wilkins; 2008.
7. Sharma A, Lanum M, Suarez-Balcazar Y. *A community needs assessment guide: a brief guide on how to conduct a needs assessment*. Chicago: Center for Urban Research and Learning and the Department of Psychology, Loyola University; September 2000. Available at: http://www.luc.edu/curl/pdfs/A_Community_Needs_Assessment_Guide_.pdf. Accessed July 6, 2009.
8. Murray S. Consumer health information. *J Can Health Libr Assoc.* 2006;27:39–40.

Advertising Health Products

LEARNING OBJECTIVES

As a result of reading this chapter, students will:

1. Explain the ways in which consumers are influenced by product advertising.
2. Describe the principle behind direct-to-consumer (DTC) marketing.
3. Illustrate the more common advertising techniques used to influence consumers.
4. Describe the constructs used in the VALS™ system.
5. Analyze the pros and cons of DTC marketing.

ADVERTISING IN AMERICA

Without advertising, consumers would not have any idea what products, services, and options are available to them. Advertising is an absolute necessity. But advertising is also an art form. Language can be used to attract, persuade, and convince consumers that one product or service is better than another. And advertisers know that Americans can be influenced. One source states that Americans see more than 16 hours of advertisements[1] every year just for pharmaceutical products. That adds up to more than $4 billion in advertising![2]

The challenge for consumers is weeding though the advertising language in an effort to determine which products are valuable and which are not. It is important to note that laws exist to protect the consumer from false or misleading advertising. More than 100 years ago the Pure Food and Drug Act was passed, followed shortly thereafter by the Sherley Amendment of that Act. Both efforts prohibited companies from making fraudulent claims about their products, or advertising those claims to the general public. There are, however, still a number of ways advertisers try to influence the consumer.

WHAT IS DIRECT-TO-CONSUMER MARKETING?

For most of the twentieth century, the marketing of health products was limited to "indirect" means. If a company wanted consumers to purchase that company's version of an anti-anxiety medicine, instead of a direct reference to the medicine, the advertisement would try to build consumer confidence in the company name.[2] This way, drug companies would attempt to get the consumer to ask for a specific company's products for whatever ailed them. It wasn't until the mid-1980s that consumers began to hear the names of specific products in an advertisement. When an advertisement makes a pitch for a specific product, it is referred to as direct-to-consumer (DTC) marketing.

HOW DOES DTC MARKETING INFLUENCE MY DECISIONS?

More than 30 years ago, Jeffrey Schrank compiled a list of the 10 most common approaches[3] in advertising used to sway consumer feelings about purchasing a product. The following sections describe five of the more common approaches seen in advertising health products and services.

The Weasel Claim

A weasel claim uses terms that make a product sound great, but in reality say nothing about the product. It is a hollow claim. For instance, if you read, "Product X is the best at reducing your cough," the term "best" is the weasel. Consumers will think that "best" must mean the cough medicine does a lot, but it doesn't. It doesn't claim to eliminate your cough, only that it is the best of some mythical comparison. Popular weasel words make the consumer feel as though the product can do magic. "Virtually everyone who used Product Y had improved function." The words "virtually" and "improved" tell the consumer nothing about the product.

The Water Is Wet

This claim makes a statement that is true to all products like it. Antibacterial soap is a simple example of this. By labeling itself "antibacterial," the soap company helps make consumer think it's a new or better or special product. The reality is that all soaps are antibacterial. They're soap!

The "So What?" Claim

The statements made in these advertisements are essentially true, but really don't mean anything related to the use of or benefit from the product. Statistical references are common in this group. "Product R has 75 percent more potassium than a banana!" OK . . . this may be true, but so what? Does that make the product better for you? Or safe? Or does it actually indicate how much 75 percent is? If a banana has 1 mg of potassium, does 1.75 mg make a big difference? Consumers need to be cautious of these types of claims—they sound great, but might mean very little.

In 1937, Edward Filene founded the Institute of Propaganda Analysis.[4] His goal was to inform Americans about the techniques used to influence the way Americans think. Many of the techniques he identified in 1937 are still prevalent in American advertising today. Two in particular are testimonials and bandwagon.

Testimonials

This technique is used to associate a product or service with someone famous, and in turn get consumers to want to "be like" that spokesperson. This technique has been used to sell everything from cars to razor blades to, yes, health products. Today, weight loss and diet programs and products rely heavily on high profile public figures to influence the public. The message is simple: "If it worked for me it can work for you." If the spokesperson is popular enough or influential enough, consumers will want to be like them. Consumers should initially ask themselves what makes this spokesperson qualified to talk about the product. The consumer also needs to consider whether the circumstances under which the spokesperson used the product will apply. Make sure you actually look at the product and its benefits, risk, costs, and whether it's really for you, instead of just looking at who advertises the product.

Bandwagon

Bandwagon advertising tries to convince the consumer to follow the crowd. If everyone else is doing "it," shouldn't you be doing "it" too? What you might hear in the advertisement would be, "How could 6000 men a day be wrong? You should try Product M too!" Or, it could be as simple as, "You don't want to be the last one to own a Product M, do you? Get yours today." The big question here for the consumer to ask is, "Why?" Let's say you choose not to hop on the bandwagon . . . what happens then? Is it possible that the crowd running along with the bandwagon has missed something about the product? A more comprehensive list of techniques is provided in **TABLE 3.1**.

WHO MAKES SURE ADVERTISERS ARE TELLING THE TRUTH?

Federal agencies are responsible for monitoring product quality and information accuracy. The Federal Trade Commission and the U.S. Postal Inspection Service are two agencies that play a role in this effort. The Federal Trade Commission has the ultimate authority to create laws regarding advertising in the United States. It establishes the standards for what is deceptive, dishonest, or misleading. The U.S. Postal Inspection Service primarily focuses on the use of the postal service to defraud consumers through faulty advertising of jobs and products.

For the most part, advertising tries to maintain its position as a self-regulated industry, and minimize governmental oversight. There are private organizations that monitor the accuracy and legitimacy of advertising. One such group is the National Advertising Review Board (NARB), whose mission is to create and implement standards of truthfulness in advertising. However, the NARB is predominantly composed of advertising agencies and professionals, with a small number of academic or former public sector professionals. The risk for bias in situations like this is great. Because of the potential for bias, organizations align themselves with groups known for their impartiality; in this case the NARB functions under the watch of the Council of Better Business Bureaus.

There are many, many agencies that watch out for the general well-being of the consumer. These are discussed more thoroughly in Chapter 18.

The Food and Drug Administration makes a distinction between types of prescription drug television advertising directed at consumers. In general, there are product claim ads and reminder ads. Product claim ads include the product name, the ailment the product is designed to address, and the risk factors associated with using the product. Reminder ads, which are shorter commercials, mention the product's name but cannot discuss the ailment, side effects, or dosing of the product. A 2007 analysis of prescription drug advertising[1] on television indicated that most ads were of the product claim variety. Almost all ads made some sort of emotional appeal (positive and/or negative), and nearly

Table 3.1
Examples of Advertising Techniques

CLAIM TYPE	DESCRIPTION	EXAMPLE
The weasel claim	Claims that appear to be substantial, but in the end are empty.	Use of Treadmill X will help control your weight.
The unfinished claim	Claims that a product has more of something, or is better, but doesn't say what the comparison is.	Using Weight Loss Product X will make you lose more weight!
The "we're different and unique" claim	Claims that no other product on the market is like it.	Only Product Z has Alpha-PQX.
The water is wet claim	The claim made for this ad can be said of any other product like it.	Hospital X will bill your insurance so you don't have to.
The "so what?" claim	Makes a claim, but there is no real indication if it has significance.	Our vitamins have twice the vitamin D as our competitor.
The vague claim	The intent or meaning of the claim is unclear, subjective, and cannot be proven.	Product X will make you feel good again.
The endorsement	Someone famous pitches the claim.	I use Product Z to test my diabetes, and you should too.
The scientific claim	Claim includes data or testing results.	Product Y burns 27 percent more fat when used daily.
The compliment the consumer claim	Claim uses flattery to entice the consumer.	You take great care of your children, and that's why you feed them Product X.
The rhetorical claim	Claim asks a question to entice an answer from the consumer.	You want to feel like the "old you" again, right?

Source: Summarized from Schrank J. *The language of advertising claims: teaching about doublespeak.* Urbana, IL: National Council of Teachers of English; 1976.

one-third used humor, while one in four ads used fantasy to make the product appealing.

The Internet has proven to be fertile ground for advertising; however, because advertising online is for the most part unregulated, this has created a new dimension to consumer protection. Two primary issues of concern are consumer privacy and behavioral advertising. The Federal Trade Commission has made several suggestions to online advertisers (who, like their alternate media counterparts, would like to remain as unregulated as possible) to enhance the protection of consumer private information. Names, contact information, credit card numbers, personal health information, and health histories can be at risk for distribution if the company collecting the information does not act in an ethical fashion. The collection of as much information as possible works to the advertiser's advantage. A dimension of online advertising that does not exist in print, radio, or television is something called *behavioral advertising*. Marketing firms can track your pattern of online use. When you visit a site online, or use a search engine, or just kill a couple hours surfing the web, your history can be traced, and in some cases sold to other Web sites. Marketing firms can then make certain you see products, in the form of pop-up ads or sidebar ads, that might interest you based on your usage pattern.

HOW DO CONSUMERS MAKE PURCHASING DECISIONS?

According to *Principles of Advertising: A Global Perspective*,[5] consumers go through five steps in making a decision about whether to purchase a product: need recognition, information search, alternative evaluation, purchase, and evaluation. Advertisers play to each of these levels of processing in their advertisements. Take for example **TABLE 3.2** regarding the purchase of a treadmill.

Beyond the process of choosing, there are certain factors that influence the decisions people make. Lee and Johnson discuss three primary factors that have an influence on whether a person is swayed by advertising. First are personal factors. These are things unique to each person such as age, sex, education, and income. Psychological influences also play a role, primarily perception, motivation, attitude, and lifestyle. Finally, social factors such as cultural background, present and perceived importance of social status, and the peer group the individual affiliates with will

Table 3.2
Stages of Decision Making and Advertising Influence

STAGE	CONSUMER BEHAVIOR	ADVERTISING APPROACH
	Issue: Purchase of a treadmill	
Need recognition	May or may not realize the need for a product.	For those who already see the need, the advertiser tells how its product can address the need. For those who do not see the need, the advertiser asks rhetorical questions. (Do you feel . . . ?)
Information search	Gathers information from self (memory), advertisement, friends, relatives, mail, and salespeople.	Descriptive ads and mailings, comparisons to other similar products.
Alternative evaluation	Determines the best option based on personal needs and potential end result.	Rational and emotional appeal.
Purchase	Buyer closes the deal: what to buy, from whom, what cost, etc.	Similar to alternative evaluation; designed to prevent consumers from changing their mind.
Evaluation	Consumer needs to feel as though it has been a good investment, and that the product will give intended results.	Designed to overcome the dissonance between wanting the product and spending the money to obtain it (buyer's remorse).

Source: Staging and descriptions summarized from Lee M, Johnson C. *Principles of advertising: a global perspective* (2nd ed.). New York: Hawthorne; 2005.

influence decision making. Clearly it is a complicated process, and advertisers may develop several approaches to promote the same product in an effort to appeal to a broad base of people.

WHAT ROLE DO EMOTIONS PLAY IN ADVERTISING?

Psychological research on the impact of emotions on personality, mood, and attitude is abundant.[6] Research is used, and even conducted, by advertising firms to determine just what emotions motivate spending. Consider a television advertisement for a drug to lower the risk of heart attack. If the company simply stated that the drug was effective and you should use it, it would not elicit much of an emotional response from the consumer. However, if the ads reference emotional scenarios such as the following, people might be more motivated to watch the commercial and get their doctors to order the product:

Scenario one: A television ad shows a person missing a daughter's wedding or a grandchild's graduation because of a heart attack. The ad then plays serene music in the background and shows visuals of how happy the family is if that family member is present for the wedding or grandchild's graduation.

Scenario two: Consider an ad for depression medication. Almost universally the ad will begin with a visual of a person suffering with depression, and by the end of the commercial show them happy, more functional, and content. This is done with great purpose; to create in the viewer a sense that the medicine being advertised can make the viewing consumer feel like the actor in the commercial.

WHAT IS THE VALS™ SYSTEM?

In 1978, SRI International released the original VALS™ system.[7] VALS (not an acronym, although it looks like one), which originally was used in the business arena, uses individual lifestyles and attitudes as predictors of consumer behavior. Over time, the system has evolved and is now focused on psychological traits, as opposed to social norms and shared values. It is owned and operated as a consulting business by an SRI Incorporated spin-off, Strategic Business Insights. VALS categorizes consumers into eight different groups based on what motivates them in their decision making (see **FIGURE 3.1**). Each group is motivated by one of three primary factors—ideals, achievement, or self-expression (see **TABLE 3.3**)—and is additionally impacted by the degree to which they have access to resources.

Believers and Thinkers are motivated by ideals. For Believers, those ideals are rooted in history and tradition. As consumers they have fewer resources, so they tend to be conservative, be loyal to a particular product, and have predictable trends in consumer choices. Believers tend to follow doctors' orders with little questioning. Thinkers' ideals still reflect a conservative trend, but these individuals are better educated, more

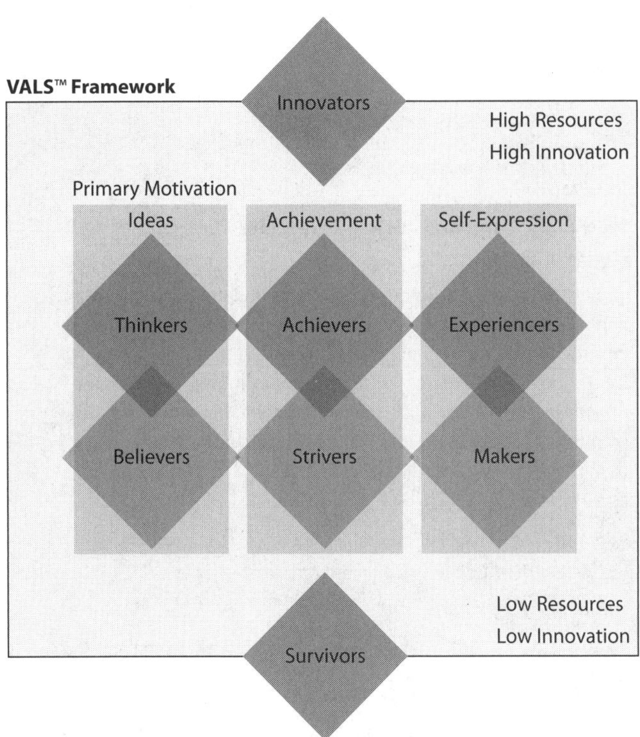

FIGURE 3.1 VALS™ Framework.
Source: Courtesy of Strategic Business Insights (SBI). http://www.strategicbusinessinsights.com/VALS.

well-off financially, and they want to have thorough and accurate information. Where Believers tend to reject change, Thinkers are more likely to keep the doors to change open, if that change seems valuable and functional.

Strivers and Achievers are driven by achievement. Strivers, on the lower end of the resource spectrum, have to be careful about covering basic needs but can also be impulsive consumers. The opinion of others is a major motivator, because Strivers want to be seen as higher on the social order than they actually are. A high percentage of Strivers smoke and suffer later in life because of it. Achievers have made their mark, and because of that want to demonstrate that they have made it. Purchasing tends to be of established names, image-related products, and products that save time. Products and services that promote predictability and stability would be desired.

Makers and Experiencers are motivated by self-expression. For Makers, self-expression is a function of building things. They value the practical and are not impressed with wealth or status. Products and services must show a value, and promote self-sufficiency. Maker men pride themselves on being strong and may be more likely to avoid medical care, thinking they can "tough it out." Experiencers are young and impulsive, and value looking good and having a good time. If the product is new and cutting edge, they want it, but as soon as the fad wanes, they are done with it and moving on.

Survivors and Innovators are two special categories in the VALS system. Survivors have few resources available to them. They may fall in the lower socioeconomic divisions of the economy, may be retired and living on a fixed income, or may live in a region that has little access to resources. Thirty-two percent of survivors are widowed. Because resources are scarce, the decisions made by these people are based on what they really need to have, not necessarily what they would like to have. Their focus on immediate needs may limit their ability to plan for the future. Health decisions in this group are high on the priority list. Innovators have plentiful resources and as such are motivated by all three of the primary motivators—image, achievement, and self-expression. Image matters, but serves as a function of expressing individuality and personality, not as a means to gain approval from others. Innovators will try anything cutting edge and new if it fits their lifestyle and allows a free expression of self. Alternative care practices would be intriguing to an Innovator. They are quick to do their own medical research and are likely to ask many, many questions of their health professional.

VALS helps medical marketers select target groups with particular affinities to particular products or services. In addition to providing insight into the lifestyles of the different VALS groups, the system also explains the different communication styles of each type so the marketer can tailor its message more effectively.

Table 3.3
VALS™ System

MOTIVATING FACTORS	VALS TYPES	RESOURCE LEVEL
Ideals, achievement, and self-expression	Innovators	Very high
Ideals	Thinkers	High
	Believers	Low
Achievement	Achievers	High
	Strivers	Low
Self-expression	Experiencers	High
	Makers	Low
Immediate needs	Survivors	Very low

Source: Adapted from SRI Business Insights.

Box 3.1
Marketing to Children

In spring 2011, a joint project incorporating the efforts of the Federal Trade Commission, Food and Drug Administration, Centers for Disease Control and Prevention, and Department of Agriculture established new voluntary guidelines[8] for the advertising industry related to the marketing of products to children. The project was designed to "advance current voluntary industry efforts by providing a template for uniform principles that could dramatically improve the nutritional quality of the foods most heavily marketed to children—and the health status of the next generation." Collaborators released two principles meant to encourage this outcome.

Principle A: Meaningful Contribution to a Healthful Diet

Foods marketed to children should provide a meaningful contribution to a healthful diet, with contributions from at least one of the following food groups:

- Fruit
- Vegetable
- Whole grain
- Fat-free or low-fat (1 percent) milk products
- Fish
- Extra lean meat or poultry
- Eggs
- Nuts and seeds
- Beans

Principle B: Nutrients with Negative Impact on Health or Weight

Foods marketed to children should be formulated to minimize the content of nutrients that could have a negative impact on health or weight. With the exception of nutrients naturally occurring in food contributions under Principle A (for example, the saturated fat and sodium naturally occurring in low-fat milk would not be counted), foods marketed to children should not contain more than the following amounts of saturated fat, trans fat, sugar, and sodium:

- *Saturated fat:* 1 g or less per reference amount customarily consumed (RACC) and 15 percent or less of calories
- *Trans fat:* 0 g per RACC
- *Added sugars:* No more than 13 g of added sugars per RACC
- *Sodium:* No more than 210 mg per serving

In the end, the government agencies involved hope these principles will be the foundation for uniform guidelines the advertising industry will follow when marketing food products to children.

HOW DID THE INFOMERCIAL BEGIN?

If you were born after 1990, infomercials may seem like they have always been on television. The truth is, they are a relatively new phenomenon. In the beginning of television, companies quickly figured out that a TV audience was a captive audience. Slowly but surely, program sponsors began placing more and more commercial material into the television programs they were sponsoring. Eventually, in the early 1950s, laws were passed regulating the number of minutes acceptable for commercials during a program. Those rules stayed in place until 1984, when then-President Ronald Reagan deregulated the cable television industry. Within weeks, 30-, 60-, and 90-minute programs for health products such as Herb-a-Life and Soloflex were on the air. Many of the original infomercials were get-rich-quick schemes, but a significant proportion focused on fitness and weight loss. Today, infomercials can be found on just about every cable network, at just about any time of day. Because many infomercials are low-budget endeavors, companies can actually spend less in advertising by taking this approach. Cowan[9] states that as the economy struggled between 2007 and 2010, the number of infomercials increased 18 percent, even as corporate advertising budgets were shrinking. See **BOX 3.1** for special guidelines for marketing aimed at children.

WHAT ARE THE HEALTH CARE FIELD ADVERTISING PRACTICES?

You will find that advertisers of health care products and services use many of the same approaches to influence consumer choice as advertisers of any other product or service. For instance, a 2007 study of hospital advertising[10] reviewed the most common appeals marketers used for the top 17 hospitals in the nation. More than 61 percent of all advertisements made some sort of emotional appeal, focusing on hope, fear, happiness, anxiety, or sympathy. Sixty percent of the advertisements reviewed made a specific reference to the hospital's status, levels of prestige, or awards received. More than half of the ads reviewed made specific reference to a disease or its symptoms. In contrast, less than 10 percent of the same reviewed ads indicated there would be less pain after the service, indicated minimal invasiveness of the procedure, used statistics to indicate successes, referred to safety, or mentioned cost.

What this study reveals is those hospitals, when competing for patients, use emotional and status-oriented appeals far more regularly than providing information about the services or the hospital. Consumers motivated by status, image, or appearance will be greatly influenced by this type of ad, yet may make a decision based on that image as opposed to the services themselves or the track record of the hospital.

WHAT IS THE COST AND EFFECT OF DIRECT-TO-CONSUMER ADVERTISING?

The bulk of research related to health advertising practices focuses on the DTC marketing of pharmaceutical products. In short, it is big business, and pharmaceutical companies make a great deal of money through DTC advertising. A Kaiser Foundation study determined that for every dollar spent on DTC marketing, pharmaceutical companies made $4.20 in profit. More than 39 million people each year report that a DTC advertisement led them to ask their medical professional about a specific drug. Because of the positive impact on sales, pharmaceutical companies now have more than 1000 lobbyists in Washington, D.C., and spend more than $150 million to influence politicians on regulatory matters.[11] It is big business.

With that much time, energy, and resources being guided toward advertising, a great deal of emphasis has been placed on the outcomes of such an effort. Simply stated, the results are mixed. Royne and Myers[12] summarized the arguments both for and against advertising pharmaceutical products directly to the consumer.

Supporters claim:

- Consumers obtain more information related to existing products.
- Information helps consumers make educated decisions.
- Advertising encourages consumers to see their doctor.
- Advertising may increase consumer knowledge of alternatives to medical treatment, or improve compliance with existing treatment.

Detractors claim:

- Advertising is promotional, not educational.
- Advertising increases demand for name-brand products instead of less expensive generic options.
- Advertising "medicalizes" normal human conditions.
- Advertising promotes brand preference and interferes with physician expertise and decision making.

Of course, not everyone reacts the same way to a pharmaceutical advertisement. Several things can influence this reaction, including degree of existing illness, history, emotional state, personal experience, and existing knowledge of the illness promoted in the ad. Thomaselli[13] reported that the percentage of consumers taking action after seeing a DTC ad is rising, from 31 percent in 1997 to 41 percent in 2006. Doohee and Begley add, however, that there are ethnic differences in how influenced consumers are. In their research,[14] advertising has a more significant influence on Hispanic and African American consumers, but those consumers were also most likely to be denied their request for a specific drug when presenting to a physician.

When all is taken into consideration, Royne and Myers[12] state the key is how the ads balance risk information with benefit information. When consumers have balanced information they can make choices in their best interest, and can initiate dialogue with their physician as opposed to demanding a particular drug.

HOW SHOULD WE ANALYZE ADVERTISING?

Experts suggest advertising should address a series of questions to help consumers make appropriate choices regarding pharmaceutical decisions. Consumers can use these suggestions to determine whether the company has provided enough information on a product to warrant a conversation with their personal physician. The following are guidelines suggested by Frosch et al.[15]:

> When a product provides information on an illness the consumer has not yet had diagnosed, and the consumer has no symptoms, the advertisement should explain the name of the condition, how prevalent the condition is, what risk factors exist for the condition (including family history, race and ethnicity, and other confounding illnesses), and lifestyle issues that might promote the illness' development. When a product provides information on a disorder, and the consumer *is* experiencing symptoms, the ad should describe the name of the condition and its prevalence, what symptoms the consumer might be experiencing, and the consequences of the condition if it were to go unaddressed. If the consumer has already been diagnosed with a condition, an advertisement should make sure it specifically states the name of the disorder.

Frosch et al. recommend that all pharmaceutical advertising address the benefits and potential risks of the drug. Benefit information should include how significant a reduction in symptoms a person should expect, how long treatment will last to get that benefit, how the medicine's benefit compares to a placebo or to lifestyle change benefit, research results of medical trials, and whether a generic alternative exists. When describing risks associated with the drug, information should be contained in a block of text distinct from the rest of the ad, narrated without distractions of noise or picture, and at a pace the consumer can understand.

When these criteria are met, the consumer can make informed decisions about choosing a drug. It then makes sense to have conversations with one's physician to determine whether the drug is the correct choice for the ailment, or if symptoms warrant testing and diagnosis related to the disorder.

CONCLUSION

Advertising has a powerful effect on consumer decision making. It is imperative that the consumer recognize this influence and make every effort to "read through" the approach taken in the advertisement, and see whether the product can have real benefit. In this way, consumers can make legitimate choices regarding their personal health and well being.

Review Questions

1. How much money did pharmaceutical companies spend on marketing in 2005?
2. What was the purpose of the Sherley Amendment and the Pure Food and Drug Act?
3. What is behavioral marketing?
4. Describe four marketing approaches commonly used in advertising.
5. Describe the stages a consumer goes through when deciding to purchase a product.
6. Write a five-sentence advertisement for a health product that makes an emotional appeal.
7. Describe the difference between Thinkers and Believers in the VALS system.
8. Describe the difference between Strivers and Achievers in the VALS system.
9. How do Innovators and Survivors fit into the VALS model?
10. What are the advantages of providing DTC marketing for health products?
11. What are the challenges to providing DTC marketing for health products?
12. If you already have been diagnosed with a disease, what should you look for when trying to determine whether an ad is telling you the "whole story" regarding its product? What if you have not been diagnosed yet?

Key Terms

advertising The act or practice of calling public attention to a product or service.

bandwagon Advertising technique where mass appeal is used to attract customers.

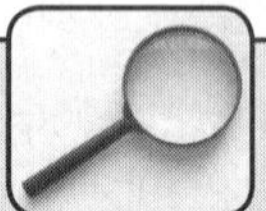

Case Study

Following are the transcripts from two hospital advertisements. Identify as many advertising techniques as you can for both ads.

Transcript for a new hospital opening in California:

Person in Ad: This is about making health care better.

Announcer: The extraordinary new Sharp Memorial Hospital is opening in January.

Person in Ad: They've thought of everything to make the nurses' jobs easier, the patient more comfortable, the family more welcome.

Announcer: It's the first hospital in San Diego where every room is a private room.

Person in Ad: And there's even a pull-out couch where family members are welcome to spend the night.

Announcer: For all that Sharp has to offer, call 1-800-82-SHARP or visit Sharp.com.

Person in Ad: You can feel the difference in these rooms.

Transcript for a children's hospital advertisement.

Kids don't use the word "impossible," so neither do we.

I guess having 50 surgical specialists performing 9,000 procedures a year might seem "impossible."

But "impossible" gets no respect around here.

And if one of those surgeries involves your child? You don't want to hear the word "impossible" either.

Our kids don't talk about impossible, so neither do we.

Children's Hospital Central California—amazing people, incredible care.

behavioral advertising Tracking a consumer's pattern of Internet use in an effort to display specific types of advertising that might appeal to those use patterns.

deregulation To remove governmental regulations and control.

direct-to-consumer Advertising sent directly to the consumer, not through a third-party provider.

infomercial A product commercial of significant length designed to look like a television show.

NARB (National Advertising Review Board) A group of advertising professionals organized to self-regulate the advertising industry.

product claim advertising A form of DTC advertising that reveals the product name and full disclosure of the product uses and side effects.

reminder advertising A form of DTC marketing that only provides the product name, without including details about its use or side effects.

Sherley amendment The section of the Pure Food and Drugs Act specifically designed to limit the amount of time commercials can be shown during a television program.

testimonial An advertising technique in which an individual client is used to share with consumers how a product or service worked for them.

VALS™ Marketing model used to design advertising to appeal to a particular group of consumers.

References

1. Frosch DL, Krueger PM, Hornik RC, Cronholm PF, Barg FK. Creating demand for prescription drugs: a content analysis of television direct-to-consumer advertising. *Ann Fam Med.* 2007;5:6–13.
2. Greene JA, Herzberg D. Hidden in plain sight: marketing prescription drugs to consumers in the twentieth century. *Am J Public Health.* 2010;100:793–803.
3. Schrank J. *The language of advertising claims: teaching about doublespeak.* Urbana, IL: National Council of Teachers of English; 1976.
4. McDonald A, Palmer L. Propaganda [Response-ible Rhetorics Web site]. December 15, 2003. Available at: http://mason.gmu.edu/~amcdonal/index.html. Accessed July 27, 2010.
5. Lee M, Johnson C. *Principles of advertising: a global perspective.* 2nd ed. New York: Hawthorne; 2005.
6. Hansen F, Christensen SR. *Emotions, advertising, and consumer choice.* Copenhagen, Denmark: Narayana Press; 2007.
7. Strategic Business Insights. U.S. Framework and VALS Types. Available at: http://www.strategicbusinessinsights.com/vals/ustypes.shtml. Accessed August 2, 2010.
8. Federal Trade Commission. Food for thought: interagency working group proposal on food marketing to children. Available at: http://www.ftc.gov/opa/2011/04/foodmarket.shtm. Accessed May 2, 2011.
9. Cowan J. The return of the infomercial. *Can Bus.* 2010;83(15):19.
10. Larson RJ, Schwartz LM, Woloshin S, Welch HG. Advertising by academic medical centers. *Arch Intern Med.* 2005;165:645–651.
11. Government Accountability Office. Prescription drugs: improvements needed in FDA's oversight of direct-to-consumer advertising. Washington, DC: GAO. December 2006. GAO-07-54
12. Royne MB, Myers SD. Recognizing consumer issues in DTC pharmaceutical advertising. *J Cons Affairs.* 2008;42:60–80.
13. Thomaselli R. DTC ads prompt consumers to see physicians. *Advert Age.* 2006;77:30.
14. Doohee L, Begley C. Racial and ethnic disparities in response to direct-to-consumer advertising. *Am J Health Sys Pharm.* 2010;67(14):1185–1190. Available from: Academic Search Premier. Accessed September 15, 2010.
15. Frosch D, Grande D, Tarn D, Kravitz R. A decade of controversy: balancing policy with evidence in the regulation of prescription drug advertising. *Am J Publ Health.* 2010;100(1):24–32. Available from: Academic Search Premier. Accessed September 15, 2010.

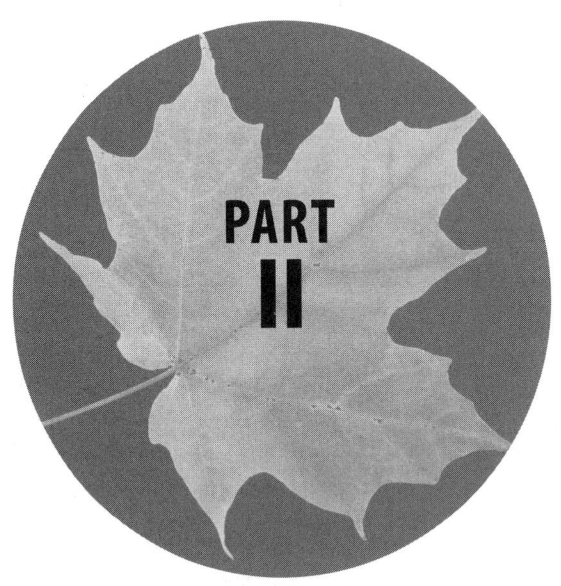

Traditional Medicine and Health Care

Cost of Health Care in the United States

LEARNING OBJECTIVES

As a result of reading this chapter, students will:

1. Discuss several ways in which healthcare may be made more affordable without limiting access to necessary care.
2. Summarize past practices that have increased healthcare costs.
3. Analyze what the health consumer can do to decrease healthcare costs.

IS THE COST OF HEALTHCARE SPIRALING OUT OF CONTROL?

Healthcare costs have risen dramatically over the past 30 years, from $253 billion in 1980 to a massive level of $2.5 trillion in 2009.[1,2] The increase from 2008 to 2009 was from $7,681 to $8,047 per U.S. resident, and in 2009, spending on healthcare comprised 17 cents of every dollar spent in the United States. **FIGURE 4.1** shows the national health expenditures for 2008.[2]

The Centers for Medicaid and Medicaid services estimate that by the year 2018, healthcare spending will be 19.3 percent of the nation's total economic output. These projections are reflected in **TABLE 4.1**.[1]

In 2009, healthcare accounted for 17 percent of the nation's gross domestic product (GDP), a percentage that is reportedly among the highest of all industrialized countries in the world.[3] Without changes to federal law, the nonpartisan Congressional Budget Office (CBO) estimated that number would rise to 25 percent by 2025.[3] In 2010, a healthcare reform law was signed by President Barack Obama. Some believe this will help make healthcare less expensive, but others disagree.

The cost of healthcare for employers rose 7.3 percent in 2009, which places a heavy burden on many companies and may result in less access to employer insurance benefits. This is what we call a catch 22 (heads I win, tails you lose). If individuals aren't offered medical benefits by their employers, they won't want to take the job. Medical benefits are certainly needed. On the other hand, if employers can't afford to pay, they go out of business and jobs are lost.

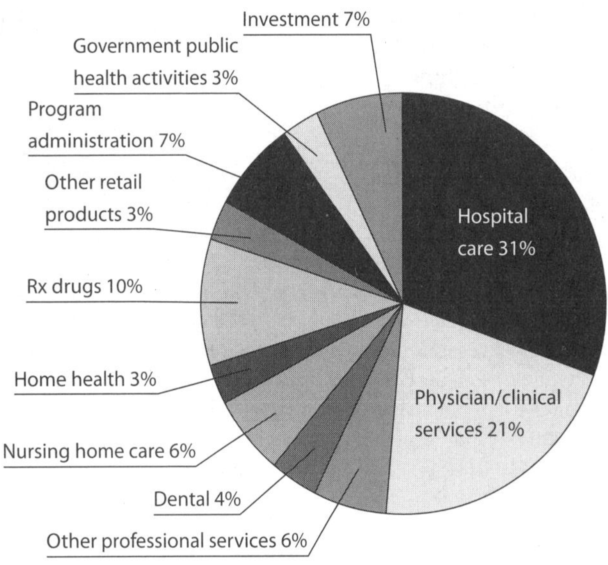

FIGURE 4.1 National health expenditures, 2008.
Source: The Kaiser Foundation, KaiserEDU.org. Medicaid: The Basics. August 2009. Available at: http://www.kaiseredu.org/tutorials/edicaidbasics2009/player.html. Accessed June 4, 2010.

Table 4.1
Projected National Health Expenditures in Trillions of Dollars

2010	2011	2012	2013	2014	2015	2016	2017	2018	2019	TOTAL 2010–2019
$2.6	$2.8	$2.9	$3.1	$3.3	$3.6	$3.8	$4.1	$4.4	$4.7	$35.3

Source: Reprinted from Centers for Medicare and Medicaid Services. Updated Extended National Health Expenditure projections, 2010-2019. Available at: http://www.cms.gov/NationalHealthExpendData/downloads/NHE_Extended_Projections.pdf. Accessed August 22, 2011.

WHAT ARE THE REASONS FOR RISING HEALTHCARE COSTS?

There is no dispute that the cost of healthcare has risen to monumental proportions. The reasons are complex and varied, but, in order to maintain a stable economy, the United States must control healthcare costs. The ballooning of healthcare costs in the United States is due to many reasons such as the following:

Waste in the healthcare system: PricewaterhouseCoopers conducted a national study[4,5] and reported that *wasteful spending* in the health system accounted for up to $1.2 trillion of the $2.2 trillion spent on healthcare in the United States, more than half of all health spending. More than 87 cents out of every dollar go directly towards paying for medical services. That is an amazing figure. Redundant, inappropriate, or unnecessary tests and procedures were identified as the largest area of wasteful spending. The study cited individuals' behavior or lifestyle as well as administrative processes as adding cost without adding value. The impact of waste is that, as healthcare costs rise, so do insurance premiums.[4,5] One could surmise that rising insurance premiums, on the other hand, drive up healthcare costs.

Unhealthy lifestyle: We, the consumers, drive up healthcare costs when we choose to engage in unhealthy lifestyles such as smoking, regularly overindulging in alcohol drinking or consuming illegal drugs, eating poorly, not exercising, not practicing stress relief techniques, and not attempting to get enough sleep at night. For example, not eating properly could result in obesity. That alone reportedly results in $147 billion in U.S. healthcare costs each year.[6] Tobacco use costs the United States $193 billion annually in direct medical costs and lost productivity.[7]

Uneducated personal health care choices: Some individuals may get the sniffles and, rather than treating themselves, rush to the doctor's office or to the emergency room. This raises healthcare costs. Others may not go to the doctor until they get a life-threatening condition or illness. This is exemplified in the following case study.

Social determinants: In the United States, the medical system is a proponent of the medical or *disease model*. This model embraces the view that many social prob-

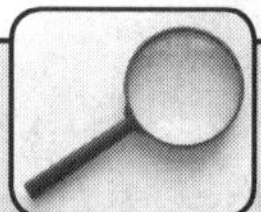

Case Study

Robert, age 48, is a long distance runner who has participated in many marathons in various states in the United States. He takes pride in eating a nutritious diet and having a body that is slender and muscular. He just completed a marathon in New York State and bested his own personal record. When he was running this marathon, he did feel some left arm tingling and numbness just as he had during his last few training runs. Robert ignores these symptoms, believing that he may have a pinched nerve in his neck. He vows that one of these days, he will take the time to get a checkup, but right now, he just doesn't have time. Robert is trying to maintain his training runs in preparation for the Hawaii marathon, and he has been under a lot of stress at work and needs to pour in some long hours into a new project. In addition, he and his wife have just had twin sons.

Questions:

1. What could be some possible scenarios as Robert continues to do all and be all?
2. What will be the impact on his future healthcare costs?
3. How will those healthcare costs affect his family?

lems such as alcoholism, obesity, drug taking, and other addictions (e.g., shopaholic, hypersexuality, gambling problems) are conditions that require medical treatment, a concept called the "medicalization of society."[8] Whether one agrees with this view or not, these treatments drive up healthcare costs.

Healthcare technologies: New technologies, such as digital imaging procedures, increase prices because they cost more than existing technologies. An MRI (magnetic resonance imaging) machine creates a strong magnetic field and combines with radio waves to form a three-dimensional image helpful in viewing the brain and other soft tissue. This has been a valuable contribution to the field of medicine. Let's use the MRI as an example of the high cost of technology. An MRI machine can range in cost between $1 and $3 million.[9] Not only does the hospital or clinic have to consider the cost of the machine, it has to have a room in which to house it and to provide all the electrical setup. Construction of the suites can cost $500,000. If an extremity MRI machine is purchased, this adds $300,000 to the cost and is only used to scan hands, feet, and knees.[9] It also costs an average of $800,000 per year to operate the scanner. The cost of hiring employees to operate these machines is high, as is the cost of repairing them when they break down. Wow. Who knew that technology could be so costly?

Facility expansion: Hospitals and clinics expand by building wings onto existing buildings or constructing new buildings on the grounds of the hospital. This cost can range in the millions of dollars. We, the consumers, eventually end up paying for these new buildings and services.[10]

Our desire for the latest treatments: Today, many treatments, including prescription drugs, are advertised on television. In response, we often go to our doctors and demand that they prescribe the medicine for us. Or, pharmaceutical representatives will visit the doctor's office and will market new drugs to the physician who, in turn, will prescribe them to their patients. These new drugs may or may not be better than the less costly older or generic drugs.

Consumer ignorance of healthcare costs: Most people who have health insurance do not know the cost of visiting their doctor, going to an emergency room, or being admitted to the hospital for medical care or surgery. We pay the copay or deductible and then don't bother to learn what the actual bill is until it is sent to us. Would we have had that knee cartilage repair if we had known what it would cost, or would we have attempted rest and physical therapy to correct the knee problem?

Government mandates: Federal and state legislation require that specific benefits or services, known as mandated benefits, be added to all health insurance plans. As a result, premiums increase. One federal mandate, the Health Insurance Portability and Accountability Act (HIPAA), although important to protect patients, nonetheless costs millions of dollars to implement.[10]

Aging population: Medical care can get very expensive as people age. By 2010, more than one in four Americans was 65 years of age or older. By the year 2020, the number of Americans 85 years or older will be 6.4 million, and the number of people 65 to 84 years of age will be 47.1 million. Medicare and Medicaid reimbursement may be in financial trouble, and the cost of long-term care and nursing home care is steadily increasing.[11]

Large amounts of money are spent on care for people in the final weeks of their lives. The 2008 National Issues Forums took place in 40 states[12] to discuss the crisis in rising healthcare costs. An aging population, use of expensive technology, and the expense of caring for people in the final weeks of life were identified as the major three causes. A study in New South Wales,[13] Australia, was cited. This study reported that, on average, inpatient costs increased greatly in the 6 months before death, from $646 per person in the sixth month to $5,545 in the last month before death. Cardiovascular diseases (43.1 percent of deaths) were associated with an average of $11,069 in inpatient costs, and cancer (25 percent of deaths) accounted for $16,853.[13] The highest average costs in the last year of life were for people who died of genitourinary system diseases ($18,948), and the highest average costs in the last month of life were for people who died of injuries ($8,913). Here in the United States, costs are even higher. CBS televised a program on the cost of dying and reported that it costs $10,000 a day to maintain a person in the intensive care unit.[14] Some people are in intensive care for weeks or even months. See the In the News feature for a further example.

As explained earlier in this chapter, there are many complex reasons for the rise in healthcare costs. Time will assess whether the new healthcare reform law will aid in decreasing healthcare costs. We, the consumers, must help by attempting to keep ourselves healthy and practicing disease prevention activities such as eating nutritiously, exercising, getting enough sleep, and obtaining health screening tests. When we do get sick, we should obtain information about treating minor conditions rather than running to the emergency room or doctor's office. It will take all of us to help solve the healthcare cost crisis.

WHAT ARE OUR MAJOR HEALTHCARE EXPENDITURES?

Physicians' services, hospital care, dental care, and eye care comprise the bulk of our healthcare expenditures. As people get older, home health care, assisted living homes,

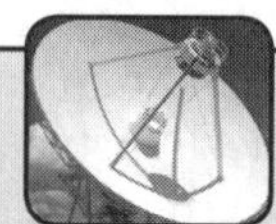

In the News

A *60 Minutes* news feature discussed the high cost of health care.[14] One example of the high cost of the last weeks before dying was exemplified by a woman, age 71 years, who was suffering from the complications of colon surgery and a hospital-acquired infection. She was unconscious in the intensive care unit at Dartmouth-Hitchcock Medical Center in Lebanon, New Hampshire, for the better part of a week. Her doctor told a CBS *60 Minutes* correspondent that it costs $10,000 a day to maintain her.

Also reported on this same program was the following case (excerpted from online at http://www.cbsnews.com/stories/2009/11/19/60minutes/main5711689_page2.shtml)[14]:

> Dorothy Glas was a former nurse who had signed a living will expressing her wishes that no extraordinary measures be taken to keep her alive. But that didn't stop a legion of doctors from conducting batteries of tests. "I can't tell you all the tests they took. But I do know that she saw over 13 specialists."[14] . . . "Neurological, gastroenterologists. She even saw a psychiatrist because they said she was depressed. And she told the psychiatrist, 'Of course, I'm depressed. I'm dying.'" When we reviewed the medical records, we discovered that there weren't 13 specialists who attended to her mother: there were 25, each of whom billed Medicare separately. The hospital told *60 Minutes* that all the tests were appropriate, and an independent physician said this case was fairly typical. Among the tests conducted was a pap smear, which is generally only recommended for much younger women, not an octogenarian who was already dying of liver and heart disease.

Questions:

1. What do you think is the reason that all those tests were performed?
2. What do you believe is the impact on the cost of healthcare?
3. What do you believe is the impact on the cost of health insurance?

and skilled nursing care become added financial problems. The next section describes how each adds to the cost of our healthcare.

Physicians' Services

In the United States, physicians and surgeons held about 661,400 jobs in 2008.[15] Primary care physicians have a median annual income of $186,044, and those practicing in medical specialties earned a median annual income of $339,738. Those physicians who are self-employed (i.e., own or partly own their own medical practice) have higher median salaries. The salaries vary according to their number of years in practice, the state or geographic region where they are practicing, and their professional reputation. Those self-employed physicians, however, do have to provide for their own health insurance and retirement pensions, and this can amount to great sums of money.

As shown in Figure 4.1 earlier in the chapter, physician/clinical services comprise 21 percent of healthcare costs.[1,2] Remember that total healthcare costs were $2.3 trillion in 2008. Twenty-one percent of $2.3 trillion is $483 billion. An astounding sum, isn't it? We all realize that national health expenditures have risen since 2008, and new graphs and charts will be published when the data are analyzed.

If physicians decide to increase their income, they may charge more for office calls and/or recommend more services per patient (e.g., lab work, blood workups, etc.). A physician fee schedule is used for reimbursement or payment from insurance companies. Current Procedural Terminology (CPT) codes are guides for setting physician fees. Medicare uses a different physician fee schedule than insurance companies; it mandated significant annual physician payment cuts for the last 10 years, which has forced many physicians to refuse patients who are on Medicare. The entire 2012 proposed Medicare Physician Fee Schedule[16] can be accessed online at https://www.cms.gov/physicianfeesched/. Physician fee schedules have served to keep physician fees fairly consistent, but also have caused conflict between physician groups, insurance companies, and the government. Physicians' practices depend on getting paid for services rendered, and their best chance of that is when their patients are insured.

At times, patients may decide to select a physician or hospital that is outside their contracted insurance network. When that happens, there is no set agreement, and doctors (providers) may charge what they want for services incurred. The insurance company, however, may not pay what the provider bills. Insurance companies that are medical preferred provider organizations (PPOs), point of service (POS) plans, high deductible health plans (HDHPs), or dental PPO plans base their amount of reimbursement on a scheduled fee basis or the usual, customary, and reasonable (UCR) schedule, also known as reasonable and customary (R&C).[17] "Usual" refers to the physician's own fees, "customary" refers to the range of fees charged by all physicians in a given region, and "reasonable" refers to a fee within a given region or area that falls below the ninetieth percentile of the customary charges. For non-network claims, the UCR

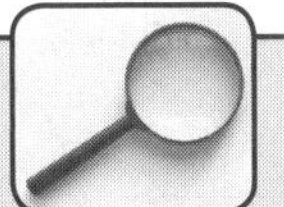

Case Study

A member is enrolled in a PPO plan that pays 90 percent of in-network charges and 70 percent of out-of-network charges. (Assume no deductibles apply.) The member is injured and needs surgery out of network, and the hospital and surgeon charges are $4,000. The carrier determines that the maximum allowable UCR charge for the surgery is $3,000. (Ninety percent of providers in the member's geographical area charge $3,000 or less for this type of surgery.) How much will the member end up paying out of his or her own pocket?

The insurance carrier will reimburse the member 70 percent of $3,000 (or $2100). The member will pay 30 percent of $3,000 ($900), *plus* the $1,000 difference between the billed charge of $4,000 and the UCR of $3,000. This additional $1,000 cost to the member is called "balance billing." In total, the member is responsible for paying $1,900 of the $4,000 billed charge, or 48 percent.

application comes first, and then coinsurance is applied. The following case study is an example provided by the ArlenGroup Employer Benefits Fact Sheet.[17]

As shown in this case study, individuals can end up paying hefty sums of money if they go out of network for treatment. Doctors also may not get the reimbursement they would ordinarily receive from an insurance company. Physicians look for other ways to supplement their income. One of those is investing in a hospital or other type of medical facility. For example, some physicians not only own their own medical practice, but also may own a hospital, a laboratory, and/or a physical therapy practice. A law known as the Anti-Referral Law[18] (also known as the Stark Law after the individual who sponsored it) is supposed to prohibit physicians from referring Medicare and Medicaid patients to a health care provider or facility with which they have a financial relationship. There are exceptions to the law, such as if a physician has an ownership interest in the entire facility rather than his or her personal specialty area (e.g., a neurologist having a financial interest in the neurology wing of the hospital). The second exception to the Stark Law is that the physician could refer the patient to the hospital if they are an active member of the hospital's medical staff. Critics use the argument that physicians who own hospitals may use poor judgment when making medical decisions. The practice may give doctors the incentive to hand pick patients who are the least sick or those who have good insurance plans and/or to prescribe unnecessary procedures.

Physicians do have great costs to maintain their practice. Malpractice insurance is one example. In 2002, obstetrics and gynecology physicians experienced a 22 percent increase in the cost of malpractice insurance, and general surgeons and internists experienced a 33 percent increase. Malpractice insurance varies among states and location within states. For example, general surgeons in Miami-Dade County, Florida, experienced a 75 percent increase between 1999 and 2002 (to $174,300). General surgeons in Minnesota saw their premiums raised by just 2 percent (to $10,140).[19] That is a substantial difference. Those physicians who pay $170,000+ in malpractice insurance will certainly be exploring ways to cover some of those costs, and more than likely, a part of that cost will come directly from patients.

Besides malpractice insurance, physicians are required to take continuing education credits that may require travel to conferences (airfare, hotel, and food expenses). They pay a lot of money to rent office space (if they don't own their own building), mortgage payments (if they do own

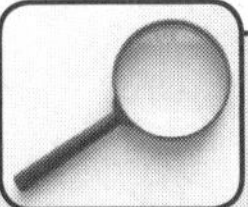

Case Study

Lydia, age 80 years, has gone to her doctor because of a middle ear infection. She is experiencing pain in her right ear, a feeling of fullness, and some loss of hearing. While in the doctor's office, Lydia also tells the doctor that she is having quite a lot of discomfort in her left hip and has been experiencing difficulty walking, especially on cold, rainy days. Dr. Brown has a major investment interest in the hospital that is attached to her office building. As treatment for Lydia's ear, Dr. Brown prescribes antibiotic ear drops and some pain medicine. She then has Lydia wheeled down the hall and over to the attached hospital to get an MRI on her "bad" left hip. There are two other hospitals in this large city.

Questions:

1. Do you feel that Dr. Brown should have discussed Lydia's options to choose where she would get her MRI procedure done?
2. How would you feel about it if the hospital had been the only one in a small community that had never before been able to raise funds for additional hospitals?

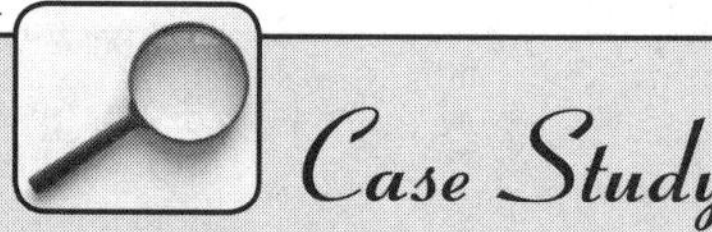

The following is an excerpt of a 2007 account of a failing hospital in Michigan.[20]

> North Oakland Medical Centers has been underwater financially, suffering an operating loss of $13.4 million in 2007. It had only 18 days' cash on hand at the end of the year, according to Standard & Poor's, and missed a payment earlier this year on $38 million in bonds issued under a lease agreement with the city of Pontiac. The Pontiac City Council has now agreed to sell the hospital property to Oakland Physicians Medical Center, an LLC formed by a consortium of physicians. The physicians expect to invest as much as $6 million toward the $11-odd million deal, and the hospital's owner, McLaren Healthcare Corp., will need to kick in $5 million.

The Michigan hospital could have closed if the Physicians Medical Center group had not taken over part of the hospital financing. Six million dollars seems like a large sum of money. Why do you suppose that the medical group put up the money? How soon do you think the group will recoup its investment? Do you believe it will eventually make money off this investment? Do you believe that the community will profit from this business venture? Why or why not?

On March 23, 2010, the practice of physician ownership in hospitals was curtailed. The Patient Protection and Affordable Care Act (the Act) was signed into law by President Obama to immediately prohibit future physician investment and caps existing physician investment in hospitals, as of the date of the Act's signing. This new piece of legislation restricts the current Stark law exception that allowed physician ownership in a hospital (the entire hospital, not just a wing of the hospital). The new legislation also states that the physicians who currently own an interest in a hospital cannot increase their interest (e.g., from 20% ownership to 30%).[21]

Questions:

1. What do you think will be the impact of the Patient Protection and Affordable Care Act on the cost of health care? Will it increase or decrease the cost? Why?

their own building), maintenance of the building, salaries of nurses and other staff, office equipment and furniture, and simple laboratory equipment (e.g., sphygmomanometers, stethoscopes, scales, etc.).

Along with the high cost of operating physician practices and decreasing reimbursement from insurance companies and Medicare, there has been an increase in physician fraud that is thought to increase health costs by $65 billion yearly. The False Claims Act was enacted so that citizens can now sue on behalf of the government to recover financial damages against people who filed a false claim for medical products and services.[22] It is also known as the whistle blower act or the qui tam actions (*qui tam* comes from the Latin phrase *qui tam pro domino rege quam pro se ipso in hac parte sequitur*, meaning "he who brings the action as well for the king as for himself"). Some overcharge the government for products sold or bill the government for services never provided. Still others cheat the government by contract fraud, defense contractor fraud, Medicare fraud, Medicaid fraud, or other public benefit fraud.[23]

Most of the fraud cases are identified as Medicare billing fraud. The definition of "fraud" has expanded to include unnecessary services, ineffective services, or non-compliance by physicians regarding Medicare requirements. Although most physicians who have patients on Medicare give them high quality care and bill only for the services provided, there are physicians who have taken advantage of a poorly regulated Medicare system. The Centers for Medicare and Medicaid Services (CMS), state and federal governmental agencies (FBI, Department of Justice, Department of Health and Human Services, Office of the Inspector General) are involved in stopping Medicare fraud.

As presented, physician services are valuable, needed, and costly. Physicians incur high costs to maintain their practices, pay office personnel salaries, and pay for malpractice insurance. There are some systems in place to curtail the cost of physician Medicare and insurance reimbursement. Much conflict, however, exists regarding ways to be fair to physicians and to healthcare consumers. The next section presents another major healthcare expenditure: hospital services.

Hospital Services

Hospitals can be classified according to the types of services they provide. For example, a hospital could be known as a trauma hospital, a women's health hospital, a military hospital, a medical school–based hospital, and so forth. Some hospitals are classified by size, based on the number of licensed beds they have. Hospitals could have from 10 beds to more than 1,500 beds. Hospitals may also be classified according to their financial base as a for-profit or nonprofit hospital.[24] Large corporations may own some for-profit hospitals, so those hospitals have to pay back a percentage of their profits to the owners (investors). And as presented earlier, some doctors own for-profit hospitals. Other hospitals are funded largely by community taxes.

As shown in Figure 4.1, 31 percent of the $2.3 trillion spent on healthcare in 2008 was spent on hospital care. That is a whopping $713 billion. The U.S. Department of Health and Human Services, Agency for Healthcare Research and Quality, has compiled statistics about hospital costs, as reflected in **TABLE 4.2**.[25]

Depending on the region, the mean or average total hospital charges ranged from $26,446.00 to $41,943.00. This figure does not reflect physician fees. The total mean or average costs ranged from $8,246.00 to $10,936.00. The Agency for Healthcare Research and Quality defines "costs" as being converted from *total charges* using cost-to-charge ratios based on hospital accounting reports from the Centers for Medicare and Medicaid Services.[25]

One of the reasons for high hospital costs is the cost of labor. The American Hospital Association (AHA) reports that labor cost increases have caused 35 percent of the overall growth in hospital costs.[26] Workforce shortages create pressure on hospitals to offer higher salaries for nurses, pharmacists, medical technicians, and other clinicians. The AHA report further claims that this rise in labor costs accounts for more than half the growth in the cost of goods that hospitals purchase and the services they offer. Other hospital costs are prescription drugs (5 percent), professional fees (5 percent), professional liability insurance (2 percent), and all others (18 percent).[26]

Other high hospital costs are due to the specialty medical machines. The following describes some of these:

- *Computerized axial tomography (CAT):* Provides detailed pictures of the body in order to help physicians more easily diagnose cancers, cardiovascular diseases, and other diseases. CAT scanning requires specialized x-ray equipment, and the scans are computerized so the pictures can be placed on a CD or printed.[27] The pictures show cross-sectional images of body parts. Depending on the model and type of machine, the selling price ranges from $500,000 to over $1 million. Operating costs may annually total $500,000.00.[28]
- *Positron emission tomography (PET):* A machine that injects a small radiopharmaceutical, FDG (a glucose analog), into the body in order to study the quality of blood flow to the heart or other tissues and to more easily detect malignancies. The machine costs $1 million to $2.5 million and has very high yearly operating costs.[29]
- *Magnetic resonance imaging (MRI):* Uses magnetic signals and radio waves to show digital pictures of nerves, muscles, ligaments, bones, and other soft tissue areas of the body.[30] The procedure involves several imaging sequences to produce several planes, image slices, or cross-sections that can aid physicians in diagnosing certain diseases earlier than other imaging techniques. Depending on the type of scanner, the cost varies, but all are expensive. For example, the 1.5-tesla scanners cost between $1 million and $1.5 million. The 3.0-tesla scanners cost between $2 million and $2.3 million. Not only does the hospital have to pay for the scanner, it also has to construct MRI suites that can cost $500,000 or more.[30]

The unfortunate thing about all this expensive (and valuable) equipment is that it becomes outdated and then needs to be replaced. Hospitals need them to attract doctors. No doctors, no patients, and then no revenue.

To decrease hospital costs, Medicare devised a method that hospitals have to follow when billing patients for services. It is dependent on physicians' diagnoses, and is called Diagnosis Related Groups (DRGs). Payment is set so that there is consistency for all Medicare patients. The CMS has now converted the DRG system to a more specific group set based on the severity of the diagnosis; it is known as Medicare Severity-DRGs (MS-DRGs).[31] Now Medicare can split a single DRG with complications into two MS-DRGs: (1) for

Table 4.2
2009 National Statistics Outcomes by Patient and Hospital Characteristics for All Discharges

		TOTAL NUMBER OF DISCHARGES	LOS, DAYS (MEAN)	CHARGES, $ (MEAN)	COSTS, $ (MEAN)	IN-HOSPITAL DEATHS
All discharges		39,434,956 (100.00%)	4.6	30,655	9,173	757,841 (1.92%)
Region	Northeast	7,663,438 (19.43%)	5.0	31,897	9,340	157,315 (2.05%)
	Midwest	8,989,260 (22.8%)	4.4	26,446	9,169	161,208 (1.79%)
	South	15,146,299 (38.41%)	4.5	27,123	8,246	296,800 (1.96%)
	West	7,635,959 (19.36%)	4.4	41,943	10,936	142,519 (1.8%)

Note: LOS, length of stay

Source: Data from HCUPnet. Healthcare Cost and Utilization Project (HCUP). 2006-2009. Agency for Healthcare Research and Quality, Rockville, MD. http://hcupnet.ahrq.gov/. Accessed June 10, 2010.

major complications (MCC), and (2) for regular complications (CC). Payment is then adjusted accordingly. The rationale for this system is that Medicare can pay less for cases that are not major complicated cases. Hospitals will have to review cases that are complicated and the hospital procedures in order to provide good care and to eliminate procedures that increase costs and patients' length of stay.[31]

Over the past 20 years, patients' length of stay in hospitals has decreased. Health insurance companies have initiated this to keep their costs down—patients go home when insurance will not cover costs. Although insurance companies' costs have decreased, patient care also has decreased. Many are forced to recuperate at home rather than in the hospital, and then suffer complications. Hospitals have lost the revenue and are forced to find other ways to make money. Many are now operating health promotion and education centers, mobile x-ray units, and ambulatory care centers.

Thus far, we have identified physician and hospital services as contributing to the high cost of healthcare. Dental services, nursing home care, in-home care, and other professional services also contribute.

Dental Services

Dental services account for 4 percent of healthcare costs. The costs of oral surgery and techniques for dealing with periodontal disease have contributed to dental care costs. Dentists also must abide by UCR fees.[17] Sometimes people who have dental bills submit a claim to their insurance company only to get a letter in return stating that the charge submitted was in excess of their UCR fees. One of the reasons is that dentists' fees vary according to geographic area of the country. Some dentists have higher expenses and then charge more. Besides the UCR fees, individuals have different dental plans, and some cover more expenses than others.

Nursing Home Care

As shown in Figure 4.1, nursing home care accounts for 6 percent of healthcare expenditures. Nursing homes may be identified as assisted living facilities or skilled nursing homes. People who do not require constant care but who can no longer live by themselves qualify for admission to an assisted living facility. Here, they are helped (assisted) with daily care such as eating, bathing, dressing, laundry, their medications, and housekeeping. They don't receive much medical care, but they can live independently until they have to be admitted to a skilled nursing facility. The average cost for a one-bedroom unit in an assisted living facility in 2009 was $33,903 annually, or $2,825 per month, but that price varied depending on the area of the country.[32] The northeast has the highest prices for both nursing homes and assisted living facilities.

A skilled nursing home must have registered nurses who can provide 24-hour care, and a licensed physician must supervise each patient's care. Many nursing homes provide custodial care in addition to skilled medical care. Custodial care means personal care: helping residents/patients bathe, dress, and eat. Residents may be living in a skilled nursing home temporarily if they are there for rehabilitation. After a course of treatment, they may return to their assisted living facility or home.

According to the AARP, the average cost of a skilled nursing home stay is $50,000 per year. Other studies show the cost for a private room may be more than $70,000 per year.[33,34] Costs vary depending on the state. For example, in Louisiana, the average cost is $50,594, compared to Connecticut where the average cost is close to $126,000.

In-Home Care

Even caring for loved ones in the home can be expensive, although depending on the circumstances the costs may not be as high as skilled nursing care or assisted living facilities. As shown in Figure 4.1, in-home care accounts for 3 percent of healthcare expenditures. Families may pay approximately $18.50 to $29.00 per hour for a home health aid.[35] If care is required 24 hours per day, the sum can get very high, and can match a nursing home's cost. If care is only needed for daytime hours, it may be the least expensive solution.

Other Professional Expenses

These services include therapists, chiropractors, optometrists, and podiatrists. According to the CMS, expenditures for these services reached $101.2 billion in 2008.[32] Thus far, the healthcare expenditures summarized have not included individuals' out-of-pocket expenses. The 2008 National Expenditures does not identify the out-of-pocket expenses that people are faced with, but there are sources that identify some of those costs.

Thus far, we have identified how most of the healthcare expenditures in the United States are spent. The major question to be answered is: In what ways could we control costs? A lot of very intelligent governmental agencies and private citizens are attempting to answer this question, but the solutions are not easy.

HOW CAN WE CONTROL HEALTHCARE COSTS?

There are many recommendations regarding how to control healthcare costs. The current administration (that of President Barack Obama) is calling for a greater emphasis on prevention of diseases, better management of chronic diseases, payment reforms to pay providers on the basis of outcomes, and research on comparative effectiveness to identify preferred diagnostic and treatment options.

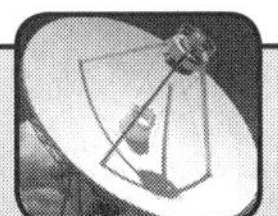

In the News

Out-of-Pocket Healthcare Spending

The *New York Times* published an article on out-of-pocket spending on March 29, 2010. A summary of this article is as follows.

The top two categories for out-of-pocket expenses in 2008 were prescription drug use and dental services. According to the Bureau of Labor Statistics, in 2008 $138.5 billion were spent in out-of-pocket healthcare expenses.[36] That sum excluded several other expenses such as health insurance premiums, nursing home care, nonprescription drugs and vitamins, topical remedies, and dressings. Out-of-pocket dental services expenditures were 22.2 percent of all out-of-pocket healthcare spending. This amount was second to prescription drug use, which is about one-third of total out-of-pocket expenses ($43 billion). **FIGURE 4.2** shows the division of expenditures.

Questions:

1. Do you think that people can continue to support out-of-pocket expenses?
2. Should insurance companies be required to insure more expenses?

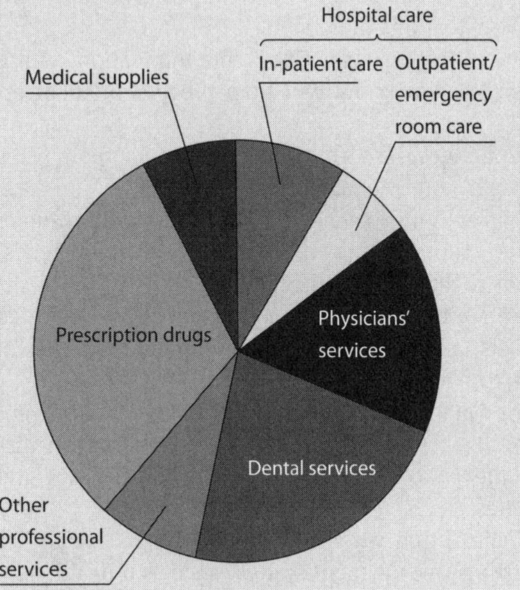

FIGURE 4.2 Aggregate out-of-pocket healthcare expenditures, 2008.
Source: U.S. Department of Labor. Bureau of Labor Statistics.

Many U.S. citizens wanted a single payer system (publicly funded and privately administered) as a part of health care reform, and although that did not happen, in 2010 a Democrat-controlled Congress passed healthcare reform legislation called the Patient Protection and Affordable Care Act (ACA). The hope is that this piece of legislation will help decrease costs. Clearly, large insurance companies have made huge profits. In the years from 2003 to 2007, profits rose 170.2 percent to $12.6 billion annually. Pharmaceutical companies also have grossed billions of dollars. For-profit hospital chains and dialysis centers are making millions and reportedly delivering worse outcomes than nonprofit facilities.[37] And yet, people are suffering with high healthcare costs.

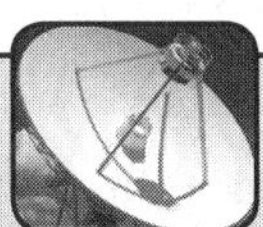

In the News

A July 2010 article in the *Baltimore Sun*, written by Dr. James Burdick, a Johns Hopkins surgeon,[38] discussed healthcare reform. He made positive comments about the appointment of Dr. Donald Berwick as the administrator of CMS. Burdick was hopeful about the ACA, describing it as open enough at present so that doctors can give input on how to decrease costs and create national treatment standards. Burdick's solutions for decreasing costs are to decrease the amount of red tape that doctors are faced with, form teams of collaborating professionals who communicate with each other, and increase electronic health records so there will eventually be a user-friendly and national record system that can send on information to the CMS. He does say that the new law is not complete, and it leaves doctors and patients relying on "insufficiently tamed private health insurance." And yet, he says it is a start to improving coverage and quality of care for millions.

Certainly, people should take self-responsibility in decreasing healthcare costs. Some tips from the BlueCross BlueShield of Illinois Web site[39] include the following:

- Keep an eye on costs. Review your own medical bills and explanations of benefits.
- Know your physician. Good communication with a physician you know will help prevent medical errors.
- Avoid unnecessary trips to the emergency room. This tip needs no explanation.
- Step up activity. Exercise is one of those prevention of disease strategies that will decrease health care needs, thereby decreasing healthcare costs.
- Take an ounce of prevention. Use seat belts, wear bike helmets, and use other safety equipment whether at work or play.
- Plan a balanced diet. Eating nutritiously will prevent becoming overweight or obese and will aid in disease prevention such as cardiovascular diseases and diabetes.

Some believe that we should use a prospective rather than a retrospective payment system, such as a health savings account (HSA). An individual would need to qualify for a low cost but high deductible health insurance plan (HDHP). Money saved from paying for a much less expensive insurance plan would go into a savings account to be used for medical care during the year.

Using alternative health care providers such as physician assistants and nurse practitioners could decrease costs. Regionalizing health services so that hospitals could share expensive equipment such as MRI and CAT scan machines also could help decrease costs. In the past, some thought that managed health care in the form of health maintenance organizations (HMOs) and the like would be the answer to decreasing healthcare costs. However, although HMOs have decreased users' personal costs, they have not decreased overall healthcare costs. HMOs offering community-based exercise programs, however, have been shown to reduce healthcare costs within the community.[40]

CONCLUSION

This chapter has presented information regarding the rising cost of healthcare, reasons for the cost, and some suggestions to decrease healthcare costs. The most important message is that all of us should take responsibility in decreasing costs while doing our part as knowledgeable health consumers.

Review Questions

1. What were the 2008 and 2009 national healthcare expenditures?
2. What are four reasons for the rise in healthcare spending?
3. How can health care be made more affordable without limiting access to necessary care?
4. What role should government play in controlling increases in the cost of care and the cost of health coverage?
5. Should individuals be responsible for the cost of their own care?
6. Are health savings accounts and high deductible insurance policies an approach that should be expanded?
7. What are the arguments for and against the Affordable Care Act and/or a nationalized health insurance system?

Suggestions for Class Activities

1. Determine the average cost of a surgical procedure. You can obtain this information from a hospital, a physician's office, or an insurance company.
2. Write a short descriptive passage about a visit to the doctor or to the emergency room (could be your visit, a relative's, or a friend's). Include the cost of the emergency room visit.
3. Visit a local nursing home and talk to the administrator. Inquire about services offered and cost per month for the typical patient in skilled nursing and in assisted living. Ask what percentage of medicare residents are accepted by the nursing home.

Key Terms

CAT (computerized axial tomography) scan An x-ray procedure aided by a computer so that cross-sectional views are obtained. Many x-ray images are taken at various bodily angles.

Current Procedural Terminology (CPT) codes Guides for setting physician fees.

gross domestic product (GDP) This is a measure of a country's overall economic output. It is the market value of all final goods and services made within the borders of a country in a year.

HDHP (high deductible health plan) A type of insurance plan that is typically cheaper than the other health plans, but has a much higher deductible (between $1,500 and $5,000). There is no coinsurance so once the deductible is paid, the remaining expenses are covered 100 percent.

Healthcare A system that offers, provides or delivers health care to individuals.

Health Care Refers to care given to a patient by medical or health professionals.

HMO (health maintenance organization) A type of health insurance provided at a lower rate and less co-pay. It requires consumers to go to a doctor in the network or expenses will not be covered.

MRI (magnetic resonating imaging) This machine creates a strong magnetic field and combines with radio waves to form a three-dimensional image helpful in viewing the brain and other soft tissue.

Patient Protection and Affordable Care Act (ACA) A health care reform law intended to expand coverage to millions of people and move the country toward a more primary care-based health care system.

PPO (preferred provider organization)/POS (point of service) A type of health insurance that provides a lower rate where-in people can use an in-network provider or pay somewhat more for an out-of-network provider. People may see specialists without a referral.

Stark Law Named after the individual who sponsored it. It is supposed to prohibit physicians from referring Medicare and Medicaid patients to a health care provider or facility with which they have a financial relationship.

UCR (Usual, Customary, and Reasonable) Used by the insurance industry to control costs. It began by reimbursing doctors 98 percent of the fee, and then went to 95 percent, 90 percent, 85 percent, 80 percent, and even lower.

References

1. Centers for Medicare and Medicaid Services. Updated and extended national health expenditures projections, 2010–2019. Available at: https://www.cms.gov/NationalHealthExpendData/downloads/NHE_Extended_Projections.pdf. Accessed July 7, 2010.
2. Kaiser Family Foundation. U.S. health care costs. Available at: http://www.kaiseredu.org/topics_im.asp?imID = 1&parentID = 61&id = 358. Accessed July 4, 2010.
3. Johnson T. Healthcare costs and U.S. competitiveness. Council on Foreign Relations. March 23, 2010. Available at: http://www.cfr.org/publication/13325/healthcare_costs_and_us_competitiveness.html. Accessed March 5, 2011.
4. PricewaterhouseCoopers. The price of excess: identifying waste in healthcare spending. Available at: http://www.pwc.com/us/en/healthcare/publications/the-price-of-excess.jhtml. Accessed July 4, 2010.
5. PricewaterhouseCoopers. PricewaterhouseCoopers cost study 2008. Available at: http://www.ahip.org/content/default.aspx?docid = 25127. Accessed July 4, 2010.
6. McKay B. Cost of treating obesity soars. *The Wall Street Journal, Life & Study*. Available at: http://online.wsj.com/article/SB10001424052970204563304574314794089897258.html. Accessed March 8, 2011
7. U.S. Department of Health and Human Services. Healthy people 2020. Leading health indicators. Available at: http://healthypeople.gov/2020/topicsobjectives2020/overview.aspx?topicid = 41. Accessed July 24, 2011.
8. Redican K, Gaffi C, Wessel T. *Dimensions of consumer health*. Englewood Cliffs, NJ: Prentice Hall; 1994.
9. Keefer A. How much do MRI machines cost? eHow. Available at: http://www.ehow.com/about_4731161_much-do-mri-machines-cost.html. Accessed July 6, 2010.
10. BlueCross BlueShield of Kansas City. Rising healthcare costs: the reasons. Available at: https://www.bcbskc.com/eprise/main/Public/Content/About_BCBSKC/News/Healthcare_Cost_Campaign/HCcosts1.html. Accessed July 1, 2010.
11. Rindfleisch T. Aging population looms over health care costs. Lacrossetribune.com. April 16, 2003. Available at: http://www.globalaging.org/health/us/healthcarecosts.htm. Accessed July 10, 2010.
12. Arizona Cooperative Extension, University of Arizona. Healthcare costs rising due to 3 reasons. July 10, 2009. Available at: http://www.extension.org/pages/Healthcare_Costs_Rising_Due_to_3_Reasons. Accessed July 10, 2010.
13. Kardamanidis K, Lim K, da Cunha C, Taylor LK, Jorm, LR. Hospital costs of older people in New South Wales in the last year of life. eMJA of Australia. *Med J Austr*. 2007;187(7):383–386.
14. CBSNews. The cost of dying. *60 Minutes*. Available at: http://www.cbsnews.com/stories/2009/11/19/60minutes/main5711689_page2.shtml?tag = contentMain;contentBody. Accessed July 15, 2010.
15. Bureau of Labor Statistics. *Occupational outlook handbook, 2010–11 edition*. Available at: http://www.bls.gov/oco/ocos074.htm#earnings. Accessed July 4, 2010.
16. Centers for Medicare and Medicaid. 2012 Medicare physician fee schedule. Available at: https://www.cms.gov/PhysicianFeeSched/01_Overview.asp#TopOfPage. Accessed July 24, 2011.
17. ArlenGroup. ArlenGroup fact sheet: usual, customary and reasonable. Available at: http://www.arlengroup.com/facts/fact_ucr.pdf. Accessed July 7, 2010.
18. Stark Law. Information on penalties, legal practices, latest news and advice. Available at: http://starklaw.org. Accessed July 7, 2010.
19. Kaiser Family Foundation. Medical malpractice policy. Available at: http://www.kaiseredu.org/topics. Accessed July 7, 2010.
20. Zieger A. Case study: midwest physicians seek hospital ownership deals. August 6, 2008. Available at: http://www.fiercehealthcare.com/story/case-study-midwest-physicians-seek-hospital-ownership-deals/2008-08-06?utm_medium = rss&utm_source = rss&cmp-id = OTC-RSS-FH0. Accessed July 7, 2010.
21. Waller Lansden Dortch & Davis. Healthcare reform bill prevents new physician ownership in hospitals. Available at: http://www.wallerlaw.com/articles/2010/03/25/healthcare-reform-bill-prevents-new-physician-ownership-in-hospitals.116887. Accessed July 7, 2010.
22. Whitney & Bogris, LLP. Medicare fraud qui tam actions. Available at: http://www.whitneybogris.com/index.php?option = com_content&view = article&id = 92&Itemid = 89. Accessed July 12, 2010.
23. Warren & Benson Law Group. Medicare fraud and other healthcare fraud. Available at: http://www.warrenbensonlaw.com/medicare-fraud/. Accessed July 24, 2010.
24. Santiago S. What are the types of hospitals, and how should I choose a hospital employer? Available at: http://healthcareers.about.com/od/whychoosehealthcare/f/HospitalFAQ.htm. Accessed July 12, 2010.
25. Agency for Healthcare Research and Quality. 2008 national statistics: outcomes by patient and hospital characteristics for all discharges. Available at: http://hcupnet.ahrq.gov/HCUPnet.jsp. Accessed July 12, 2010.
26. Davis C. Labor costs are key driver of hospital cost growth. [FierceHealthcare Web site]. Available at: http://www.fiercehealthcare.com/story/labor-costs-are-key-driver-hospital-cost-growth/2010-03-15. Accessed July 12, 2010.

27. RadiologyInfo.org. CT—Head. Available at: http://www.radiologyinfo.org/en/info.cfm?pg=headct. Accessed July 12, 2010.
28. Yoo I-S. Autopsy minus the scalpel [*USA Today* Web site]. Available at: http://www.usatoday.com/tech/news/techinnovations/2004-03-22-autopsy-usat_x.htm. Accessed July 13, 2010.
29. Bay Area Cancer Network Online. Positron emission tomography (PET) scan, PET/CT & vitamin B-12. Available at: http://www.babcn.org/images/news/petscan.htm. Accessed July 13, 2010.
30. Wikipedia. Magnetic resonance imaging. Available at: http://en.wikipedia.org/wiki/Magnetic_resonance_imaging. Accessed July 13, 2010.
31. Dotson P. AAWC alert! Changes to Medicare hospital payment 2007–2008. Available at: http://www.aawconline.org/medicare-payment.shtml. Accessed July 13, 2011.
32. National Coalition on Health Care. CMS report on 2008 national health care expenditures. Available at: http://nchc.org/facts-resources/cms-report-2008-national-health-care-expenditures. Accessed July 14, 2010.
33. Carter R. Study shows nursing home and assisted living costs grow in 2009. Available at: http://www.nursing-home-neglect.com/study-shows-nursing-home-and-assisted-living-costs-grow-in-2009. Accessed July 14, 2010.
34. Wang D. The average cost of nursing home care. Available at: http://www.ehow.com/about_5426391_average-cost-nursing-home-care.html. Accessed July 14, 2010.
35. Slobac C. Cost of home health care [Disabled World Web site]. June 13, 2010. Available at: http://www.disabled-world.com/disability/caregivers/home-care-costs.php. Accessed July 13, 2011.
36. Rampell C. Business out-of-pocket health care spending [*New York Times* Web site]. Available at: http://economix.blogs.nytimes.com/2010/03/29/out-of-pocket-health-care-spending/. Accessed July 9, 2010.
37. The Lund report: unlocking our healthcare system. Single payer healthcare only way to control costs. June 2009. Available at: http://lund.server274.com/resource/single_payer_healthcare_only_way_to_control_costs. Accessed July 11, 2010.
38. Burdick J. A leader for health care reform [*Baltimore Sun* Web site]. July 11, 2010. Available at: http://www.baltimoresun.com/news/opinion/oped/bs-ed-berwick-medicare-20100711,0,1104987.story. Accessed July 20, 2010.
39. BlueCross BlueShield of Illinois. Bringing health care costs under control. Available at: https://www.bcbsil.com/abbott/bringing_health.htm. Accessed July 10, 2010.
40. Edwards M. Healthcare costs might decrease with an HMO fitness program [That's fit Web site]. Available at: http://www.thatsfit.com/2007/01/19/healthcare-costs-might-decrease-with-an-hmo-fitness-program/. Accessed July 10, 2010.

Traditional Medical and Health Care

LEARNING OBJECTIVES

As a result of reading this chapter, students will:

1. Identify the steps that should be taken to improve the U.S. healthcare delivery system.
2. Assess potential problems that will be faced 20 years from now if the medical system is not improved.
3. List and describe several measures that must be implemented to contain healthcare delivery system costs.
4. Analyze the complexities of the U.S. healthcare delivery system and how they impact health.
5. Distinguish between osteopathic and medical doctors' educational training.

WHAT ARE THE COMPLEXITIES OF THE U.S. HEALTHCARE DELIVERY SYSTEM?

The healthcare industry in the United States is very complex, and due to a myriad of reasons, delivery of health care to U.S. citizens is suffering. Ownership of the healthcare system is largely in private hands, although governmental entities at the state, county, and federal level own many of the health facilities. Coordination of care among doctors and hospitals is rare, specialist care is favored over primary care, and costs are increasing at an amazing rate. Health insurance coverage among children under 18 years of age and adults ages 18–64 years has dropped from 1999 to 2009.[1] Please see **FIGURES 5.1** and **5.2**. During the same time

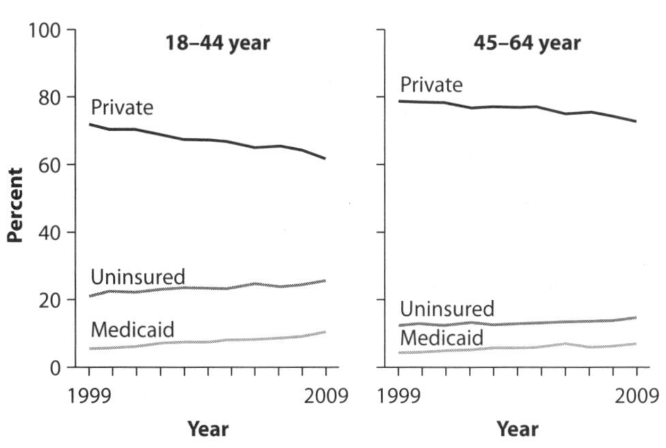

FIGURE 5.1 Health insurance coverage among adults.
Source: National Center for Health Statistics. Health, United States, 2010: With Special Feature on Death and Dying. Hyattsville, MD. 2011.

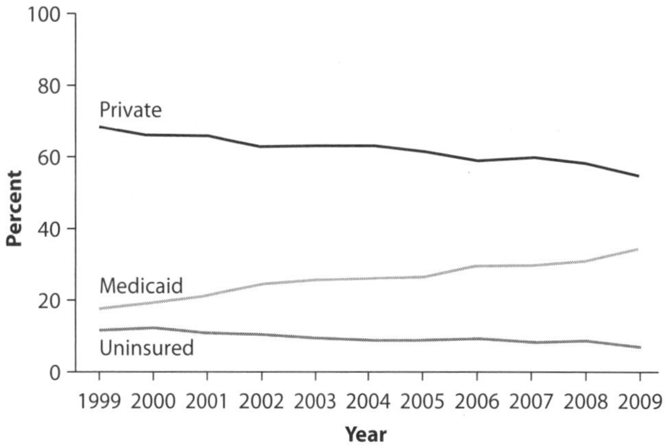

FIGURE 5.2 Health insurance coverage among children under 18 years of age.
Source: National Center for Health Statistics. Health, United States, 2010: With Special Feature on Death and Dying. Hyattsville, MD. 2011.

period, personal health care expenditures have increased. Please see **FIGURE 5.3**, which depicts the expenditures by source of funds.[1]

Just over 59 percent of Americans receive health insurance through an employer, a drop from 1999 when it was at 64 percent.[2] That percentage may decline even more, and the employee's expected contribution to these plans varies widely. As a result, a significant number of people cannot obtain health insurance through their employer or are unable to afford individual coverage.[2] The mean health insurance costs per worker hour for employees with access to coverage from 1999 to 2010 shows an increase from $1.60 per hour to $3.35 per hour (see **FIGURE 5.4**).

The U.S. Census Bureau estimated that 16.7 percent of the U.S. population, or 50.7 million people, were uninsured at some time in 2010.[3] Approximately 38 percent of the uninsured are in households earning $50,000 or more per year.[4] Despite the most severe economic downturn in 80 years, healthcare spending in the United States rose an estimated 5.7 percent to $2.5 trillion in 2009.[5] At the current rate of growth, healthcare costs are predicted to nearly double to $4.5 trillion in 2019.[5] At that point, they will account for 19.3 percent, or almost one-fifth, of our gross domestic product (GDP). Of that, approximately 45 percent was government expenditure.[4]

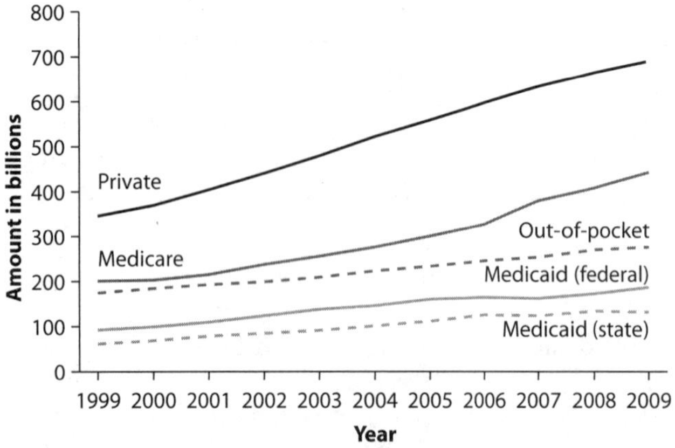

FIGURE 5.3 Personal health care expenditures, by source of funds.
Source: National Center for Health Statistics. Health, United States, 2010: With Special Feature on Death and Dying. Hyattsville, MD. 2011.

The World Health Organization (WHO) ranked the overall performance of the U.S. healthcare system as thirty-seventh out of 191 countries worldwide, and ranked the United States at number 1 for expenditure per capita.[6] Our problems may be due to a variety of reasons. We have a healthcare system that has not optimized operations at hospitals and regional networks, and a system that has not developed performance measures regarding quality and scope of medical care.[7] The Institute of Medicine[7] proposes the following six quality criteria with which to improve the U.S. healthcare delivery system:

- Safety
- Effectiveness
- Patient-centeredness
- Timeliness
- Efficiency
- Equity of health care for all

Adding to the poor quality of our healthcare delivery system has been the lack of utilization of existing science and technology. Examples offered by Sainfort[7] are in the areas of genomics, sensor technologies, nanotechnologies, and information and communication technologies. The committee on the Quality of Healthcare in America identified several key areas in which information technology could contribute to an improved delivery system[8]:

- Access to medical knowledge base
- Computer-aided decision support systems
- Collection and sharing of clinical information
- Reduction in medical errors
- Enhanced patient and clinician communication

Another factor that has increased health care delivery problems has been changing mortality patterns. By 2025, the group of individuals age 65 or older is projected to increase to 20 percent of the entire population from the

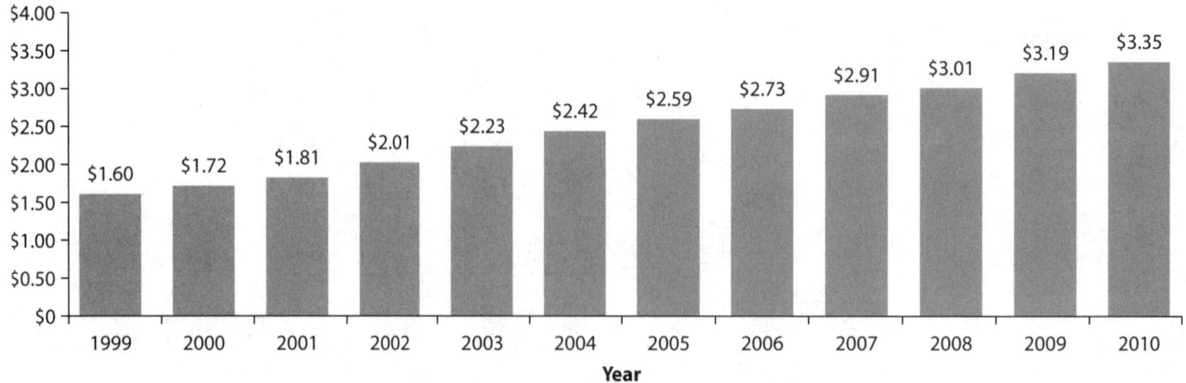

FIGURE 5.4 Mean health insurance costs per worker hour for employees with access to coverage, 1999–2010.
Source: The Henry J. Kaiser Family Foundation. Kaiser Family Foundation calculations base on data from the National Compensation Survey, 1999-2010, conducted by the Bureau of Labor Statistics. Available at: http://www.kff.org/insurance/snapshot/employer-health-insurance-costs-and-worker-compensation.cfm.

current 14 percent.[3] The consequence is that people with chronic medical conditions (e.g., diabetes, dementias, arthritis) will be surviving longer and will need medical care for even more years. It will be extremely beneficial, therefore, to improve the U.S. healthcare delivery system. Let's now turn to the medical/healthcare programs that are currently in place.

WHAT ARE THE CURRENT HEALTHCARE PROGRAMS?

Medicare and Medicaid

The Centers for Medicare and Medicaid Services (CMS) is a component of the U.S. Department of Health and Human Services. Medicare is the largest health insurance program in the United States. It covers nearly 40 million Americans including people who are age 65 or older, some disabled people under age 65, and people of all ages with end-stage renal disease (permanent kidney failure treated with dialysis or a transplant).[9] See **BOX 5.1** for important details about Medicare.[9]

Medicaid is a medical assistance program for people under the age of 65 who have limited income and assets. Persons receiving a Supplemental Security Income (SSI) check automatically qualify for Medicaid. The cost of Medicaid grew an estimated 9.9 percent in 2009, which puts an increased burden on states even though they receive federal aid.[10] Medicaid will pay for certain goods and services. It is important to note that there are eligibility requirements and limitations on what is covered under Medicaid. Some examples of services for which regular Medicaid will pay can be seen in **BOX 5.2**.[10]

Box 5.1

Medicare Services

Medicare Part A

Part A is hospital insurance. Most people don't pay a premium for Part A because they or a spouse already paid for it through their payroll taxes while working. It helps cover inpatient care in hospitals, including critical access hospitals, and skilled nursing facilities (not custodial or long-term care). It also helps cover hospice care and some home health care.

Medicare Part B

Part B is medical insurance. Most people pay a monthly premium for Part B. Medicare Part B helps cover doctors' services and outpatient care. It also covers some other medical services that Part A doesn't cover, such as some of the services of physical and occupational therapists, and some home health care.

Prescription Drug Benefits

Medicare prescription drug coverage is insurance. Private companies provide the coverage. Beneficiaries choose the drug plan and pay a monthly premium. Like other insurance, if a beneficiary decides not to enroll in a drug plan when they are first eligible, they may pay a penalty if they choose to join later.

Box 5.2

Medicaid Services

- Doctor's visits
- Certain dentures
- Eye care services due to injury or disease
- Hospital bills, laboratory, and x-ray services
- Most prescription medicines
- Personal care services
- Transportation for medical appointments
- Rehabilitation services
- Medical equipment
- Medicare premiums, deductibles, and co-payments for certain persons with Medicare

State Children's Health Insurance Program

The State Children's Health Insurance Program (SCHIP) was created in 1997 to provide matching funding to states to provide health care coverage to children age 18 years or younger whose families' income was too high to qualify for Medicaid but too little to afford health insurance. The level was determined to be approximately twice the federal poverty level, or about $41,000 in 2007.[11]

Veteran's Health Administration

The Veteran's Health Administration (VA) provides care for U.S. military veterans. The VA offers many benefits for veterans based upon discharge from active military service other than dishonorable conditions.[12] Services include education, vocational rehabilitation, home loans, and survivor benefits. Those related to health care delivery services include life insurance, disability compensation, and burial allowances. Disability compensation is a benefit paid to a veteran because of injuries or diseases that happened while he or she was on active duty, or were made worse by active military service. It is also paid to certain veterans disabled from VA health care. The benefits are tax-free.[12]

TRICARE

TRICARE is the Department of Defense's healthcare insurance program for active duty service members, retired ser-

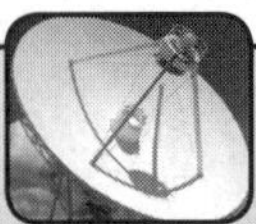

In the News

Healthcare reform legislation (Patient Protection and Affordable Care Act) was approved by Congress in 2010. Because of that, many people were apprehensive that Medicare benefits would be reduced. There are no cuts to the traditional Medicare benefit, however, there are spending cuts in Medicare Advantage,[14] a program that uses private firms such as Humana and UnitedHealth Group to deliver Medicare benefits. Medicare Advantage has cost the federal government 10 percent more than traditional Medicare.[14] "Many of the providers offer extra coverage and some of those extras could be dropped as Medicare Advantage subsidies are brought more in line with the cost of traditional Medicare benefits."[14] To give companies time to make needed changes, Medicare Advantage payment rates are frozen in 2011 and then will be gradually reduced so that by 2019, costs will be closer to traditional Medicare program costs and will save the government $117 billion between 2010 and 2019. Enrollment in Medicare Advantage is expected to drop from 13.9 million enrollees to 9.1 million enrollees in 2019.[14]

People also began to question if the new healthcare reform bill would bring any benefits to Medicare. Reuter's explains that Medicare would improve the prescription drug program by closing a significant coverage gap. The gap has been known as the "doughnut hole." After people get $2,700 of prescription drug benefits, they have to pay for their own prescriptions until they have paid $6,154. Medicare coverage would then begin again after that.[15] However, in 2010, people who fell into the doughnut hole got a $250 rebate, and in 2011 got a 50 percent discount on brand-name drugs. By 2020, people will be covered for 75 percent of their prescription drug costs.[16]

vice members, and their dependents. It is also available for activated National Guard or Reserve members. TRICARE offers several healthcare programs including TRICARE Pharmacy, TRICARE Dental (United Concordia), and TRICARE for Life.[13]

WHAT INSTITUTIONS ARE CARING FOR THE SICK?

Hospitals

When people get sick, need surgery, or need mental health services, they usually go to hospitals. Some hospitals are public (nonprofit) and some are private (for-profit). A public hospital is owned by the government and receives government funding. People may receive care free of charge. In 2007, of the roughly 5,010 nonfederal, short-term, acute care community hospitals in the United States, approximately 2,923 (58 percent) were nonprofit.[16] Nonprofit hospitals are often affiliated with a religious denomination and have a charitable purpose. See **TABLE 5.1** for a list of the different types of hospitals in existence in 2009 from data taken in the 2009 annual survey of U.S. hospitals.

Major Medical Centers

Many large cities not only have several hospitals, but also have major medical centers. Those associated with a medical school are often part of a conglomerate of health care services. Health care conglomerates are composed of hos-

Table 5.1
U.S. Hospitals, November 2009

TOTAL NUMBER OF ALL U.S. REGISTERED* HOSPITALS	5,795
Number of U.S. community** hospitals	5,008
Number of nongovernment not-for-profit community hospitals	2,918
Number of investor-owned (for-profit) community hospitals	998
Number of state and local government community hospitals	1,092
Number of federal government hospitals	211
Number of nonfederal psychiatric hospitals	444
Number of nonfederal long-term care hospitals	117
Number of hospital units of institutions (prison hospitals, college infirmaries, etc.)	15

Note: * Registered hospitals meet AHA's criteria for registration as a hospital facility.[16] **Community hospitals defined as all nonfederal, short-term general, and other special hospitals (obstetrics and gynecology; eye, ear, nose, and throat; rehabilitation; orthopedic; and other specialty services.[16]

Source: American Hospital Association. Fast Facts on US Hospitals. Available at: http://www.aha.org/aha/resource-center/Statistics-and-Studies/fast-facts.html. Accessed August 12, 2011.

Box 5.3
Major U.S. Medical Centers

- Cleveland Clinic
- Mayo Clinic
- Texas Medical Center
- Massachusetts General
- New York Presbyterian Hospital
- UC, San Francisco Medical Center
- Ronald Reagan UCLA Medical Center
- Duke University Health System
- Johns Hopkins Hospital

pitals, clinics, and research facilities that either include, or are affiliated with, a medical school. Major medical centers are considered the crown jewels of health care in the United States. See **BOX 5.3** for a sample list of major medical centers. Medical centers vary greatly in their organization, the services they provide, and their ownership and operation.[1]

WHO PROVIDES THE CARE?

Physician: Primary Care Provider and Specialists

A variety of health professionals provide primary care, nursing care, and specialty care. The primary care provider is the person first seen for checkups and health problems. This person may be a *medical doctor (MD)* or a *doctor of osteopathic medicine (DO)*. Both may specialize in internal medicine or family practice. In addition to primary care specialists, some physicians specialize in an advanced practice; for example, a pediatrician specializes in the care of children and an obstetrician or gynecologist specializes in women's health care and prenatal care. Physicians may specialize in surgery or in neurology. Some may become ophthalmologists (eye doctors) or podiatrists (foot care doctors). There are also nonphysician health care providers, which are identified next.

Nonphysician Health Care Providers

A *nurse practitioner (NP)* is a registered nurse who has obtained advanced education and clinical training; these days, most obtain a master's or doctorate degree in nursing practice studies.[16] The NP may work independently or collaboratively on a health care team. The NP may specialize in family medicine, geriatrics, or other areas. NPs take health histories and provide complete physical examinations, diagnose and treat many common acute and chronic problems, interpret laboratory results and x-rays, prescribe and manage medications, and perform other therapies.[17] They may provide health teaching and counseling to support healthy lifestyle behaviors and prevent illness, and are expected to refer patients to other health professionals as needed.

Another type of health care provider is the *physician assistant (PA)*, who can also provide many services and works under the guidance of a physician. A typical course of training would be a 33-month, graduate curriculum in the basic sciences, medicine, clinical skills, public health and epidemiology, health care administration, and psychosocial and behavioral sciences.[17] Students first complete a bachelor's degree as well as a set of program prerequisites.

PAs may be the principal care providers in rural or inner-city clinics where a physician is present for only 1 or 2 days each week. In such cases, the PA confers with the supervising physician and other medical professionals as needed and as required by law. Just as with the NP, the PA may provide diagnostic, therapeutic, and preventive health care services, as delegated by a physician. They may take medical histories, examine and treat patients, order and interpret laboratory tests and x-rays, and make diagnoses.[18] They also treat minor injuries by suturing, splinting, and casting. Physician assistants also may prescribe certain medications.

WHO ARE THE ORTHODOX OR TRADITIONAL PHYSICIANS?

Allopathic Physician

The allopathic physician is considered the traditional medical doctor (MD). The training of MDs takes many years.[19] Prospective MDs must first get an undergraduate BS or BA degree, usually in biology, chemistry, or physics, while maintaining at least a 3.5 GPA. They usually take the Medical College Admissions Test (MCAT) examination before graduating from college, and to be considered for medical schools, will need to make a score of 27 or above. There are only 132 accredited 4-year medical schools in the United States, so the process to get accepted into one of them is quite rigorous.[19]

Medical school includes 4 years of preclinical and clinical aspects. After medical school, graduates enter a residency program (graduate medical education). The residency may be 3 to 7 years or more depending on the specialty area. For example, family practice, pediatrics, and internal medicine require 3-year residencies whereas general surgery requires a 5-year residency. According to the American Medical Association,[19] the first year of the residency may be considered an internship, although the term is no longer used. After medical school and residency, doctors then have to obtain a license to practice, which requires completing a series of exams. Most physicians will then opt to become board certified in their specialty areas. Moreover, physicians who desire to become more highly specialized in an area may complete a fellowship that could take 1 to 3 additional years. The learning does not stop there. Even after all these years of training, while in practice, physicians are required to obtain continuing medical education credits every year. Although the figure changes each year, currently, there are approximately 788,000 active MD physicians.[19]

Osteopathic Physician

Doctors of osteopathic medicine (DOs) practice a "whole person" approach to health care by not just treating specific symptoms. Osteopathic physicians are also considered traditional physicians. Osteopathic physicians understand how all the body's systems are interconnected and how each one affects the others. They believe that the musculoskeletal system reflects and influences the condition of all other body systems and believe that disease and its symptoms may be caused by disturbances of bones, muscles, or ligaments.[20]

Andrew Taylor Still was a medical doctor who founded osteopathic medicine in 1874. He was antagonistic toward drug and surgical practices of his day. He was especially disillusioned with blood-letting practices. Dr. Still believed that adequate functioning of the body depended on uninterrupted nerve and blood supply to tissues, so he began to use spinal manipulation to remove interference. Thus began the practice of osteopathy, and in 1892, the American School of Osteopathy at Kirksville, Missouri, was founded. Currently, there are 26 colleges of osteopathic medicine in the United States.[21]

To become a doctor of osteopathy, individuals must complete a 4-year undergraduate degree including specific science courses. Just as applicants for medical schools must do, applicants for osteopathy schools must take the MCAT. In addition, osteopathic medical schools typically require applicants to participate in a personal interview.[20]

The curriculum at osteopathic medical schools consists of 4 years of academic and clinical studies, and emphasizes preventive medicine and comprehensive patient care. Clinical studies concentrate on teaching doctoral students how to use osteopathic principles and osteopathic manipulative treatment to diagnose and treat patients. After completing osteopathic medical college, DOs obtain graduate medical education through internships, residencies, and fellowships that range from 3 to 8 years of training. During this time, DOs may specialize in any area of medicine, the same as a medical doctor (e.g., family medicine, general internal medicine, and pediatrics, or specialized disciplines such as surgery, radiology, oncology, psychiatry, and sports medicine).

Although many people are not familiar with the educational background and requirements of osteopathic physicians, they are fully trained physicians who prescribe drugs, perform surgery, and use accepted methods to maintain and restore health. Currently, there are approximately 55,000 licensed DOs in the United States, and about 60 percent of them practice as primary care doctors.[21]

WHAT IS THE FLEXNER REPORT?

In 1906, Abraham Flexner was commissioned by the Carnegie Foundation and the American Medical Association's Council on Medical Education to review 155 medical schools and their educational curriculum.[22] Flexner was not a doctor; he was a secondary school teacher and principal for 19 years in Louisville, Kentucky. His report was published in 1910 and is known as the Flexner Report.[22,23] Flexner found discrepancies among medical schools in terms of length of program and types of courses. Some medical students had never attended college. The Flexner Report rank ordered the medical schools and triggered much-needed reforms in their standards, organization, and curriculum. As a result of the study, certain schools closed and others were reorganized and restructured. By 1926, the AMA had a monopoly over the education and licensing of physicians.[24] Thereafter, all medical schools in the United States were based at universities and the curriculum became consistent and rigorous among all medical schools.

HOW SHOULD I CHOOSE OR FIRE A PHYSICIAN?

Thus far in this chapter, we have discussed the healthcare delivery system and identified several health professionals and physicians. Now, let's discuss how to choose a physician and, if necessary, how to fire one. Finding a good

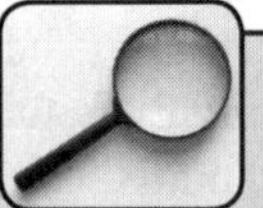

Case Study

Ann has lived all of her life in a large city in Illinois. She has just graduated from college and has accepted a job in a neighboring state. Ann has moved to a large, strange city where she knows no one, although she met a few people when she interviewed for the job. One of the major tasks that Ann wants to do is to find a family doctor and a gynecologist.

Questions:

1. What steps must Ann take to find competent physicians?
2. How can Ann verify that the physicians she selects have adequate medical training and years of experience?
3. If Ann's doctors do not provide adequate care for her, what options does she have?

physician is one of the most important health consumer functions that individuals and families need to perform.

Finding and Selecting a Physician

People want to find a doctor with whom they can develop trust and faith; therefore, identifying a potential doctor may take some research. Whatever methods you use to find a physician, the most important step is determining which criteria are important (e.g., clinical training, experience, board certification, plus interests and expertise in a specialized area). For some people, the age and sex of the physician are important. For many people, it is also important to choose a physician whose philosophy of care is in keeping with their own.

As you are attempting to select a physician, you might want to consider the setting of the physician's office. Determine if you would like a small, more intimate setting or if you would be agreeable to seeing a physician whose practice is within a large clinic setting. The location of the office is another important criterion. If you live in a large city (e.g., Chicago or Houston), you might want to select a physician whose office is close to your home or work.

Now that you have determined certain important criteria, there are other factors that need to be considered. For instance, if a person accepts a health maintenance organization (HMO) insurance plan, a list of physicians associated with that particular HMO is identified. With traditional insurance plans and preferred provider organization (PPO) health insurance, a wider physician selection is offered. Nonetheless, choices are available.

One of the ways that people select a physician is to use the telephone book. They just arbitrarily select a physician without knowing much about the person. This is definitely not the best way to select a physician. Some people rely on the recommendation of a physician by an acquaintance or friend. This is a moderately good way for you to select a physician. Some try researching the physician online, and this is another good method of narrowing your search. Many physicians today do have a personal Web site or one maintained by the hospital or clinic with which the physician is associated. Another database you could examine is the American Board of Medical Specialties' (ABMS) Compendium of Certified Medical Specialists.[24] Most communities and cities have an online Directory of Medical Specialists[25] where people can obtain information about all physicians in the area. You could also check the American Medical Association's online Doctor Finder Directory.[26]

However you find your physician, it is important to check to determine whether a prospective doctor is affiliated with a hospital accredited by the Joint Commission. The Joint Commission accredits approximately 4,168 general, children's, long-term acute, psychiatric, rehabilitation and specialty hospitals, and 378 critical access hospitals, through an accreditation program.[27] Approximately 82 percent of the nation's hospitals are currently accredited by the Joint Commission. Also, check the American Hospital Association's Guide to the Health Care Field,[28] which is an encyclopedic hospital directory of health care and hospital systems profiles.

As you can see, it is not an easy job to select a physician. You have to decide which personal criteria are important and then make a responsible choice. It is wonderful that today many helpful databases are available—but only if we take the time to access them.

Firing a Physician

There are times when you might encounter problems with your physician. Perhaps you have to wait a long period of time before getting in to see the doctor. Perhaps the doctor seemed rushed and eager to get out of the examination room. Perhaps the doctor did not take time to adequately answer your questions. Perhaps he or she refused your right to get a second opinion. The main point to consider is that if you have one isolated incident, keep your doctor. But if you have consistent problems, it is your right to find another physician. Start the search using many of the techniques discussed in the previous section. Ask a friend or other health care provider. Check credentials. Look for a board-certified physician. When you have selected your new physician, ask in writing to have your records transferred to your new doctor.

As shown, to find a doctor that you will be comfortable with, you must conduct a careful and thoughtful research process. Once you have found a physician, you need to be knowledgeable about your rights as a patient.

WHAT ARE OUR RIGHTS?

Patients do have the right to be competently cared for, and many patient's bills of rights have been formulated. For example, there are mental health bills of rights, hospice patients' bills of rights, insurance plan bills of rights, and so forth. The following lists the American Medical Association (AMA) bill of rights[29] and the U.S. Advisory Commission on Consumer Protection and Quality in the Health Care Industry patient's bill of rights.[30]

The AMA wrote a bill of rights within its Code of Medical Ethics. The rights are as follows[29]:

- The right to receive information from physicians and to discuss the benefits, risks, and costs of appropriate treatment alternatives
- The right to make decisions regarding the health care that is recommended by the physician
- The right to courtesy, respect, dignity, responsiveness, and timely attention to health needs
- The right to confidentiality
- The right to continuity of health care
- The basic right to have adequate health care

In 1998 the U.S. Advisory Commission on Consumer Protection and Quality in the Health Care Industry created its patient's bill of rights[29] to reach three major goals: (1) to help patients feel more confident in the U.S. health care system; (2) to stress the importance of a strong relationship between patients and their health care providers; and (3) to stress the key role patients play in staying healthy by laying out rights and responsibilities for all patients and health care providers. The following eight key areas were delineated[30]:

- *Information for patients:* You have the right to accurate and easily understood information about your health plan, health care professionals, and health care facilities.
- *Choice of providers and plans:* You have the right to choose health care providers who can give you high-quality health care when you need it.
- *Access to emergency services:* If you have severe pain, an injury, or sudden illness that makes you believe that your health is in danger, you have the right to be screened and stabilized using emergency services.
- *Taking part in treatment decisions:* You have the right to know your treatment options and take part in decisions about your care. Parents, guardians, family members, or others that you choose can speak for you if you cannot make your own decisions.
- *Respect and nondiscrimination:* You have a right to considerate, respectful care from your doctors, health plan representatives, and other health care providers that does not discriminate against you.
- *Confidentiality of health information:* You have the right to talk privately with health care providers and to have your health care information protected. You also have the right to read and copy your own medical record. You have the right to ask that your doctor change your record if it is not correct, relevant, or complete.
- *Complaints and appeals:* You have the right to a fair, fast, and objective review of any complaint you have against your health plan, doctors, hospitals or other health care personnel. This includes complaints about waiting times, operating hours, the actions of health care personnel, and the adequacy of health care facilities.
- *Consumer responsibilities:* In a healthcare system that protects consumers' or patients' rights, patients should expect to take on some responsibilities to get well and/or stay well (for instance, exercising and not using tobacco). Patients are expected to do things like treat health care workers and other patients with respect, try to pay their medical bills, and follow the rules and benefits of their health plan coverage. Having patients involved in their care increases the chance of the best possible outcomes and helps support a high quality, cost-conscious healthcare system.

The previous lists of patient's rights demonstrate that we do have protection, but, when necessary, we must choose *to exercise* our rights. If our rights are taken from us, one option is to sue the hospital or physician. The problem is that often people instigate malpractice lawsuits that are not necessary and are started for financial gain.

WHAT IS MEDICAL MALPRACTICE AND HOW HAS IT IMPACTED INSURANCE COSTS?

Medical malpractice is professional negligence by act or omission by a health care provider in which care provided deviates from accepted standards of practice in the medical community and causes injury or death to the patient.[30] There are many legitimate reasons for medical malpractice suits. Doctors may fail to diagnose a disease, misdiagnose it, or do something to cause a patient's death (e.g., medication error). Doctors may make a mistake when conducting surgery or delivering a baby. In fact, one in five Americans has experienced medical errors directly or has a family member who has suffered a medical error.[31] The consequence is that doctors may find themselves in court.

Because of the large number of malpractice suits, malpractice insurance rates have risen so high that it has caused a crisis among doctors, who must be insured in order to practice. They complain that medical malpractice lawsuits have gone out of control and that settlements are too large. Almost 60 percent of liability claims against doctors are dropped, withdrawn, or dismissed without payment.[30] The problem is that those cases cost an average of more than $22,000 to defend in 2008, up from the $18,000 average in 2007. Of the cases that go to trial, over 90 percent found that physicians were not negligent. The cost of going to trial, however, was on average $110,000 in 2008.[32]

Doctors are not the only ones sued for malpractice. It could be a practicing nurse working at a retirement home or any health care professional who does not treat according to the standards of their field. Just because a suit has been started does not mean that the doctor or health care professional is guilty as charged. Malpractice has to be proven in court, and many times the cases are settled before they ever reach court. In fact, it has been estimated that 9 out of 10 cases are settled out of court.[32]

It could be that some health professionals and doctors are at fault. Perhaps they have a history of either poor care or poor doctoring. It could be a failure of state boards to weed them out. It could be, however, that many cases were started out of pure greed by people or insurance companies. Frivolous cases (cases without merit) cause the cost of malpractice insurance to explode and have also caused a shortage of doctors in specialty areas that seem to get many lawsuits, such as obstetrics and gynecology.

THE INFORMED CONSUMER: APPLYING THE CONCEPTS LEARNED TO YOUR DAILY LIFE

Now that you have learned some facts about the U.S. healthcare delivery system and the health care professionals who are available, how can you apply these concepts to your daily life?

You will be graduating from college and will find it necessary to use the healthcare delivery system. Perhaps you will get married and have a family. It will be important to find a family physician, and if you are a female, a gynecologist. If you get pregnant, you will need to find an obstetrician. How will you get insurance? What means are available to you to get insurance? What would be the criteria that you would use to find your physicians? Would you use an MD or a DO? If you moved from one state to another, what means would you use to locate a competent doctor? You will one day be faced with decisions like these; therefore, now is the time to begin thinking about what you would do. Good luck with all your future decisions.

CONCLUSION

As shown in this chapter, the U.S. healthcare system is complex. There are many professionals who can give us care, and we have defined who the orthodox physicians are. We have a huge responsibility to select our physicians with care and to know when to fire our doctors. It is up to us. Are you up to the challenge?

Suggestions for Class Activities

1. Discuss a newspaper report about an incompetent physician or dentist and the appropriateness of the disciplinary action taken. (You could find this on the Internet or access newspaper archives.)
2. Interview one or two physicians about their philosophy regarding healthcare costs and what they would do to solve healthcare delivery problems. Prepare a written summary.
3. Interview one or two physicians or nurses and ask their view about nationalized health insurance programs and the Patient Protection and Affordable Care Act. Prepare a written summary.

Review Questions

1. What are three reasons that the U.S. healthcare delivery system has problems?
2. What are three current U.S. healthcare programs? Do you believe they are adequate? Why or why not?
3. From reading the *In the News* section of this chapter, what are three misperceptions about the impact of the Patient Protection and Affordable Care Act on Medicare?
4. What is an allopathic doctor?
5. What is the main difference in the academic preparation of an allopathic versus an osteopathic physician?
6. What is the philosophy of an osteopathic physician?
7. In what ways did the Flexner Report change the training of medical doctors?
8. As learned in this chapter, how would you proceed if you wanted to find and select a physician?
9. What reasons would lead you to fire your physician?
10. What are three patients' rights?
11. How have malpractice suits impacted healthcare costs?

Key Terms

allopathic physician A traditional or orthodox physician who is a medical doctor (MD).

dementias Gradual and progressive decline in cognitive and reasoning skills plus loss of memory. The most common is Alzheimer's disease.

genomics A recent scientific discipline that strives to define and characterize the complete genetic makeup of an organism.

health care conglomerates Comprised of hospitals, clinics, and research facilities that either include, or are affiliated with, a medical school.

information and communications technology (ICT) An umbrella term that includes any communication device or application including radio, television, cellular phones, computer and network hardware and software, and satellite systems. Also includes services and applications associated with them, such as videoconferencing and distance learning.

nanotechnologies The study of the controlling of matter on an atomic level. Generally nanotechnology (or nanotech) deals with structures that are 100 nanometers or smaller in at least one dimension, and involves developing materials or devices within that size.

nurse practitioner (NP) A registered nurse who has obtained advanced education and clinical training. Most obtain a master's or doctorate degree in nursing practice studies.

osteopathic physician (DO) A traditional or orthodox physician who has similar training as the medical doctor but who has advanced studies in the interconnection of the muscles, bones, and nerves.

physician assistant (PA) A professional who can also provide many health care services and works under the guidance of a physician.

sensor technologies Devices such as a photoelectric cell that receives and responds to a signal or stimulus.

References

1. National Center for Health Statistics. *Health, United States, 2010: with special feature on death and dying*. Hyattsville, MD: NCHS; 2011.
2. Kaiser Family Foundation. Employer Health Benefits 2010 Annual Survey. Average premiums for single and family coverage, 1999-2010. Available at: http://facts.kff.org/chart.aspx?ch = 1545. Accessed May 26, 2010
3. U.S. Census Bureau. Income, poverty, and health insurance coverage in the United States. Available at: http://www.census.gov/prod/2010pubs/p60-238.pdf. Accessed May 26, 2010.
4. Terry K. Health spending hits 17.3 percent of GDP in largest annual jump [CBS Interactive Business Network Web site]. Available at: http://industry.bnet.com/healthcare/10001674/health-spending-hits-173-percent-of-gdp-in-largest-annual-jump/. Accessed May 25, 2010.
5. Truffer C, Keehan S, Smith S, et al. Health spending projections through 2019: the recession's impact continues. *Health Aff*. 2010;29(3):522–529.
6. World Health Organization. World Health Organization assesses the world's health systems. June 21, 2000. Available at: http://www.who.int/ing-pr-2000/en/pr2000-44.html. Accessed May 25, 2010.
7. Sainfort F. Healthcare delivery systems in the United States. *Eng Enterp*. 2004 Summer:6–9.
8. Institute of Medicine, Committee on Quality of Health Care in America. *Crossing the quality chasm: a new health system for the 21st century*. Washington, DC: National Academies Press; 2001.
9. Centers for Medicare and Medicaid Services. CMS programs and information. Available at: http://www.cms.gov. Accessed May 25, 2010.
10. Advocacy Center. Medicaid. Available at: http://www.advocacyla.org/tl_files/publications/Medicaid.pdf. Accessed June 1, 2010.
11. SourceWatch. State Children's Health Insurance Program (SCHIP) (U.S.). Available at: http://www.sourcewatch.org/index.php. Accessed June 1, 2010.
12. U.S. Department of Veterans Affairs. Veterans services. Available at: http://www.va.gov/landing2_vetsrv.htm. Accessed June 2, 2010.
13. Military.com. TRICARE Standard Overview. Available at: http://www.military.com/benefits/tricare/tricare-standard/tricare-standard-overview. Accessed June 2, 2010.
14. Health Affairs Health Policy Brief. Medicare Advantage Plans. Available at: http://www.healthaffairs.org/healthpolicybriefs/brief.php?brief_id = 48. Accessed July 24, 2011.
15. Reuters. Q + A: How does healthcare overhaul affect Medicare? March 22, 2010. Available at: http://www.reuters.com/article/idUSTRE62J1FS20100322. Accessed July 10, 2010.
16. American Hospital Association. Fast facts on US hospitals. American Hospital Association Hospital Statistics, 2011 edition. Chicago: Health Forum;2010. Available online at: http://www.aha.org/research/rc/stat-studies/fast-facts.shtml. Accessed September 19, 2011.
17. Mayo Clinic. Nurse practitioner career overview. Available at: http://www.mayo.edu/mshs/np-career.html. Accessed July 9, 2010.
18. U.S. Department of Labor, Bureau of Labor Statistics. Physician assistants. Available at: http://www.bls.gov/oco/ocos081.htm. Accessed July 9, 2010.
19. American Medical Association. Requirements for becoming a physician. Available at: http://www.ama-assn.org/ama/pub/education-careers/becoming-physician.shtml. Accessed July 15, 2010.
20. American Osteopathic Association. Osteopathic medicine. Available at: http://www.osteopathic.org/index. Accessed May 24, 2010.
21. American Association of Colleges of Osteopathic Medicine. What is osteopathic medicine? Available at: http://www.aacom.org/about/osteomed/pages/default.aspx. Accessed May 24, 2010.
22. MedicineNet.com. Flexner report . . . birth of modern medical education. Available at: http://www.medicinenet.com/script/main/art.asp?articlekey = 8795. Accessed May 28, 2010.
23. Carnegie Foundation for the Advancement of Teaching. Medical education in the United States and Canada bulletin number four (the Flexner report). Available at: http://www.carnegiefoundation.org/publications/medical-education-united-states-and-canada-bulletin-number-four-flexner-report-0. Accessed May 28, 2010.
24. Olakanmi O. The AMA, NMA, and the Flexner Report of 1910. Available at: http://www.ama-assn.org/ama1/pub/upload/mm/369/flexner.pdf. Accessed May 28, 2010.
25. American Board of Medical Specialties. *The official ABMS directory of board certified medical specialists, 2009*. St. Louis, MO: Elsevier Saunders; 2009.
26. American Medical Association. DoctorFinder. Available at: https://extapps.ama-assn.org/doctorfinder/. Accessed May 28, 2010.
27. Joint Commission. Facts about hospital accreditation. Available at: http://www.jointcommission.org/assets/1/18/Hospital_Accreditation_1_31_11.pdf. Accessed July 24, 2011.
28. American Hospital Association. American Hospital Association guide to the health care field. 2009.
29. American Cancer Society. Patient's bill of rights. What is the patients' bill of rights. Available at: http://www.cancer.org/docroot/MIT/content/MIT_3_2_Patients_Bill_Of_Rights.asp. Accessed May 26, 2010.
30. President's Advisory Commission on Consumer Protection and Quality in the Health Care Industry. Consumer bill of rights and responsibilities. November 1997. Available at: http://www.hcqualitycommission.gov/cborr/. Accessed May 27, 2010.
31. Wikipedia. Medical malpractice. Available at: http://en.wikipedia.org/wiki/Medical_malpractice. Accessed July 8, 2010.
32. American Medical Association. The case for medical liability reform. Available at: http://www.ama-assn.org/ama1/pub/upload/mm/-1/case-for-mlr.pdf. Accessed July 24, 2011.

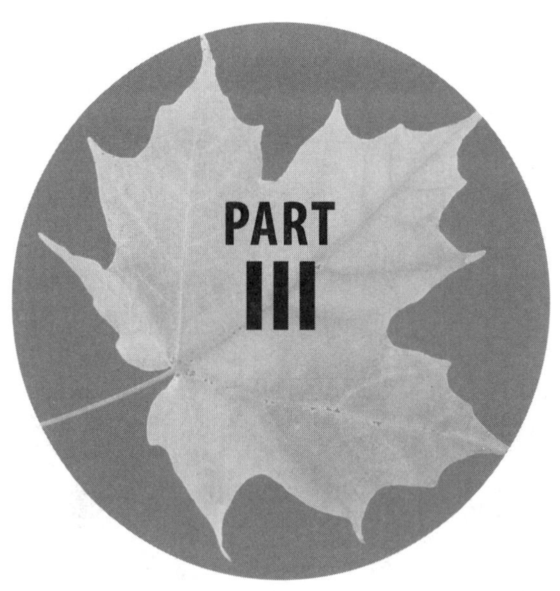

Complementary and Alternative Medicine and Health Care

Integrative Medicine, CAM, and Health Care

LEARNING OBJECTIVES

As a result of reading this chapter, students will:

1. Assess the impact of integrative medicine on health care in the United States.
2. Analyze why some traditional health care professionals might be opposed to alternative practitioners.
3. Explain how the government has fostered the growth of alternative medicine.
4. Describe the role of the health consumer in taking self-responsibility for health care choices.

WHAT IS INTEGRATIVE MEDICINE?

Integrative medicine units are being implemented into hospitals all over the nation, and the term "integrative medicine" is now becoming more familiar. Many people, however, are uncertain about the definition of integrative medicine. The National Center for Complementary and Alternative Medicine (NCCAM), a center within the National Institutes of Health (NIH), defines integrative medicine as "medicine that combines treatments from conventional medicine and complementary and alternative medicine (CAM) for which there is evidence of safety and effectiveness."[1] Integrative medicine encompasses holistic healing methodologies because it focuses on the patient, a system that focuses on healing the whole person—mind, body, and spirit. Integrative medicine combines the best of Western and Eastern medicine and makes use of all appropriate therapeutic approaches and evidence-based global medical modalities to achieve optimal health and healing.[2]

The knowledge and use of complementary and alternative medicine is an important aspect of integrative medicine that helps attain a more in-depth understanding of the nature of illness, healing, and wellness. Integrative medicine has been described by Snyderman and Weil[2] as a movement driven by consumers who sought alternative healing methods. Eventually, integrative medicine gained the attention of academic health centers. In May 2004, an outcome of the integrative medicine and alternative health care movement was the formation of a national consortium, the Consortium of Academic Health Centers for Integrative Medicine.[3] The membership consists of 44 highly reputable academic centers and is supported by membership dues and grants from partners such as the Bravewell Collaborative. Some of those academic centers are located at very impressive universities and/or medical centers: Stanford University, University of Arizona, University of California at Los Angeles and San Francisco, University of Colorado at Denver School of Medicine, John Hopkins University, Duke University, and Mayo Clinic (see **TABLE 6.1**).

Another outcome of the integrative medicine movement was a national summit convened by the Bravewell Collaborative and the Institute of Medicine in February 2009 to explore integrative medicine's potential to improve the U.S. healthcare system.[4] A quote from the summit chair, Ralph Snyderman, MD, Chancellor Emeritus of Duke University School of Medicine, describes how he views integrative medicine: "The integrative approach flips the healthcare system on its head and puts the patient at the center, addressing not just symptoms, but the real causes of illness. It is care that is preventive, predictive and personalized."[4]

As described, integrated medicine may be bringing a change to how medical professionals and individuals view

Table 6.1
Consortium of Academic Health Centers for Integrative Medicine, United States

Arizona
University of Arizona, Program in Integrative Medicine

California
Stanford University, Stanford Center for Integrative Medicine
University of California, Irvine, Susan Samueli Center for Integrative Medicine
University of California, Los Angeles, Collaborative Centers for Integrative Medicine
University of California, San Francisco, Osher Center for Integrative Medicine

Colorado
University of Colorado at Denver School of Medicine, The Center for Integrative Medicine

Connecticut
University of Connecticut Health Center, Programs in Complementary and Integrative Medicine
Yale University, Integrative Medicine at Yale
Integrative Medicine Center at Griffin Hospital

Hawaii
University of Hawaii-Manoa, John A. Burns School of Medicine, Department of Complementary and Alternative Medicine

Illinois
Northwestern University Feinberg School of Medicine, Northwestern Memorial Physician's Group Center for Integrative Medicine
University of Illinois at Chicago School of Medicine

Kansas
University of Kansas, Program in Integrative Medicine

Maryland
Johns Hopkins University, School of Medicine, Center for Complementary and Alternative
University of Maryland, Center for Integrative Medicine

Massachusetts
Boston University School of Medicine, Program in Integrative Cross Cultural Care
Harvard Medical School, Osher Institute
University of Massachusetts Medical School, Center for Mindfulness

Michigan
University of Michigan, Integrative Medicine

Minnesota
Mayo Clinic, Complementary and Integrative Medicine Program Research
University of Minnesota, Center for Spirituality and Healing

New Jersey
University of Medicine and Dentistry of New Jersey, Institute for Complementary & Alternative Medicine

New Mexico
University of New Mexico, Health Science Center

New York
Albert Einstein College of Medicine of Yeshiva University, Continuum Center for Health and Healing, Program in Integrative Medicine
Columbia University
Richard and Hinda Rosenthal Center for Complementary & Alternative Medicine

North Carolina
Duke University, Duke Integrative Medicine
University of North Carolina at Chapel Hill, Program on Integrative Medicine
Wake Forest University School of Medicine, Center for Integrative Medicine

Ohio
The Ohio State University, Center for Integrative Medicine
University of Cincinnati College of Medicine

Oregon
Oregon Health and Science University, Women's Primary Care and Integrative Medicine, Center for Women's Health

Pennsylvania
Thomas Jefferson University, Jefferson Myrna Brind Center of Integrative Medicine
University of Pennsylvania, CAM at Penn
University of Pittsburgh, Center for Integrative Medicine

Tennessee
Vanderbilt University, Vanderbilt Center for Integrative Health

Texas
University of Texas Medical Branch, UTMB Integrative Health Care

Vermont
University of Vermont College of Medicine, Program in Integrative Medicine

Washington
University of Washington, UW Integrative Health Program

Washington, DC
George Washington University, Center for Integrative Medicine
Georgetown University, School of Medicine

Wisconsin
University of Wisconsin-Madison, UW Integrative Medicine Program

Source: Courtesy of the Consortium of Academic Health Centers for Integrative Medicine

health and the treatment of illness. Now that the meaning of integrative medicine has been introduced, where does one go to get integrated medical care and what are the integrated medicine organizational structures? The following addresses these questions.

WHERE ARE INTEGRATIVE MEDICINE CLINICS LOCATED AND WHAT ARE THEIR ORGANIZATIONAL STRUCTURES?

Most integrative medicine clinics are located in a hospital setting. Integrative medicine, however, may be implemented at doctor's offices or clinics. Some doctors set up an integrative medicine network within a community as they refer their own patients to alternative practitioners (e.g., chiropractors, acupuncturists, massage therapists). Integrative medicine structural models have some common characteristics. They embrace the best of both scientific-based medicine and evidence-validated alternative methods. They aim for a patient-centered and interdisciplinary mix of traditional and alternative medical treatments. They may involve individual case management of patients while using several types of healing practitioners. For example, an integrative medicine clinic in Sweden involved a senior researcher, a doctoral student, a general practitioner, and eight complementary therapy providers [massage therapists, naprapath (treats connective tissue disorders), shiatsu therapists (Japanese massage and bodywork), an acupuncturist, and a qi gong therapist (energy healing)].[5]

In 2002, McKinsey and Company, a management consulting company, conducted a million-dollar study (pro bono) for the Bravewell Collaborative to explore how existing integrative medicine clinics operated and how they could network, share information, conduct clinical research, and more successfully serve clients.[6] The study revealed that integrative medicine clinics operated according to different organizational models, had different approaches, were financed differently, and offered different services. They recommended that Bravewell Collaborative develop a network among the leading U.S. integrative clinics. Results of the study and recommendations have subsequently aided the development of integrative clinical care. Impressive Web sites for many integrative clinics can be found online (see **BOX 6.1**).

To illustrate the use of integrative medicine clinics, please refer to the following case study.

Box 6.1
Integrative Medicine Clinics: Online Descriptions

The UPMC Center for Integrative Medicine, located at UPMC Shadyside in Pittsburgh, provides services intended to complement—not replace—more conventional medical treatments. From age-old therapies, such as acupuncture and naturopathic approaches, to mind–body methods, such as biofeedback and relaxation therapies, our staff work with each patient to determine which services are most appropriate.

Duke Integrative Medicine is a state-of-the-art healing environment. We provide medical care that combines the very best scientific medicine with evidence-based complementary therapies. Our team of expert physicians and nurses and professionally trained therapists works in partnership with each of our patients to offer individualized, whole person care.

Integrative Medicine specialists at UW Health in Madison, Wisconsin, offer services that draw from both conventional and complementary medicine. Dedicated to helping you achieve your highest potential for wellness, we have a healing-oriented philosophy that focuses on less invasive therapies to help remove barriers that may be blocking the body's ability to heal.

Source: Courtesy of UPMC; Wellness & Writing Connections www.wellnessandwritingconnections.com; and UW Integrative Medicine Program

WHAT HAS BEEN THE HISTORY OF RESISTANCE TO ALTERNATIVE MEDICINE AND INTEGRATED CARE?

Historically, the traditional or orthodox field of medicine (i.e., biomedicine) rigorously opposed and ridiculed many CAM therapies.[7] A part of the opposition may have stemmed from the belief that the client's (patient's) role was to be compliant, to not question, and to be accepting of what the doctor prescribed.[8] The physician's role was to be the authoritative and all-knowing figure in the client–doctor relationship. Disease was only considered to be the result of a pathogen entering the body, and treatments of disease consisted mainly of treating the symptoms with medications (e.g., antibiotics for bacterial infections) and surgery. Doctors did not typically sit with patients and explain ways in which they could help themselves in the healing process.

The acquisition and the healing of diseases, however, is a complicated process and often requires more than traditional therapies.[2,6–11] Many alternative health practices help an individual to self-heal (e.g., meditation, biofeedback, imagery, and more). Healing requires a harmony of the mind, body, and spirit[2,6–11] and a healthy lifestyle (good nutrition, physical exercise, stress management, restful sleep, etc.). Positive health practices will aid the person who does get ill and will help them achieve a higher level of wellness faster. One of the most important concepts to understand is that people heal in different ways; that is, what works well for one person may not work for another. For instance, in Ayurvedic medicine, a natural healing system, treatment is based upon a person's dosha or body constitution. According to Ayurvedic medicine, there are three doshas—Vata, Pitta, and Kapha, and each is supposedly composed of two of the five elements that make up the universe: space, air,

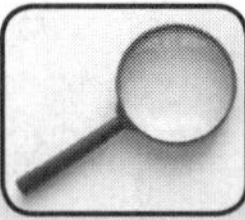

Case Study

Tom lives in Madison, Wisconsin, and is a graduate student in business at the University of Wisconsin. Over spring break, Tom went skiing at a ski resort in the Upper Peninsula of Michigan. He fell while skiing and is now experiencing a great amount of lower back pain and muscle spasms. Tom went to health services on campus and was seen by the university physician. A series of x-rays and an MRI was done. No spinal disc injury was apparent by x-ray, so the doctor diagnosed Tom with spinal facet joint injury. Facet joints are the bony projections on the back of the spine. The doctor told Tom that his injury would require rest, heat, and nonsteroidal anti-inflammatory drugs. Furthermore, the doctor told Tom that the university had an Integrative Medicine unit where he could seek some sort of alternative therapy that might help with the muscle spasms and pain. The doctor recommended that Tom see an acupuncturist or the campus chiropractor. Acupuncture is a Chinese technique that involves placing very tiny needles in certain areas of the body to decrease pain from an injury. Tom doesn't know that much about either therapy and is somewhat apprehensive about them.

Questions:

1. Where could Tom acquire information about both therapies including results of scientific research studies?
2. What could Tom's doctor say to alleviate Tom's concerns?
3. Where could Tom gain more information about the campus Integrative Medicine clinic?

fire, water, and earth. An individual may be primarily one of the three or a combination of the three. After diagnosing the type of dosha and the reason for disrupted body harmony, the Ayurvedic medicine physician will prescribe the treatment accordingly. More about Ayurvedic medicine is described in Chapter 8.

Through the years, however, many biomedical and osteopathic physicians began embracing a holistic lifestyle, and based on research evidence, they began to promote therapies such as meditation, yoga, nutritional supplements, and massage as beneficial. Currently, many more orthodox physicians are now acknowledging the usefulness of select CAM therapies (e.g., chiropractic medicine, meditation, yoga, massage, biofeedback, acupuncture) and have participated in planning and implementing integrative medicine clinics in their hospitals.[7]

WHO WERE THE EARLY PIONEERS PROMOTING CAM THERAPIES AND INTEGRATIVE MEDICINE?

Several key biomedical physicians have paved the way for the acceptance of several CAM therapies. A few early pioneers are described in the following sections.

Herbert Benson, MD

The first is Dr. Herbert Benson (see **FIGURE 6.1**), a cardiologist and professor at Harvard Medical School. In the late 1960s, Dr. Benson conducted research using monkeys that linked stress to physical health. At that time, this idea was contrary to existing medical thought.[12] Later Dr. Benson and a colleague, Robert Wallace, researched the effects of Transcendental Meditation (TM) on blood pressure. Benson and Wallace found that subjects who practiced TM, and who were able to change thought patterns, experienced decreases in their metabolism, rate of breathing, and heart rate, and had slower brain waves. They believed the technique was useful for treating conditions such as insomnia, anxiety, hypertension, and chronic pain. Dr. Benson studied other meditative techniques (e.g., diaphragmatic breathing, repetitive prayer, qi gong, tai chi, yoga, progressive muscle relaxation, jogging, and even knitting) that he found also produced a relaxed state. He labeled it the "relaxation response," which is the foundation of mind–body medicine. In 1975, Dr. Benson published a book, *The Relaxation Response*, and since then has published 10 other books focusing on the mind–body connection. He is currently Director Emeritus of the Benson-Henry Institute (BHI) and Mind/Body Medical Institute Associate Professor of Medicine, Harvard Medical School.

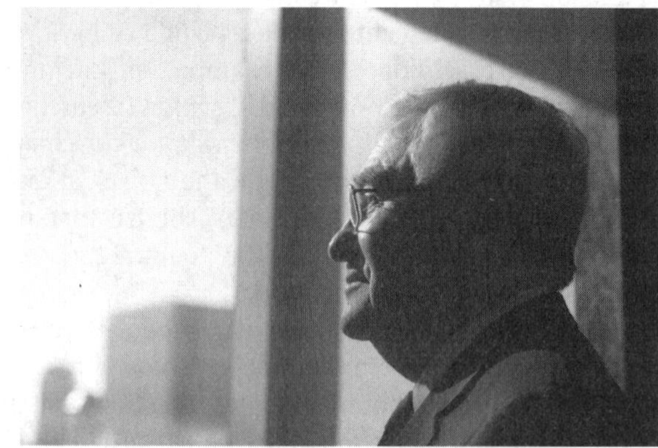

FIGURE 6.1 Herbert Benson, MD

David Eisenberg, MD

Another key individual is Dr. David Eisenberg, who was the first U.S. medical exchange student to the People's Republic of China. There he mastered Chinese and attended the Beijing College of Traditional Chinese Medicine while learning Eastern healing modalities (e.g., acupuncture, tai chi). In 1993, he was the medical advisor to the PBS series, *Healing and the Mind* with Bill Moyers. Dr. Eisenberg became an MD specializing in internal medicine and joined the faculty at Harvard. He directed two large national U.S. surveys on the use of CAM therapies; wrote a text, *Encounters with Qi*; and has published many scientific data-based research studies. Currently, Dr. Eisenberg is the Director of Harvard Medical School's Osher Research Center, and is the Program Director of Integrative Medicine at Brigham and Women's Hospital in Boston, Massachusetts.[13]

Bernard Siegel, MD

An early pioneer is Dr. Bernard (Bernie) Siegel (**FIGURE 6.2**), a physician who graduated with honors from Cornell University Medical College. Dr. Siegel practiced medicine for many years and was a general and pediatric surgeon until he retired. He spent much of his life teaching techniques to help cancer patients use their own body energy to help in the healing process, techniques such as meditation and positive imagery. He also believes in using humor as a healing technique. To further his belief in patients' self healing power, he founded ECaP (Exceptional Cancer Patients) a type of individual and group therapy support that uses drawings, dreams, positive imagery and other holistic methods. Dr. Siegel has published several best-selling books promoting holistic healing methods, including *Love, Medicine and Miracles*; *Peace, Love & Healing*; and *How to Live Between Office Visits*.[14]

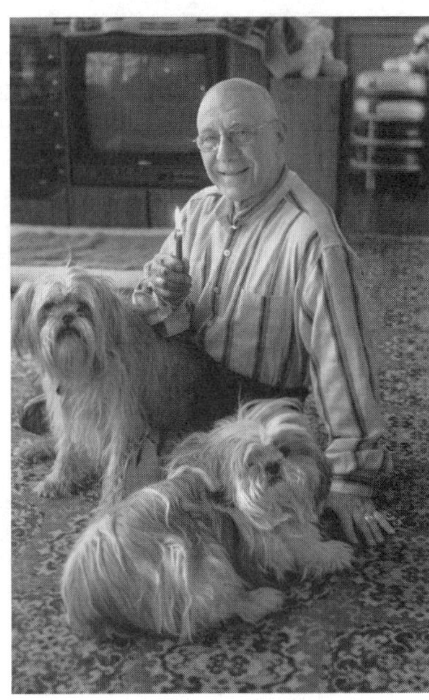

FIGURE 6.2 Bernard (Bernie) Siegel, MD

Andrew Weil, MD

Perhaps one of the best known key pioneers is Andrew Weil, MD, a Harvard-trained physician (**FIGURE 6.3**). Dr. Weil became a clinical professor at the University of Arizona Medical Center in 1983. While there, he established the Foundation for Integrative Medicine, and in 1994, Dr. Weil founded the Program in Integrative Medicine. Now, it is known as the Arizona Center for Integrative Medicine, and Dr. Weil is the program director.[15] Through his speeches, television appearances, and writings by way of news articles and texts, Dr. Weil's views about CAM therapies and integrative medicine have gained widespread acceptance. His Web site features "Ask Dr. Weil," a popular venue accessed by individuals wanting information about CAM therapies, including botanicals.

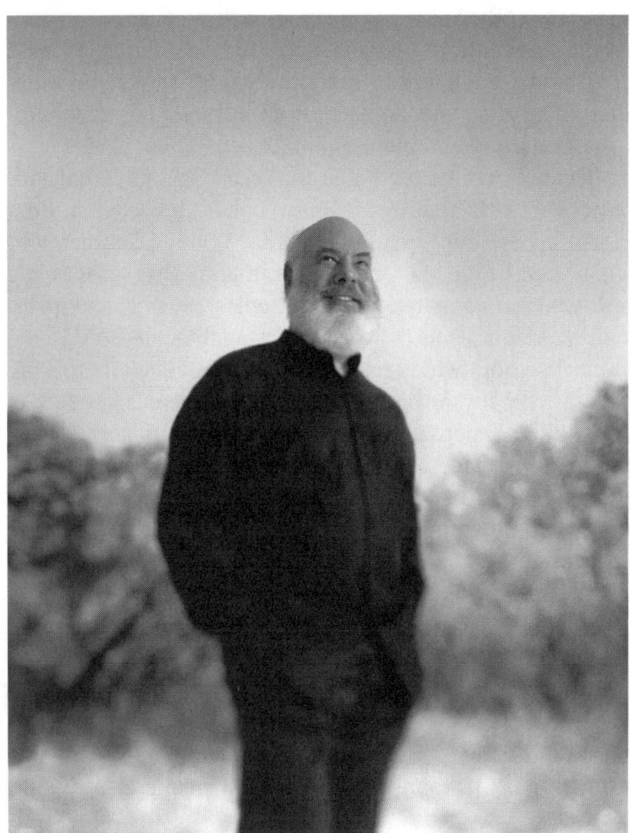

FIGURE 6.3 Andrew Weil, MD

Deepak Chopra, MD

Dr. Deepak Chopra (see **FIGURE 6.4**) has done much to promote integrative medicine. Dr. Chopra is an Indian-trained biomedical physician who also completed an internship and several residencies and fellowships at university-affiliated medical centers in Boston.[11] He is cofounder of the Chopra Center for Wellbeing, where he serves as the director of education.[11] The center offers training programs in physical,

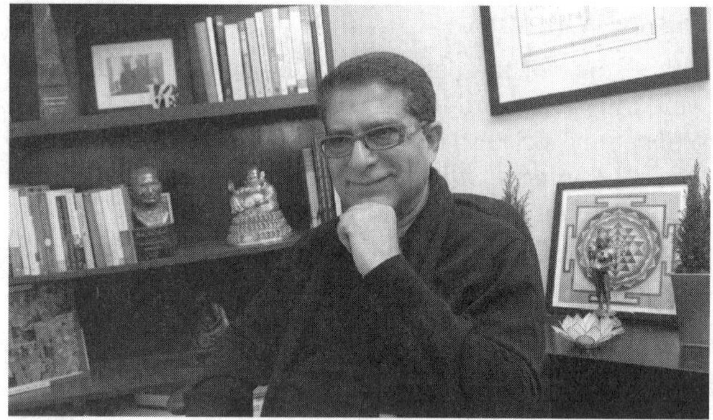

FIGURE 6.4 Deepak Chopra, MD

emotional, and spiritual healing. Dr. Chopra gives workshops utilizing Ayurvedic medicine modalities and practical tools of mind–body healing such as energy healing, guided meditation, visualization, and writing exercises.[11] Dr. Chopra is the author of more than 50 books and more than 100 audio, video, and CD-ROM titles. He has been published on every continent and in dozens of languages.

Because of these reputable and respected individuals, integrative medicine programs have been established at dozens of institutions, including the Mayo Clinic; Georgetown, Duke, and Columbia Universities; and at Drs. Eisenberg's and Weil's alma mater, Harvard Medical School. The medical profession seems to be selectively embracing CAM in the clinical setting, which has benefited patients by increasing access to many forms of alternative therapies/medicine. An additional potential benefit is that patients going to orthodox physicians will be more likely to disclose the CAM therapies that they are using, especially herbal medicines that could potentially interact with prescription drugs.

Moreover, a sign that physicians are more accepting of CAM therapies is that they are referring their patients to alternative practitioners such as chiropractors, massage therapists, acupuncturists, and other types of alternative practitioners. Over 50 percent of conventional physicians in the United States use or refer patients for some CAM treatments.[16,17] Other professions (e.g., psychotherapy) are also beginning to incorporate certain alternative therapies within the treatment regimen.[17] Often, these alternative medicine advocates are featured in news articles.

WHAT ARE THE HISTORICAL MILESTONES OF INTEGRATIVE MEDICINE?

Development of Wellness Programs

The journey to integrative medicine began with the development of wellness programs in which people became more proactive about preventing diseases and taking responsibility for their own health. During the 1950s, there were only a few wellness programs. Halbert Dunn was one of the first to develop employee wellness programs in the 1950s.[19] Several wellness programs were developed during the 1960s and 1970s, and "wellness" became a buzzword as people became aware of the benefits of exercise and nutrition in preventing high cholesterol levels, heart attacks, and stroke.

During the 1980s, additional wellness programs were being developed, such as the 1982 "wellness awareness" training program developed by Teamster leaders in Orange County, Florida, so that they could decrease the cost of their union's health insurance program.

During the 1990s, even more companies began to develop wellness programs as an incentive to their employees to lose excess pounds and to quit smoking.

Development of Health Promotion Programs

A 1990 study by Dean Ornish, MD, showed that lifestyle changes can eventually reverse heart disease.[20] This study gave legitimacy to wellness programs, and they proliferated in the 1990s and 2000s. By this time, the programs began to be called "health promotion programs" because many more strategies than educational programs were being incorporated into the programming (e.g., use of media, health fairs, laws, etc.). In addition to worksites, schools, universities, medical centers, hospitals, community health departments, and state health departments were implementing health promotion programs. The importance of wellness and health promotion programs is that people began to be enthusiastic about the value and benefits of a healthy lifestyle. People began to investigate ways to make themselves

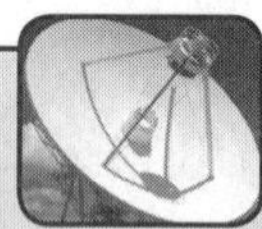

In the News

The *New York Times* has published several articles featuring Dr. Weil and Dr. Chopra. A *New York Times*[18] article published in June 2010 featured a story about a new magazine called *MyMag*, developed to produce single-issue magazines as marketing tools for celebrities. The *New York Times* article reported that in May 2010, *MyMag* featured Deepak Chopra. Chopra stated that he would donate his share of the revenue to charity. According to the news article, the celebrities choose what goes inside. Dr. Chopra included material from the hip-hop journal *Wax Poetics* and photos of him recording his Sirius radio show. "I'm not doing this to get into the media business," Dr Chopra said via e-mail. "I'm simply creating a new channel through which I can connect to people."[18]

feel better through rest, stress management, exercise, and better eating habits. All of this paved the way for a natural progression of examining other treatment modalities, many of which came from European and Eastern countries.

At the governmental level, two extremely important developments occurred: the establishment of the National Center for Complementary and Alternative Medicine and the formation of the White House Commission on Complementary and Alternative Medicine Policy.

National Center for Complementary and Alternative Medicine

The establishment of the National Center for Complementary and Alternative Medicine (NCCAM) is one of the most important milestones that gives scientific credence to select CAM practices.[1] This National Institutes of Health (NIH) center was first created in 1992, but began as the Office of Alternative Medicine (OAM). At that time, the U.S. Congress passed legislation (Public Law 102-170) to provide $2 million to establish the OAM to assess the worth of promising unconventional medical practices. By 1999, Congress updated the status of the OAM to become NCCAM. The purpose of the NCCAM is to "conduct scientific research on the diverse medical and health care systems, practices, and products that are not generally considered part of conventional medicine."[1] In May 2004, the NCCAM announced its findings from a large national survey about Americans' use of CAM. This was a part of the 2002 National Health Interview Survey. In December 2008, the NCCAM released data regarding children's use of CAM and assessed trends in adult CAM use. In July 2009, the NCCAM revealed the results of a 2007 national study regarding the amount of money Americans spend on CAM annually: nearly $34 billion out-of-pocket, of which about two-thirds was for self-care. Please see Appendix 6.A for the entire time line of the NCCAM.

The White House Commission on Complementary and Alternative Medicine Policy

In March 2000, President Clinton appointed 20 people (physicians, registered nurses, PhDs, CAM practitioners) to the White House Commission on Complementary and Alternative Medicine Policy. The commission was to make legislative and administrative recommendations to aid public policy in ensuring the safety of products and practices that had been, or might be, labeled "CAM" and to identify potential benefits for the public. After 18 months of reviewing a thousand papers on CAM use and listening to over 700 testimonies about CAM, several recommendations about the role of the federal government emerged.[21] They are summarized as follows: The federal government should disclose research findings; ensure the safety of products; help assess the appropriate levels of training of various CAM practitioners and the research regarding their practice; aid in evaluating the different ways that states are regulating CAM practitioners; and facilitate dialogue among CAM and conventional providers, scientists, and the public. The report also emphasized that states can take a leadership role in the regulation of CAM practitioners and orthodox practitioners who incorporate CAM into their practices.

WHAT CHANGES HAVE OCCURRED IN MEDICAL CARE AND EDUCATION?

The White House Commission on Complementary and Alternative Medicine Policy is advocating that the education and training of conventional health professionals should include CAM and that the training of CAM practitioners should include conventional health care.[21] Medical schools throughout the country have ongoing initiatives in integrative medicine. As previously discussed, 10 medical schools formed the Consortium of Academic Health Centers for Integrative Medicine. Many changes occurred from the 1990s to the 2000s.

A study by Wetzel in 1998 concluded that 64 percent of medical schools offered courses on CAM, although 68 percent were stand-alone electives and only 31 percent were part of required courses.[22] Topics were chiropractic, acupuncture, homeopathy, herbal therapies, and mind–body techniques. In response to the 2000–2001 Liaison Committee on Medical Education Annual Medical School Questionnaire, the White House Commission on Complementary and Alternative Medicine Policy found that data from all 125 allopathic medical schools indicate that, although no medical school requires a separate CAM course, 91 schools (73 percent) include CAM in required conventional medical courses, 64 (51 percent) offer CAM as a stand-alone elective, and 32 (26 percent) include CAM as part of an elective. All results may be seen in **TABLE 6.2**.

Additionally, 10 medical schools received curriculum grants from the NIH.[20] Examples of medical schools that have integrated CAM curriculum into their programs are Tufts Program in Evidence-Based Medicine, University of Michigan Medical School, the Oregon Health and Science University, the University of Washington School of Medicine, and Bastyr University in Seattle, Washington. Many other professions (including psychology, social work, nursing, and pharmacy) have advocated that CAM be included in the curriculum.[16] Students enrolled in pharmacy school seem to be positive about CAM curricula and expressed a desire to have CAM curricula integrated beginning in the first year rather than waiting until later in their education.[23]

Several health professionals have outlined CAM educational curricula needs: (1) focus on critical thinking and critical reading of the literature, (2) identify thematic content and express topics in clear language, (3) formulate concise learning objectives, (4) include an experiential component, (5) promote a willingness to communicate profes-

Table 6.2

CAM Topics Included in Required or Elective Courses at Medical Schools Accredited by the Liaison Committee on Medical Education

TOPIC	REQUIRED COURSE ONLY	ELECTIVE COURSE ONLY	BOTH
Acupuncture	18	54	28
Herbal medicine	28	45	33
Homeopathy	17	48	18
Manual healing techniques	15	50	11
Meditation	13	53	17
Nutritional supplement therapy	30	42	36
Spirituality	25	43	35

Source: ©2000-2001 Liaison Committee on Medical Education Annual Medical School Questionnaire. Available at: http://www.whccamp.hhs.gov/pdfs/fr2002_chapter_4.pdf. Accessed August 12, 2011.

sionally with CAM clinicians, and (6) teach students to talk with patients about alternative therapies.[24,25] Brokaw et al. advocate that CAM studies should emphasize a critical evaluation of the scientific literature, should enlist the involvement of basic science departments, and should avoid advocacy of unproven therapies.[26] Furthermore, the Society of General Internal Medicine (SGIM) has outlined its view of what CAM education should be in a position paper published in 2008.[27]

In this paper, the SGIM laid out primary goals for physicians regarding CAM practices so that they could better understand the basic theories, benefits, risks, evidence basis for therapies, and how to adopt a nonjudgmental attitude about CAM to enhance their patient–doctor relationships. Secondary goals of the SGIM were to help patients integrate CAM and conventional therapies at appropriate times.

WHAT CHANGES HAVE OCCURRED IN INSURANCE COVERAGE FOR CAM CARE?

Insurance companies have expanded coverage to include the services of alternative practitioners. According to Pelletier and Astin,[10] just about every insurance carrier offers some form of CAM coverage. Some health plans cover acupuncture, traditional Chinese medicine, homeopathy (provided by a licensed physician), naturopathy, and massage whereas others offer only chiropractic care.[28,29] Additionally, many state legislatures have begun to mandate insurance coverage (e.g., Washington State mandates chiropractic coverage). Insurance companies do recognize that more people are seeking out alternative practitioners and are responding to that by offering health insurance.

As evidence of changing views about insurance coverage for CAM practices, a national survey study by Wolsko et al. demonstrated that a large percentage of individuals would sign with a company that offered health insurance. When presented with a choice of two insurance plans that were otherwise equivalent, participants in a study were asked if they would choose the insurance plan offering CAM benefits or not.[30] Among eligible respondents, 69 percent reported that they would be more likely to sign up with that insurance plan, 25 percent were indifferent, and 6.5 percent said that they would be less likely to sign up with that insurance plan. When CAM is offered on an experimental basis to patients, however, only a small percentage of covered patients tend to access CAM.[31] The insurance business is highly competitive; therefore, it makes sense that insurance companies would be willing to offer CAM insurance if it increases the chance of people selecting their company.

It is true that a large percentage of individuals are seeking CAM practitioners and would like health insurance coverage, but is it cost effective? In an article written by John Weeks in 2002, the American Chiropractic Association (ACA) bet the Medicare administration that they would save money, or at least the amount of money spent would be cost neutral, if Medicare would fund chiropractic services.[32] Medicare invested $50 million to implement a 2-year pilot study. An analysis of the study found that chiropractic was indeed saving money in three of the four sites studied. The fourth site, however, was Chicago, Illinois, where Medicare lost money. Because the ACA lost the "bet," Medicare is retrieving the amount of money spent on the study by now reimbursing chiropractors less than before the study. The ACA is contesting the results because they believe that Chicago's results were due to measurement errors, and that three of the four sites demonstrated a savings.

A program that Medicare has agreed to cover is Dr. Dean Ornish's lifestyle program. His many years of clinical research demonstrated that comprehensive lifestyle changes (e.g., exercise, nutrition) may begin to reverse even severe coronary heart disease without using drugs or surgery.[33] Dr. Ornish conducted a more recent randomized controlled study that demonstrated how comprehensive lifestyle changes may stop or reverse the progression of prostate cancer. His explanation is that comprehensive lifestyle changes affect gene expression, "turning on" disease-preventing genes and "turning off" genes that promote cancer and heart disease.

Although the government-sponsored Medicare program is quite selective about CAM funding, private insurance companies will compete if there is evidence of profitability.[30] Companies want to be sure that they will save money on use of complementary therapies relative to conventional therapies. Meanwhile, a benefit of potential increased insurance coverage may motivate CAM practitioners to standardize their diagnostics and treatments in order to receive reimbursement.

WHAT IS THE FUTURE OF INTEGRATIVE MEDICINE?

The term "integrative medicine" is catching on in medical circles, and medical schools are integrating CAM courses into their curricula. Medical doctors and other health care professionals are learning more about holistic ways of healing and holistic lifestyles. Dr. Weil believes that the future of integrative medicine will be strong. He reasons that "unprecedented numbers" of patients are seeking out alternative practitioners because of the following: (1) they are dissatisfied with conventional medicine; (2) there is a divide between what patients expect of doctors and what medical schools are trained to do; (3) patients want more than medicine (prescriptions) and surgery; (4) patients want someone who will sit down and talk to them; (5) they want someone to talk with them about dietary supplements; and (6) patients want someone who will be sensitive to them if they ask about Chinese medicine.[33]

Physicians are learning much more about traditional Chinese medicine and how to incorporate acupuncture into their practices. New kinds of health institutes are being built such as healing centers (hybrids between spas and clinics) that address lifestyle issues. Centers for the practice of meditation are proliferating. There is broader insurance coverage for CAM practices and more innovative research. Lay people as well as physicians are learning more about botanicals, their functions and effects.

Postdoctoral fellowships are being instituted. As an example, the Bravewell Collaborative, the National Institute of Nursing Research, and the National Institutes of Health Clinical Center are sponsoring a BNC Fellowship for research in integrative medicine.[34] Fellows will attend the University of Arizona's Program in Integrative Medicine and will become involved in an integrative medicine–related research project at the NIH campus in Bethesda, Maryland.

New and innovative proposals related to integrative medicine are being formulated. One proposal is that a new NIH institute be formed: a National Institute of Healing. This type of institute or center could investigate all healing phenomena, spontaneous remissions of cancer, and other diseases. Some are proposing that a National Registry of Healing, classified by disease, should be developed. Also related to integrative medicine will be its future impact on encouraging and pressuring the Food and Drug Administration (FDA) to better regulate and standardize herbal supplements and botanicals.[35] The future of integrative medicine appears to be bright. We all should hope that whatever occurs, integrative medicine will be evidence-based and truly used in ways that optimize health.

WHAT ARE PATIENT RESPONSIBILITIES WHEN USING INTEGRATIVE MEDICINE CLINICS AND SELECTING ALTERNATIVE HEALTH CARE MODALITIES?

Integrative medicine clinics are being implemented in many hospitals and universities across the nation. We should be responsible consumers of our health care when making decisions about using integrative medicine clinics and when selecting alternative health care therapies. We can do much to advance safe integrative medicine practices by researching a particular integrative medicine clinic. Certainly, the number and type of traditional and alternative practitioners should be identified. We should learn the academic background of each individual. Often, the backgrounds of all physicians and therapists may be obtained online or in brochures or pamphlets produced by the clinic.

It is our responsibility to also research all of the "natural and holistic approaches" to health and healing offered by the site. Certainly, anyone who uses herbal supplements, or is engaging in an alternative therapy, should inform their family physician. If you believe that you will use, or are using an alternative therapy, you should ask your health insurance company if it covers any alternative therapies. Most of all, you should be an informed consumer of both traditional and alternative therapies.

THE INFORMED CONSUMER: APPLYING THE CONCEPTS LEARNED TO YOUR DAILY LIFE

Thus far you have received some information regarding the meaning of integrative medicine and some of the past resistance to it.

- Do you feel that this resistance was legitimate? Why or why not?
- If you are asked to be a student member of a committee at your university to explore the viability of developing an integrative medicine clinic, what advice would you offer to fellow committee members?
- Do you think the university group healthcare plans should cover integrative medicine practices?
- What information could you give committee members about the NCCAM?
- Do you think that faculty, staff, and students at your university would be accepting of an integrative medicine clinic? Why or why not?

CONCLUSION

This chapter was intended to raise your awareness and knowledge about integrative medicine, the development of integrative medicine clinics, and the early pioneers who advocated for alternative medicine. A historical time line of events leading to a more holistic type of health care was also presented. Hopefully, you will become a responsible consumer of your own health care when the time comes for you to select your physicians and other health care providers.

Suggestions for Class Activities

1. Research your county (parish) or several cities in your county (parish) to assess if there are any established integrative medicine clinics.
2. Visit an integrative medicine clinic and report on your findings.
3. Conduct a short knowledge and attitude survey on your campus related to integrative medicine and report the findings to your class.

Review Questions

1. What is the definition of integrative medicine?
2. What are integrative medicine clinics?
3. What have been the reasons for past resistance to alternative medicine and integrated care?
4. Who were the early pioneers promoting CAM and integrative medicine?
5. List and describe three historical milestones of integrative medicine?
6. Do you believe the Presidential Commission and/or the establishment of the NCCAM helped to expand CAM therapies? If so, how?
7. What changes have been made in medical care and medical education related to CAM?
8. How has insurance coverage for CAM care changed through the last 20 years?
9. What is the future of integrative medicine?
10. Should, we, as health consumers (or patients), take responsibility regarding alternative health care? If yes, what should we be responsible for?

Key Terms

acupuncture A traditional Chinese medicine treatment that uses stainless steel needles at specific points in the body to increase the flow of life energy known as Qi or Chi.

allopathic medicine A system in which medical doctors and other health care professionals (such as nurses, pharmacists, and therapists) treat symptoms and diseases using drugs, radiation, or surgery. Also called biomedicine, conventional medicine, mainstream medicine, orthodox medicine, and Western medicine.

Ayurvedic medicine (Ayurveda) A traditional system of medicine of India. The word Ayurveda is a Sanskrit word that means *Science of Life* or *Sciences of Lifespan*.

biofeedback The technique used to train people to control their own involuntary body processes such as heart rate, respirations, and even brain waves. It requires watching a monitor of some sort in order to change the rate using mental control.

biomedical physician or scientist These physicians apply research in many fields related to life sciences or body processes (anatomy and physiology, biology, pathology). They research the process of disease causation and attempt to find new treatment modalities.

biomedicine The application of the principles of the natural sciences, especially biology and physiology, to clinical medicine.

botanicals Substances obtained from plants.

Bravewell Collaborative Founded in 2002 by a small group of leading philanthropists dedicated to transforming the culture and delivery of health care and improving the health of the public through integrative medicine.

chronic Refers to an illness or medical condition that is characterized by long duration or frequent recurrence.

complementary and alternative medicine A group of diverse medical and healthcare systems, practices, and products that are not generally considered to be part of conventional medicine (NCCAM Definition).

consumer A person who buys and uses goods. In this text, it means the person who buys and uses health-related goods.

dosha In Ayurvedic medicine, a dosha is one of three energies that make up one's constitution: Vata, Pitta and Kapha.

facet joints Are synovial joints that help support the weight and control movement between individual vertebrae of the spine. Facet joints are at the back on either side of the spinal column, between the discs and the vertebral bodies. The bony prominences of each vertebra form a joint with the vertebrae above and below. The role of the facet joints is to limit excessive movement and provide stability for the spine.

holistic health Refers to the physical, emotional, spiritual, social, and mental domains of health. All should be seen as making up the whole person.

integrative medicine Combines treatments from conventional medicine and CAM for which there is evidence of safety and effectiveness.

naturopathic medicine A system of medical practices that relies on more natural healing methods (herbs, massage, exercise). It encompasses a belief in the body's ability to heal itself.

orthodox medicine Medical system that uses traditional medical practices such as drugs, surgery, or radiation to prevent or treat disease. It may be referred to as conventional medicine, mainstream medicine, and Western medicine.

pathogen A disease causing germ such as bacteria, virus, or fungus.

Qi Life energy in the body. In Chinese medicine and others, the belief is that if Qi is blocked, disease will occur.

Qigong A type of energy therapy that uses movement, breathing techniques, and meditation to enhance and move Qi throughout the body. This is purported to improve health and overall life energy.

randomized controlled study A study in which the people involved are drawn from a population by random and then assigned to a treatment protocol by a random draw.

transcendental A belief in the supernatural. A belief in miracles. A belief in the spiritual.

transcendental meditation A technique wherein people repeat a phrase to help themselves relax during medication. Also known as TM.

References

1. National Center for Complementary and Alternative Medicine. Health info page. 2009. Available at: http://nccam.nih.gov/health/whatiscam/overview.htm. Accessed April 10, 2010.
2. Snyderman R, Weil AT. Integrative medicine: bringing medicine back to its roots. *Arch Intern Med*. 2002;162(4):395–397.
3. Bravewell Collaborative. Consortium of Academic Health Centers for Integrative Medicine. 2010. Available at: http://www.imconsortium.org/members/home.html. Accessed April 12, 2010.
4. Bravewell Collaborative. The Summit on Integrative Medicine and the Health of the Public. 2010. Available at: http://www.bravewell.org/transforming_healthcare/national_summit. Accessed April 8, 2010.
5. Sundberg T, Halpin J, Warenmark A, Falkenberg T. Towards a model for integrative medicine in Swedish primary care. *BMC Health Serv Res*. 2007;7:107. Available at: http://www.biomedcentral.com/1472-6963/7/107. Accessed April 15, 2010.
6. Bravewell Collaborative. The McKinsey report. 2010. Available at: http://www.bravewell.org/transforming_healthcare/models_for_change/McKinsey_Report/. Accessed April 15, 2010.
7. Baer H. *Toward an integrative medicine: merging alternative therapies with biomedicine*. Walnut Creek, CA: AltaMira Press; 2004.
8. Eliopoulos C. *Integrating conventional and alternative therapies: holistic care for chronic conditions*. St. Louis, MO: Mosby; 1999.
9. Eisenberg D, Delbanco TL, Ettner SL, et al. Trends in alternative medicine use in the United States, 1990–1997: results of a follow-up national survey. *JAMA*. 1998;180:1569–1575.
10. Pelletier K, Astin J. Integration and reimbursement of complementary and alternative medicine by managed care and insurance providers: 2000 update and cohort analysis. *Alt Ther Health Illness*. 2002;8(1):38–39, 42, 44.
11. Chopra Center. Deepak Chopra, MD: co-founder of the Chopra Center for Wellbeing. 2009. Available at: http://www.chopra.com/aboutdeepak. Accessed April 24, 2010.
12. Benson-Henry Institute for Mind Body Medicine. About the Benson-Henry Institute for Mind Body Medicine. 2009. Available at: http://www.mgh.harvard.edu/bhi/about/. Accessed April 24, 2010.
13. Harvard Medical School Osher Research Center. David M. Eisenberg, MD. 2010. Available at: http://www.osher.hms.harvard.edu/peoplebio.asp?name=eisenberg. Accessed April 24, 2010.
14. Siegel B. Accept, retreat and surrender: How to heal yourself. 2010. Available at: http://www.shareguide.com/Siegel.html. Accessed April 24, 2010.
15. American Academy of Achievement. Andrew Weil, MD. February 26, 2010. Available at: http://www.achievement.org/autodoc/page/wei1bio-1. Accessed April 24, 2010.
16. Levine M, Weber-Levine M, Mayberry R. Complementary and alternative medical practices: training, experience, and attitudes of a primary care medical school faculty. *J Am Board Fam Pract*. 2003;16(4):318–326.
17. Boucher T, Lenz S. An organizational survey of physicians' attitudes about and practice of complementary and alternative medicine. *Altern Ther Health Med*. 1998;4(6):59–65.
18. Clifford S. Back in magazines, with stars [*New York Times* Web site]. May 9, 2010. Available at: http://www.nytimes.com/2010/05/10/business/media/10deepak.html?ref=deepak_chopra. Accessed June 21, 2010.
19. Employee Wellness. Employee wellness programs: economic considerations. Available at: http://www.employee-wellness.org. Accessed May 4, 2010.
20. Ornish D, Brown SE, Scherwitz LW. Can lifestyle changes reverse coronary heart disease. *Lancet*. 1990;336:129–133.
21. White House Commission on Complementary and Alternative Medicine Policy. Chapter 4: education and training of health care practitioners. Available at: http://www.whccamp.hhs.gov/fr4.html. Accessed April 7, 2010.
22. Wetzel M, Eisenberg D, Kaptchuk T. Courses involving complementary and alternative medicine at US medical schools. *JAMA*. 1998;280(9):784–787.
23. Tiralongo E, Wallis M. Integrating complementary and alternative medicine education into the pharmacy curriculum. *Am J Pharm Educ*. 2008;72(4):74. Available at: http://www.ajpe.org/view.asp?art=aj720474&pdf=yes. Accessed April 7, 2010.
24. Frenkel M, Frye A, Heliker D, et al. Lessons learned from complementary and integrative medicine curriculum change in a medical school. *Med Educ*. 2007;41(2):205–213.
25. Kligler B, Gordon A, Stuart M, Sierpina V. Suggested curriculum guidelines on complementary and alternative medicine: recommendations of the society of teachers of family medicine group on alternative medicine. *Fam Med*. 1999;31:30–33.
26. Brokaw JJ, Tunnicliff G, Raess BU, Saxon DW. The teaching of complementary and alternative medicine in U.S. medical schools: a survey of course directors. *Acad Med*. 2002;77(9):876–881.
27. SGIM CAM Interest Group. Position statement on CAM education. July 5, 2008. Available at: http://www.sgim.org/userfiles/file/SGIM%20CAM%20Statement%207-5-08.pdf. Accessed May 6, 2010.
28. Pelletier KR. *The best alternative medicine: what works? What does not?* New York: Simon & Schuster; 2000.
29. Ernst E. *The desktop guide to complementary and alternative medicine: an evidence-based approach*. London, UK: HarcourtLimited; 2001.
30. Wolsko PM, Eisenberg DM, Davis RB, Ettner SL, Phillips RS. Insurance coverage, medical conditions, and visits to alternative medicine providers: results of a national survey. *Arch Intern Med*. 2002;162(3):281–287.
31. Hess DJ. Complementary and alternative medicine: utilization patterns and CAM social movements, integrative medicine and epistemic politics, research and evaluation, regulatory

politics. Available at: http://science.jrank.org/pages/63327/complementary-alternative-medicine.html#ixzz0kjAI9SpZ. Accessed April 29, 2010.

32. Weeks J. Medicare pilot shakes out as $50-million high stakes game for chiropractors. April 3, 2010. Available at: http://theintegratorblog.com/site/index.php?option=com_content&task=view&id=644&Itemid=189. Accessed April 10, 2010.
33. Bunk S. Is integrative medicine the future? Reiman-Weil debate focuses on scientific evidence issues. *Scientist*. 1999;13(10):1.
34. National Institute of Nursing Research, National Institute of Health, U.S. Department of Health and Human Services. The BNC fellowship. Available at: http://www.ninr.nih.gov/Training/TrainingOpportunitiesIntramural/BNCFellowship.htm. Accessed April 29, 2010.
35. Fontanarosa P, Rennie D, DeAngelis C. The need for regulation of dietary supplements—lessons from ephedra. *JAMA*. 2003;289:1568–1570. (doi:10.1001/jama.289.12.1568).

APPENDIX 6.A

Time Line: Development of the NIH National Center for Complementary and Alternative Medicine (selected entries).

October 1991—The U.S. Congress passes legislation (Public Law 102-170) that provides $2 million in funding for fiscal year 1992 to establish an office within the National Institutes of Health (NIH) to investigate and evaluate promising unconventional medical practices. Dr. Stephen C. Groft is appointed acting director of the new Office of Alternative Medicine (OAM).

October 1992—Dr. Joseph J. Jacobs is appointed first director of the OAM.

June 1993—The NIH Revitalization Act of 1993 (P.L.103-43) formally establishes the OAM within the Office of the Director, NIH, to facilitate study and evaluation of complementary and alternative medical practices and to disseminate the resulting information to the public.

October 1996—A Public Information Clearinghouse is established.

November 1996—The OAM is designated a World Health Organization Collaborating Center in Traditional Medicine.

October 1998—NCCAM is established by Congress under Title VI, Section 601 of the Omnibus Appropriations Act of 1999 (P.L. 105-277). This bill amends Title IV of the Public Health Service Act and elevates the status of the OAM to an NIH Center.

February 1999—The U.S. Secretary of Health and Human Services (HHS) signs the organizational change memorandum creating NCCAM, making it the twenty-fifth independent component of NIH. The NCCAM director is vested with broad decision-making authority, especially concerning financial and administrative management and fiscal and review responsibility for grants and contracts.

May 1999—The NCCAM Trans-Agency CAM Coordinating Committee (TCAMCC) is established by the NCCAM director to foster the center's collaboration across the HHS and other federal agencies. This committee supersedes a trans-agency committee established by the NIH director in 1997.

August 1999—The National Advisory Council on Complementary and Alternative Medicine (NACCAM) is chartered.

September 2000—NCCAM's first strategic plan is published.

February 2001—NCCAM and the National Library of Medicine launch CAM on PubMed, a comprehensive Internet source of research-based information on CAM.

May 2004—NCCAM and the National Center for Health Statistics of the U.S. Centers for Disease Control and Prevention announce findings from the largest nationally representative survey to date on Americans' use of CAM (part of the 2002 National Health Interview Survey).

January 2005—The National Academies' Institute of Medicine releases a report, *Complementary and Alternative Medicine in the United States*, that was requested by NCCAM and federal partners. The report focuses on the scientific and policy implications of the widespread use of CAM.

February 2005—NCCAM publishes its second strategic plan, *Expanding Horizons of Health Care: Strategic Plan 2005–2009*, following a year-long process of input from the public, staff, and groups of outside experts.

November 2006—The center's founding director, Dr. Stephen E. Straus, steps down and becomes senior advisor to NIH Director Dr. Elias A. Zerhouni. Dr. Ruth L. Kirschstein is named acting director of NCCAM.

May 2007—NCCAM establishes a Complementary and Integrative Medicine Consult Service at the NIH Clinical Center.

January 2008—Dr. Josephine P. Briggs is named second Director of NCCAM.

June 2008—NCCAM launches "Time to Talk," an educational campaign to encourage patients and their health care providers to openly discuss the use of CAM.

December 2008—An NCCAM-supported supplement on CAM in the 2007 National Health Interview Survey yields the first nationally representative data on children's use of CAM and on trends in adult CAM use.

February 2009—NCCAM marks its tenth anniversary with a year of special events: an inaugural Stephen E. Straus Distinguished Lecture in the Science of Complementary and Alternative Medicine and NCCAM's 10th Anniversary Research Symposium, Exploring the Science of Complementary and Alternative Medicine, highlighting advances in the field of CAM research.

July 2009—The first nationally representative figures are released on how much Americans spend on CAM, from a nationwide government study co-funded by NCCAM. In 2007, they spent nearly $34 billion out-of-pocket on CAM, of which about two-thirds was for self-care.

Source: NIH National Center for Complementary and Alternative Medicine. The NIH Almanac. http://www.nih.gov/about/almanac/organization/NCCAM.htm#legistation

Complementary and Alternative Health Care: Historical Foundations of Holistic Healing

LEARNING OBJECTIVES

As a result of reading this chapter, students will:

1. Describe the prevalence of CAM use and identify the amount of money spent on CAM products or practices.
2. Identify several barriers to CAM use.
3. Distinguish between healing and the healer's role.
4. Assess how CAM has affected health care in the United States.
5. Analyze how past holistic healing modalities and healing professionals have influenced present-day medicine.
6. Relate the concept of shopping for health and using complementary and alternative medicine.

WHAT IS THE PREVALENCE OF CAM USE?

Dr. David Eisenberg led two national landmark survey studies in the 1990s and found that consumer visits to alternative practitioners (APs) increased from 34 percent in 1993[1] to 47.3 percent in 1997.[2] More recent numbers were reported at the National Center for Complementary and Alternative Medicine (NCCAM) Web site.[3] These results are from the 2007 National Health Interview Survey (NHIS) conducted by the National Center for Health Statistics at the Centers for Disease Control and Prevention (CDC). The NHIS is an annual in-person survey that contains a section related to CAM use. Findings revealed that, in the United States, of 23,393 adults age 18 years or older, 38.3 percent (about 4 in 10) used some form of complementary and/or alternative medicine (CAM).[3] This was an increase from 36 percent reported in 2002. Of 9,417 children age 17 years or younger, approximately 12 percent (about 1 in 8) were reported to be using CAM.[3] See **FIGURE 7.1**.

CAM use was reportedly greater among the higher educated, people with higher incomes, and women.[3] The type of therapies most utilized were meditation, massage therapy, deep breathing exercises, and yoga. Popular natural products used were fish oil, glucosamine, echinacea, and flaxseed.

Two studies assessing CAM use by college students are described next. Of 997 students participating in a southern university survey study,[4] about 53 percent reported knowledge of CAM therapies and 50 percent of students reported employing at least one CAM therapy in the last year. More females and older students used CAM. The most commonly used CAM therapies in this study were massage (30.9 percent), herbal supplements (19.6 percent), yoga

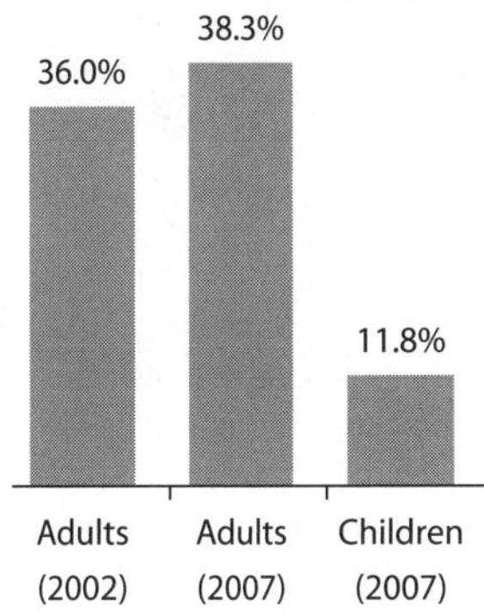

FIGURE 7.1 CAM use by U.S. adults and children.
Source: Barnes PM, Bloom B, Nahin R. CDC National Health Statistics Report #12. Complementary and Alternative Medicine Use Among Adults and Children: United States, 2007. December 2008.

(16.2 percent), aromatherapy (14.9 percent), meditation (14.2 percent), and chiropractic (14.1 percent). A small percentage used faith healing (5.5 percent) and reflexology (2.9 percent).[4] The most commonly used herbal supplements were creatine (12.8 percent), protein bars (12.8 percent), Metabolife (7.6 percent), Xenadrine (7.4 percent), ginseng (7.3 percent), gingko biloba (6.4 percent), Hydroxycut (4.6 percent), echinacea (2.2 percent), calcium (2.4 percent), Stacker 2 & 3 (2 percent), valerian (1.9 percent), St. John's wort (1.5 percent), kava kava (1.3 percent), herbal teas (1.2 percent), several types of vitamins and minerals, and 103 other supplements with percentages ranging from 0.2 to 0.7 percent. Most were body building supplements, immune boosters, and herbs to treat anxiety or insomnia.

Of 1,383 college students participating in a second study, a majority (n = 913, 66 percent) reported using CAM therapies, with higher use found among older students and female students.[5] Of the participants, 43 percent had used high-dose vitamin/nutritional supplements and 42 percent had used herbal medicines, but no breakdown on the type of vitamin, supplement, or herb was given.

There are also several studies assessing CAM knowledge and use among nurses. A recent publication[6] reported that clinical nurse specialists at a large Midwestern academic medical center used several CAM therapies personally and professionally, including humor, massage, spirituality/prayer, healing touch, acupuncture, and music therapy. After reading the results of these studies, we can ascertain that CAM is used by a wide variety of populations.

HOW MUCH MONEY HAS BEEN SPENT ON CAM?

Using alternative therapies is not inexpensive—Americans spent $33.9 billion[7] on CAM in 2006, even though their insurance policies would not cover some or all of their expenses. This was out-of-pocket money spent on alternative modalities such as herbal supplements, meditation, chiropractic care, and acupuncture. Reportedly, $22 billion of the $33.9 billion was spent on self-care costs such as CAM products, classes, and materials and $11.9 billion on approximately 354.2 million visits to CAM practitioners.[7] Based on the usage reports and the amount of money that people are spending on CAM, we can assume that in the future, there will be an increase in CAM use and costs.

WHY DO PEOPLE SEEK ALTERNATIVE FORMS OF MEDICAL CARE?

People may choose to use an alternative therapy or supplement in addition to their conventional treatment, or some may use an alternative therapy instead of traditional medicine. The reasons why people seek alternative forms of medical care vary. Some people select a therapy because its philosophy is compatible with their own beliefs about health care, or because they feel the alternative therapy relates with their personal values and spiritual beliefs regarding the nature of their illness.[8] People may want to feel a greater sense of control over their own treatment and seek out a doctor who will allow them choices. They may want to feel empowered to make some of their own health care decisions.[8] Some people are just plainly dissatisfied with conventional treatment. The following case study exemplifies some of these reasons.

Many individuals who use CAM tend to be innovative and at the cutting edge of cultural change. They are very interested in the environment and the world and possess a great sense of spirituality. Kaptchuk & Eisenberg[9] wrote about the persuasive appeal of CAM and identified four major elements.

The first element is the association of CAM with *nature*, a metaphor for many alternative medicines or therapies. For example, food that is labeled as organic rather than processed is desirable. CAM therapies are supposedly more natural than artificial and pure rather than synthetic.

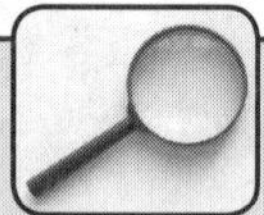

Case Study

Amy was raised in a small city in Indiana and has had a traditional medical doctor who served as her physician since she was a young girl. She is now 27 years old and has moved to another state. The medical doctor that she saw in this new city seemed cold and impersonal. He gave her little time in the office and did not ask her how she felt about taking medicine that he prescribed for her health problems. A friend convinced Amy to go see a more holistic doctor, a naturopathic physician. Amy made an appointment and went to the new physician the next week. He spent a lot of time with Amy getting to know her and to diagnose her health problems. In addition, the naturopathic physician gave her several treatment options. Rather than being perceived as impersonal and ineffective, Amy felt the naturopathic physician was warm and understanding, and she liked feeling empowered to make treatment choices.

Questions:

1. Are the qualities of being warm and understanding ones that you would treasure in a doctor?
2. Do you like the idea of being given treatment choices or options? Why or why not?

The second element is identified as vitalism, or the body's capacity to heal itself. The enhancement or balancing of life forces, qi, or psychic energy is a main theme and belief in the concept of vitalism. These life forces are not a physical force but are related to an energy within the body that is capable of healing. For patients, there is intuitive appeal in this noninvasive notion of healing from within.

The third element is science.[9] Alternative medicine's scientific process may match the steps of biomedical scientific techniques, but it depends greatly on observation. Alternative medicine is a more person-friendly science that embraces the concept of holism (connectedness of physical, mental, spiritual, emotional health). Sickness is viewed as a result of a weakened body that has fallen into an unbalanced condition. As such, it is remedied by overall strengthening of the body's natural resistance to disease. The human experience becomes the central element of CAM science rather than being marginalized. A person would not be told that their condition is "all in their head." In other words, the person is treated, not just the symptom or the disease.

A fourth element is the aspect of spirituality[9]—this does not refer particularly to religiosity, although for some, it may. Religion or spiritual experiences become important as people view health, illness, and healing. CAM offers a satisfying unification of the physical and spiritual because it bridges the gap between the domain of medical science and religion or spirituality, and the patient is allowed to make connections with nature and the universe.

Several theories have been posed regarding underlying motives for using CAM. One of these is that patients using CAM may be essentially neurotic, and therefore, are drawn towards the touching/talking approach of many therapies. Because CAM practitioners mainly see people with chronic diseases, it could be likely that neurosis levels are high in their patients. It could also be that people with high levels of stress (e.g., stress from having cancer) may seek out CAM practitioners. Another underlying motive is that people who have a better understanding of the workings of the human body are attracted to CAM therapists because diagnosis and treatment involve them more in the process. Some individuals may believe their condition is not serious enough to make an appointment to see their medical doctor (MD) and, therefore, see an alternative practitioner. Some individuals may seek out an alternative practitioner if they fear the side effects of traditional medical treatments.

Despite the limitations of the existing literature on the motives for CAM use, a few consistent findings have emerged. It is clear that, in general, CAM does not replace orthodox medical care. Rather, it serves as a substitute in some particular situations and as an adjunct in others. Some individuals simply will not use an alternative therapy when not considered appropriate for the condition in question.

WHAT ARE THE BARRIERS TO CAM USE?

There are several barriers to CAM use. Although insurance coverage is increasing for CAM therapies, there are still many that are not covered by insurance companies. Therefore, expense is a barrier. Another barrier is lack of knowledge. Many people do not have knowledge of alternative practices and are skeptical about their efficacy. They may also fear that alternative therapies are harmful. Of 485 students attending a west coast university, 22.7 percent reported that the cost of the therapy was a barrier, 19.7 percent reported that competence of the provider was a barrier, and 16.5 percent reported that possible danger or harm to the user was a barrier.[10]

HOW DO PHYSICIANS FEEL ABOUT CAM?

As discussed in Chapter 1, many MD and osteopathic (DO) physicians are embracing holistic care and CAM modalities. Research has shown that over 50 percent of conventional physicians in the United States use or refer patients for selective CAM treatments.[11,12] Most perceive them as having efficacy,[9] are interested in learning more about the therapies, and have generally positive attitudes toward alternative medical practices.[8,9] Additionally, as discussed in Chapter 6, many hospitals are adding integrated medicine programs, and insurance companies have expanded coverage to include services of alternative practitioners.[13] Other professions (e.g., psychotherapy) are also beginning to incorporate certain alternative therapies within the treatment regimen.[14] The American Medical Association has issued a proclamation to all members encouraging them to become involved in the scientific evaluation of alternative medicine.

In sum, we have determined that a lot of people are using CAM and that, without insurance, it is costly. People have varying reasons for using alternative medicine, and certainly there are barriers preventing CAM usage. Here in the United States, our medical doctors are beginning to engage in CAM educational classes, are conducting research studies of CAM therapies, and are becoming skilled in selective CAM modalities (e.g., acupuncture). It seems that people who use CAM want to be a part of the healing process. So what does the word "healing" really mean, and what is the role of the healer?

WHAT IS HEALING AND WHAT IS THE HEALER'S ROLE?

There is a distinction between the word "healing" and the word "cure." People with chronic illnesses may realize that they cannot be cured of the disease, but they want to feel as well as they possibly can, given the limitations of the disease. They consider factors other than the "elimination" of the disease, such as the kinds of adjustments they need to make in order to live with the disease. Healing means to use the mind, body, and spirit to control disease, promote a sense of well-being, and enhance the quality of life. A sense of well-being, comfort, and an integration of the body–mind–spirit are important characteristics of the healing process. On the other hand, the healer role is an important aspect. The healer is the one who restores health or makes a person whole again. Compassion, empathy, touch, and caring are all significant aspects of the healer's role. Scientific knowledge and skill in performing caregiving activities are important foundations to a healing relationship between the healer and the patient.

Clinicians and health care professionals use various healing approaches such as nurturing and caring, facilitating practices, assisting with transitions, promoting and restoring balance of mind, and encouraging optimal functioning and quality of life. The healer needs to develop personal attributes in the area of respecting clients, listening, providing time, and trusting intuition. The healer needs to recognize his or her own strengths and limitations. In addition, the healer's role is to model positive health practices and to understand the role of the body, mind, and spirit in the healing process. Lastly, the healer must recognize that the quality of self that he or she offers may be more significant to the healing process than the procedures that are performed.

The next portion of this chapter will help you understand some historical aspects of alternative and traditional healing modalities and the progression to current health consumer actions.

WHAT AND WHO ARE THE KEY HISTORICAL HEALING MODALITIES, EVENTS, AND PROFESSIONALS IMPACTING CURRENT HEALING THOUGHT?

Healing methods have been around since ancient times. The following is a historical overview of healing practitioners and methodologies that will include shamanism, Greek Asclepion institutions, Chinese medicine, Ayurvedic medicine, and early Christian healing. An overview of key events occurring during the scientific healing revolution and the impact of psychology and spirituality on present-day medicine also is presented.

Shamanism

Primitive tribes considered illness the work of evil spirits. The tribes, therefore, selected masters of the healing tradition who were known as medicine men, witch doctors, seers, or shamans.[15] The word "shaman" literally means "he (or she) who knows."

To aid healing of tribe members, the early shamans used various types of communication with the spiritual world that included singing, dancing, storytelling, and drawing.[15,16] Many achieved altered states of consciousness to assist in their healing rituals. Prehistoric paintings on cave walls and ceilings in France and Spain dating back some 32,000 years are thought by some researchers to have been the work of shamans. A social anthropologist, David Lewis-Williams,[17] has proposed that Cro-Magnon (the earliest modern people in Europe) shamans made some of the paintings. They would enter dark caves and, while in a trance state, paint images of their visions. The paintings were of strange patterns and lines, and later included animals. Lewis-Williams interprets images from a cave in Lascaux, France, as hallucinogenic sequenced experiences.[17] See **FIGURE 7.2** for a sample cave painting picture from Patagonia, Argentina.

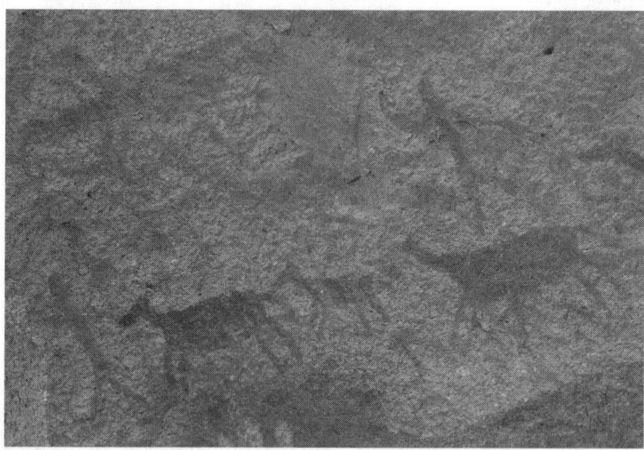

FIGURE 7.2 Cave painting from Patagonia, Argentina.

Anthropological studies have proven that many shamanic cultures used hallucinogenic substances to enter the "Otherworld."[17] The shaman was thought to be aided in this voyage to the Otherworld by particular animals who were the "spirit guides." Other ways in which shamans entered a trance state were to fast, place themselves in isolation for long periods of time, use sensory deprivation, and even undergo torture.

> The shaman acts as intermediary between the world of men and the gods, and has the power to descend into the realms of the dead. His spirit is believed to journey forth from his body, which remains in a state of trance. Sometime the long journey which it takes is described by him in a chant. Sometimes he induces the conditions of ecstasy by beating his drum or by an elaborate and exciting dance.[16]

In summary, there are three key features of shamanism[15]:

1. Shamans can voluntarily enter altered states of consciousness.
2. In these states, they may experience themselves journeying to other realms.

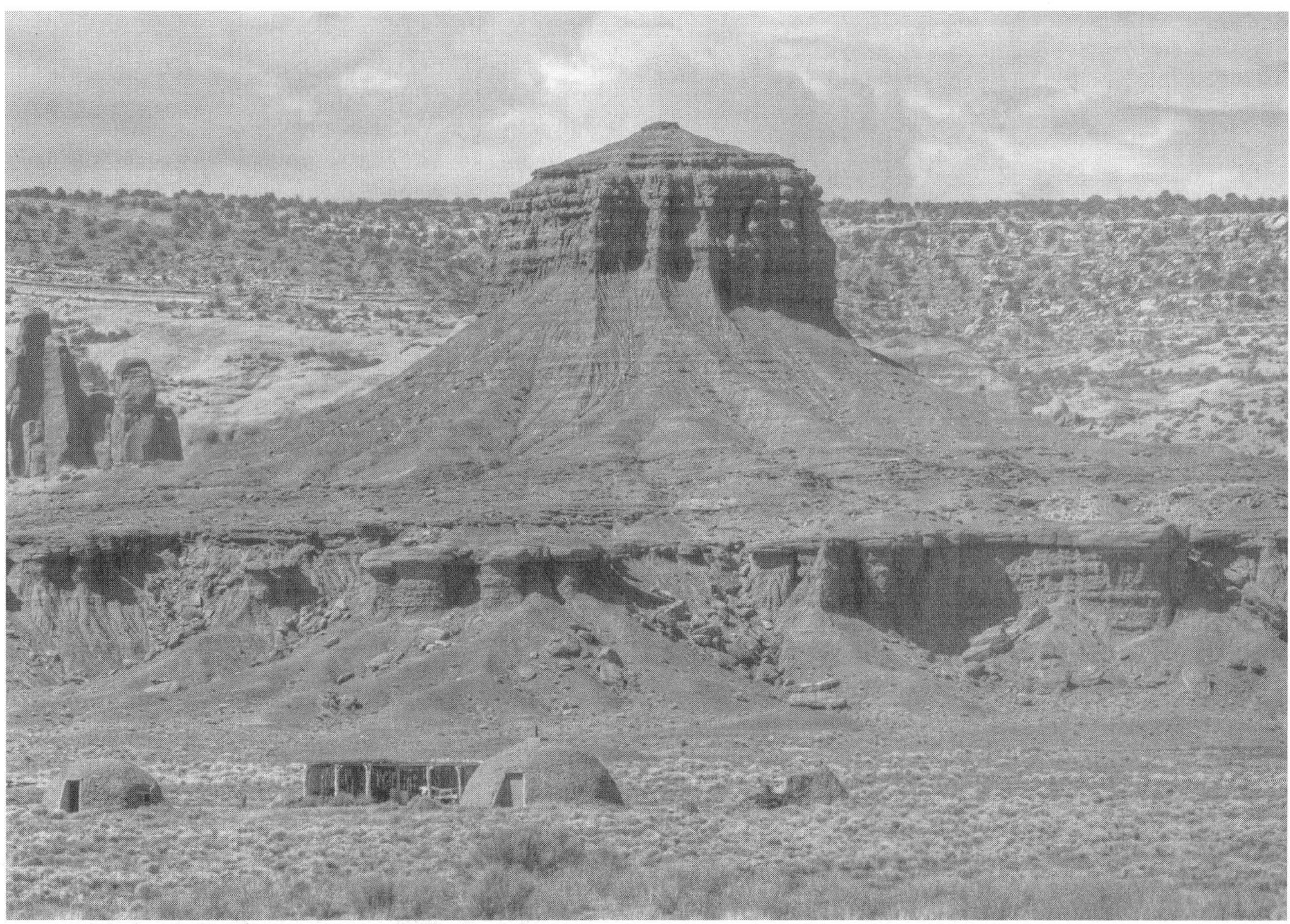

FIGURE 7.3 Native American ceremonial sweat lodge, Monument Valley, Utah.

3. They use these journeys to acquire knowledge or power and to help people in their community.

Their communication with the spiritual world help shamans gain a position of respect and power within their tribes. Shamans do not separate the body, mind, and soul, but see these parts as an integrated whole. Even though modern medicine has spread throughout the world, many cultures continue to rely on shamans for healing. In Native American groups, only the shaman has the power to communicate with gods or spirits. The shaman is considered a mystic, a poet, a sage, and a healer. This person is usually extraordinary in appearance and in acting talents. They use drumming, singing, fasting, dancing, spinning, and sweat lodges. The sweat lodge, which is built as a ceremonial sauna, is used for a purification ceremony.[18] See **FIGURE 7.3** for a picture of a Native American ceremonial sweat lodge in Monument Valley, Utah.

Greek Asclepions

The Asclepions (also spelled Asklepions) were sanctuaries of healing and had their roots in ancient Greece on the island of Kos (also spelled Cos).[19] They were named after Asclepius, the Divine Physician, who was worshipped as the god of medicine. Asclepius was said to be the son of Apollo and the Nymph Coronis, and is often shown in pictures as standing with a long wooden staff with a long snake entwined around it[19,20] (see **FIGURE 7.4**).

Early Asclepions were built in areas of natural beauty throughout Greece. They created a healing environment that addressed the physical, mental, and spiritual aspects of individuals. Before people could enter the Asclepions, they had to undergo Katharsis (catharsis) or purification.[21] This consisted of a series of cleansing baths and purging, accompanied by a cleansing diet. Purification could last several days. Once admitted to the healing centers, the healers utilized music, dream interpretations, drama, massage, humor, baths, herbs, and rest as treatments.[21]

Greek and Roman Influences on Healing

The foundation of modern medicine is thought to come mostly from ancient Greek physicians, although both Greek and Roman physicians had a tremendous influence

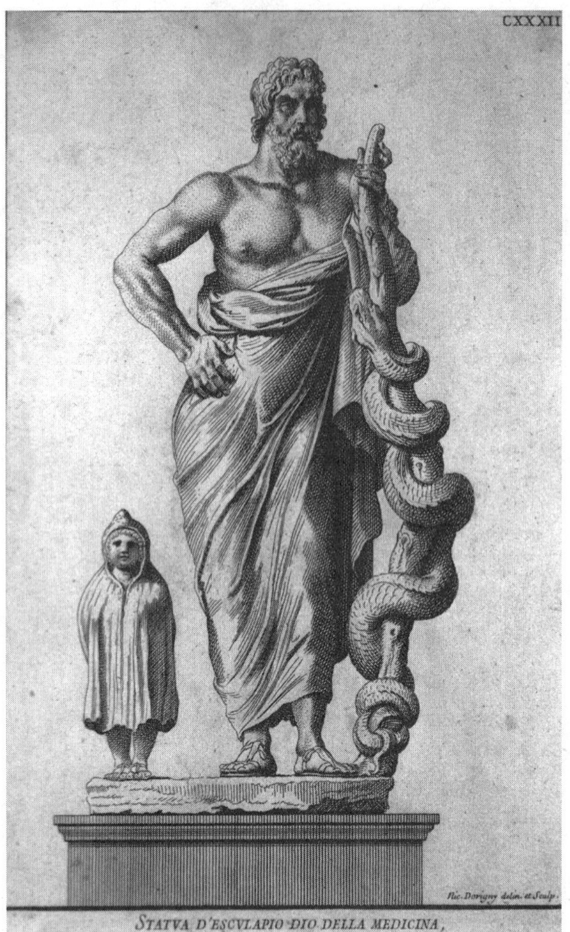

FIGURE 7.4 Asclepius with his serpent-entwined staff.

on medicine. Probably the most famous physician of all is Hippocrates, who lived from 460–377 BCE and is known as the father of modern medicine. He was born on an Aegean island named Cos,[22] and his father was also a physician. Hippocrates spent much of his early years on Cos at a local Asclepion. Hippocrates founded the Hippocratic school of medicine, and even today, new MDs pledge the Hippocratic Oath. From the Greeks came other great physicians such as Galen (great anatomical knowledge), Soranus (study of gynecology), and Dioscorides (books on herbal medicines). The Greeks had an extensive knowledge of herbs and herbal properties and used them when treating illnesses.

Greek healing methodologies influenced Roman medicine, and Roman methods influenced the Greeks. Because the Romans knew that poor hygiene was linked to disease and death, public bath houses and other similar public hygienic facilities were built.[23] Other influences from the Romans came through their use of surgical tools. Some that were used in ancient Rome were scalpels, hooks (as probes for dissection and raising blood vessels), bone drills, forceps, catheters, vaginal specula, and surgical saws for amputations and surgeries.[23]

Chinese Medicine

At one time Chinese medicine was thought to have begun during the time of Qin (221–206 BC), but based on manuscripts excavated in 1973 from Tomb Three of the Mawangdui site at Changsha, Hunan, most of the standardization of Chinese medicine occurred during the Western Han dynasty (206 BC–220 AD).[24] Knowledge of healing was recorded in the *Huangdi Neijing* (*The Yellow Emperor's Inner Canon*);[24,25] and knowledge of pharmacology was recorded in the *Shennong Jing (Classic of Shennong)* and Shennong Bencao Jing (Herbal Classic of Shennong). More on the contributions of Shennong, known as the Divine Farmer, follows in Chapter 9. A third important medical classic is the *Nanjing* (*Classic of Difficult Issues*), which explains medical theory and practice more clearly than the *Huangdi Neijing*.

In general, herbal medicines and acupuncture therapy are the two aspects most associated with Chinese medicine. However, acupuncture as we know it today (inserting steel needles into body parts) was not mentioned in the Mawangdui manuscripts. Although there is no mention of acupuncture needles, early Chinese doctors did use stone probes to open up boils and abscesses.[24,25] The acupuncture needling technique is not believed to have been used before 168 BC.[24]

Early Chinese medicine physicians recognized the movement of life energy or *qi*. They believed that illness occurs when energy flow is blocked. Acupuncture and herbal medicines are used to unblock energy so that it can flow more freely through the body. Chinese medicine is used today, and is increasing in popularity in U.S. and western medicine.

Ayurvedic Medicine

Ayurvedic medicine is the traditional system of medicine of India. The word "Ayurveda" means the "science of life" or "sciences of lifespan." It is the oldest healing system of all, and may have begun sometime between 5,000 and 10,000 years ago. Ayurvedic medicine is a holistic healing system that may have influenced ancient Chinese medicine and the humoral medicine practiced by Hippocrates in Greece. Some call it the "mother of all healing."[26] The early healers of India were known as sages or seers, and they were the ones who began to systemize healing after having identified "Veda," the knowledge of how our world works.[27] The secrets of sickness and health were communicated to the sages through deep mediation and were written down over 2,000 years ago in the four main Vedas (Ric, Sama, Yajur, and Atharva), which are sacred texts of India. The Ric is said to be the oldest surviving book of any Indo-European language.[28] All that the sages learned was organized into the Indian healing system called Ayurveda. The *Charaka samhita* text was written 2,000 years before the microscope was invented, and yet it listed 20 different microscopic organisms that can cause disease and discussed how disease spreads. The *Sushrutha samhita* text (300–400 AD) offered information about surgery, surgical equipment, suturing, and the importance of hygiene.[27]

Ayurvedic healing techniques promote unity of the mind, body, and spirit. Similar to Chinese medicine, the Ayurvedic belief is that when energy fields are blocked, they cause illness; however, in Ayurvedic medicine, the energy fields are identified as chakras.

Ayurvedic medicine went through a period of decline in India during the British rule, but in 1947, when India gained its independence, Ayurveda again grew in importance and new schools of medicine were established. More on Ayurvedic medicine may be found in Chapter 8, which describes various methods of using Ayurveda to treat illness.

Early Christian Healing

The Bible is used as evidence of the spiritual dimension to restoring physical health. Jesus Christ was known as a healer and worker of miracles, someone who healed people both physically and spiritually. Early Judean beliefs held that people who had sinned or who were evil became sick, and that health and healing stemmed from repentance and divine forgiveness. (Judea was a kingdom ruled by the Herods and was part of the Roman province of Syria.) To heal the sick, a ceremonial practice called anointing was used.

In early biblical times, both laypeople (men and women) and priests used anointing to heal the sick using oils such as frankincense and myrrh. It involved dipping a finger in the oil and touching the person either on the forehead or on another body part. By the middle ages, anointing became used solely by male Catholic priests, and rules were set as to who could and could not anoint. After the Reformation in the 1500s, the use of anointing (laying on of hands) by most of the newer Christian denominations sharply decreased in scope and breadth. Anointing has returned somewhat in the present day. The Roman Catholic Church uses blessed oil for final anointing or at the time of last breath. The Anglican Church allows anointing when visiting the sick, and in the Lutheran tradition, anointing is used after a silent laying on of the hands. The belief that anointing is superstitious is waning, and many groups want to restore the practice as a sign of hope for those suffering spiritually as well as emotionally or physically.[29]

An example of an 1800s Christian healer is Mary Baker Eddy (1821–1910), the founder of Christian Science.[30] She had grown up in ill health most of her life. When she was in her early forties, she became a patient of a New England healer, Phineas Parkhurst Quimby.[30] At the time, Mrs. Eddy was an invalid, but after undergoing one week's treatment by Mr. Quimby, she was "cured." During the ensuing years, Eddy worked with Quimby and began to write and give public lectures on Quimby's healing process. Several years later, Eddy had an accident and almost died. Quimby himself had died earlier, so she used Quimby's healing methods to heal herself. She called this the "Science of Christianity," and later named it Christian Science, a healing methodology that didn't use medicine, and that was based on the healing methods of Phineas Quimby. When Mrs. Eddy was 88 years old, she founded the *Christian Science Monitor*.[30] In 1995, Mary Baker Eddy was elected to the National Women's Hall of Fame as the only U.S. woman to found a worldwide religion.

Scientific Healing Revolution

The Scientific Revolution occurred during the 1800s. Physicians and nurses began separating themselves from the early healing practices and moved toward scientific practices. R. T. H. Laennec invented the stethoscope in France in 1816, a new technology that helped fight tuberculosis, said to be the single worst disease of the urban landscape. If contracted, the chances of survival were about 60 percent. Another new technology was further perfection of the microscope by Carl Zeis in Germany. Zeis worked with others to solve disease problems at the cellular level. On a greater scale, the position of Public Health Officer was created and the person assigned or hired to that position, along with civil engineers, worked to improve the deplorable sanitary conditions in major cities.[31]

Cholera was another horrific epidemic. In 1849, approximately 7000 people died in London from cholera. In 1883, the organism causing cholera (Vibrio cholerae, a comma shaped bacterium) was identified in water by Robert Koch via the microscope and subsequently was contained by public health officials. Great gains also were made during the 1800s in cellular biology and public health. Public health laws were passed in order to protect people from epidemic diseases.[31]

The scientific revolution not only encompassed new technology and new public health laws, but also distinguished some individuals who became notable for saving lives through public health practices. Florence Nightingale was one of those people (see her photo in **FIGURE 7.5**). She was born to wealthy British parents, and she is named after the city in which she was born, Florence, Italy.[32]

Nightingale had to overcome prejudice and convince her wealthy parents to allow her to become a nurse, a practice associated with working class women. In the 1850s, Russia invaded Turkey, and Britain and France went to Turkey's aid (Crimean War). A newspaper in London published stories about typhus, cholera, and dysentery among the servicemen. The government allowed Nightingale to travel to Turkey and to take 30 other nurses with her. They found deplorable, unsanitary conditions—soldiers in bloody, dirty uniforms and unwashed. Her efforts at sanitizing the service hospitals and aiding the wounded rapidly turned around the

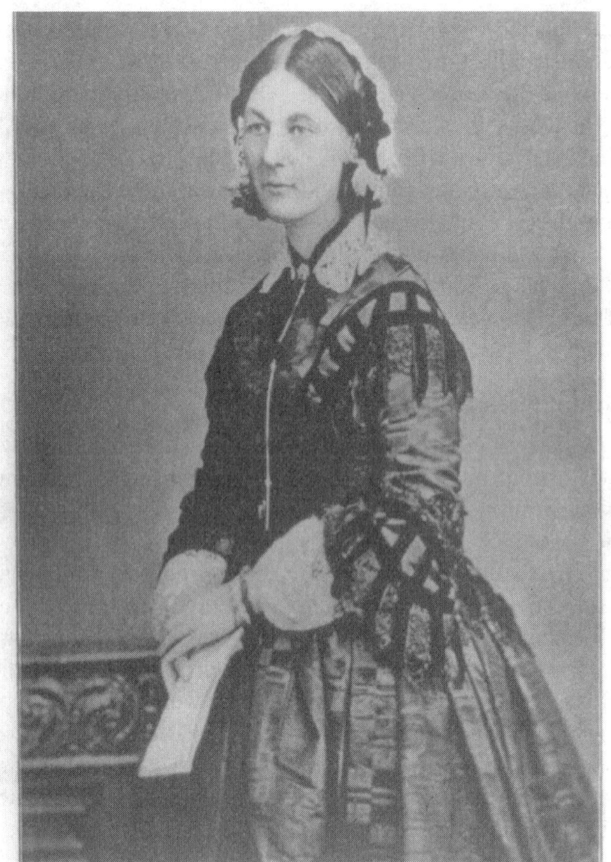

FIGURE 7.5 Florence Nightingale.

death toll in the Crimean War. On the base of the Turkish army barracks that served as British military base and hospital, a Florence Nightingale museum has been established in Istanbul, Turkey.[32] Nightingale will always be remembered as having promoted a holistic approach to caring for the wounded and ill.

Psychology and Spirituality

It is impossible to discuss a history of healing without pointing out the impact of psychology and spirituality. In the 1960s and 1970s health care began being sensitive about the importance of mind, body, and spirit in healing. Theoretical frameworks began describing various paradigms or theories; the decision of which theory to use was based solely on the unique characteristics and preferences of the clinician. An early holistic psychological theory is Gestalt psychology. The word means "unified whole."[33] Gestalt therapy was founded by Frederick (Fritz) and Laura Perls in the 1940s. It is a theory characterized by the phrase "the whole is greater than the sum of its parts"—hence, "wholistic" or "holistic." In other words, the theory speaks to mental health as being dependent on the rest of the human experience: social, emotional, physical, and sexual. It is most famous for the Gestalt "laws" of perception, which attempted to describe which properties of visual elements make them appear to belong together as an entity.

Currently, holistic psychology builds on Gestalt, transpersonal, and psychosynthesis psychological theory. It involves adopting, adapting, and using techniques to effect personal change, transformation, and healing. It is a psychology that is no longer one-dimensional but reveals a multidimensional, yet unique, individual. It seems to be a psychology that complements our new attention to alternative healing methods. Through the years, many psychology theories have been developed,[34] and clinicians select a model that aligns with their views about mental health (i.e., behavioral, cognitive, developmental, humanist, personality, and social psychology). An example of a personality theory is Freud's psychoanalytical theory. On the other hand, behaviorists align more with behavioral or cognitive-behavioral theories.

Spirituality models are being developed and are evolving. Some align spirituality and religion whereas others show a distinct difference. It has been difficult to assess spirituality because the meaning of spirituality is different and personal from individual to individual. For example, some individuals feel most spiritual when they are sitting in church but others feel spiritual when walking a beach looking at the ocean or skiing down a mountain.

Most theoretical frameworks include the concepts of self-discovery, relationships, and eco-awareness.[35] A literature review found that the self, others, and God provide the key elements within a definition of spirituality. Identified within those three key elements were emerging themes such as meaning, hope, relatedness/connectedness, beliefs/belief systems, and expressions of spirituality.[36] In particular, the nature of God was viewed as taking many forms and, essentially, is whatever an individual takes to be of highest value in his or her life. The authors concluded that the themes that emerged could be used as a framework for future exploration of the concept of spirituality.[36]

A look at some historical events that have impacted healing through the ages is important in that it shows us where we were and helps us assess what the future may bring. As you can see, a holistic approach to healing seems to be valued throughout history and is valued today. This can be exemplified by the many professional associations that have provided high standards and principles of practice and use the word "holistic" in their name (i.e., American Holistic Nurses Association, American Holistic Medical Association, and American Holistic Health Association).

Both alternative medicine and traditional (western) medicine will continue to complement each other more and more through the oncoming years. We, the health care consumers, need to make careful choices and utilize the best of both.

IS CAM SCIENTIFICALLY LEGITIMATE OR IS IT QUACKERY?

CAM as Scientific

Most of the scientific research on selective forms of alternative medicine practices are being conducted at the National Center for Complementary and Alternative Medicine (NCCAM).[3] At present, the NCCAM funds four research centers: Centers of Excellence for Research on CAM, Centers for Dietary Supplements Research: Botanicals, Developmental Centers for Research on CAM, and International Centers for Research on CAM.[3] Each funds specific research and are presented in **BOX 7.1**.

The NCCAM publishes the results of studies on its Web site and provides links to research that is ongoing or completed on specific topics. To give one example, the NCCAM provides a link on yoga to many research studies used to assess the effect of yoga on a variety of conditions (e.g., pediatric headaches, post-traumatic stress disorder, fatigue and sleep in cancer, eating disorders, menopausal hot flashes).

Box 7.1

NCCAM Funds Four Research Centers

Centers of Excellence for Research on CAM: Research on acupuncture (Massachusetts), antioxidants (Oregon, North Carolina), botanicals (Montana, South Carolina, Illinois, New York, California), energy medicine (Pennsylvania), mind–body/meditation (California, Wisconsin), and traditional Chinese medicine (for alcohol and drug abuse in Massachusetts, arthritis in Maryland, and Chinese herbal therapy in New York).

Centers for Dietary Supplements Research: Botanicals: Research of botanicals in six areas: age-related diseases (Indiana), metabolic syndrome (Louisiana), women's health (Illinois), immuno-modulators (New York), lipids (North Carolina), and dietary supplements (Iowa).

Developmental Centers for Research on CAM: These centers collaborate with CAM schools and conventional biomedical research institutions. Research on acupuncture (Massachusetts), botanical medicine (Minnesota, Washington), chiropractic manipulation (Iowa, Kansas, New York), mind–body medicine (Oregon), and osteopathy (Arizona, Texas).

International Centers for Research on CAM: Research on botanicals (International Center for Indigenous Phytotherapy Studies: HIV/AIDS) and, traditional Chinese medicine for functional bowel disorders (Massachusetts).

Also listed at the Web site are the following study results (some positive and some not):

- A study indicates ginkgo biloba does not reduce the risk of cancer.
- Tai chi and qi gong show some beneficial health effects.
- A two-year study of knee osteoarthritis pain reports similar outcomes with glucosamine and chondroitin, Celecoxib and placebo.
- Fish oil enhances the effects of green tea on Alzheimer's disease in mice.
- A study shows green tea may repair DNA damage caused by UV radiation.
- Stress management may enhance immune function in people with HIV.

The NCAAM Web site also provides links to PubMed CAM research studies that have been published in various scientific journals. Dhikav and others published two studies on yoga in *Journal of Sex Medicine*: "Yoga in Male Sexual Functioning: A Noncomparative Pilot Study" and "Yoga in Female Sexual Functions." Another link was to an Oxford journal, *Evidence-Based Complementary and Alternative Medicine*. An example of a research study published in the journal is, "Using Complementary and Alternative Medicines to Target the Host Response During Severe Influenza." Two Chinese herbs were studied for protection of mice against influenza.[37] NCCAM's Web site is a repository for CAM information, past and ongoing research, information regarding grants and training programs, plus links to other CAM sites.

CAM research is ongoing. Some results will be promising, some will demonstrate effectiveness, and some will identify CAM practices that are not effective. Every day, we learn something new about CAM, a practice or a medicine (herb or supplement). We need to study the research and then make intelligent choices. The In the News box shows two news articles published in July 2010 that exemplify the importance of reading, studying, and analyzing information regarding CAM and other healing modalities.

CAM as Quackery

The most publicized source of CAM criticism comes from Quackwatch (www.quackwatch.com),[38] a Web site operated by Stephen Barrett, MD. Quackwatch reports on its Web site that it is affiliated with the National Council Against Health Fraud, an organization that Barrett has been a member of for many years. Barrett and others (e.g., Rosemary Jacobs, William T. Jarvis) hold the view that there is no alternative medicine, only scientifically proven, evidence-based medicine that is supported by data-driven studies. Barrett writes that the alternative movement is a type of societal trend that is rejecting science as a method of determining truth, and that the movement supports pseudoscience over science.[38] His case in point is a section he wrote on "Science

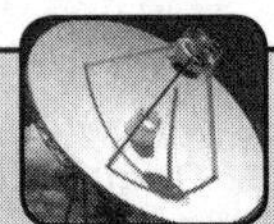

In the News

Features on CAM Studies

An article published in *Medical News Today*, "Questioning the Safety and Effectiveness of Herbal Dietary Supplements,"[39] stated that millions of people are taking herbs and plant-based supplements, placing themselves at risk because the supplements may not be safe or effective. Most of the concern regards contaminants such as toxic metals (lead and mercury) or pesticides that may be contained within the supplements. Another concern was that the plants may be toxic or interact with prescribed drugs. The U.S. Food and Drug Administration now requires all supplement manufacturers to test their products for contaminants.

A second article reported the results of a study assessing different meditation techniques to treat stress disorders.[40] The authors claim that doctors are increasingly prescribing meditation to patients for stress-related disorders, but they should have a better understanding of the type of meditation to recommend. Meditation techniques were identified as Tibetan Buddhist (loving kindness and compassion), Buddhist (Zen and Diamond Way), and Chinese (qi gong) traditions. Researchers found that there was a difference in effect depending on the type of meditation technique.

versus Vitalism." As discussed earlier in this chapter, Chinese traditional medicine and Ayurvedic medicine are based on the principle of vitalism (a life force within the body). Barrett claims that vitalists pretend to be scientific, but they really reject scientific methods and regard "personal experience, subjective judgment, and emotional satisfaction as preferable to objectivity and hard evidence."[38] One section under Quackwatch is titled "Questionable Products, Services and Theories." Over 100 topics are listed alphabetically, from acupuncture to chiropractic, homeopathy, naturopathy, therapeutic touch, and so forth, either condemning or questioning each as quackery. In fact, Barrett is so passionately against alternative medicine that he wrote an article in Quackwatch pointing out reasons why the NCCAM should be defunded.[38]

After reading the preceding sections on "CAM as Scientific" and "CAM as Quackery," perhaps, as a health consumer, you could ponder and answer the following questions:

1. Do you believe that CAM research should continue? If so, why?
2. Do you believe that funding for CAM research at the NCCAM should be withdrawn? If so, why?
3. If funding were withdrawn from the NCCAM, and for all those sites across the United States that are conducting CAM research, how would research continue?
4. If Dr. Barrett believes that healing modalities need to be tested scientifically and proven effective (evidence based), and if he is calling upon defunding of our major national research center (NCCAM), how does he expect to learn what really works and what doesn't?
5. What can you do as a health consumer to advocate for the scientific study of any medical or healing treatment, whether it is labeled alternative or traditional?

CONCLUSION

This chapter is intended to give you an overall look at CAM in terms of how many people are using CAM, who they are, and the costs involved. A brief history of healing was introduced so that you could relate those historical events and professionals to current medical practices. Moreover, those practices that we "Westerners" call *alternative* are in actuality healing methods that have been used for centuries. Perhaps, as we study more about CAM practices, we will learn some beneficial information from our predecessors.

Suggestions for Class Activities

1. Visit a health food store:
   a. Describe the kinds of products sold, product claims (to improve health or intended use), and product prices.
   b. Ask the proprietor and salespeople what their educational background is and what kind of training they received in order to sell products and herbs.
   c. Bring a sample or two back from the health store (if not expensive) and show to your classmates. (Samples could be a food product such as potato chips, an energy bar, or soap.)

d. Prepare a written report of your findings.

2. Research more in depth one of the historical figures presented. Prepare a report and present it to your classmates.
3. Research modern day Asclepions. (Where located, services offered, looks of the building and grounds, cost for clients). Prepare a report and present it to your classmates.

Review Questions

1. What is the prevalence of CAM use?
2. Who are the greatest users of CAM?
3. What is the cost of CAM use?
4. What is a definition of "healing"?
5. What are three characteristics of the healer's role?
6. What is the role of the shaman?
7. What main characteristic is similar in shamans all over the world and in various cultures?
8. What is an Asclepion?
9. How have the Greeks and Romans contributed to medicine and healing?
10. How long have Ayurvedic and Chinese medicine been practiced?
11. Who was the most revered Judaean early healer?
12. What was Mary Baker Eddy's contribution to healing?
13. Describe how Florence Nightingale impacted healing practices.
14. How have psychology and spirituality impacted healing?
15. Is it correct to say that CAM users are "shopping for health"?
16. What is the name of the national CAM research center?
17. What is the name of the quackery Web site presented in this chapter?

Key Terms

anointing Involves dipping a finger in oil and touching a person either on the forehead or on another body part as a part of religious ceremony.

Asclepions Sanctuaries of healing. They had their roots in ancient Greece on the island of Kos.

Ayurvedic medicine A traditional system of medicine of India. The word Ayurveda is a Sanskrit word that means *Science of Life* or *Sciences of Lifespan*.

Christian Science A healing methodology that does not use medicine. Mary Baker-Eddy founded Christian Science and based it on the healing methods of Phineas Quimby.

echinacea A genus of herbaceous flowering plants in the daisy family, *Asteraceae*. It is an herb used to fight infections, especially upper respiratory conditions such as the common cold.

flaxseed A member of the genus *Linum* in the family *Linaceae*. It is a blue flowering plant that contains rich oily seeds. It is recommended for general well being and digestive health.

glucosamine It is a natural compound found in healthy cartilage. Glucosamine sulfate is used for arthritic conditions.

organic Agriculture conducted according to certain standards, especially the use of only naturally produced fertilizers and non-chemical means of pest control.

prevalence Measure of how much of a disease or condition there is in a population at a particular point in time.

psychic energy The concept that the human mind can create, transmit and receive energy that can be utilized for healing purposes.

Qi (Chi) According to TCM, Qi is a bodily energy that flows through unseen channels in the body called meridians. Illness is believed to occur when Qi is blocked.

seer Masters of the healing tradition. A person who knows.

shamanism An anthropological term referencing a range of beliefs and practices regarding a person (shaman) who is believed to be able to communicate with the spiritual world.

spirituality A belief in a higher power; a way to find meaning and hope in one's life; awareness of purpose and meaning in life.

sweat lodge Used for a purification ceremony; a place built as a ceremonial sauna lodge.

References

1. Eisenberg D, Davis R, Ettner S, et al. Trends in alternative medicine use in the United States, 1990–1997: results of a follow-up national survey. *JAMA*.1998;1280:1569–1575.
2. Eisenberg D, Kessler R, Norlock F, Calkins D, Delbanco T. Unconventional medicine in the United States—prevalence, costs, and patterns of use. *JAMA*. 1993;328(4):246–252.
3. National Center for Complementary and Alternative Medicine. The use of complementary and alternative medicine in the United States. Available at: http://nccam.nih.gov/news/camstats/2007/camsurvey_fs1.htm. Accessed July 17, 2010.
4. Synovitz L, Gillan W, Wood R, Nordness M, Kelly J. An exploration of college students' complementary and alternative

medicine use: relationship to health locus of control and spirituality level. *Am J Health Educ.* 2006;37(2):84–93.

5. Chng C, Neill K, Fogle P. Predictors of college students' use of complementary and alternative medicine. *Am J Health Educ.* 2003;34(5):267–291.
6. Cutshal S, Derscheid D, Miers A, et al. Knowledge, attitudes, and use of complementary and alternative therapies among clinical nurse specialists in an academic medical center. *Clin Nurs Spec.* 2010;24(3):125–131. Available at: http://www.nursingcenter.com/library/JournalArticle.asp?Article_ID=1002829. Accessed July 15, 2010.
7. Nahin, RL, Barnes PM, Stussman BJ, Bloom B. *Costs of complementary and alternative medicine (CAM) and frequency of visits to CAM practitioners: United States, 2007.* Hyattsville, MD: National Center for Health Statistics; 2009.
8. Astin J. Why patients use alternative medicine. *JAMA.* 1998;279(19):1548–1553.
9. Kaptchuk T, Eisenberg D. The persuasive appeal of alternative medicine. *Ann Intern Med.* 1998;129(12):1061–1065
10. Gaedeke R, Tootelian D, Holst C. Alternative medicine among college students. *J Hosp Market.* 1999;3(1):107–118.
11. Levine M, Weber-Levine M, Mayberry R. Complementary and alternative medical practices: training, experience, and attitudes of a primary care medical school faculty. *J Am Board Fam Pract.* 2003;16(4):318–326.
12. Boucher T, Lenz S. An organizational survey of physicians' attitudes about and practice of complementary and alternative medicine. *Altern Ther Health Med.* 1998;4(6):59–65.
13. Wetzel M, Eisenberg D, Kaptchuk T. Courses involving complementary and alternative medicine at US medical schools. *JAMA.* 1998;280(9):784–787.
14. Bassman L, Uellendahl G. Complementary/alternative medicine: ethical, professional, and practical challenges for psychologists. *Pro Psychol Res Pract.* 2003;34(3):264–270.
15. Walsh R. *The world of shamanism: new views of an ancient tradition.* Woodbury, MN: Llewellyn; 2007.
16. Davidson H, Ellis R. *Gods and myths of northern Europe.* New York: Penguin; 1964.
17. Coppens P. Cave paintings: entrancing the otherworld. *Frontier.* 2003;9:6. Available at: http://www.philipcoppens.com/cavepaintings.html. Accessed July 10, 2010.
18. Wikipedia. Picture of Hupa Sweat House. Available at: http://en.wikipedia.org/wiki/File:Hupa_Sweat_House.jpg. Accessed August 9, 2011.
19. Asklepion. Picture of Asclepius Purchased from Pixmac at: http://www.pixmac.com/picture/white+marble+classic+statue+of+asclepius+isolated+on+black+background/000061901311. Accessed July 19, 2010.
20. MythNet Picture Gallery. Picture of Asclepius. Available at: http://www.classicsunveiled.com/mythnet/html/pics10.htm. Accessed July 19, 2010.
21. Greek Medicine.net. The Asclepions: sanctuaries of healing. Available at: http://www.greekmedicine.net/mythology/asclepions.html. Accessed July 19, 2010.
22. The Role of Women in the Art of Ancient Greece. Ancient Greek medicine: index of ancient Greek medicine. Available at: http://www.fjkluth.com/gmed.html. Accessed July 19, 2010.
23. Wikipedia. Medicine in ancient Rome. Available at: http://en.wikipedia.org/wiki/Medicine_in_ancient_Rome. Accessed July 20, 2010.
24. Galambos I. *The origins of Chinese medicine—The early development of medical literature in China.* 1966.
25. Purify Our Mind. History of traditional Chinese medicine. Available at: http://www.purifymind.com/HistoryMed.htm. Accessed July 20, 2010.
26. Health Education Alliance for Life and Longevity. History of Ayurveda. Available at: http://www.heall.com/body/altmed/treatment/ayurveda/history.html. Accessed July 20, 2010.
27. Bradford, N. (ed.). *The one spirit encyclopedia of complementary health.* London: Hamlyn; 2000.
28. Florida Vedic College. The history of Ayurveda. Available at: http://www.floridavediccollege.edu/ayurveda/history.htm. Accessed July 15, 2010.
29. Smith LL. What happened to Christian anointing—How did we lose it in history? Available at: http://ezinearticles.com/?What-Happened-to-Christian-Anointing---How-Did-We-Lose-it-in-History?&id=1416033. Accessed July 12, 2010.
30. Mary Baker Eddy: founder of Christian Science. Available at: http://marybakereddy.wwwhubs.com. Accessed July 12, 2010.
31. McVeigh, DP. Public health and technology during the 19th century. Available at: http://www.ilt.columbia.edu/projects/bluetelephone/html/health.html. Accessed July 9, 2010.
32. Spartacus Educational. Biography of Florence Nightingale. Available at: http://www.spartacus.schoolnet.co.uk/REnightingale.htm. Accessed July 15, 2010.
33. Yontef G. Gestalt therapy: an introduction. *Awareness, Dialogue, and Process.* Gouldsboro, ME: Gestalt Journal Press; 1993.
34. Cherry K. Psychology theories. Available at: http://psychology.about.com/od/psychology101/u/psychology-theories.htm. Accessed July 15, 2010.
35. Delaney C. The spirituality scale: Development and psychometric testing of a holistic instrument to assess the human spiritual dimension. *J. Holist Nurs.* 2005;23(2):145–167. Available at: http://jhn.sagepub.com/content/23/2/145.abstract. Accessed August 9, 2011.
36. Dyson J, Cobb M., Forman D. The meaning of spirituality: a literature review. *J Adv Nurs.* 1997;26(6):1183–1188.
37. Alleva L, Charles C, Clark I. Using complementary and alternative medicines to target the host response during severe influenza. *Evid Based Complement Alt Med.* 2010;7(4):501–510.
38. Barrett S. Quackwatch: Your guide to quackery, health fraud, and intelligent decisions. Available at: http://www.quackwatch.com. Accessed July 24, 2010.
39. *Medical News Today.* Questioning the safety and effectiveness of herbal dietary supplements. July 23, 2010. Available at: http://www.medicalnewstoday.com/articles/195593.php. Accessed July 21, 2010.
40. *Medical News Today.* Results vary with different meditation techniques. July 21, 2010. Available at: http://www.medicalnewstoday.com/articles/195403.php. Accessed July 21, 2010.

Alternative Medical Systems: Ayurvedic Medicine and Its Practices

LEARNING OBJECTIVES

As a result of reading this chapter, students will:

1. Explain the foundation of Ayurvedic medicine principles.
2. Compare and contrast Ayurvedic and Western medicine disease causation beliefs.
3. Assess the validity of the general guidelines for treating dosha imbalances.
4. Analyze what should be the minimum standard for the sale of over-the-counter Ayurvedic medicines.

WHAT IS AYURVEDIC MEDICINE?

As presented in Chapter 7, the word, "Ayurveda" is a Sanskrit word that means "science of life." It is derived from two roots: *Ayur* meaning "life" and *Veda* meaning "knowledge or science." The practice of Ayurvedic medicine had its origins in India 5,000 to 10,000 years ago, making it the oldest healing science known. Ayurvedic healing methods were first taught and passed down orally, and were eventually written down several thousand years ago, although much of the material is inaccessible.[1] Ayurvedic medicine places equal emphasis on body, mind, and spirit, and strives to restore the innate harmony of the individual.[2] To promote healing, life stresses must be alleviated and the natural flow of energy within people must be balanced so that the body's immune system will be enhanced, thus able to defend more against disease. The basic life force in the body is *prana*, and is similar to the Chinese notion of *chi*. Today, those practicing Ayurvedic medicine maintain that it is not a substitute for Western medicine but complements it.

Proponents of Ayurveda medicine consider it helpful for several conditions such as alleviating side effects of cancer chemotherapy; recovering from the effects of surgery, because it encourages healing; and aiding chronic, metabolic, and stress-related conditions.[3] Surgery is no longer common for Ayurvedic practitioners, although it was historically. Ayurveda first focuses on naturalistic healing methods.[1]

WHAT ARE THE MAIN AYURVEDA PRINCIPLES?

Four main principles are identified in Ayurveda: Principle of Inner Balance, Principle of Universal Cosmos (Five Elements), Principle of Body Energies (Doshas), and Principle of Disease Causation.

Principle of Inner Balance

As mentioned, Ayurvedic principles are based on a holistic view of healing. One of the Ayurvedic principles is to maintain inner balance.[1] It places major emphasis on maintaining health by preventing disease and illness. Diet, exercise, positive lifestyle, and balancing one's life (physically, mentally, emotionally, and socially) are encouraged. Ayurvedic science holds that each person is unique and has a different pattern of energy that comprises or makes up that person's constitution.[1,4] That constitution stays with the person throughout life.

Both internal and external factors may be responsible for upsetting balance within an individual, thereby upsetting that person's constitution. Examples that may cause imbalance are diet and food choices, differing seasons and weather, social relationships, and work-related stresses. In Ayurvedic thought, the diagnosis needs to focus on finding the source of the interrupted balance, and treatment will strive to bring a person back to his or her original constitution.

Principle of Universal Cosmos: Five Elements

According to Ayurvedic thought, every human being is a creation of the cosmos and universal consciousness.[4] The universe consists of five elements (or *tattwa*) that form the sum and substance of the physical universe as well as serve as the building blocks of nature and they originate from, and are composed of, an energy called prana. The five elements are: (1) earth (*Prithvi*), (2) water (*Apa*), (3) fire (*Tejas*), (4) air (*Vayu*), and (5) ether or space (*Akash*). All five elements are thought to be present in all cells of the body.[3] Every substance in our world is made up of a combination of the tattwa, and all substances can be classified according to their predominant element. The tattwa combine to make the seven tissues (*dhatu*) that give the body its structure—plasma, blood, muscle, lipid, bone, and nervous and reproductive systems. Tattwa also make up the different tastes of sweet, salty, sour, pungent, bitter, and astringent.

Prana is the prime moving force in the body and the universe. The word prana is composed of two parts: pra means foreword or before and ana means breath.[4] Ayurvedic philosophy holds that there are five pranic forces that govern body movement and function: prana, udana, samana, apana and vyana.[4] Prana provides the elements with energy and gives them power to become the building blocks for all bodily functions. The five elements are described[4] in **BOX 8.1**.

Box 8.1

Definitions of the Five Elements

Ether represents the space or field in which everything happens. At the same time, it is the source of all matter and represents the distance among matter. Sound and nonresistance is a chief characteristic of ether.

Air is matter in a gaseous form. It is moving and dynamic. All energy transfer reactions require oxygen within the body. Air is also required for fire to burn. Air has no form.

Fire is powerful because it can change solids into liquids and gases and back again. Energy (fire) within our bodies binds atoms together and changes food that we eat into fat (stored energy) and muscle. Fire also is responsible for our nervous reactions, our feelings, and even our thought processes. Fire has a form but no substance.

Water is the liquid state and represents change. No living thing can survive without water. The human body is largely composed of water. Bodies contain blood, lymph, and other fluids that circulate throughout the body and in between cells of the body. Those fluids help to carry away waste, regulate body temperature, and carry hormonal information throughout the body. The blood contains our disease protection properties (immune system). Water is seen as a substance but has no stability.

Earth represents the solid state of matter. Earth is represented in our bodies as the bones, teeth, cells, and tissues. Earth is considered a stable substance. It manifests stability, permanence, and rigidity.

Principle of Body Energies (Dosha)

Ayurveda holds that the five elements make up the body's constitution, which is identified as *dosha*. There are three mental doshas and three body doshas.[2] The three body doshas are *vata* (movement), *pitta* (transformation), and *kapha* (structure).[5] Each individual is composed of a combination of the three, although different people have different ratios of the three doshas. Each person's combination of doshas (or body constitution) is established at birth. In males, the energy is called *Purusha*, choiceless passive awareness. Female energy is called *Prakruti*, choiceful, active consciousness. Most sources don't distinguish the gender energies and use the term Prakruti for both genders. When there is imbalance in the body elements (vata, pitta, or kapha), disease occurs because of a lack of proper cellular function. In Indian terminology, the imbalance is called *Vikruti*.[4]

Vata, pitta, and kapha can exist in varying combinations, but usually one of the three is predominant. According to Ayurveda, there are seven body types: mono-types (vata, pitta, or kapha predominant), dual types (vata-pitta, pitta-kapha, or kapha-vata), and equal types (vata, pitta, and kapha in equal proportions). (See **BOX 8.2** for examples of combinations.) When all of the types are evenly distributed, a person is said to be "tri-doshic."[6] These individuals are more likely to remain in balance, because the ratio of vata, pitta, and kapha is nearly even. They will tend to have lifelong good health and a good immune system, but because they don't have a "lead" dosha to start with, when they get out of balance, they have to work harder to balance all three doshas.

Characteristics of Vata, Pitta, and Kapha

The characteristics of vata, pitta, and kapha vary quite a bit, and are described in the following sections.

Box 8.2

Dosha Combinations

Vata	Vata-kapha
Pitta	Pitta-vata
Kapha	Pitta-kapha
Vata-pitta	

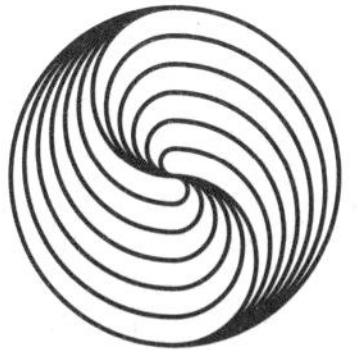

FIGURE 8.1 Vata sign.

Vata. Vata is composed of space and air. The images found for vata incorporate the sense of air, and are shown in **FIGURE 8.1**.

Vata is the subtle energy associated with movement and is located in the brain, large intestine, pelvic cavity, bones, skin, ears, and thighs.[6,7] Vata governs breathing, blinking muscle and tissue movement, heartbeat, and cellular activity. According to Ayurveda, vata is the most important dosha because it leads the other doshas. More than half of all illnesses are vata disorders. If vata is kept in balance, pitta and kapha will stay in balance.[6–8]

Attributes of vata types are dry, light, cold, rough, subtle, mobile, clear, and astringent[6–8] (see **BOX 8.3**).

According to Ayurveda, the body type of vata people tends to be thin, which is somewhat analogous to the Western description of the endomorph body shape. They have a tendency to have cold hands and feet and hate cold weather. A person with a predominant vata personality has a quick mind, and is flexible and creative.[4,6,7] Vata types grasp concepts quickly, but then forget them quickly. Vatas are usually "on the move"; their energy vacillates back and forth. They walk, talk, and think fast. Their sleeping patterns are erratic, and they seek adventuresome activities. They seem to like foods such as salads and raw vegetables but also balance that by eating foods that are cooked. The tastes best associated with vata are sweet, sour, and salty foods.

In Balance: Vata promotes creativity and flexibility. Vata types have normal sleep patterns.

Out of Balance: Vata types may experience psychological disorders of fear, anxiety, and various phobias. Movements for eating, digestion, and elimination are disturbed. They may have insomnia, or light or interrupted sleep.[7,8]

Common vata disorders[1,4,6,7] include flatulence, tics, twitches, aching joints, dry skin and hair, nerve disorders, constipation, and mental confusion. Vata types tend to have neurological, muscular, and rheumatic diseases.[4,8] Vata in the body tends to increase with age and is exhibited by the drying and wrinkling of the skin. Vata types should avoid excessive stimulation like drinking caffeine and watching television. Vata people should dress warmly and eat warm, moist, slightly oily, heavy foods.[6,7] They should attempt to maintain a constant daily schedule and obtain regular sleeping habits and meals.

Pitta. The pitta dosha is made up of fire and water. The image for pitta incorporates this sense. When looking at the image, you can see the fire on top and water on the bottom (see **FIGURE 8.2**).

Some say the pitta dosha is "digestive fire" or *agni*. The pitta dosha is located in the small intestine, stomach, sweat glands, blood, skin, and eyes. In Ayurveda, good digestion is the key to good health. When digestion is poor, a substance called *ama* is produced, and may be seen in the body as a white coating on the tongue but can also be lining the colon and clogging blood vessels.[9] Agni, when working normally, will maintain good digestion and ensures that the body's waste products, *malas* (sweat, urine, feces), are working efficiently. Pitta governs digestive functions such as absorption, assimilation, nutrition, metabolism, and body temperature, but it also governs the ability to digest

Box 8.3

Vata Qualities and Manifestations in the Body

QUALITIES	MANIFESTATIONS IN THE BODY
Dry	Dry skin, hair, lips and tongue; dry colon, tendency toward constipation; hoarse voice
Light	Light muscles, bones, thin body frame; light, scanty sleep; tendency to be underweight
Cold	Cold hands and feet; poor circulation; hates cold and loves hot; stiffness of muscles
Rough	Rough cracked skin, nails, hair, teeth, hands, and feet; cracking joints
Subtle	Subtle fear, anxiety, and insecurity; fine goose pimples; minute muscle twitching, fine tremors; delicate body
Mobile	Fast walking and talking; doing many things at once; restless eyes, eyebrows, hands, and feet; unstable joints; many dreams; loves traveling but does not stay long at one place; swinging moods, shaky faith, scattered mind
Clear	Clairvoyant; understands immediately and forgets immediately; clear, empty mind; experiences void and loneliness
Astringent	Dry choking sensation in the throat; hiccoughing, burping; loves oily foods and mushy soups; craves sweet, sour, and salty tastes; tendency toward constipation

FIGURE 8.2 Pitta sign.

ideas and gain an understanding of true reality. A person with a dominant pitta body type usually has a medium build, is strong, has stamina and endurance, and maintains a stable body weight,[8] which is analogous to the Western mesomorph body type. Qualities of the pitta type include hot, sharp, light, sour, oily, spreading, bitter, pungent, red, and yellow[8] (see **BOX 8.4**).

Pittas are generally very intelligent and quick-witted, but may be overly critical. They tend to possess little patience and a short temper, and may erupt from time to time.[1]

In Balance: Pitta promotes understanding and intelligence. There is strong and complete digestion, healthy facial tone and coloration, and stimulated and open intellect.[8–10]

Out of Balance: Pitta arouses anger, hatred, and jealousy. Pittas tend to have incomplete digestion; variable, blotchy skin color; an unhealthy appearance; and cognitive reasoning is impaired.

Likely diseases in pitta types are inflammatory diseases such as boils, abscesses, ulcers, irritable bowels, hemorrhoids, and diarrhea. Pitta people should not push themselves too hard,[8] should avoid artificial stimulants and alcohol, should regularly meditate, and should sleep and work in cooler rooms.

Kapha. Kapha is made of earth and water. The image for kapha incorporates water on the top of the image and earth on the lower half (see **FIGURE 8.3**).

Kapha supplies water for all body parts and systems. It lubricates joints, moisturizes skin, and maintains immunity. It is the energy that forms the body structure and provides support for the bones, muscle, and insulating fat.[1,6–10] It gives people stamina and physical strength. Kapha is located in the chest, lungs, and the spinal fluid surrounding the spinal cord.

Kapha people have heavy bones, muscles, and fat. The body type is analogous to the Western ectomorph body type. Their tendency is to be overweight, and they have slow metabolism and digestion. The skin may be cool and clammy, the eyes big and liquid looking, and their hair thick and wavy. Qualities of kapha are heavy, slow, cool, oily, liquid, hard, soft, dense, static, viscous, cloudy, slimy, sweet, and salty[9,10] (see **BOX 8.5**).

Kaphas are slow to pick up new ideas but have great long-term memory. They are slow to start new projects. They tend to be slow at everything they do, contrary to vatas who are always on the run. They move slowly, eat slowly, act slowly, think slowly, and are slow to anger. Kaphas tend to be forgiving, loving, and compassionate. A person with a dominant kapha metabolic body type is easy-going, laid back, and relaxed.

Box 8.4

Pitta Qualities and Manifestations in the Body

QUALITIES	MANIFESTATIONS IN THE BODY
Hot	Good digestive fire; strong appetite; body temperature tends to be higher than average; hates heat; tendency toward grey hair with receding hairline or baldness; soft brown hair on the body and face
Sharp	Sharp teeth, distinct eyes, pointed nose, tapering chin, heart-shaped face; good absorption and digestion; sharp memory and understanding; irritable; probing mind
Light	Light/medium body frame; does not tolerate bright light; fair shiny skin, bright eyes
Oily	Soft oily skin, hair, and feces; sensitive to deep-fried food (which may cause headache)
Liquid	Loose liquid stools; soft delicate muscles; excess urine, sweat, and thirst
Spreading	Rashes, hives, acne, inflammation all over the body or in certain areas; wants to spread his or her name and fame all over the country
Sour	Sour acid stomach, acidic pH; sensitive teeth; excess salivation
Bitter	Bitter taste in the mouth; nausea; vomiting; repulsion toward bitter taste; cynical
Pungent	Heartburn, burning sensations in general; strong feelings of anger and hate
Red	Red flushed skin, eyes, cheeks, and nose; red color aggravates
Yellow	Yellow eyes, skin, urine, and feces; jaundice; overproduction of bile; yellow color aggravates

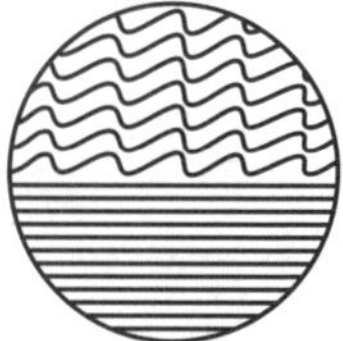

FIGURE 8.3 Kapha sign.

In Balance: This is expressed as love, calmness, and forgiveness. They appear strong and calm.

Out of Balance: This may lead to attachment, greed, and envy. They appear dull and lethargic.

Likely diseases in kapha people include respiratory, asthma, allergy, and sinusitis problems. Kapha people need stimulation such as physical activity and new life experiences. They need to avoid sweet and heavy foods but need hot and spicy foods.[6–10]

If you are interested in finding out what your dosha is, please complete a dosha questionnaire, like the one found in **BOX 8.6**.[11]

Subdoshas

Each of the doshas has five subdoshas. See **BOX 8.7** for the subdoshas and their function.[12]

The concept of doshas and their subdoshas has been scientifically tested. Alex Hankey[13–15] tested the concepts by conducting a statistical (factor) analysis of the results of completed prakriti (Ayurveda body type) questionnaires. He found that dosha qualities and functions describe individual differences in physiology. Hankey used a different approach to test for regulatory functions of the organs and found they were equated with the three doshas. He also used an electrophysiological approach that indicated that dosha differences influence fundamental cellular functions and, ultimately, tissue function.

As previously stated, according to Ayurveda, health exists when all aspects of the body are in proper balance; disease occurs when that balance is disturbed. According to Ayurveda philosophy, out of balance doshas or subdoshas leads to disease conditions. Excess vata, for example, might lead to arthritis, anxiety, and fatigue.[6,7,9] Excess kapha, on the other hand, is said to cause obesity and diabetes.[6,7,9,10]

Principle of Disease Causation

Besides the belief that an imbalance in the dosha causes body dysfunction and disease, Ayurveda identifies four main causes of disease: mental factors, lifestyle habits, dosha imbalance, and metabolic toxins.[9,10] Mental factors begin with an emotional imbalance or stress in an individual. If individuals are stressed, it will lead to unhealthy lifestyles and worsening mental stresses. Lifestyle habits include lack of exercise, substance-taking habits, poor dietary behaviors,

Box 8.5

Kapha Qualities and Manifestations in the Body

QUALITIES	MANIFESTATIONS IN THE BODY
Heavy	Heavy bones and muscles; large body frame; tends to be overweight; grounded; deep heavy voice
Slow	Walks and talks slowly; steady appetite and thirst with slow metabolism and digestion
Cold	Cold clammy skin; repeated colds, congestion, and cough; desire for sweets and cold drinks
Oily	Oily skin, hair, and feces; lubricated, unctuous joints and other organs
Liquid	Congestive disorders; edema; excessive salivation; mucus
Hard	Firmness and solidity of muscles; compact, condensed tissues
Smooth	Smooth skin; gentle, calm nature; smoothness of organs; smooth, gentle mind
Dense	Dense pads of fat; thick skin, hair, nails, and feces
Soft	Soft pleasing look; love, care, compassion, kindness, and forgiveness
Static	Loves sitting, sleeping, and doing nothing
Viscous	Viscous, sticky, cohesive quality causes compactness, firmness of joints, muscles, tissues, and organs; loves to hug; is deeply attached in love and relationships
Cloudy	Mind is cloudy and foggy in the morning; often desires coffee as a stimulant to start the day
Slimy	Excess salivation; slow digestion; attachment
Sweet	Anabolic action of sweet taste stimulates sperm formation, increasing quantity of semen; craving for sweets
Salty	Helps digestion and growth; gives energy; maintains osmotic condition; craving for salt; water retention

Box 8.6

Naturally Healthy with Ayurveda Dosha Questionnaire[11]

Identify your birth dosha with our questionnaire. When answering each question, do so from a general viewpoint throughout your life. Print this page and place an X on only one answer per question.

Body size:	____ Thin	____ Medium	____ Muscular
Weight change:	____ Irregular	____ Regular	____ Can skip meal
Energy level:	____ Bursts	____ Constant	____ Low
Digestion:	____ Irregular	____ Quick	____ Slow
Nails:	____ Brittle, tend to break	____ Medium, well-defined and strong	____ Thick
Skin type:	____ Thin, dry	____ Smooth	____ Thick, oily
Physical activity:	____ Always active	____ Moderate	____ Not much
Personality:	____ Vivacious, talkative	____ Intense, strong personal view	____ Laid back
Memory:	____ Good short-term	____ Medium accurate	____ Slow to remember
I am most likely to feel a room:	____ Cold	____ Hot	____ Cool
I typically sleep:	____ Restlessly throughout night	____ Soundly	____ Too much
Speech:	____ Talkative, fast	____ Articulate, strong	____ Slow, melodious
In my activities, I tend to be:	____ Bored easily	____ Precise	____ Slow
I typically have:	____ Joint pains	____ Headache	____ Congestion
Total dosha:	____ *VATA*	____ *PITTA*	____ *KAPHA*

Add Xs in each column and place the total at the bottom of each column. The column with the highest score is your predominant dosha.

poor sleep patterns, and unsafe sexual practices. Previously discussed was the concept of dosha imbalance (imbalance of vata, pitta, kapha, or one of the combinations). The fourth cause of disease is metabolic toxins that accumulate in the body because of the byproducts of metabolism and presence of other toxins. Treatment is based on the cause of the disease and is discussed later in this chapter.

WHAT TYPES OF DIAGNOSTIC METHODS ARE USED IN AYURVEDA?

Determination of Dosha Type

First, the Ayurvedic physician or practitioner will determine the body dosha type by administering a dosha questionnaire or orally asking selective questions to determine dosha. Next, a test to determine dosha balance (prakriti) or imbalance (vikruiti) may be administered.

Health and Family History and Physical Exam

Once the dosha and either balance or imbalance have been established, two main methods of diagnosis are determining the history of illness and examining the patient.[16] First, a complete health and family history will be taken. Next, an Ayurvedic physician or practitioner will conduct a physical examination of the body, much as a Western physician (MD or DO) does. This may include palpating the body, or listening to the heart, lungs, and intestines with a stethoscope. In addition, the Ayurvedic physician or practitioner will conduct an examination much different than a Western physician. This will include examining in detail the pulse, tongue, lips, eyes, and nails to aid in diagnosing wellness or illness. Observation is used more than laboratory testing, but the Ayurvedic physician will utilize blood, stool, and urine laboratory testing. A systemic examination will follow, which includes examination of the body systems (digestive system, respiratory system, heart and circulatory system, nervous system, urinary system, musculoskeletal system, reproductive system, skin and hair, and eyes).[16] The following gives an overview of the pulse, tongue, facial, nail, lip, and eye diagnoses.

Pulse Diagnostic Technique

Ayurvedic doctors use the pulse to describe the balance (or imbalance) of the three doshas and to diagnose a body illness such as a heart condition. The Ayurvedic technique of pulse-taking may have been derived from Chinese medical theory. A radial artery pulse is felt with the first three fingers, the index, middle, and ring fingers, and the pulse is taken from both wrists.[17] There are three aspects to the pulse:

Snake pulse (Vata): The position of the index finger denotes the vata dosha. When vata is strong in the constitution, the index finger will feel the pulse strongly. The pulse will be irregular and thin, moving in waves like the motion of a serpent.

Frog pulse (Pitta): The middle finger denotes the pulse corresponding to the pitta dosha. When the person has a predominant pitta constitution, the pulse under the middle finger will be stronger. Ayurveda describes this pulse as "active, excited, and moves like the jumping of a frog."

Swan pulse (Kapha): When the throbbing of the pulse under the ring finger is most noticeable, it is a sign of a kapha constitution. The pulse feels strong and its movement resembles the floating of a swan. Hence, this pulse is called swan pulse.

Tongue Diagnostic Technique

An Ayurvedic physician would examine the size, shape, surface, margins, and color of the tongue. The tongue is mapped much like the feet in zone therapy, that is, different areas of the tongue are thought to correspond to different organs of the body[18] (see **FIGURE 8.4**).

A blemish, discoloration, or coating on some part of the tongue is used to indicate a body problem.[17,18]

- *Pale tongue:* Anemic condition or lack of blood in the body
- *Blue tongue:* Indication of heart disease
- *Whitish tongue:* Indication of kapha imbalance and mucus accumulation
- *Red or yellow-green tongue:* Indication of pitta imbalance
- *Black or brown tongue:* Indication of vata imbalance
- *Coating on the tongue:* Indication of toxins in the stomach, or small or large intestine (see **FIGURE 8.5** for a coated tongue)

Facial Diagnosis

Ayurveda holds that the face mirrors the mind and that disorders and/or disease may be indicated by wrinkle pattern,

Box 8.7
Subdoshas and Their Function

SUBDOSHAS	LOCATION	DIRECTION	FUNCTION
Vayus **(Vata)**			
Prana	Senses, brain, throat, chest	Inward	Intake
Udana	Chest, throat	Upward	Output
Samana	Small intestine	Balancing	Absorption
Vyana	From heart outward to whole body, especially extremities	Outward	Circulation
Apana	Pelvis	Downward	Regulates pelvic holding in and letting go
Pittas			
Sadhaka	Brain and heart	Inward	Inner combustion or fire
Alochaka	Eyes	Upward	Receive light
Pachaka	Stomach, liver/spleen	Equalizing	Digestion, discrimination
Bhrajaka	Stomach	Outward	Digestion, warmth and sunlight
Ranjaka	Liver	Downward	Warmth in blood
Kaphas			
Tarpaka	Brain, heart, nerves	Inward	Calmness, stability, happiness
Bodhaka	Tongue, sensory in head	Upward	Taste, knowledge, perception
Kledaka	Stomach (alkaline), and mucous lining	Balancing	Liquefies food
Sleshaka	Joints, limbs, and skin	Outward	Cohesion and ease of movement
Avalambaka	Chest, heart, and lungs	Downward	Lubrication

Source: Reprinted from Rafael T. Ayurveda for the Childbearing Years. *Wise Womanhood.* 2009: 4.

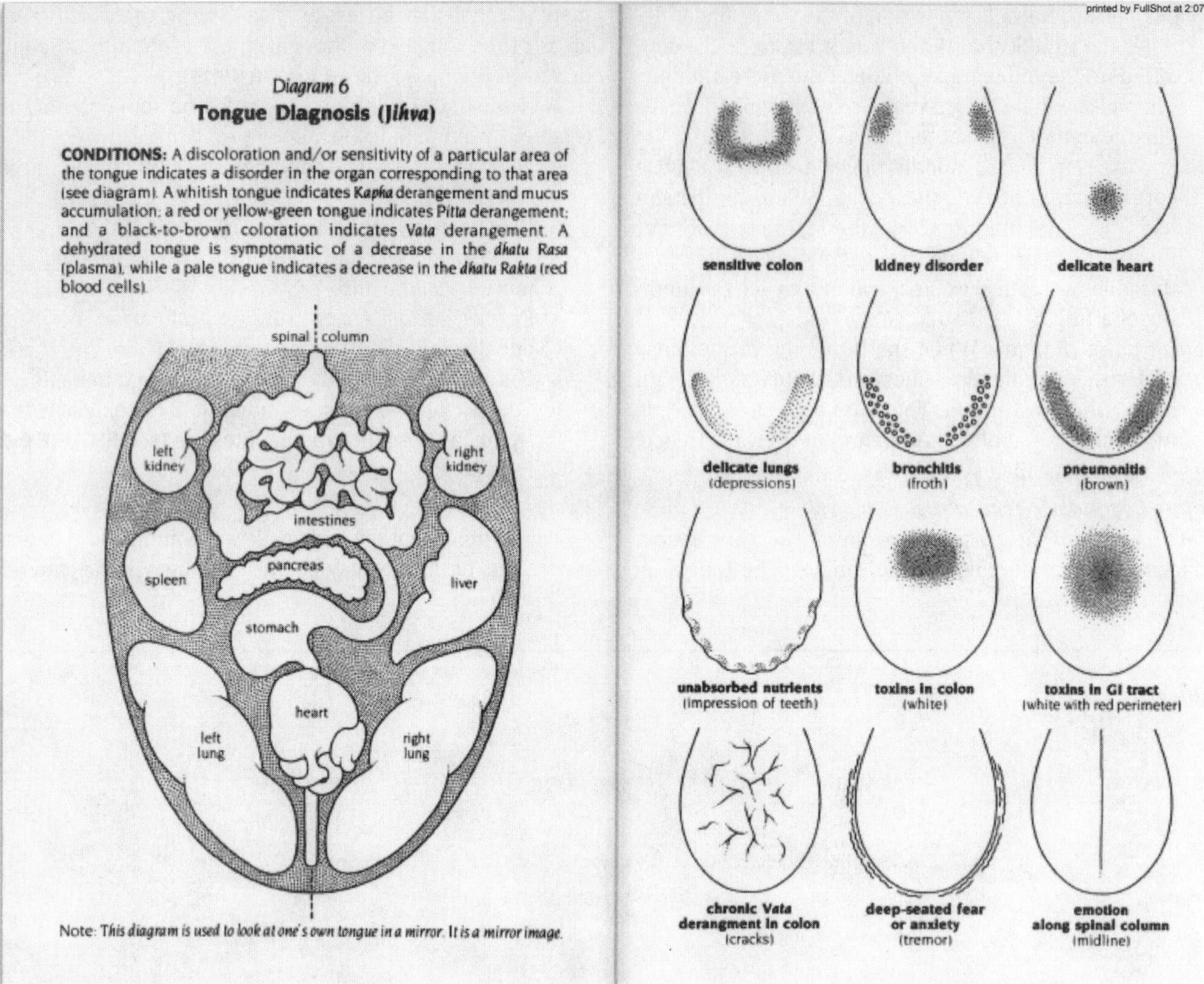

FIGURE 8.4 Tongue mapping.

Source: Reproduced with permission from "Ayurveda: The Science of Self-Healing, A Practical Guide" by Dr. Vasant Lad. Lotus Press, a division of Lotus Brands, Inc. P.O. Box 325, Twin Lakes, WI 53181, USA, www.lotuspress.com.

looks of the eyelids and eyes, appearance and shape of the nose, and appearance of the lips.[17]

Wrinkles:

- *Horizontal wrinkles on forehead:* Indicate deep-seated anxiety and worry

Eyelids and eyes:

- *Lower eyelid fullness:* Indicates impaired kidneys
- *Excessive blinking:* Indicates nervousness, anxiety, or fear and is vata imbalance
- *Drooping upper eyelid:* Indicates sense of insecurity, fear, or lack of confidence and is vata imbalance
- *Prominent eye:* Indicates thyroid gland dysfunction
- *Yellow conjunctiva:* Indicates a weak liver
- *Small iris:* Indicates weak joints
- *White ring around the iris:* Indicates an excessive intake of salt or sugar
- *Prominent white ring:* Indicates joint degeneration with potential for arthritis and joint pain

Nose:

- *Butterfly-like nose discoloration:* Indicates malabsorption of iron or folic acid and may indicate a digestive disorder.
- *Shape of the nose:* Indicates the dosha. Sharp nose is pitta, crooked nose is vata, and blunt nose is kapha.

Lips:

- *Dry and rough lips:* Indicate dehydration or vata imbalance
- *Pale lips:* Indicate anemia
- *Repeated attacks of inflammatory patches along the margins of the lips:* Indicate the presence of herpes and a chronic pitta derangement

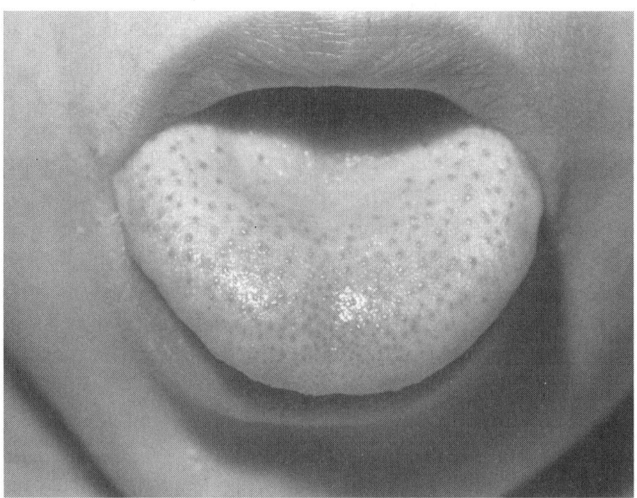

FIGURE 8.5 Coated tongue.

- *Multiple pale brown spots on the lips:* Indicate poor digestion or worms in the colon
- *Yellow lips:* Indicate jaundice
- *Blue lips:* Indicate or may signal heart problems[18]

Once the diagnosis has been established, the Ayurvedic physician or practitioner will recommend therapy or treatment.

WHAT ARE THE MAJOR AYURVEDIC THERAPIES?

Several types of treatment are recommended in Ayurveda. Treatment is usually comprehensive and customized. The health program is based on maintaining prakruti (balanced dosha constitution) and focuses on healing Vikruti (imbalanced dosha constitution).

General Guidelines for Balancing Vata, Pitta, and Kapha

See **BOXES 8.8**, **8.9**, and **8.10** for balancing guidelines. See **BOX 8.11** for overall treatments.[1]

Ayurvedic treatments are categorized into six major treatment concepts[19,20]:

1. *Shodhanam:* Cleansing
2. *Shamanam:* Balancing
3. *Pathya vyavastha:* Prescription of diet and activity
4. *Nidan parivarjan:* Avoidance of disease-causing and aggravating factors
5. *Rasayana:* Rejuvenation
6. *Satvajaya:* Mental hygiene/psychotherapy

Before Shodhanam therapy begins, Ayurveda recommends precleansing procedures called *purva-karma*,[19,20] which prepare the body for Shodhanam.

Box 8.8
General Guidelines for Balancing Vata

- Keep warm
- Keep calm
- Avoid cold, frozen, or raw foods
- Avoid extreme cold
- Eat warm foods and spices
- Keep a regular routine
- Get plenty of rest

Box 8.9
General Guidelines for Balancing Pitta

- Avoid excessive heat
- Avoid excessive oil
- Avoid excessive steam
- Limit salt intake
- Eat cooling, nonspicy foods
- Exercise during the cooler part of the day

Box 8.10
General Guidelines for Balancing Kapha

- Get plenty of exercise
- Avoid heavy foods
- Keep active
- Avoid dairy
- Avoid iced food or drinks
- Vary your routine
- Avoid fatty, oily foods
- Eat light, dry food
- No daytime naps

Purva-karma Therapy

Two main treatments are utilized to carry out purva-karma: *Snehan* and *Swedan*. Snehan is given both internally and externally. In *internal Snehan*, patients are given medicated edible oil or medicated edible butter in a dose prescribed by the Ayurvedic therapist (e.g., two spoonfuls). Nothing else is taken by mouth on that day.[19,20] The mixture is called *ghee* or *sneha* and is best if made from cow's milk. The intention of internal Snehan is to enhance later *Pancha-*

Box 8.11

Ayurveda Treatments: General Summary

- A dosha-specific natural diet custom suited for you
- Therapeutic nutritional supplements
- Healing botanical herbs and spices
- Detoxification of accumulated toxins
- Ayurvedic bodywork and massage
- Rejuvenation therapy to delay aging and promote energy
- Yoga
- Daily routines
- Understanding of a healthy lifestyle

karma procedures in order to rid the body of impurities. *External Snehan* is carried out by medicated ghee body massage, given every few days for a week or more. Ghee is also known as clarified butter, and is prepared by simmering unsalted butter until all water is evaporated. It will become a clear, golden liquid. The liquid may then be mixed with herbs. The skin absorbs part of the medicated oil and carries it to the bloodstream.[20,21] See **FIGURE 8.6** for photo of person receiving body massage with ghee.

The second purva-karma treatment is Swedana therapy or Swedan. This is the use of dry or wet fomentation or heat therapy to facilitate sweating. It can be given in many ways: sunbathing, in a sweat box, pouring warm water on the body, a steam bath, or sitting in a tub of warm water. The water may contain milk, herbs, or medicated oil. According to individual needs, Swedan can be whole body therapy or just focus on a diseased part of the body. Swedan reportedly liquefies toxins and increases the movement of toxins into the gastrointestinal tract.[20,21] Once purva-karma procedures are completed, Shodhanam therapy begins.

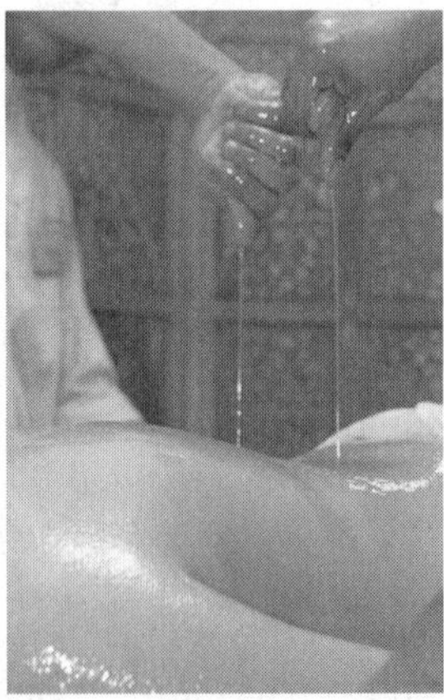

FIGURE 8.6 Ghee body massage.

Shodhanam Therapy

Shodhanam therapy involves five procedures grouped under a term called Panchakarma treatment.[22] *Pancha* in Sanskrit stands for *five* and *Karma* stands for *therapeutic measures*, so *Panchakarma* means five types of therapeutic measures. Panchakarma is a comprehensive system of knowledge and practices to purify the body of toxins and restore it to balance with the laws of Mother Nature.[22,24] The therapies are intended to balance the doshas, relieve stress, and rid the body of toxins. A recommendation is that while a person is undergoing Panchakarma treatment they should also be on a special diet that is monitored by a doctor.[22,24] The following describes the five procedures intended to rid the body of toxins:

Vamana: First is forced vomiting. It is intended to remove kapha toxins collected in the body and respiratory tract. It is given to people with a kapha imbalance by a daily treatment that is supposed to loosen and mobilize toxins.

Virechana: Second is forced purging. This therapy is intended to remove *pitta* toxins that accumulate in the liver and gallbladder by completely cleansing the gastrointestinal tract. Benefits of Virechana include helping to root out chronic fever, diabetes, asthma, skin disorders such as herpes, paraplegia, hemiplegia, joint disorders, digestive disorders, constipation, hyperacidity, vitiligo, psoriasis, headaches, elephantiasis, and gynecological disorders.[23,24]

Basti: Third is medicated enema or colonic irrigation. Basti is intended to eliminate loosened vata dosha, which is predominantly located in the colon and bones, but also supposedly cleanses the body of toxins from all three doshas.[22,23,24] The treatment involves the introduction of medicinal substances, such as herbal oils and decoctions in a liquid medium, into the rectum of the person. Medicated oil or ghee and an herbal decoction are given as an enema to cleanse the colon and increase the muscle tone. This procedure is usually applied for 8 to 30 days, based on the medical condition of a person. It reportedly benefits hemiplegia, paraplegia, colitis, cervical spondylosis, irritable bowel syndrome, constipation, digestive disorders, backache and sciatica, hepatomegaly and splenomegaly, obesity, hemmorhoids, sexual arousal problems, and infertility.[22,23,24]

Nasya: Fourth is nose or sinus cleaning. Nasya treatment is intended to cleanse kapha toxins from the head and neck region. Some use a neti pot to pour salt water through the nose to combat chronic sinus problems (water irrigation). Medicated oil may also be administered through the nose for up to 30 days, depending on the medical condition of a person. Nasya reportedly benefits trigeminal neuralgia, Bell's palsy, memory, eyesight, insomnia, elimination of excess mucus, hyperpigmentation in the face, premature graying of hair, clarity of voice, headaches of various origin, hemiplegia, loss of smell and taste, frozen shoulder, migraine, stiffness of the neck, nasal allergies, nasal polyps, neurological dysfunctions, paraplegia, and sinusitis.[23]

Raktamokshana: Fifth is procedures to detoxify the blood. This may include bloodletting or the use of certain herbs to cleanse the blood. It is not advisable during general Panchakarma, and most Ayurveda centers do not offer Raktamokshana due to the high risk of infection involved in blood cleansing.[22,23,24]

A study at the Institute of Science, Technology and Public Policy at Maharishi University of Management in Fairfield, Iowa, in collaboration with a special laboratory at Colorado University, demonstrated that classical Panchakarma treatment eliminated up to 50 percent of the detectable toxins in the blood. This particular study found that PCB and DDE are entering the food chain, causing high levels of those chemicals to appear in the blood in the general population. With the Panchakarma treatments, a large proportion of these fat-soluble toxins were reported to be eliminated from the body.[25]

As shown, Shodhan therapy requires quite a lot of time. First there is a week of pre-preparation called purva-karma, and then, depending on individual needs, panchakarma therapy could last a week or more. In addition, Shodhan therapy could be harsh on the body because it is intended to be a thorough cleansing. The purpose is to drive imbalanced doshas out of the body. The next therapy discussed in this chapter, Shamana, is much milder.

Shamana Therapy

Shamana therapy is intended to achieve a balanced state in the body[26] and to alleviate symptoms of disease.[27] This intervention focuses on the spiritual dimensions of healing,[3] and is much milder than Shodhan therapy; however, according to Ayurvedic thought, it is not as long lasting. Kulkami[26] describes seven Shamana procedures as follows:

1. *Deepan (creating appetite):* Consuming food or mild medicines that help in empowering agni (digestive fire or digestive enzymes). This includes consuming ghee, oil, spices, hot drinks and warm food. Improving deepan helps achieve dosha balance.
2. *Pachan (digesting):* Pachan is an aid to digest toxins (ama). This is a preferred treatment in digestive disorders. People are encouraged to eat foods such as dry ginger and sweet kernel, which help digestion when eaten after lunch or dinner.
3. *Kshudha-nigrah (hunger control/fasting):* This is a treatment for dosha imbalance and involves total, partial, or selective fasting. Avoiding food for a period of time or changing lifestyle can provide rest to the digestive tract.
4. *Trushna-nigrah (thirst control):* This treatment helps when water retention is a problem. In the case of generalized edema or ascites, if water intake is monitored, the urinary tract gets an opportunity to clear the accumulated fluid from the body.
5. *Vyayam (exercises):* This is the prescribed treatment in conditions like obesity and diabetes. It helps to re-establish balance without medicines or with the lowest possible dose.
6. *Atap-seva (sun bath):* This is a preferred treatment in vata disorders. It is recommended for many skin disorders and uses solar energy as a medicine. This treatment also works well in cases of arthritis pain and rheumatic conditions.
7. *Marut-seva (consumption of fresh air):* This is the prescribed treatment for tuberculosis, asthma, and other lung conditions. Breathing fresh air helps lung function and provides energy within the respiratory system. (Known as sitting in the wind/breathing exercises—*pranayama*.)

Pathya Vyavastha Therapy

This treatment is a prescription of diet and activity.[28] Patients might be encouraged and taught yoga, but all forms of physical activity are recommended in order to enhance the effects of therapeutic measures. A nutritious diet is prescribed in order to stimulate agni and optimize digestion. In our society, we identify certain foods as healthy and others as unhealthy. In Ayurveda, what's good for one person is bad for another and vice versa. For example, a person tending toward an excess of vata might be advised to avoid raw vegetables but consume nuts and seeds in abundance.[28] Someone with an excess of kapha would be given the opposite recommendation. The foods recommended may also change depending on the season. In Ayurvedic medicine, individuals are given specific details about the optimal ways to prepare and consume foods.

Nidan Parivarjan Therapy

This treatment focuses on helping individuals change their lifestyles to avoid known disease-causing factors (e.g., smoking, alcohol and other drug use, diet).[28]

Rasayana Therapy

In Ayurveda, *Rasayana* means that which nourishes the body and boosts immunity. It is also called rejuvenation therapy,[29] and focuses on promoting strength and vitality. It may involve the use of herbs or drugs, diet, and a changed lifestyle. One source refers to Rasayana therapy as the use of Panchakarma techniques.[29,30] Although we found no scientific documentation, Ayurveda purports that the benefits of Rasayana are many (e.g., more youthful skin, higher resistance to disease, improved intelligence, improved attitude about life, better sense of well-being).

Satvajaya Therapy

Satvajaya is psychotherapy or mental health counseling for those needing it. It might involve helping people to restrain from overindulging in alcohol or other drugs, or it might involve helping people to improve their memory or gain self-concept and self-esteem. One of its therapies is the use of meditation.[28]

Thus far, most of the Ayurveda therapeutic modalities have been very holistic, in that the body and mind are addressed in the treatment plan. Shodhanam (Panchakarma) could be challenging, and if not monitored well, could be harmful because of dehydration or electrolyte imbalances. The other treatments are certainly utilized in western medicine as well as Ayurvedic medicine.

WHAT HERBS OR PLANTS ARE USED IN AYURVEDIC MEDICINE?

More than 600 herbal formulas and 250 single-plant drugs[31] are used in Ayurvedic medicine. Ayurvedic pharmaceuticals form a branch of Ayurveda that deals with the collection and selection of drugs.[32] The practice studies the preparation, preservation, mode of administration, and dosage specifications. Many processing techniques of crude drugs are carried out and tested, much like Western pharmaceutical companies do. For example, trituration (reducing to a powder or diluting a medicinal powder) is used. Some crude drugs are treated by heating them or placing them in liquid. Some are preserved (stored) in various types of containers, and the effect of using various types of containers are tested. Drugs are also formulated in various ways, including distillations, ointments, powders, pills, medicated oils, and so forth.[33] The drugs are scientifically tested. There is a preclinical stage of testing a drug, after which comes a drug development period that is composed of four phases of clinical studies.[32] After Phase III, the drug is either approved for safety and efficacy or rejected. Phase IV and V studies are conducted while the drug is being marketed.

According to a survey conducted by the NCCAM,[31] more than 200,000 people in the United States had used Ayurvedic medicine in the previous year. Please see **TABLE 8.1** for the plants and herbs used in Ayurvedic medicine and their intended uses.[34,35]

Some Ayurvedic medicines have been scientifically tested according to Western standards, but many have not. There have been concerns about toxicity, formulations, interactions, and evidence of scientific testing on these medicines. One study[33] found that nearly 21 percent of Ayurvedic medicines tested had detectable levels of lead (most common), mercury, or arsenic. Some over-the-counter drugs manufactured in South Asia use fillers for some of these herbs that may contain lead, mercury, and/or arsenic.[31] Adverse drug reactions to other Ayurvedic medicines have been reported,[36] but may be due to inadequate preparation of the drug. The NCCAM reports that health officials in India and other countries have taken steps to address these concerns.

We are neither recommending nor condemning these plants for medicinal use. We do recommend that if you want to try an herb that is listed to treat yourself for any condition that you may have, please do so under the guidance of your family doctor.

On the other hand, scientific testing here in the United States has shown favorable results for turmeric (curcumin)[37] and *Salvia lavandulaefolia* (Spanish sage).[38] Turmeric has been used for thousands of years to treat many different illnesses. It is used as a food coloring and gives Indian curry its color and flavor. It is also used in mustard and in butter

Case Study

You live in a large city on the West Coast of the United States. You have learned information regarding some of the Chinese medicine healing practices such as acupuncture and have participated in some energy work (tai chi). Since you were in your twenties, you have suffered with digestive disorder problems and have been diagnosed with irritable bowel syndrome, a condition that causes you a lot of abdominal pain after eating. A friend suggested that you go see an Ayurvedic medicine doctor or practitioner for treatment.

Questions:

1. Where would you find out the credentials of an Ayurvedic medicine doctor or practitioner?
2. If the doctor suggested that you undergo Shodhanam treatment, which of the five would you agree to?
3. What could be some therapeutic and/or ill effects from Shodhanam treatment?
4. Which of the Shamana therapy treatments would you want prescribed, and why?

Table 8.1
Ayurvedic Plants/Herbs and Their Uses[34,35]

Amalaki (Ami) is an herb made from the Indian gooseberry (*Embilica officinalis* or *Phyllanthus emblica*). It is usually used in juice form and is supposed to help promote longevity. Some test tube studies suggest that it has antioxidant, antibacterial, and anti-inflammatory properties. It is used in Ayurvedic medicine to rebuild and maintain new tissues and increase red blood cell count. It is considered helpful in cleansing the mouth, strengthening teeth, and nourishing the bones, and is the highest natural source of vitamin C. It is one of three herbs used in *triphala*, the primary Ayurvedic tonic for maintaining health.

Arjuna (*Terminalia arjuna*, bark extract) is another herb that is supposed to have antioxidant properties. In Ayurveda, it is used as a cardiac tonic, and is traditionally given to support circulation and oxygenation of all tissues. It is often combined with *ashwagandha*, *brahmi*, and *guggul* in heart formulas.

Ashoka is Sanskrit for "without sorrow." The bark, flowers, and seeds of the Ashoka plant are used. It is used in Ayurveda as an aid for heavy menstrual periods due to uterine fibroids. It is also used to help maintain proper function of the female reproductive system.

Ashwagandha means "winter cherry." It is made from a small evergreen perennial shrub that grows to 1.5 meters tall and is found in dry areas of India and as far west as Israel. In Sanskrit, it means "the sweat or smell of a horse" because the roots smell like a horse. It is sometimes referred to as Indian ginseng, making reference to its nervous system tonic actions. In Ayurveda, it is used as an antioxidant, antibacterial, and antianxiety herb. It is purported to have aphrodisiac properties.

Bacopa is said to aid mental acuity and has antianxiety properties. It has also been used to help epilepsy.

Bhringaraj is used on the head to lessen premature graying of hair, balding, and bald spots. The herb is ground into a powder and added to an oil. It is also thought to be a liver tonic that is helpful for chronic hepatitis.

Bibitaki is used as a laxative to cleanse the bowels. It is also used as a gargle for sore throats because of its heating and soothing properties. It is one of three herbs used in *triphala*, the primary Ayurvedic tonic for maintaining health.

Bitter melon is said to regulate the body's ability to process sugars by suppressing the neutral response to the stimuli of sweet tastes.

Boswellia (frankincense) has been used extensively in Ayurveda for its anti-inflammatory effects and joint support, such as in rheumatoid arthritis, bursitis, tendonitis, or osteoarthritis.

Brahmi has been used as a tonic for improving memory, relieving stress and anxiety, and increasing mental alertness. It has been used for epilepsy and premature aging. It is considered the primary Ayurvedic nerve and cardiac tonic. It is also available in oil form.

Chitrak is a pungent herb used to support liver function, improve digestion, and remove toxins from the GI tract.

Chyavanprash is a famous herbal jam made from amalaki fruit, one of the highest sources of vitamin C. It is fortified with over 20 herbs to rejuvenate and strengthen the immune system. It is used in Ayurveda as a longevity tonic.

Cilantro and coriander are powerful aids to digestion. They come from the same plant: cilantro comes from the first or vegetative stage of the plant's life cycle and coriander is the dried seed of cilantro. According to Ayurveda, allergies result from improper digestion and an accumulation of ama (toxic substances) in the body. By enhancing digestion, cilantro and coriander work to alleviate the root cause of allergies.

Coleus forskohlii has been a part of Ayurvedic medicine for centuries. An extract from the plant is used to treat hypothyroidism, heart disease, and respiratory disorders.

Cumin is the seed of a small plant and is supposed to aid digestion and help flush toxins out of the body. Sprinkle ground, dry-roasted cumin on fresh yogurt, add salt to taste, and enjoy at lunch.

Dandelion and dandelion root are regarded as a liver tonic. It is used for people who suffer from mild fluid retention, such as may occur in PMS.

Fennel is said to be extremely good for digestion. In India, eating a few fennel seeds after a meal is a common practice. Fennel is a cooling spice.

Garcinia cambogia extract is used as an ephedra-free diet aid. It contains biologically active phytochemicals such as hydroxycitric acid and antioxidants. It supports normal appetite levels and metabolism and storage of carbohydrates and fats to maintain normal body weight.

Gokshura has diuretic properties and is useful in renal stones, painful urination, and kidney dysfunction. It is also used to support proper function of the urinary tract and prostate.

Gotu kola is used to promote wound healing and slow the progress of leprosy. It was also reputed to prolong life, increase energy, and enhance sexual potency. The best-documented use of gotu kola is to treat chronic venous insufficiency, a condition closely related to varicose veins.

Guduchi is a bitter tonic that has diuretic properties and is supposed to help remove urinary stones. It is also touted as enhancing immune resistance to diseases and as being protective of liver function.

(*Continues*)

Table 8.1
Ayurvedic Plants/Herbs and Their Uses[34,35] (Continued)

Guggul (aka guggulu) is made from the sap or gum resin of the mukul myrrh tree. Historically it was used for its antiseptic and deep penetrating actions in the treatment of elevated blood cholesterol and arthritis. It is often used as a carrier and combined with other herbs to treat several specific conditions. It is traditionally used for arthritis, skin diseases, pains in the nervous system, obesity, digestive problems, infections in the mouth, and menstrual problems.

Gymnema is commonly referred to as "Gurmar, the destroyer of sugar." It is traditionally used in formulas to control blood sugar levels in the body. It is a member of the milkweed family. Leaves of the herb are chewed as a therapy for diabetes mellitus, snakebites (root powder), fever, cough, hemorrhoids, and urinary disorders.

Haritaki is used for many conditions. Topically as a paste, it is used for wounds and hemorrhoids. In a gargle, it is used for oral ulcers and sore throat. It is used internally as a digestive aid and for diarrhea. It is also used to aid coughing and asthma. It is one of three herbs used in *triphala*, the primary Ayurvedic tonic for maintaining health.

Holy basil is considered a sacred plant by the Hindus in India and is often planted near shrines. It is used for the common cold, asthma, bronchitis, and earache.

Kutki is a bitter and pungent herb used to support proper function of the liver and spleen. One of the chemicals in kutki, picroliv, is in Phase II clinical trials in India to support claims that it is a powerful liver protectant.

Manjista is considered one of the best blood purifying herbs in Ayurveda. It is thought to detox blood and dissolve plaque in the blood. It is used as an immune regulator and has antioxidant properties.

Neem is considered one of the best healing and disinfectant agents for skin diseases and an anti-inflammatory for joint and muscle pain. The Neem tree has been called the village pharmacy, because its bark, leaves, sap, fruit, seeds, and twigs have so many diverse uses in the traditional medicine of India. Poets called it *Sarva Roga Nivarini*, "The One That Can Cure All Ailments."

Phyllanthus amarus An herb used to treat jaundice and thought to be effective for treating hepatitis B. Despite numerous test tube and animal studies showing efficacy against the hepatitis B virus, *it did* not generally do well in human trials.

Phyllanthus embilica is commonly known as Indian gooseberry. It is supposed to decrease blood cholesterol and blood glucose levels.

Shatavari root is traditionally used to support women's health by restoring hormonal balance in women during the menstrual cycle and menopause. It is also used as an aid for stomach ulcers, inflammation, and chronic fevers.

Turmeric is a widely used tropical herb in the ginger family. The active ingredient in turmeric is curcumin. Its stalk is used in both food and medicine, yielding the familiar yellow ingredient that colors and adds flavor to curry. Turmeric is believed to have anti-inflammatory, antiseptic, and antibacterial properties. It is used to strengthen the overall energy of the body, relieve gas, dispel worms, improve digestion, regulate menstruation, dissolve gallstones, and relieve arthritis.

Tylophora indica (*T. asthmatica*) is a climbing perennial plant indigenous to India, where it grows wild in the southern and eastern regions. The leaves and roots have laxative, emetic, and expectorant properties. It is supposed to be a remedy for asthma (hence the name, *T. asthmatica*). However, the studies that found it effective were poorly designed, and a better designed study found no benefits. It is still recommended for some of its other traditional uses, including hay fever, bronchitis, and the common cold.

and cheese to enhance yellow color. Turmeric is used as an anti-inflammatory, to treat digestive and liver problems, and stimulates the production of bile by the gallbladder. Scientists at M.D. Anderson Cancer Center in Texas found that turmeric was helpful in potentiating the antitumor effects of a drug used for pancreatic cancer.[39] See **FIGURE 8.7** for a photograph of a turmeric plant and root.

WHAT MINERALS AND METALS ARE USED IN AYURVEDIC MEDICINE?

Several metals and minerals are purified or refined for use in Ayurvedic medicine.[22] These include gold, silver, copper, lead, tin, iron, sand (from river banks), lime, red chalk, gems, salts, red arsenic, and mercury. There are references to the uses of rasa (mercury), metals, and gems in the classical Ayurvedic texts, the *Charaka* Samhita and *Sushruta Samhita*. Within the classical texts, all the adverse reactions to medicines when prepared or used inappropriately are described.[36] To gain a brief understanding of the Ayurvedic preparation and use of metals, an explanation of gold follows.

Gold has been used since Ayurvedic medicine began. It supposedly has many purposes, including to promote longevity, combat aging, and treat impotency. It is used in Ayurvedic medicine as a tonic and an anti-infective, combats liver and heart disease, and currently is used for rheumatoid arthritis. The preparation of gold involves several complicated steps described by Mishra,[22, p86] which are simplified and paraphrased as follows:

The leaves of gold are heated, and when red hot, are dipped in a special oil. This process is repeated seven times. The same process is repeated using buttermilk, cow's urine, strongly processed herbs (decoction), rice made into sour gruel, and radish. The leaves are then dried by heat. The gold is then carefully measured along with other ingredients and placed in an earthenware container and mixed with another ingredient called latex of *Calotropis gigentea*. The mixture is titrated, made into a paste, and dried in the sunlight. This process is repeated 7 to 14 times using fresh latex. A portion of the mixture is poured into liquefied metallic gold in a closed earthen pot and heated to above 1000°C. The mass disintegrates into a red-brown powder, which is collected and becomes the gold drug.

We have given you an account of how one particular metal (gold) is processed into a medicine. Again, we are neither promoting nor condemning these medicines, but hopefully, having presented a brief explanation of Ayurvedic medicines, you will become more motivated to explore further and to assess the literature for scientific research that may have been conducted. One study conducted found that all metal-containing products exceeded one or more standards for daily intake, although the U.S.-based American Herbal Products Association showed a lower level of toxic metals.[33] We, the consumer, need to make careful choices when we are selecting and buying our over-the-counter medicines, including Ayurvedic medicines.

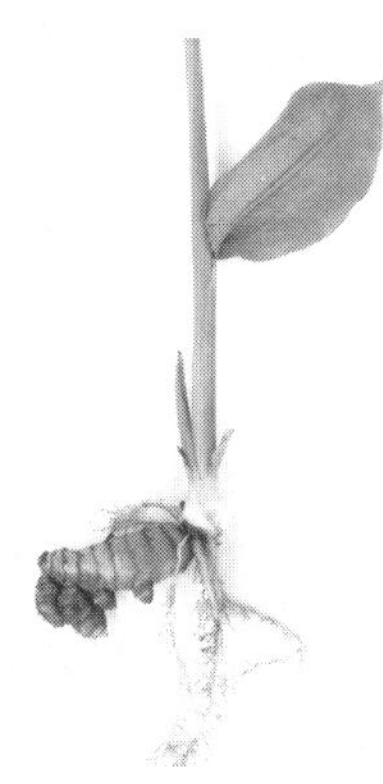

FIGURE 8.7 Turmeric plant and roots.

There are concerns about the use of silver. For example, colloidal silver, a traditional Ayurvedic remedy, is considered a powerful germicide, but when taken in excessive amounts can be toxic to all human tissue. If taken, only about 50 mcg can be excreted per day. The rest is deposited under the skin and tissues as silver sulfide and can cause permanent gray-black staining of the skin and mucous membranes. Excess colloidal silver can cause arteriosclerosis and could damage organs.[41] Colloidal silver can react with other drugs and cause even greater side effects. Because of this, the U.S. Food and Drug Administration refuses to approve the use of colloidal silver supplements for medicinal purposes.[41]

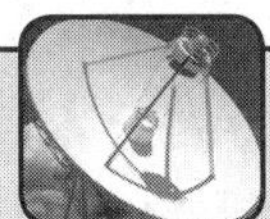

In the News

An article published on August 4, 2010, in TopNews[40] online concerned Ayurvedic medicines and lead content. A middle-aged man in Sydney, Australia, took Ayurvedic medicine that was produced in India. After consuming the medicine for several months he started having pain and vomiting. He was admitted to a hospital, where doctors found high levels of lead (2.3 percent) in his blood. Also, his blood report showed a significant amount of mercury and arsenic.

Although the news article was disconcerting, there was a lot of missing information, including

- Reason for taking the medication
- Identification of the medication
- Dosage recommended
- Length of time the medication was recommended to be taken
- Whether the individual followed the recommended dosage and length of time
- Whether the individual was under a doctor's care
- The general health of the individual
- Whether the individual was taking other medications

1. What other information do you think might be missing from this news article?
2. What impact do you think such an article has on Ayurvedic medicine?

It is extremely important that we, as health consumers, analyze and assess what we read in the newspapers, what we read online, and what we hear on television.

WHAT DOES THE NCCAM REPORT ABOUT AYURVEDA?

According to the NCCAM,[31] there is not enough scientific evidence to vouch for the effectiveness of Ayurvedic practices, and so it is calling for more rigorous research. Most clinical trials have been small, had research design problems, lacked appropriate control groups, or had other problems. On the NCCAM[31] Web site, examples of Ayurvedic medicine research include studies of:

- Herbal therapies, including curcuminoids (substances found in turmeric), used for cardiovascular conditions
- A compound from the cowhage plant (*Mucuna pruriens*), used to prevent or lessen the side effects from Parkinson's disease drugs
- Three botanicals (ginger, turmeric, and boswellia) used to treat inflammatory disorders such as arthritis and asthma
- Gotu kola (*Centella asiatica*), an herb used to treat Alzheimer's disease

WHAT IS THE NATIONAL INSTITUTE OF AYURVEDIC MEDICINE (NIAM)?

The National Institute of Ayurvedic Medicine (NIAM) is located in Brewster, New York. The NIAM was established in 1982 by Scott Gerson, MD, the nation's only medical doctor to hold a PhD in Ayurveda as well as a conventional allopathic medicine degree. Gerson wrote his doctoral paper, Panchakarma Chikitsa (detoxification therapy), which was approved in 2003 by both the University of Poona and Tilak Ayurved Mahavidyalaya. Dr. Gerson's medical practice is at the NIAM, where he has combined Ayurveda and conventional medicine for more than 15 years. The institute is the largest holder of Ayurveda data and information in the United States.[42]

One can take a certificate course in Ayurveda at the NIAM, which is a 3-year program. Candidates for the program must have completed 2 years of college or university study and have graduated from a school of medicine, nursing, oriental medicine, nutrition, physical therapy, massage, social work, or other allied health discipline. The following gives more detail about various ways to become an Ayurvedic physician or practitioner.

WHAT IS THE TRAINING OF AN AYURVEDIC MEDICINE DOCTOR OR PRACTITIONER?

In India, the highest degree one can obtain in Ayurveda is the PhD. Students can get a Bachelor of Ayurvedic Medicine and Surgery (BAMS) in a 5 ½-year program of study. The postgraduate programs lead to the Doctorate in Ayurveda. Graduates can get employment as medical officers/doctors at government and private Ayurvedic hospitals or open their own practices.[43]

In 2004, the National Ayurvedic Medical Association established educational standards in the United States. There is no widely accepted licensure for the practice of Ayurvedic medicine in the United States; however, there are several schools that offer extensive training. The types of training programs offered in the United States are:

- *Correspondence programs:* Some include Internet study and others include reading textbooks required by the instructor. Testing and credit hours vary. The National Ayurvedic Medical Association does not recognize correspondence course hours toward national certification.
- *Full-time training programs:* Two examples of this type of program are at the California College of Ayurveda (18-month course) and the Ayurvedic Institute in New Mexico (16-month course).
- *Weekend training program:* There are about 10 weekend training programs; the length varies from 12 weekends to 24 weekends.
- *Short-term seminar courses:* Many of these are introductory courses, although some focus on a specific treatment modality.
- *Internship programs:* Internship programs were started at the California College of Ayurveda, but today several schools offer them. Student interns may simply observe an Ayurvedic practitioner or actually engage in Ayurvedic practices under the direct observation of an Ayurvedic doctor or practitioner.

See **BOX 8.12** for places to receive Ayurveda training in the United States.

Box 8.12
Ayurveda Training in the United States

Ayurvedic Institute
11311 Menaul NE
Albuquerque, NM 87112
Phone: 505-291-9698
Web site: http://www.ayurveda.com

California College of Ayurveda
1117A East Main Street
Grass Valley, CA 95945
Enrollment: 866-541-6699
General Information: 530-274-9100
Web site: http://www.ayurvedacollege.com

American Institute of Vedic Studies
PO Box 8357
Santa Fe, NM 87504-8357
Phone: 505-983-9385
Web site: http://www.vedanet.com

CONCLUSION

A great deal of information about Ayurvedic medicine has been included in this chapter, but it clearly has offered only a brief summary of its practices. Please keep in mind that because a practice is termed "alternative" does not mean that it is not effective. On the other hand, we should not believe that all alternative practices are, indeed, effective. We, as health consumers, need to be willing to investigate all forms of healing practices and make our decisions about our health and lifestyles based on knowledge of what is safe and efficacious.

Suggestions for Class Activities

1. With a partner, research five Ayurvedic herbs listed in this chapter to assess whether there are any published scientific studies that show benefits or harmful effects from the herbs.
2. Practice the Ayurvedic method of taking a pulse using three fingers.
3. Take the Dosha questionnaire and, according to Ayurvedic principles, determine the type of dosha you are.

Review Questions

1. What is the meaning of the word "Ayurveda"?
2. From what country does Ayurvedic medicine originate?
3. What are the five elements?
4. What does dosha mean?
5. What are the three doshas? Describe two characteristics of each.
6. What is prana?
7. What is the meaning of agni and ama?
8. What diagnostic methods are used in Ayurveda, and how do they compare with traditional Western diagnostic methods?
9. Compare and contrast shamanam and shodhanam treatment.
10. What is snehan treatment?
11. What is panchakarma treatment? Describe three of the five types of panchakarma.
12. What is the status of scientific research on Ayurvedic medicines?
13. What is the NIAM?
14. What is the academic training of Ayurvedic practitioners, and where in the United States could a person receive Ayurvedic medicine training?

Key Terms

Ayurveda Sanskrit word that means life science or science of life.

Ayurvedic medicine A form of holistic alternative medicine that is the traditional system of medicine of India. It may have influenced ancient Chinese medicine and the humoral medicine practiced by Hippocrates in Greece.

basti Medicated enema or colonic irrigation.

constitution Pattern of energy that comprises or makes up a person.

dosha Five elements space (akasha), air (vayu), fire (agni), water (apu), and earth (prithvi) make up the body's constitution called dosha. There are three doshas: Vata, Pitta, and Kapha.

five elements (or tattwa) Earth, water, fire, air, and ether or space.

ghee A mixture also known as sneha made from cow's milk into an edible oil or medicated butter.

malas Waste products such as urine, feces, or sweat.

nasya Nose or sinus irrigation.

neti pot Used to give nose or sinus irrigation, usually using a mild salt solution.

panchakarma treatment Five types of cleansing therapy (vomiting, purging, colonic cleansing, nose and sinus cleansing, and blood detoxification).

pathya vyavastha treatment Use of diet and activity.

prakriti Dosha balance.

prana Energy.

pulse taking There are three types of pulses: snake pulse, which denotes vata dosha; frog pulse, which denotes pitta dosha; and swan pulse, which denotes kapha dosha.

purva-karma treatment Precleansing procedures before shodhanam or shamanam treatment. It involves snehan and swedan treatments.

raktamoksha Detoxifying the blood by bloodletting or using certain herbs.

Salvia labandulaefolia Plant known as Spanish sage. Used for healing purposes.

satvajaya treatment Use of mental hygiene/psychotherapy.

seven tissues (dhatu) Plasma, blood, muscle, lipid, bone, nervous system, and reproductive system.

shamanam treatment A balancing treatment.

shodhanam treatment A cleansing treatment using five procedures; called panchakarma treatment.

snehan treatment Internally it involves ingesting medicated edible oil or butter; externally it is medicated body massage.

swedan treatment Use of dry or wet fomentation or heat therapy to facilitate sweating.

tri-doshic Having fairly equal characteristics of vata, pitta, and kapha.

turmeric A plant that contains curcumin. Used for healing purposes.

vamana Forced vomiting.
vikruiti Dosha imbalance.
virechana Forced purging.

References

1. Lad V. Ayurveda: A brief introduction and guide. Available at: http://www.sahej.com/ayurveda_intro.html. Accessed September 23, 2011. Ayurveda: a brief introduction and guide.
2. Mishra L, Singh BB, Dagenais S. Ayurveda: a historical perspective and principles of the traditional healthcare system in India. *Altern Ther Health Med.* 2001;7(2):36–42.
3. Pelletier K. *The best alternative medicine: what works? What does not?* New York: Simon & Schuster; 2000.
4. Ancient Synergy. Dosha questionnaire. Available at: http://www.ancientsynergy.com/7.html. Accessed July 2, 2010.
5. The Chopra Center. Ayurveda: the science of life. Available at: http://www.chopra.com/ayurveda. Accessed July 2, 2010.
6. Coffey L. What's your dosha? Tridoshas. Available at: http://www.whatsyourdosha.com/trdoshas.html. Accessed July 2, 2010.
7. Blue Lotus Ayurveda. The three doshas in Ayurveda: vata, pitta, and kapha. Available at: http://www.bluelotusayurveda.com/doshas.html. Accessed July 3, 2010.
8. Alternative Medicine Health Care. Available at: http://health.indiamart.com/ayurveda/vata-dosh.html. Accessed July 2, 2010.
9. Bradford N (ed.). *The one spirit encyclopedia of complementary health.* London: Hamlin; 2000.
10. Lad V. An introduction to Ayurveda. Available at: http://www.healthy.net/scr/article.aspx?Id = 373. Accessed July 9, 2010.
11. Chopra Center. The dosha quiz. Available at: http://doshaquiz.chopra.com. Accessed July 14, 2010.
12. Rafael T. Ayurveda for the childbearing years: A primer. Table B: The subdoshas. Boulder, Terra Rafael; 2009. P. 4.
13. Hankey A. Establishing the scientific validity of tridoshas: doshas, subdoshas and dosha prakritis. *Ancient Sci Life.* 2010;29(3).
14. Hankey A. A test of the systems analysis underlying the scientific theory of Ayurveda's tridosha. *J Altern Complent Med.* 2005;11(3):385–390.
15. Hankey A. The scientific value of Ayurveda. *J Altern Complement Med.* 2005;11(2):221–225.
16. Ayurvedic-Medicines.org. Diagnosis by Ayurveda. Available at: http://www.ayurvedic-medicines.org/ayurveda/diagnosis.htm. Accessed July 3, 2010.
17. Holistic online.com Pulse diagnosis. Available at: http://www.holisticonline.com/ayurveda/ayv-diag-pulse.htm. Accessed July 3, 2010.
18. Institute for Optimum Nutrition. Tongue diagnosis. Available at: http://www.ion.ac.uk/information/onarchives/tonguediagnosis. Accessed July 3, 2010.
19. AyurvedaYoga. Purva karma. Available at: http://www.ayurvedayogatraining.com/purvakarma. Accessed July 2, 2010.
20. Kulkami S. Aurveda purva-karma [Health Information Network]. Available at: http://www.nzhealth.net.nz/ayurveda/purva-karma.shtml. Accessed July 6, 2010.
21. Kerala Ayurvedics.com. Purva karma before panchakarma in Ayurveda. Available at: http://www.keralaayurvedics.com/diseases-diagnosis-and-treatment/treatments/panchakarma/purva-karma-before-panchakarma-in-ayurveda.html. Accessed July 2, 2010.
22. Mishra L, Singh BB, Dagenais S. Healthcare and disease management in Ayurveda. *Altern Ther Health Med.* 2001;7(2):44–50.
23. Ilovelndia.com. Panchakarma treatment. Available at: http://ayurveda.iloveindia.com/panchakarma/index.html. Accessed July 5, 2010.
24. Ayurveda Retreat. Panchakarma. Available at: http://www.ayurveda.org/panchkarmadetox.html. Accessed July 13, 2010.
25. Herron R. Detoxification. *Altern Ther Health Med.* 2002;8(5):93–103.
26. Kulkarni S. Shaman [Health Information Network]. Available at: http://www.nzhealth.net.nz/ayurveda/shaman.shtml. Accessed July 5, 2010.
27. Indianetzone. Shamana chikitsa, Auyrveda. Available at: http://www.indianetzone.com/6/shamana.htm. Accessed July 5, 2010.
28. dreddyclinic.com. About Ayurveda. Available at: http://www.dreddyclinic.com/ayurvedic/ayurvedic.htm. Accessed July 14, 2010.
29. YgoY. Rasayana therapy in Aurveda—Benefits. Available at: http://ayurveda.ygoy.com/2009/08/08/rasayana-therapy-in-ayurveda-benefits/. Accessed July 14, 2010.
30. Prokerala Health & Beauty. Ayurveda rejuvenation therapy, anti aging treatment and panchakarma. Available at: http://www.prokerala.com/health/ayurveda/rasayana-ayurveda-rejuvenation.htm. Accessed July 14, 2010.
31. National Center for Complementary and Alternative Medicine. Ayurvedic medicine: an introduction. Available at: http://nccam.nih.gov/health/ayurveda/introduction.htm#ususe. Accessed July 10, 2010.
32. Lavekar GS. Scientific validation of drug development and clinical research in Ayurveda. Central Council for Research in Ayurveda and Siddha; 2006. No 61-65. AYU No.5 66–84.
33. Saper RB, Phillips RS, Sehgal A, et al. Lead, mercury, and arsenic in U.S. and Indian-manufactured Ayurvedic medicines sold via the Internet. *JAMA.* 2008;300(8):915–923.
34. Ayurvedic Center. Historical uses of Ayurvedic herbs. Available at: http://www.holheal.com/ayurved4.html. Accessed July 10, 2010.
35. Premila MS. *Ayurvedic herbs: a clinical guide to the healing plants of traditional Indian medicine.* New York: Haworth Press; 2006.
36. Modha J. Adverse drug reaction of Ayurveda medicines [Boloji.com]. Available at: http://www.boloji.com/ayurveda/av078.html. Accessed July 14, 2010.
37. Aggarwal B, Sundaram C, Malani N, et al. Curcumin: the Indian solid gold. *Adv Exp Med Biol.* 2007;595:1–75.
38. Tildesley NT, Kennedy DO, Perry EK, et al. *Salvia lavandulaefolia* (Spanish sage) enhances memory in healthy young volunteers. *Pharmacol Biochem Behav.* 2003;75(3):669–674.
39. Kiefer D. Novel turmeric compound delivers much more curcumin to the blood [Life Extension]. 2007. Available at: http://www.lef.org/magazine/mag2007/oct2007_report_curcumin_02.htm. Accessed July 2, 2010.
40. Pathania A. Ayurvedic medicine containing lead causes ill-effect [TopNews]. Available at: http://topnews.us/content/224260-ayurvedic-medicine-containing-lead-causes-ill-effect. Accessed July 3, 2010.
41. Valentino S. Colloidal silver side effects [EzineArticles]. Available at: http://ezinearticles.com/?Colloidal-Silver-Side-Effects&id = 353791. Accessed July 15, 2010.
42. Vedic Society. The National Institute of Ayurvedic Medicine, New York, USA. Available at: http://www.panchakarma.com/the-national-institute-of-ayurvedic-medicine-new-york-usa-p-342.html. Accessed July 14, 2010.
43. Ponmelil VA. About Ayurveda, medicine higher studies in India. Available at: http://education.newkerala.com/india-education/About-Ayurveda-Medicine-Higher-Studies-in-India.html. Accessed July 15, 2010.

Alternative Medical Systems: Traditional Chinese Medicine

LEARNING OBJECTIVES

As a result of reading this chapter, students will:

1. Assess why people are skeptical about the efficacy of medical systems different from Western traditional medical practice.
2. Explain how traditional Chinese medicine could co-exist with and complement Western traditional medicine.
3. Analyze the impact that traditional Chinese medicine may have on future U.S. medical practices.
4. Describe four steps that consumers could take in making a decision about whether or not to use traditional Chinese medicine treatments.

WHAT IS TRADITIONAL CHINESE MEDICINE (TCM)?

The oldest written records of a Chinese medicine system originated about 2,800 years ago, although evidence of Chinese medical practices such as surgical tools, dietary medicine, and herbal formulas were evident centuries before.[1] In an e-mail conversation (August 21, 2010), S. Dharmananda clarified that during the early period, Chinese medicine was not known as traditional Chinese medicine because there was nothing to contrast it to such as modern medicine. It was known as *Zhong Yi*; *Zhong* is short for *Zhong Guo* (central country, meaning China) and *Yi* means medicine.

Ancient traditional Chinese medicine (TCM) was a complex, empirical natural science that was an integral part of the culture of China that is now referred to as Daoism.[1] At about 100 CE (AD) the doctrines of TCM were laid out in the *Huangdi Neijing* (also spelled Huang Di Nei Jing), *Yellow Emperor's Canon of Internal Medicine or Yellow Emperor's Inner Canon.* It included physiology, pathology, prevention, diagnosis, meridian theory, acupuncture, and other treatments.[2,3]

Western influence caused a decline in TCM, but after the Communists took power in 1949, they sent researchers out to the countryside to interview and learn from the old practitioners. At that time, there were little or no medical services, and TCM was cheaper to use than modern medicine. Thus began the resurgence of traditional Chinese medicine, not only in China, but also in the West. Modified forms of TCM also are practiced in other parts of the East and Southeast Asia. Today, many Chinese medical doctors and practitioners are trained in traditional Chinese medicine as well as Western medical thought and theory.

Rather than focusing on specific parts of the body affected by disease or injury, TCM is based on a holistic approach to health care; therefore, remedies are prescribed to treat the entire body. Chinese medicine focuses on treating the root cause of illnesses, not just their symptoms. Acupuncture, acupressure, herbal medicines, qi gong, tai chi, Chinese psychology, massage, dietary therapy, and exercise are mainstream TCM treatment modalities. According to results from the *2007 National Health Interview Survey,* about 3 million U.S. adults reported having used acupuncture in the previous year.[4] Internationally, TCM is widely used in China, Japan, and Korea,[5] and is also becoming popular in Europe and the Americas.

Four main theories constitute the basis of traditional Chinese medicine: the theory of *qi* (*chi*), meridian theory, the theory of yin-yang, and the theory of the five elements. The following sections present these theories and their application to medicine.

WHAT IS THE THEORY OF QI (CHI)?

At the heart of TCM is the concept of a vital energy the Chinese call qi (chi), pronounced *chee*. Qi is also known as vital breath, vital force, life force, vital power, moving power, and so forth. Qi energy manifests simultaneously on a spiritual as well as physical level, and it is in a constant state of change.[6] According to Chinese philosophers, qi is the force that animates humans as well as the entire universe, and it unites the heavens and earth. It flows along the surface of the body and through the body's organs.[5] One of the ways that TCM is used to treat disease is to overcome blockages in the circulation of qi. According to the Chinese, qi takes many forms and functions within the body, and is derived from two main sources: the air we breathe and the food we eat.[7] Qi is believed to flow through the body by way of channels, or meridians, that correspond to particular organs or organ systems. Each organ, in turn, has its own characteristic qi. According to TCM, there is a liver qi, kidney qi, and other forms of qi. For instance, nutritive qi is thought to exist within the body and nourishes it; defensive qi exists more externally (but is still within the body) and serves to protect the body.[6]

WHAT IS THE THEORY OF MERIDIANS?

In TCM, qi is thought to flow throughout the body both externally and internally through channels called meridians. According to Chinese belief, there are 12 major meridians that link to 12 vital organs, plus 6 minor meridians that link to other areas of the body. Six of the major meridians are linked to yin and six are linked to yang. (A discussion of yin-yang follows this section.) The meridians form a network that crisscrosses throughout the body linking organs, skin, flesh, muscles, and bones. The qi circulates through the meridians from internal organs out through major meridian branches to smaller ones. The meridians supposedly go out to the outside of the body in the skin and then return to the internal body, much like the pattern of blood vessels and nerves.[7] The meridians can be thought of as rivers of energy with the main purpose of transporting qi throughout the body. See **FIGURE 9.1**.

According to TCM, the meridians have a dual role. One is to prevent harmful energies (e.g., bacteria and viruses) from entering the body; the second is to indicate the presence of harmful energy already inside the body, indicated by body symptoms such as aches, pains, heat, or cold. Any type of

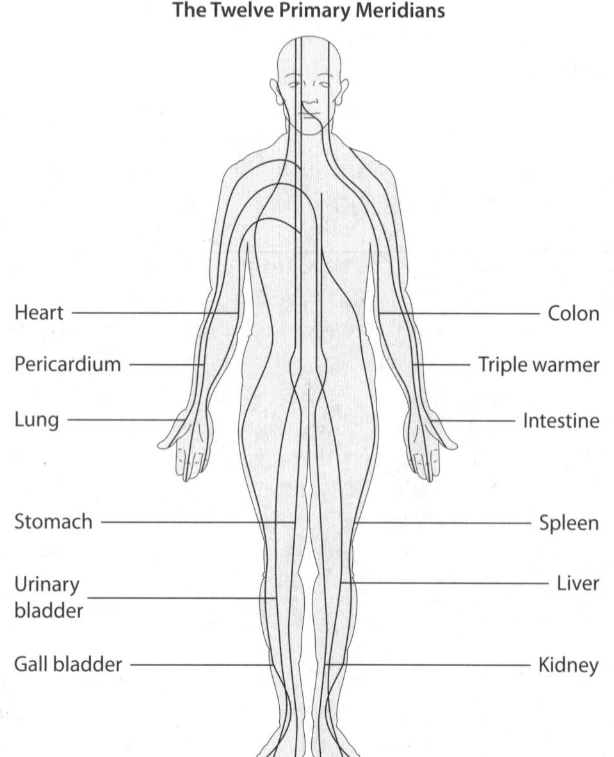

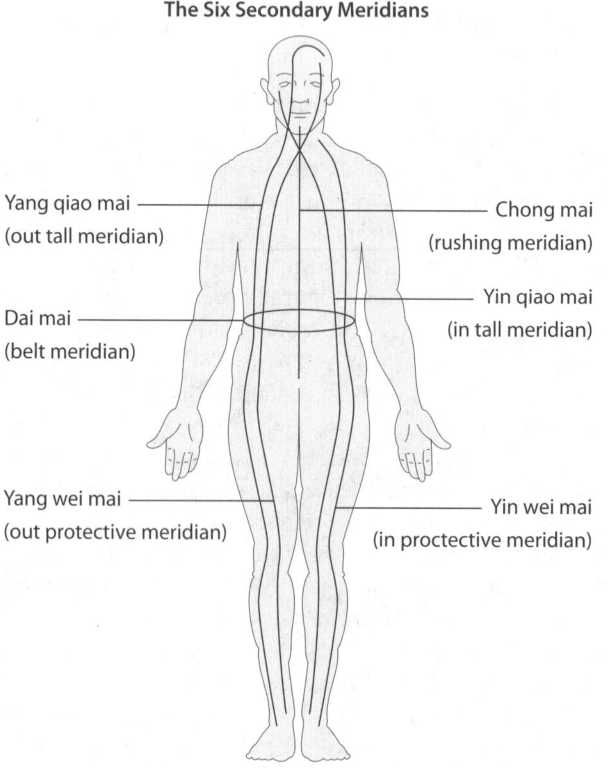

FIGURE 9.1 Twelve primary meridians and six secondary meridians.

"disease" is a sign that the energy within the meridian system is out of balance. When a meridian is blocked, one part of the body is getting too much qi and enters a state of excess or overactivity, while another part of the body or organ is getting too little and becomes deficient in qi and appears underactive.[7] Along the meridians are highly charged energy points, which are called pressure points in Western medicine or *tsubo* in Japanese. Stimulating different tsubo (e.g., using acupuncture) is supposed to affect qi movement and correct an energy imbalance. Meridian points connected to major organs are the lung meridian, large intestine meridian, spleen meridian, stomach meridian, heart meridian, small intestine meridian, urinary bladder meridian, pericardium (lining over the heart) meridian, liver meridian, gall bladder meridian, and triple heater meridian. The pericardium meridian (yin) is paired with the triple heater meridian (yang). The triple heater meridian heats three sections of the body[6]: the upper section is the head and neck area, the middle section is the chest area, and the bottom section is in the naval area. The triple heater meridian regulates the flow of energy in these three regions.[6] For more information on meridians, you can access many charts online.

Thus far, we have discussed the theory of a particular energy called qi that moves within and throughout the body within channels called meridians. When qi is blocked, disease occurs. According to the Chinese philosophers and medical doctors, qi is not the only factor determining wellness and illness. The next theory in the grand scheme of traditional Chinese medicine is the theory of yin-yang.

WHAT IS THE THEORY OF YIN AND YANG?

The theory of yin and yang is the basis of ancient Chinese philosophy and has been applied to traditional Chinese medicine thought and practice. The first references to yin-yang date back to the Zhou dynasty (about 1000–770 BCE).[6] TCM belief is that everything is composed of two opposing but complementary energies—yin and yang. Even though yin and yang are opposite, one cannot exist without the other; therefore, they are never separate. This intertwined relationship is expressed in the classic yin-yang symbol (see **FIGURE 9.2**).

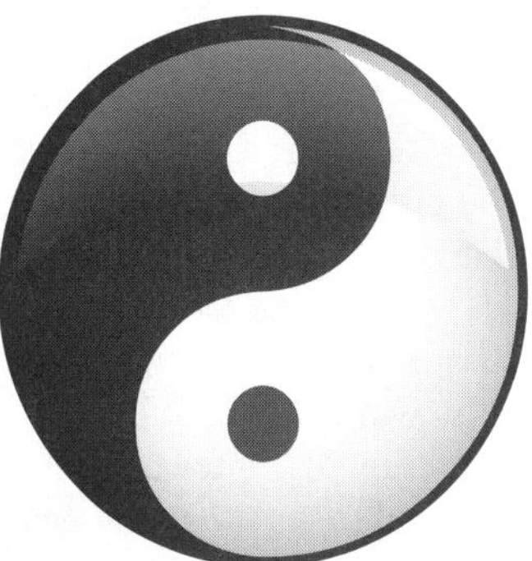

FIGURE 9.2 Yin-yang symbol.

The outer circle represents "everything," and the black and white shapes within the circle represent the interaction of two energies, called yin (black) and yang (white). They are not completely black or white, just as things in life are not completely black or white, and they cannot exist without each other. The yin-yang symbol expresses the interaction between these two forces; the two spots denote that each principle contains the seed of its opposite, which it will produce through interacting with its opposite.

Yin and yang are in a constant state of dynamic balance; when one becomes unbalanced, the other changes proportion and achieves a new balance. TCM belief is that there is no absolute yang or absolute yin. Yin and yang are manifested everywhere, and all movement and changes are in between them. The Chinese call these movements life. The designation of yin or yang is said to be relative to, or in comparison with, some other related condition, that is, yin and yang describe relationships.[6,7] For example, yin originally meant the dark side of the mountain, and yang meant the sun side. On the body, the yang meridians are on the side that is normally in the sun (the back), and the yin meridians are on the shadow side (the front). But, early morning can be said to be yang in comparison to late afternoon, which is more yin. A man is more yang than a woman, but a young woman is more yang than an old woman. See **BOX 9.1** for yin-yang characteristics.[6]

The theory of yin-yang is reflected in medicine as the opposing yin-yang of human body structures, the opposing yin-yang character of the organs, and the opposing yin-yang symptoms that occur with illness. For example, yin organs are those that store the fluids extracted by yang organs (blood, body fluids, qi). The yin organs are

Box 9.1
Yin-Yang Characteristics

YIN CHARACTERISTICS	YANG CHARACTERISTICS
Earth	Heaven
Female	Male
Matter	Energy
Darkness	Light
Shade	Brightness
Cold	Warm
Winter	Summer
Passive	Active
Sweet	Salty

of vital importance for the body, because weakness of the yin organs often leads to death. On the other hand, the yang organs play an important role in digestion and, if necessary, can even be removed without causing death.[6] Every yin organ is related to a yang organ with a similar function (e.g., lung/large intestine for excretion and inhalation; spleen/stomach for storage; kidney/bladder for purifying). The area above the waist is said to be yang and is affected by yang pathogenic factors such as the wind. The area below the waist is said to be yin and affected by yin pathogenic factors such as dampness.[6] See **BOX 9.2**.

Another principle holds that yin and yang continue to change and to succeed each other. As each force reaches its extreme, it becomes the other, thus producing a never-ending cycle. For example, as day (yin) progresses, it eventually becomes night (yang), and then the cycle repeats in an eternal cycle of reversal.[6] TCM holds that all phenomena have within them the seeds of their opposite state, that is, sickness has the seeds of health, health contains the seeds of sickness, wealth contains the seeds of poverty, and so on. According to TCM, one is never really healthy because health contains the principle of its opposite, sickness.

The application of qi and yin-yang to medicine is beginning to unfold, but cannot be complete without a discussion of the theory of the five elements.

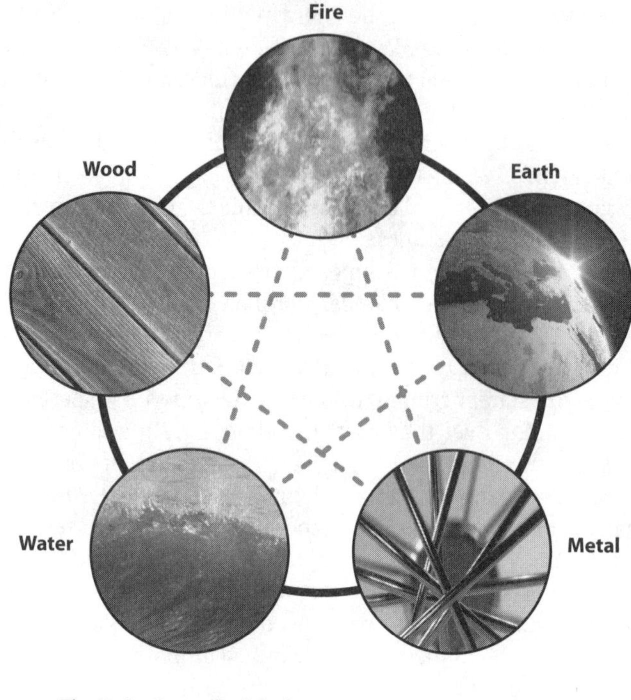

FIGURE 9.3 Five elements symbol.

WHAT IS THE THEORY OF THE FIVE ELEMENTS?

The theory of the five elements is another ancient philosophical concept used to explain the physical universe. The first recorded reference to the five elements dates back to the Warring States Period (476–221 BCE).[6] The theory marked the beginning of Chinese "scientific" medicine because the healers now observed nature and set out to find patterns within it to apply in interpreting disease states. The five elements are identified as water, fire, wood, metal, and earth; all are found in the natural environment and are used to interpret the relationship between the physiology and pathology of the human body and nature.[8] See **FIGURE 9.3**.

Box 9.2

Yin and Yang Organs

Yin Organs	Yang Organs
Lung	Large intestine
Spleen	Stomach
Kidney	Bladder
Heart	Small intestine
Liver	Gallbladder

In TCM, the five elements have basic qualities. Water moistens downward. Fire flares upwards. Wood can be bent and straightened. Metal can be molded and can harden. Earth permits sowing, growing, and reaping.

The five elements are also seen as stages of a seasonal cycle.[8] Wood corresponds to spring and is associated with birth because that is the time for growth. Fire corresponds to summer and is associated with growth, radiating, and flourishing. In late summer (earth) everything is ripening. In autumn (metal), the forces return to the earth. In winter (water) life is directed to the inside and associated with storage.

The five elements are also described as movements. Wood is seen as outward movement in all directions. Metal is inward movement. Water represents a downward movement, and fire represents upward movement. Earth is seen as a neutral movement, or stability.

An interrelationship exists among the five elements. In a *generating sequence*, wood generates fire, fire generates earth, earth generates metal, metal generates water, and water generates wood.[6] In a *controlling sequence*, wood controls earth, earth controls water, water controls fire, fire controls metal, and metal controls wood.[6] There also are other documented interrelations, but those mentioned should give an idea regarding the interrelationships. When applied to medicine, an example of the five elements during a controlling sequence is spleen controls the kidneys, lungs control the liver, and kidneys control the heart.[6]

Table 9.1
Five Elements and Yin-Yang Chart

Yin-Yang	Wood	Fire	Earth	Metal	Water
Seasons	Spring	Summer	Late summer	Autumn	Winter
Directions	East	South	Center	West	North
Colors	Green	Red	Yellow	White	Black
Tastes	Sour	Bitter	Sweet	Pungent	Salty
Climates	Wind	Heat	Dampness	Dryness	Cold
Zodiac animals	Tiger, rabbit	Snake, horse	Ox, dragon, goat, dog	Monkey, rooster	Pig, rat
Animals	Fish	Birds	Humans	Mammals	Shell-covered
Celestial animals	Dragon	Phoenix	Serpent	Tiger	Tortoise
Grains	Wheat	Beans	Rice	Hemp	Millet
Yin organs	Liver	Heart	Spleen	Lungs	Kidneys
Yang organs	Gallbladder	Small intestine	Stomach	Large intestine	Bladder
Sense organs	Eyes	Tongue	Mouth	Nose	Ears
Emotions	Anger	Joy	Worry	Grief	Fear
Emotional	Hot temper	Hysteria	Depression	Self-pity	Phobias
Form	Tall/rectangular	Angular/pyramid	Flat/square	Round/circular	Irregular/wavy
Sounds	Shouting	Laughing	Singing	Crying	Groaning
Danger	Rot, disease	Conflagration, fire	Collision, falling	Wounding	Flooding
Activity	Creativity, relationships with children	Intellect, schooling, fame	Estate, house, home	Commerce, success, trade	Travel, writing, communication

The five elements constantly move and change and are dependent on one another. The visceral organs, as well as other body organs, are thought to have similar properties to the five elements and interact physiologically and pathologically just as the five elements do. **TABLE 9.1** shows the categorization of phenomena[8] according to the five elements.

As shown in the table, the five elements are also associated with body shapes.[9]

- *Wood type:* Slender and tall body shape
- *Fire type:* Pointed head and chin, small hands, with curly or a small amount of hair
- *Metal type:* Square and broad shoulders, strong body type, and a triangle-shaped face
- *Earth type:* Large head, larger body and belly, strong legs, and a wide jaw
- *Water type:* Round face and body with a longer than normal torso

From examining Table 9.1 and the relationship of the five elements with body type, one can perceive that the five elements of nature correspond with, among other things, body parts, sensations, and colors. The theory of the five elements reinforces basic concepts in Chinese medicine regarding the wholeness of body, mind, and spirit and the importance of maintaining harmony with nature and balance within the body.

Now that we have explored the theories that comprise the basis of Chinese medicine, let's examine several TCM diagnostic methods.

WHAT ARE TCM DIAGNOSTIC METHODS?

Of course, there are similarities between TCM and traditional, Western diagnostic methods, but there also are some differences.

Observation of the Patient

Just like traditional physicians, TCM doctors and practitioners observe and examine the body with their eyes and listen to body sounds with a stethoscope. However, they also listen to the voice and the breath, and they note the smell of the breath, skin, secretions, or excretions.[5,9] The sound of the voice, such as hoarseness or an unusually loud voice, indicates certain body deficiencies or illnesses. Body odors such as halitosis might indicate a stomach disorder. Rancid odors are supposedly related to liver problems. Scorched or burned odors are related to the heart, and putrid odors are related to the kidneys.[9]

As a part of the physical examination, the entire body appearance is noted and related to one of the five element body types. Other body observations might include noting if a person appears very skinny (emaciated) or very large, the size of their thighs, hair loss, musculoskeletal problems, and any changes in muscles, tendons, blood vessels, skin, and bones. If an abnormality is found, the doctor will determine whether it is due to an excess or deficiency of yin or yang. TCM doctors also observe their patients' spirit, called *Shen*. The Shen is supposed to exhibit qualities such as vitality and mental, emotional, and spiritual well-being and is thought to show in the eyes, complexion, and state of mind.[9]

Tongue Diagnosis

As with Ayurvedic medicine, traditional Chinese medicine doctors or practitioners will examine the tongue, which aids in their diagnosis. They observe the color (normal is pink or light red), shape, features (texture, spots, numbness, deviated), moisture (dry or wet), coating (white, powder, yellow, gray, black), coat thickness, cracks (short ones, long ones, transverse, irregular), and coat root (rooted coating cannot be scratched off).[9] Again, the doctors will examine the tongue to determine whether there is an excess or deficiency of yin and yang (see **FIGURE 9.4**).

Pulse Diagnosis

During the physical examination, TCM doctors or practitioners use pulse diagnosis. Various sources differ, but there are approximately 29 different pulse qualities. Each of the 29 has a designated Chinese name. Pulses are felt on both the left and right wrist at three radial artery sites on each wrist and at three depths (superficial, middle, and deep).[5,10]

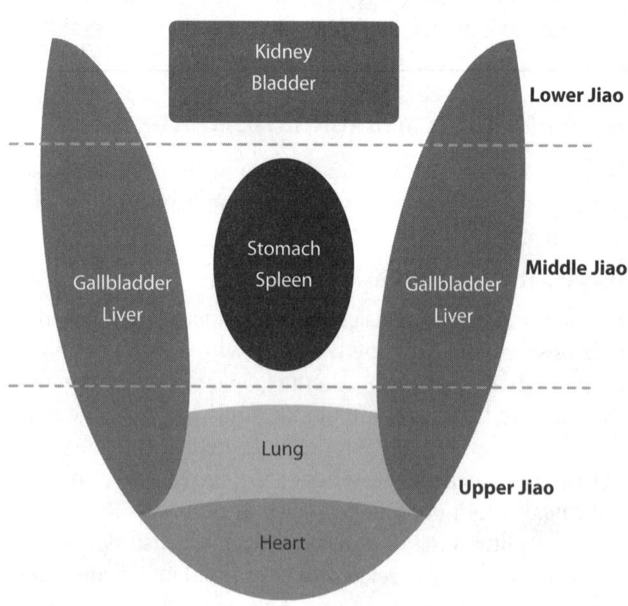

FIGURE 9.4 Tongue chart.

Pulse Taking Practice

To feel a pulse, use the middle three fingers of your left hand to feel the right pulse and vice versa for the left pulse reading. The second finger should rest just below the wrist crease on the thumb side. The other two fingers will rest next to this. Press with all three fingers gently and then deeper until you feel a pulse. What you are trying to do is feel for the quality of the pulse as well as the count. Press harder until you don't feel a pulse, and then ease off until you feel it again. Now see if the quality has changed. See **FIGURE 9.5** for an image of pulse taking.

As in the other diagnostic methods, general deficiency and excess of yin and yang are identified by the pulse diagnosis. See **BOX 9.3** for main pulse descriptions.[9]

Eight Guiding Principles

The TCM practitioner or doctor may also use the Eight Guiding Principles when making a diagnosis to differentiate energetic imbalances in the body. These consist of the four polar opposites: yin/yang; cold/heat; deficiency or excess energy, blood, or fluids; and interior/exterior.[6] A cold diagnosis would involve a slowed metabolism, low grade fever, pale skin, and chills whereas a heat diagnosis would result from a high fever and reddened or flushed skin. Interior means pathogens that enter the body whereas exterior means pathogens that cause problems on the skin or hair. A lack of blood or other body fluids would cause a deficiency whereas swelling, because of too much fluid in the body or too much qi energy, would cause an excess diagnosis. If either yin or yang becomes too dominant, the practitioner would attempt to treat that condition.

Medical History

Just as in traditional Western medicine, TCM doctors or practitioners use questioning as a diagnostic tool. They will interview a patient about past medical history, origin of the problem, living and environmental conditions, current and past emotional issues, and eating patterns and diet, and

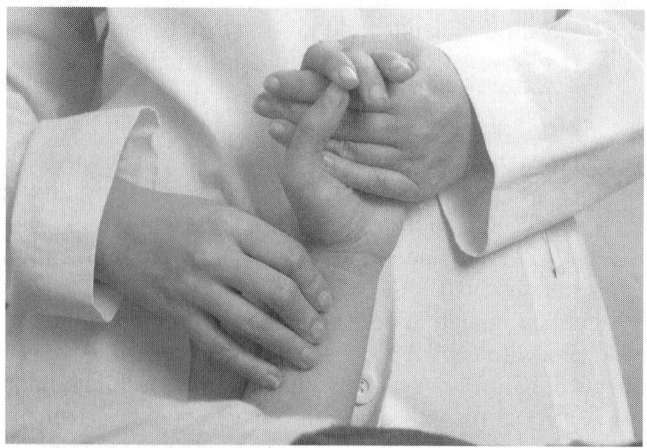

FIGURE 9.5 Pulse taking.

Box 9.3

Traditional Chinese Medicine Pulse Descriptions

- *Fu mai* (floating, superficial)
- *Hong mai* (surging, flooding)
- *Ge mai* (leathery, drum skin, tympanic, hard)
- *Kou mai* (hollow or scallion stalk, green onion)
- *Ru mai* (soft or soggy)
- *San mai* (scattered)
- *Xu mai* (forceless, empty, deficient)
- *Chen mai* (deep)
- *Fu mai* (hidden)
- *Lao mai* (firm, confined)
- *Ruo mai* (weak)
- *Chi mai* (slow)
- *Huan mai* (slowed down, moderate, or relaxed)
- *Se mai* (choppy, hesitant)
- *Jie mai* (knotted, bound)
- *Shi mai* (excess, full, replete, forceful)
- *Hua mai* (slippery, rolling)
- *Jin mai* (tight, tense)
- *Chang mai* (long)
- *Xuan mai* (wiry, taut)
- *Wei mai* (minute, faint, indistinct)
- *Xi mai* (thready, thin)
- *Duan mai* (short)
- *Dai mai* (regularly intermittent)
- *Shuo mai* (rapid)
- *Ji mai* (racing, swift, hurried)
- *Cu mai* (rapid-irregular, skipping, abrupt)
- *Dong mai* (moving, throbbing, stirring)
- *Da mai* (large, big)

ask specific questions related to all the body systems (e.g., circulatory, respiratory, nervous, etc.).[9]

After all the diagnostics are completed and a diagnosis is made, treatments are prescribed. One TCM source, *The Chinese Medical Sampler*, likened the planning of treatment to a tree. That relationship is paraphrased[11] as follows:

> The reason that the person goes to the doctor or practitioner is the presenting complaint or problem. That represents one branch of the tree. Other signs and symptoms represent the other branches of the tree. The underlying cause of the illness is represented by the main root of the tree, and factors contributing to the illness are represented by other tree roots. After assessing all the branches and roots, three possible types of treatment are selected.
>
> - Treat the branches—making the patient comfortable.
> - Treat the root—restoring health.
> - Treat both the root and the branches—the branches are interfering to the point that reducing their effects is a high priority.[11]

Just as in Western medicine, Chinese medicine doctors and practitioners have to plan and make priority decisions before starting a treatment program. As previously mentioned, the treatment modalities used are acupuncture, acupressure, herbal medicines, qi gong, tai chi, Chinese psychology, massage, diet, and exercise. A few of those are presented in the next section.

WHAT ARE TCM TREATMENT MODALITIES?

In TCM, the mainstream treatments are acupuncture and acupressure, herbal medicines, diet, and exercise. Because there is a myriad of information regarding each, they will be introduced separately.

What Are Acupuncture and Acupressure?

Acupuncture is the insertion of stainless steel needles into the skin at specific points on the body called acupuncture points to affect the flow of qi (energy) through body channels or meridians.[12–15] The needles used are sterilized or are sterile, disposable needles. They are about the thickness of a human hair and would fit inside the body of a hypodermic needle used for drawing blood.[12] They range from 0.16 mm to 0.38 mm in thickness, and the tip is conical, allowing it to penetrate tissues separating muscle fiber without causing damage.[12,13] The shape and size of the needle make the insertion relatively painless (see **FIGURE 9.6**).

Acupressure is an ancient healing method that uses a finger to find key points (trigger points) on the surface of the body. As with acupuncture, the object is to promote the flow of qi energy and to stimulate the body's own immune system. Gentle and firm pressure of the hands and even the feet are used to stimulate the trigger points, which are the same points used in acupuncture. A major difference between acupressure and acupuncture is that people can be taught to apply acupressure on their own bodies. It may be effective in helping to relieve such conditions as headaches, eyestrain, sinus problems, neck pain, muscle aches, and lower backaches.

How Acupuncture Works

How acupuncture works is still not fully known. Although the TCM explanation is that acupuncture affects the flow of qi, some studies from the early 1980s found that it stimulated the release of endorphins, the body's natural feel-good chemicals.[14] Others believe that acupuncture stimulates the body's immune system and affords protection against disease.[13,15]

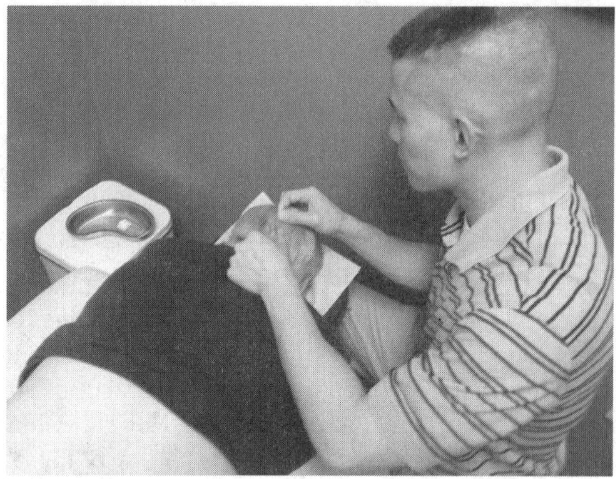

FIGURE 9.6 Scalp acupuncture by Kenneth K. Chow, Dipl OM, DNM, CBP, Baton Rouge, LA.

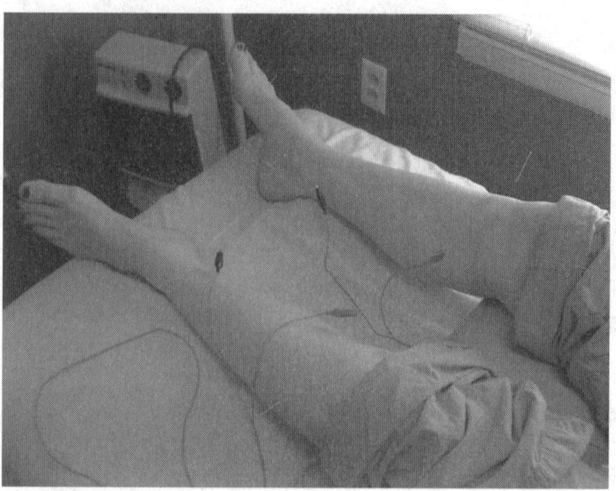

FIGURE 9.7 Electro-acupuncture by Kenneth K. Chow, Dipl OM, DNM, CBP, Baton Rouge, LA.

Methods of Giving Acupuncture

Besides needling technique, acupuncture may be given in several other ways[2,14,15,17,18]:

- *Electro-acupuncture:* Mild electrical pulses are relayed via acupuncture needles to various trigger points in the skin (see **FIGURE 9.7**).
- *Trigger-point acupuncture:* Needles are inserted at a location that is distant from the affected organ or body part. Qi energy is channeled through nerves.
- *Laser acupuncture:* Rays or laser beams are used in place of the acupuncture needles to facilitate the trigger point.
- *Acupuncture point injection:* Sterile syringes are used to inject medication such as vitamins and herbal products into the system via trigger points.
- *Moxibustion:* Heat is used at acupuncture points. The herb *Artemisia*, also known as mugwort, a type of chrysanthemum, is burned near the body to create heat in the meridian and increase the flow of energy and blood. It may be directly applied on the skin, rolled up and placed on the needle, or used as a stick of moxa that can be held over the desired area to be treated.
- *Cupping:* A round glass cup is heated and kept upside down over an area of the body, creating a vacuum that will keep the cup attached to the skin. The purpose is to promote blood circulation or energy and to open skin pores so that toxins are flushed out. See **FIGURE 9.8** for a photo of cupping.
- *Injection:* Sterile water, saline, procaine, morphine, or vitamins are injected into the meridian points.
- *Earlobe needling:* Needles or staples are used in ear acupuncture points.

The Japanese, Koreans, and Vietnamese have also developed their own forms of acupuncture with modifications such as needleless and trigger point acupuncture, which will be discussed in a later section.

Early Acupuncture Techniques

The earliest acupuncture tools were sharp pieces of bone, stone (bian stone), or flint used to scratch or prick acupuncture points. Bian stone needles were excavated from ruins in China dating back to the New Stone Age (4,000–10,000 years ago).[15] As time went on, early needles were made from bamboo and bone, but those were thicker than modern needles, and more than likely caused discomfort. Metal needles

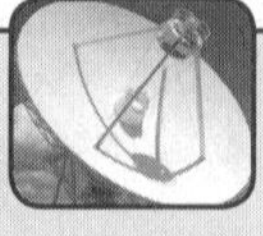

In the News

In a *Wall Street Journal* article entitled "Decoding an Ancient Therapy: High-Tech Tools Show How Acupuncture Works in Treating Arthritis, Back Pain, Other Ills," Melinda Beck explored acupuncture, how it works, and whether it was effective. A growing body of research now suggests that it may stimulate blood flow and tissue repair at the needle sites. Acupuncture may also send nerve signals to the brain area that regulates the perception of pain. Neuroimaging studies showed a calming effect on the area of the brain that registers pain, and Doppler ultrasound showed that acupuncture increased blood flow. Thermal imaging showed that it also could decrease inflammation.[16]

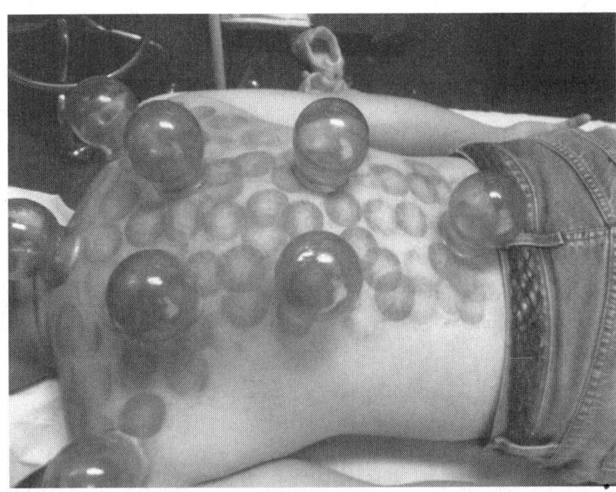

FIGURE 9.8 Cupping by Kenneth K. Chow, Dipl OM, DNM, CBP, Baton Rouge, LA.

were employed at the advent of the Iron Age and Bronze Age. Early metals used were iron, copper, bronze, silver, and gold. It was not until the twentieth century that stainless steel needles were used; these are still used today.

Wang Weiyi, a famous physician during the Song Dynasty (960–1279) wrote a text, *The Illustrated Manual on Points for Acupuncture and Moxibustion*, in which he identified 657 acupuncture points. He also created two bronze statues to illustrate meridians and acupuncture points.[15] During the Ming Dynasty (1568–1644), new developments in acupuncture occurred. The technique was refined; moxa sticks were used for indirect treatment; and extra points outside the main meridians were identified.

Acupuncture Treatment Process

To give acupuncture, the client is either seated or asked to lie on a cot or table, much as one does when getting a massage. Usually, 3–15 long, thin, solid, sterile disposable or stainless steel needles are placed in various locations on the body according to the meridians, not necessarily at the anatomic site of symptoms. The acupuncturist may insert and remove the needles quickly or leave them in for longer periods of time, often with the application of heat or electrical impulses.[14] In order to stimulate qi, the needles are twirled once when placed in the skin and then left in for approximately 20 to 40 minutes.

Acupuncture Styles

There are several different styles of acupuncture. Although acupuncture originated in China, it has spread to Korea, Japan, Vietnam, Europe, and the Americas; thus, various styles have evolved.

- *Traditional Chinese acupuncture:* This is the most common form studied and practiced in the United States. Traditional Chinese acupuncture uses thicker needles and deeper insertion than the Japanese style. A deep, radiating sensation is sought with each needle. In the hands of master Chinese practitioners, this technique is not very painful, though it can cause soreness.[19]
- *Japanese acupuncture:* The Japanese style of acupuncture uses fewer and thinner needles with less stimulation. Kanshinho is a guiding tube insertion method developed by the famous seventeenth-century blind acupuncturist Waichi Sugiyama. The guiding tube method drastically decreases the pain associated with the initial insertion of the needle and is now used by practitioners worldwide.[20]
- *Five element acupuncture:* Even though the concept of the five elements exists in all classical forms of acupuncture, five element acupuncturists focus more on the energetic, spiritual, and emotional components of health. One of the five elements (fire, earth, metal, water, or wood) is diagnosed as a cause of a patient's disorder. The practitioner analyzes where the energetic blocks are through the use of acupuncture. Five element acupuncturists generally use thinner needles with more subtle stimulation than TCM practitioners.[21]
- *Korean acupuncture:* Korean acupuncture uses points in the hand that correspond to areas of the body and bodily symptoms. Korean acupuncture placed a great deal of emphasis on the five elements theory and takes into account a person's body type and constitution.[12]
- *Auricular acupuncture:* This is acupuncture that uses points in the ears that correspond to areas of the body and bodily symptoms. It is more commonly used for pain control and drug, alcohol, and nicotine addictions.[22] For some people, auricular acupuncture offers a pleasurable alternative to using needles on other parts of the body.[12]
- *Medical acupuncture:* Medical acupuncture is performed by a Western medical doctor. The definition from the American Board of Medical Acupuncture is "Medical acupuncture is a medical discipline having a central core of knowledge embracing the integration of acupuncture from various traditions into contemporary biomedical practice. A Physician Acupuncturist is one who has acquired specialized knowledge and experience related to the integration of acupuncture within a biomedicine practice."[21]
- *Veterinary acupuncture:* This is acupuncture used on animals.[22,23] Some conditions that acupuncture is used for in animals are arthritis and hip dysplasia, back pain and disc disease, incontinence and urinary retention, some types of nerve damage, and chronic painful conditions.[23]
- *Trigger point therapeutic treatments:* Trigger points are specific areas in the muscles where stabbing pain,

weakness, tingling, or aching pain is felt. Pressure is applied at those points, or needles may be inserted. Massage therapists and physical therapists as well as acupuncturists may use trigger points.[12]

Side Effects of Acupuncture

In general, adverse reactions to acupuncture are minimal, although case reports of complications do exist. Bleeding rarely occurs. Infection is minimized by most practitioners through the recommended use of sterile disposable needles. Allergic reaction to the stainless steel needles is also rare. Pain varies by patient, but treatment is usually painless or slightly painful. Some patients report that their symptoms temporarily increased rather than decreased after having acupuncture. For patients receiving auricular treatments, the possibility of inflammation of the cartilage (chondritis) exists, although it is rare.[11]

Acupuncture Research

Some of the diseases that have been treated with acupuncture are headaches, menstrual cramps, dental pain, tennis elbow, fibromyalgia, osteoarthritis, stroke rehabilitation, asthma, addiction, postoperative nausea, lower back pain, gynecological problems, gastrointestinal ailments, and carpal tunnel syndrome. One meta review study found that moxibustion, acupuncture, and laser acupoint stimulation were effective in the correction of breech presentation.[17]

Acupuncture research is ongoing here in the United States. The National Center for Complementary and Alternative Medicine (NCCAM) has funded several studies that have shown positive results.

- A landmark study of the use of acupuncture for osteoarthritis of the knee showed that acupuncture provided pain relief and improved function of the knee.[24] This study was the largest Phase III clinical trial of acupuncture and was funded by the NCCAM and the National Institute of Arthritis and Musculoskeletal and Skin Diseases at the National Institutes of Health.
- A study of the use of acupuncture to help symptoms of post-traumatic stress disorder (PTSD) involved 73 people who were divided into three treatment groups: acupuncture, cognitive-behavioral therapy, and a control group. Even though the study is considered small, the results showed that acupuncture provided treatment effects similar to the cognitive-behavioral group, and both of those groups were superior to the control group.[25]
- Preliminary results of a study on the use of acupuncture given as a complement to in vitro fertilization (IVF) showed that it increased the odds of achieving pregnancy.[26]
- Acupuncture or simulated acupuncture treatments were better than usual care in managing low back pain in a study conducted by Group Health Center for Health Studies in Seattle and funded by the NCCAM.[27] The trial enrolled 638 adults with chronic lower back pain, who were assigned to one of four groups: individualized acupuncture, standardized acupuncture, simulated acupuncture (no real penetration of the skin), and usual traditional back care. The three acupuncture groups all improved their dysfunction scores significantly more than the group receiving traditional care. The researchers noted that the finding indicates something unknown but meaningful is taking place during acupuncture treatments, whether using simulated or real needling.
- Transcutaneous electrical acupoint stimulation (TEAS) uses skin electrodes to apply electrical stimulation to acupuncture points. A study by Meade et.al found that of 48 participants who had received TEAS as an adjunctive treatment for opioid use during a detoxification program, 29 percent at two weeks post discharge began taking opioid drugs again, compared with 65 percent of participants who did not receive TEAS. Further, study participants receiving TEAS were more than two times less likely to have not used any drugs. Limitations of the study are the small number of participants and brief duration of treatment.[28]

Other studies utilizing acupuncture for pain relief,[29] tension headaches,[30] and cancer pain in rats[31] also showed promising results. Please see **BOX 9.4** for a list of topics on the Internet Health Library Web site related to research on the use of acupuncture.[32]

Thus far, the research studies presented have been those that show promising or positive results. There are, however, many other reports that have cast doubt on the effectiveness of acupuncture. The Cochrane Collaboration has 12 centers around the world and 10,000 health expert volunteers who engage in reviews of evidence-based clinical studies.[33] Hundreds of those reviews have been published and thousands are stored in the Cochrane Collaboration library. The reviews of acupuncture research have concluded that any perceived benefit of acupuncture for the following conditions has been a placebo effect: for smokers trying to quit, cocaine dependence using auricular acupuncture, inducing labor, epilepsy treatment, Bell's palsy, chronic asthma, stroke rehabilitation, breech presentation, depression, carpal tunnel syndrome, irritable bowel syndrome, schizophrenia, and many other conditions.[33] The Cochrane Collaboration also criticized the quality of many of the clinical trial studies. On the positive side, the Cochrane Collaboration found that there were some conditions in which acupuncture was found to be effective. Some of those are pelvic and back pain during pregnancy, lower back pain, headaches, postoperative nausea and vomiting, chemotherapy-induced nausea and vomiting, neck disorders, and bedwetting.[33]

Prevalence, Training, Certification, and Licensing of Acupuncturists

According to the NCCAM,[34] about 3.1 million U.S. adults and 150,000 children had used acupuncture in 2006. This

Box 9.4

Web Pages about Acupuncture Research Related to Body Disorders and Diseases

- Acupuncture and Acne
- Acupuncture and Alcoholism
- Acupuncture and Angina
- Acupuncture and Ankylosing Spondylitis
- Acupuncture and Apoplexy Patients
- Acupuncture and Arteriosclerosis
- Acupuncture and Asthma
- Acupuncture and Back Pain
- Acupuncture and Bell's Palsy
- Acupuncture and Brain Hemorrhage
- Acupuncture and Bronchial Asthma
- Acupuncture and Cataract
- Acupuncture and Cerebral Infarction
- Acupuncture and Cerebral Palsy
- Acupuncture-Acupressure and Children Undergoing Tonsillectomy
- Acupuncture and Chronic Neck Pain
- Acupuncture and Chronic Spinal Pain Syndromes
- Acupuncture and Cold/Flu
- Acupuncture and Constipation
- Acupuncture and Crohn's Disease
- Acupuncture and Dental Pain
- Acupuncture and Depression
- Acupuncture and Dermatitis
- Acupuncture and Diarrhea
- Acupuncture and Eczema
- Acupuncture, Moxibustion Therapy and Female Urethral Syndrome
- Acupuncture and Frozen Shoulder
- Acupuncture and Gout
- Acupuncture and Hayfever
- Acupuncture and Hypothyroidism
- Acupuncture and Infertility
- Acupuncture and Insomnia
- Acupuncture and Irritable Bowel Syndrome
- Acupuncture and Post-operative Nausea and Vomiting
- Acupuncture and Metatarsalgia
- Acupuncture and Migraine
- Acupuncture and Peripheral Arterial Disease
- Acupuncture and Postoperative Vomiting in Children
- Acupuncture and Polycystic Ovaries
- Acupuncture and Rheumatoid Arthritis
- Acupuncture and Stomach Carcinoma Pain
- Acupuncture and Substance Abuse
- Acupuncture and Tendonitis
- Acupuncture and Tennis Elbow
- Acupuncture and Tinnitus
- Acupuncture and Varicose Eczema
- Acupuncture and Wound Healing
- Autogenics, Acupuncture and Chronic Pain

estimate came from the 2007 National Health Interview Survey (NHIS), which included a comprehensive survey of CAM use by Americans. Between the 2002 and 2007 NHIS, acupuncture use among adults increased by an estimated 1 million people.[35]

The number of acupuncturists is rapidly growing, and was projected to quadruple by 2015. The American Association of Acupuncture and Oriental Medicine (AAOM) reports that there are 15,000 to 17,000 practicing professional acupuncturists in the United States.[36] The number of nonprofessional acupuncturists is estimated to be between 12,000 and 30,000. A variety of clinicians incorporate acupuncture into their practices, including chiropractors, dentists, medical doctors, naturopaths, osteopaths, physical therapists, podiatrists, and veterinarians.

Since its inception in 1982, the National Certification Commission for Acupuncture and Oriental Medicine (NCCAOM) has certified close to 10,000 Diplomates in Acupuncture, Chinese Herbology, and Asian Bodywork Therapy. The degrees received vary, including licensed acupuncturists (LAc), Oriental medical doctors (OMD), and physician acupuncturists (MD or DO).[35]

Currently, there are approximately 3,000 acupuncturists with medical degrees practicing in the United States.[36] The regulation and licensing of acupuncturists in the United States is state dependent; most states require a health professional degree such as being a medical doctor, doctor of osteopathy, chiropractor, dentist, podiatrist, naturopath, physician assistant, or registered nurse. Here in the United States, there are nonphysician and physician acupuncturists.

Nonphysician Acupuncturists

The education, testing, and licensing of nonphysician acupuncturists varies by state. Most states require that applicants who are trained in the United States, must have graduated from a program accredited by the Accreditation Commission for Acupuncture and Oriental Medicine (ACAOM). The typical education standard for an acupuncturist is between 2,000 and 3,000 hours of training at an independently accredited master's degree 4-year school. ACAOM's professional requirements are stated in the *ACAOM Accreditation Manual* as follows[35,p4]:

> 1.2.1. Master's-Level and Master's Degree Programs The professional program in acupuncture shall be at least three academic years in length and follow at least two years of accredited postsecondary education.
>
> The professional program in Oriental medicine shall be at least four academic years in length and follow at least two years of accredited postsecondary education.

The program of study covering acupuncture and herbal medicines covers history; theory (e.g., qi, yin-yang, five elements); acupuncture and point/meridian theory; diagnostic skills; treatment planning; treatment techniques, equipment, and safety; counseling and communication skills; ethics and practice management; biomedical clinical sciences; Oriental herbal studies; and other Oriental medicine modalities (body work, exercise/breathing therapy, diet counseling).[35]

The ACAOM administers a qualifying exam for certification as a Diploma in Acupuncture (Dipl. Ac.), although particular licensing requirements vary by state. Typically, a licensing board will also require that the applicant pass the NCCAOM certification examination. Once certified, acupuncturists can apply for a license. The NCCAOM published a table in January 2001 that outlines how various states use its certification examination in their acupuncturist licensing requirements.[35] Only a few states require the supervision of a physician for the almost 11,000 practicing nonphysician acupuncturists.

Physician Acupuncturists

Most states recognize acupuncture as being within the scope of practice for licensed physicians, but state regulations vary. Although some states allow physicians to practice acupuncture without additional education, most states require between 200 and 300 hours of specialized training in acupuncture, and in some cases they must pass an examination. The American Board of Medical Acupuncture[36] has published standards set by the World Health Organization and the World Federation of Acupuncture and Moxibustion Societies.

> 4.2.1 For licensed graduates of modern Western medical colleges, who already have had education and training in anatomy, physiology, neurology, and all the other basic and clinical sciences involved in medical diagnosis and treatment, training in acupuncture can be accomplished following a different training pathway for them to master acupuncture as a special medical modality.
>
> The theoretical part and objectives of this acupuncture training are parallel to those described in the complete training section, and the acupuncture core syllabus will be the same. ... The whole course should be devoted to acquiring the knowledge and skill in acupuncture as well as the related basic theory for at least 200 hours of formal training. By the end of the course the participants should be able to integrate acupuncture into their medical practices. The proficiency of training and practice should be evaluated through an official examination by health authorities to ensure safety, competence, and efficacy.

A table published by the American Academy of Medical Acupuncture (AAMA) in 1999 outlines various state requirements.[36] This table can be viewed at http://www.medicalacupuncture.org/acu_info/licensure.html.[37]

The AAMA is the only acupuncture society in North America composed solely of physicians but will accept members from diverse backgrounds. The World Federa-

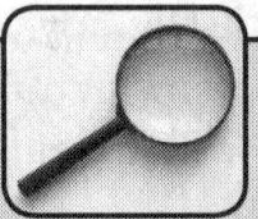

Case Study

Blake is having a great deal of hip and back pain. He used to run a lot and still plays tennis, which he does not want to give up. His private medical doctor has told him that the MRI showed he has a pinched sciatic nerve from a herniated disc. The doctor has suggested that Blake have back surgery to remove the disc and stabilize the vertebrae. He is very concerned about having this done. A friend suggested that Blake should try other means to treat the condition and specifically said he should try acupuncture. Blake has heard about acupuncture but he has a fear of needles.

Questions:

1. What would you suggest Blake could do to learn more about acupuncture as a treatment for back pain?
2. Where would he find a person or doctor who would be a professionally trained acupuncturist?
3. Do insurance companies pay for acupuncture?

tion of Acupuncture-Moxibustion Societies set the training guidelines and membership requirements.[37] Requirements for admission to the AAMA include possessing an active MD or DO license (or equivalent) to practice medicine under U.S. or Canadian jurisdiction; completion of a minimum of 220 hours of formal training in medical acupuncture (120 hours didactic, 100 hours clinical), or the equivalent in an apprenticeship program acceptable to the Membership Committee; and 2 years of experience practicing medical acupuncture.

The American Board of Medical Acupuncture (ABMA) was formally established in 2000 as an independent entity within the American Academy of Medical Acupuncture.[36] Its mission is to promote safe, ethical, efficacious medical acupuncture to the public by maintaining high standards for the examination and certification of physician acupuncturists as medical specialists. A physician who desires certification by the ABMA must complete a formal course of study and training designed for physicians that, at a minimum, meets the guidelines and standards set forth by the World Health Organization and the World Federation of Acupuncture and Moxibustion Societies (WFAS). Programs must be a minimum of 200 hours of acupuncture-specific training, post–medical school, of which 100 hours should be clinical. Currently, 200 AAMA members have qualified for ABMA Board Certification.

As shown in the preceding sections, becoming an acupuncturist requires knowledge about the body's anatomy and physiology as well as the basic tenets of Chinese medicine. The study of herbal medicine is included within the curriculum of most acupuncture programs. Even though this text includes a separate chapter on herbal medicines, a brief overview of Chinese herbal medicine is presented next.

WHAT IS HERBAL MEDICINE THERAPY?

Traditional Chinese herbal medicine (CHM) is the study and use of plants and plant parts. Here in the United States, herbal products are classified as dietary supplements. Different parts of plants are brewed, stewed, and squeezed to make the medicine.[38] For example, the roots of ginseng, Chinese gromwell, and Taiwan Angelica are used. Dried ginger and lily bulb are from the rhizome of plants. Additionally, leaves, flowers, seeds, and even grass and vines are used in making herbal medicines.[39] Before being prescribed, each person is evaluated according to Chinese medicine theory (previously described in this chapter), and then a specialized formula made up of one or several herbs is prescribed for that person.[38]

History

Some say that Chinese usage of herbal medicine dates back to 3494 BCE. The Chinese people say that the founder of herbal medicine is Shen Nong (also spelled Shennong), the legendary emperor who lived during that time. He is also known as the Divine Cultivator/Divine Farmer by the Chinese people because he taught people how to farm.[40] To determine the nature of different herbal medicines, Shen Nong would ingest various kinds of plants to assess how they affected his own body. To find the appropriate herbs for pain or illness, Shen Nong is said to have tasted a hundred herbs including 70 toxic substances in a single day. Because there were no written records, the discoveries of Shen Nong were passed down verbally for 2,000 years from generation to generation.[41] See **FIGURE 9.9** for an image of Shen Nong.

Another pioneer, considered the most famous of China's ancient herbal doctors, was Zhang Zhongjing (or Zhang Ji). His text, *Shang Han Za Bing Lun* (*Treatise on Cold Damage*), contained over 100 effective formulas, many of which are still used today.[38] An early herbalist, Tao Hongjing, reorganized the *Shen Nong Ben Cao Jing* (the earliest Chinese herbal materia medica). He added 365 new herbs, which brought the total number of herbs to 730 and divided the herbs into categories and "qualities," which he recorded in a book. This early classic greatly impacted the study of herbs in future generations. The earliest Tang dynasty herbal dictionary is thought to be entirely based on it.[38] In other

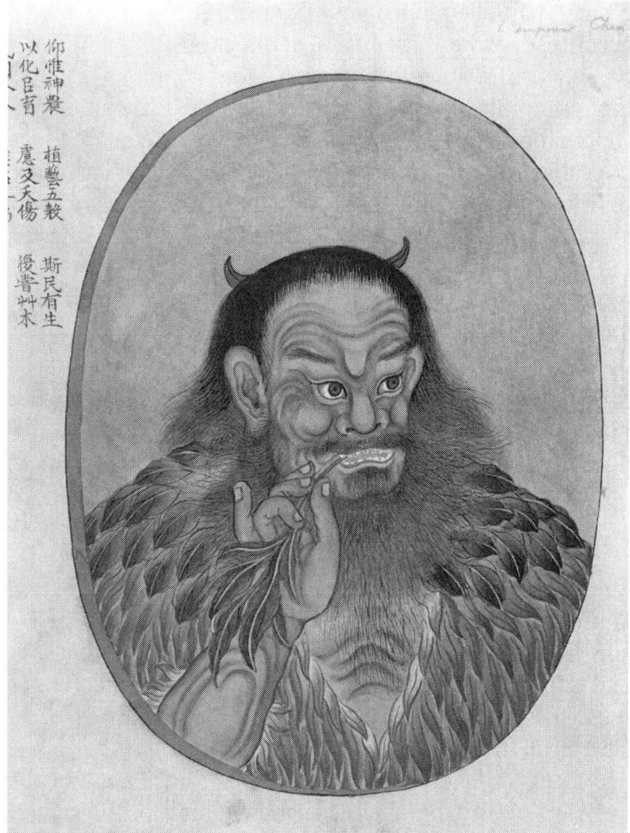

FIGURE 9.9 Shen Nong.

classic texts, there are early written accounts from 180 BCE that describe herbs still used today in Chinese medicine.[5]

Safety Issues

There are approximately 6,000 different medicinal substances listed in the Chinese pharmacopoeia; about 600 different herbs are used today.[42] Because herbal medicines are considered dietary supplements, the manufacturer does not have to prove the product's safety and effectiveness before it is marketed.[34] According to federal regulation of dietary supplements, manufacturers are expected to make sure their products are safe by processing them consistently and by meeting quality standards. Good manufacturing practices (GMP) regulations went into effect in 2008 for large companies and was phased in for small companies in 2010.[34] GMP delineates what manufacturers should be doing to make their products safe.

Many Chinese herbs are available over the counter; however, other than remedies for minor ailments, they may not be safe for public use.[43] Chinese herbs should be prescribed by a qualified practitioner who has made a full diagnosis, making the remedies safe for everyone.[43] The problems that have occurred have been because an unqualified practitioner has prescribed the herbs and may have prescribed them in an untraditional way or the herb was made with poor quality control. In rare instances (1 in 10,000 experiences), an allergic reaction from using the herbs might occur (e.g., an herb used for skin diseases).[43] If individuals have poor digestive functions, a more common reaction is a gastrointestinal response, which might include constipation or diarrhea, nausea, or bloating. It could be that the side effect may occur if the herbal formula is not quite right for the needs of the individual.[44] A suggestion is to look for a practitioner who is registered with the Register of Chinese Herbal Medicine.[45] These practitioners are fully informed about herbals and their safe use and they will follow detailed guidelines and a code of practice produced by the Register.[43] Keep in mind, however, that even though the Chinese herbal doctor or practitioner may prescribe the herbs, it is the Chinese herbal pharmacist who prepares and dispenses them, even though he or she is not registered to practice herbal medicine.[43]

Herbal Properties and Classification

Many Chinese herbs have been shown to have antibiotic, antifungal, and anticancer properties. In TCM, herbal medicine is used along with acupuncture in treating illnesses and is thought to strengthen people for acupuncture. Herbal medicine is also prescribed to balance the body.[38,43] The classification of herbs is quite varied. They may be classified as upper, middle, and lower. Upper herbs are thought to expel illnesses, but their strength and function are gentle. It might take months or years for these herbs to have an effect. Middle herbs are thought to cure illness. If taken to eliminate suffering, they are to be used quickly, but if taken to increase life span, they should be taken gradually. Lower herbs are used to attack the organism causing the illness and are to be taken short term.[46]

Herbs also may be classified according to direction. There are herbs that work up, down, outward, and inward. Herbal medicines that work from inside out are considered yin (preparations taken internally) and those that work from outside in are yang (e.g., ointments used on the skin).

Herbs also may be classified according to temperature. There are herbs that warm and those that cool. An example of a cold herb might be *zhi mu* or the *Anemarrhena* rhizome, which is used to lower a high temperature due to a fever; the correct dosage would ensure it is not brought too low.[42] Hot herbs are used for severe and often acute internal coldness. Warm herbs are thought to create movement and warmth.[47]

Chinese pharmacists have also categorized and identified herbs based on their taste. *Sour* tasting herbs are indicated for use in prolonged cough, chronic diarrhea, urinary incontinence, and other conditions related to hypometabolism (underperformance).[42] In TCM, these diseases are seen as deficiencies or cold patterns. *Bitter* herbs are commonly used for the acute stage of infectious diseases, as well as the patterns of damp-heat or damp-cold, such as in arthritis. They are identified as herbs that descend, dry, and detoxify.[47] *Sweet* herbs are thought to tone and harmonize many body systems such as the digestive, respiratory, immune, and endocrine systems. They are thought to promote urination. Sweet tasting herbs inhibit pain due to muscle constriction and are commonly used for treating dry cough and dysfunction of the gastrointestinal tract such as spleen and stomach disharmony. *Spicy* herbs are thought to disperse and circulate qi and have an overall effect of activating and enhancing metabolism. They are thought to vitalize the blood to promote good blood circulation and stimulate the sweat glands to perspire. Spicy herbs are commonly used in the treatment of external patterns (catching a cold). *Salty* herbs detoxify (e.g., sore throat),[47] purge, and open the bowels. In addition, salty herbs have the function of softening firm masses and fibrous adhesions; therefore, they are often indicated for sores, inflammatory masses, cysts, and connective tissue proliferation.[42] Finally, herbs may be classified as related to yin (sour, bitter, and salty tastes) and yang (acrid, sweet), or as herbs that tonify or stagnate.[43]

Forms of Herbal Preparations

Usually, it is not one herb but a combination of herbs mixed together that achieves the desired effect. A decoction (concentrated tea or soup) is the traditional way to prepare herbal medicine. The practitioner weighs out a day's dosage of herbs and combines them in a bag. Enough bags are given for the length of days required. The patient will boil a bag each day for 30–60 minutes and consume it several times during that day.

Herbs also may be given as granulated herbs or highly concentrated powdered extracts. First, the herbs are prepared in the same manner as the decoction, but then they are dehydrated to leave a powder residue. The powders are mixed together for each patient in a custom formula. The patient will take it home and boil it for consumption, in effect, re-creating the decoction.[42]

Premade formulas may consist of 4 to 20 herbs mixed according to a formula and then delivered as pills, tablets, capsules, powders, alcohol extracts, or water extracts. Some herbs are also made into a paste and applied to the skin.[40] Please see **TABLE 9.2** for 15 commonly used Chinese herbs, reprinted with permission from S. Dharmananda.[41]

Table 9.2
Fifteen Most Commonly Used Chinese Herbals

Astragalus (huangqi)	The long tap roots of astragalus are, today, the most commonly used herb material in China. Astragalus normalizes immune responses (used for immune deficiency, allergies, and autoimmunity), benefits digestive functions, and treats disorders of the skin from burns to carbuncles. Astragalus is used as a promoter of the functions of several other herbs, such as salvia and tang-kuei (mentioned below). It is used in the treatment of AIDS and hepatitis, for chronic colitis, senility, and cardiovascular diseases. Cancer patients who take this herb can often avoid the white blood cell deficiencies (leukopenia) that occur with chemotherapy. The root is rich in polysaccharides and flavonoids that produce the beneficial effects. Astragalus may be used by itself, usually as a liquid extract, or in combination with other herbs in the form of teas, pills, or tablets. Dosage is from 1–60 grams per day, depending on the application and form. Caution: Some individuals may experience flatulence and abdominal bloating from use of astragalus.
Atractylodes (baizhu)	The rhizomes of atractylodes are considered very important to the treatment of digestive disorders and problems of moisture accumulation. The herb helps move moisture (and nutrients) from the digestive tract to the blood, reducing problems of diarrhea, gas, and bloating, and helps move moisture from the body tissues to the bladder for elimination, alleviating edema. The herb is frequently included in tonic prescriptions, and the herb is rarely used by itself. Dosage is from 200 milligrams in capsules and tablets to 15 grams per day in the form of decoction. Caution: Persons suffering from a hot and dry condition may experience worsening of those symptoms if large amounts of atractylodes are used.
Bupleurum (chaihu)	The thin roots of bupleurum are one of the most frequently used herbs in the Japanese practice of Oriental medicine. Doctors in Japan have found it useful in the treatment of liver diseases, skin ailments, arthritis, menopausal syndrome, withdrawal from corticosteroid use, nephritis, stress-induced ulcers, and mental disorders. The roots are rich in saponins that reduce inflammation and regulate hormone levels. The herb is not used by itself, but rather in formulas with about four to twelve ingredients, made as teas, pills, or tablets. Dosage ranges from a few hundred milligrams of powder to about 15 grams in tea per day. Caution: Some individuals may experience dizziness or headaches from use of bupleurum.
Cinnamon (guizhi and rougi)	The twigs (guizhi) and bark (rougi) of this large tropical tree are said to warm the body, invigorate the circulation, and harmonize the energy of the upper and lower body. Modern studies demonstrate that cinnamon reduces allergy reactions. Traditionally, cinnamon twig is used when the peripheral circulation is poor and cinnamon bark is used when the entire body is cold. If the upper body is warm and the lower body is cold, then cinnamon will correct the imbalance. Cinnamon is usually cooked together with other herbs to make a warming tea, or powdered with other herbs to make a pill or tablet that regulates circulation of blood. Dosage is 0.3–3 grams of bark and up to 9 grams of twig per day. Caution: Large amounts of cinnamon are irritating to the liver and should not be used by those with inflammatory liver disorders.
Coptis (huanglian)	This rhizome (underground stem) is one of the most bitter herbs used in Chinese medicine. It is rich in alkaloids that inhibit infections and calm nervous agitation; it is usually combined with other bitter-tasting herbs, such as phellodendron, scute, and gardenia, to promote these actions. Examples of its many uses include treatment of skin diseases, intestinal infections, hypertension, and insomnia. Coptis is a close relative of an extremely bitter and very useful American herb, goldenseal. Because of its taste, coptis is most often used in the form of pills or tablets. Typical dosage is from a few hundred milligrams of powder to 3 grams in decoction per day. Caution: Regular use of coptis in large dosage may cause diarrhea.

(Continues)

Table 9.2
Fifteen Most Commonly Used Chinese Herbals (Continued)

Ginger (jiang)	The fibrous rhizome of this herb is highly spicy and said to benefit digestion, neutralize poisons in food, ventilate the lungs, and warm the circulation to the limbs. Today, ginger is commonly used as a spice in cooking; as a medicine it has been shown helpful in counteracting nausea from various causes including morning sickness, motion sickness, and food contamination. Many herbalists use ginger in the treatment of cough (it acts as an expectorant) and common cold. Ginger is used in making teas and the powder is encapsulated for easy consumption. Typical dosage is from a few milligrams used as an assistant in herb formulas to about 3 grams per day in making decoctions. Instant tea granules (sugar or honey base) are available. Caution: Persons who suffer from dryness—dry cough, thirst, dry constipation, etc.—may find that ginger worsens the condition.
Ginseng (renshen)	The root has long been cherished as a disease-preventive and a life preserver. It calms the spirit, nourishes the viscera, and helps one gain wisdom. Modern applications include normalizing blood pressure, regulating blood sugar, resisting fatigue, increasing oxygen utilization, and enhancing immune functions. Traditionally, the root is cooked in a double boiler to make a tea, used either alone or with several other herbs. Today, teas can be made quickly from carefully prepared extracts in liquid or dry form; ginseng powder is made into tablets or encapsulated, and ginseng formulas are available in numerous forms for easy consumption. Typical dosage is 0.5–3.0 grams. Higher doses may be used over the short term for specific therapeutic actions: in China 30 grams is recommended to treat shock (sudden hypotension). Caution: Excessive consumption of ginseng can lead to nervousness and may produce hormonal imbalance in women.
Hoelen (fuling)	This herb is a large fungus that grows on pine roots. It is used to alleviate irritation of the gastro-intestinal system and, like atractylodes, it helps transport moisture out of the digestive system into the blood stream and from the various body tissues to the bladder. When bits of the pine root are included in the herb material it is called fushen; the combination of the fungus and pine produces a mild sedative action. This herb, because it is quite mild, is mostly used in making decoctions or dried decoctions, with a dosage equivalent of about 10–15 grams per day. The herb is non-toxic and rarely causes any adverse effects.
Licorice (gancao)	The roots have an extremely sweet taste (but are also bitter) and are said to neutralize toxins, relieve inflammation, and enhance digestion. In Europe, a drug has been made from licorice extract that heals gastric ulcers. Licorice is used by Chinese doctors in the treatment of hepatitis, sore throat, muscle spasms, and, when baked with honey, for treatment of hyperthyroidism and heart valve diseases. Traditionally, licorice is thought to enhance the effectiveness of herb formulas and is used to moderate the flavor of herb teas; as a result, it is found in about one-third of all Chinese herb prescriptions. Licorice powder is encapsulated for easy consumption or mixed with other herbs and tableted. Dosage is from very small amounts (a few hundred milligrams) to 15 grams per day in decoction used to treat viral hepatitis. Caution: Excessive consumption of licorice over an extended period to time can cause sodium/potassium imbalance with symptoms of tachycardia and/or edema.
Ma-huang (mahuang)	The stem-like leaves when taken in a dose of several grams stimulate perspiration, open the breathing passages, and invigorate the central nervous system energy. It has been shown that most of these effects are due to two alkaloid components, ephedrine and pseudoephedrine, both of them having been made into modern drugs (for asthma and sinus congestion, respectively). In addition, the stimulating action of ma-huang has led to its use as a metabolic enhancer (burns calories more quickly) for those who are trying to lose weight. Ma-huang also has anti-inflammatory actions useful in treating some cases of arthralgia and myalgia. Ma-huang can be made into a tea, or used in extract form; powdered ma-huang is rarely used. Dosage range is 1–9 grams/day, usually in two or three divided doses. Caution: The stimulant effect of ma-huang can cause insomnia and agitation; persons with very high blood pressure may find this symptom worsened by use of ma-huang.
Peony (baishao and chihshao)	The root of this common flower is used to regulate the blood. It relaxes the blood vessels, reduces platelet sticking, nourishes the blood, and promotes circulation to the skin and extremities. The root of both wild and cultivated peonies are used. The wild peony yields "red peony" (chihshao), a fibrous root that is especially used for stimulating blood circulation. The cultivated peony yields "white peony" (baishao), a dense root that nourishes the blood. Peony is often combined with tang-kuei, licorice, or other herbs mentioned here to enhance or control their effects. The dosage range is from 0.5–15 grams per day. Peony rarely causes any adverse reactions.

Table 9.2
Fifteen Most Commonly Used Chinese Herbals (Continued)

Rehmannia (dihuang)	The root of this herb is a dark, moist herb that is extensively used to nourish the blood and the hormonal system. It is frequently used in the treatment of problems of aging, because of its ability to restore the levels of several declining hormones. There are two forms of the herb that are currently used: one, designated shengdihuang or raw rehmannia, is given to reduce inflammation and is included in many formulas for autoimmune disorders; the other is designated shoudihuang or cooked rehmannia, and is used as a nourishing tonic. Often, the two forms are combined together in equal proportions to address inflammatory problems that are related to the lack of adequate levels of regulating hormones. The herb is mainly used in making decoctions or dried decoctions, with a dosage of 10–30 grams per day. Caution: Persons with weak digestion and tendency to experience loose stool or diarrhea may find that this herb, especially cooked rehmannia, worsens those symptoms.
Rhubarb (dahuang)	This large root was one of the first herbs that the Western world imported from China. It serves as a very reliable laxative, and also has other benefits: enhancing appetite when taken before meals in small amounts, promoting blood circulation and relieving pain in cases of injury or inflammation, and inhibiting intestinal infections. Rhubarb also reduces autoimmune reactions. The impact of rhubarb is influenced by how it is prepared; if it is cooked for a long period of time, the laxative actions are reduced but other actions are retained. Typical dosage is 0.5–3 grams per day. Caution: Rhubarb, alone or in formulas, should not be used by those with irritable bowel conditions, as it may cause cramping and diarrhea.
Salvia (danshen)	The deep red roots of this Chinese sage plant have become an important herb during the past two decades even though it was used for centuries before that. It is applied in almost all cases where the body tissues have been damaged by disease or injury; thus, it is given for post-stroke syndrome, traumatic injury, chronic inflammation and/or infection, and degenerative diseases. It is best known for its ability to promote circulation in the capillary beds—the so-called microcirculation system. In addition, salvia lowers blood pressure, helps reduce cholesterol, and enhances function of the liver. It may be consumed alone or with other herbs, in wines, teas, pills, or tablets; dosage is 1–20 grams per day. Salvia rarely causes any adverse reactions.
Tang-kuei (danggui)	The root has been long respected as a blood-nourishing agent. It has its highest rate of use among women because tang-kuei will help to regulate uterine blood flow and contraction, but when employed in complex formulas it can be used by both men and women to nourish the blood, moisten the intestines, improve the circulation, calm tension, and relieve pain. Tang-kuei is frequently said to have estrogenic effects, but this is not a valid claim. The recommended dosage for tang-kuei is 0.5–9 grams per day. Tang-kuei may be made as a tea or cooked with chicken to make soup (the taste is quite strong), but it is often used today as a powder, encapsulated or made into tablets, alone or with other herbs. Caution: Some individuals find that tang-kuei causes nausea or loose stool.

Source: Courtesy of Institute for Traditional Medicine.

Chinese Herbal Medicine Research Results

Chinese herbal medicines have been studied by the NCCAM for use in cancer, heart disease, diabetes, and HIV/AIDS.[34] The following list presents studies reported by the NCCAM of some of the herbs listed in Table 9.2:

- *Astragalus:* Historically used in Chinese medicine to support and enhance the immune system. There is not an abundance of research, however, regarding astragalus for any health condition because high-quality clinical trials (studies in people) are generally lacking. Some preliminary evidence indicates that astragalus, either alone or in combination with other herbs, may have potential benefits for the immune system, heart, and liver, and as an adjunctive therapy for cancer. At this writing, NCCAM-funded investigators are studying the effect of astragalus on the immune system.
- *Cinnamon (guizhi and rougi):* The twigs and bark are said to improve circulation, reduce allergy attacks, and harmonize the upper and lower body. No research at NCCAM.
- *Ginger (jiang):* Ginger has been used to aid digestion, neutralize poisons in food, and counteract nausea. It has also been used for rheumatoid arthritis, osteoarthritis, and joint and muscle pain. The NCCAM reports that some studies suggest that the short-term use of ginger can safely relieve pregnancy-related nausea and vomiting, but are mixed on whether ginger is effective for nausea caused by motion, chemotherapy, or surgery. In addition, the studies are unclear as to whether

ginger is effective in treating rheumatoid arthritis, osteoarthritis, or joint and muscle pain. Ongoing studies are investigating the general safety and effectiveness of ginger's use for health purposes, as well as its active components and effects on inflammation. Also, ongoing studies are investigating the effects of ginger dietary supplements on joint inflammation, rheumatoid arthritis, and osteoporosis.

- *Ginseng (renshen):* The root has been used for numerous conditions and support for overall health. Modern applications include normalizing blood pressure, regulating blood sugar, resisting fatigue, increasing oxygen utilization, and enhancing immune functions. Studies reported at the NCCAM have shown that Asian ginseng may lower blood glucose, and indicate possible beneficial effects on immune function. Most evidence is preliminary (based on small clinical trials). Ongoing research is studying the herb's potential role in treating insulin resistance, cancer, and Alzheimer's disease.
- *Licorice (gancao):* Licorice contains a compound called glycyrrhizin (or glycyrrhizic acid). The roots have an extremely sweet taste (but are also bitter) and are said to neutralize toxins, relieve inflammation, enhance digestion, heal gastric ulcers, and treat hepatitis. The NCCAM reports that an injectable form of licorice extract—not available in the United States—has been shown to have beneficial effects against hepatitis C in clinical trials, but an oral form has not been studied. The NCCAM reports that more research is needed before reaching any conclusions and that not enough reliable data has been collected to determine whether licorice is effective for any condition.

The following Chinese herbs have been researched and reported on in journals and texts other than at the NCCAM Web site:

- *Atractylodes (baizhu):* The rhizomes of atractylodes are considered very important to the treatment of digestive disorders and problems of moisture accumulation. The herb has also been investigated for possible antitumor properties. A laboratory research study of baizhu indicated that the herb causes apoptosis (programmed cell death) of human leukemia cells.[48] A study on rats to assess gastric emptying and intestinal propulsion indicated that baizhu promoted gastrointestinal motility.[49] Besides *Atractylodes macrocephala*, there are several other species of *Atractylodes*, including *carlinoidses, chinensis, comosa, cuneata, erosodentata, japonica, koreana, ovata,* and *rubra*.[50] Japonica was shown to have hypoglycemic (lowering blood sugar) and anti-inflammatory actions.[51] See **FIGURE 9.10** for an image of *Atractylodes macrocephala*.[52]
- *Ma-huang:* Ma-huang is a tall shrub with many branches that grows mostly in the desert. This herb was used in Chinese medicine for 500 years to treat asthma. It contains two alkaloid components, ephedrine and pseudoephedrine, which are used as modern drugs for treating asthma and sinus congestion. The stimulating action of ma-huang led to its use as a metabolic enhancer (burns calories more quickly) for those trying to lose weight. Adverse reactions to ma-huang were heart-related: sudden deaths, strokes, mini-strokes, rapid heartbeat, and heart attacks. In 2000, the FDA issued a warning about the use of ma-huang in dietary supplements, and in 2004 banned the use of *Ephedra sinica* and active ephedrine alkaloids.[53] The plant, however, is not banned and certain species of ma-haung may be found in medicines today.[54] There is scientific evidenced that ma-huang combined with caffeine is an effective weight loss product (but has dangerous side effects), and is effective for asthma and chronic obstructive pulmonary disease.[55]

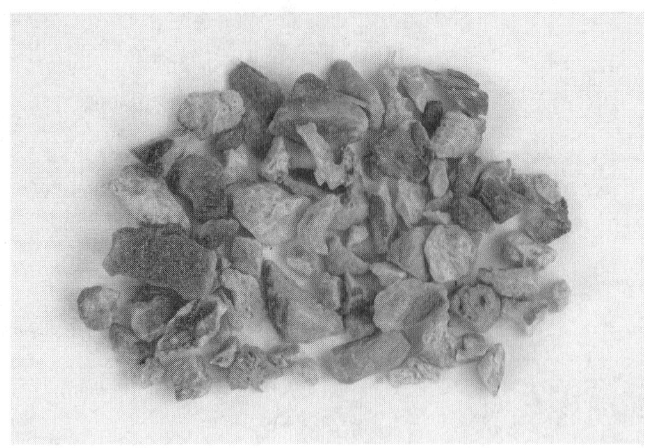

FIGURE 9.10 *Atractylodes macrocephala.*

- *Peony (baishao and chihshao):* The root of this common flower is used to regulate the blood. It relaxes the blood vessels, reduces platelet sticking, nourishes the blood, and promotes circulation to the skin and extremities. Numerous studies of the effects of the peony root have been conducted, and results show that the white peony root has a strong antispasmodic effect as well as analgesic, sedative, and anticonvulsive effects. A decoction of the root has bacteriostatic action on staphylococcus. A tea made from the dried crushed petals has been used as a cough remedy and for the inflammation from arthritis.[56]
- *Rhubarb (dahuang):* This root has laxative effects, promotes circulation, and inhibits intestinal infections. No U.S.-based studies were found, but there are Chinese-based research studies. In a study of 60 patients with liver cirrhosis, a decoction of rhubarb and peony showed an effective rate of 90 percent in treating liver

cirrhosis, in comparison to another medicine that had 73.33 percent effectiveness.[56] Other studies showed the effectiveness of rhubarb for cancer,[56,57] pregnancy-induced hypertension,[58] and hepatitis (liver disease).[59] See **FIGURE 9.11**.

- *Salvia (danshen):* Chinese sage plant. Proponents of salvia claim it is beneficial when body tissues have been damaged by disease or injury (e.g., post-stroke syndrome, traumatic injury, chronic inflammation and/or infection, and degenerative diseases). It promotes circulation, lowers blood pressure, helps reduce cholesterol, and enhances function of the liver. The research studies on salvia are inconclusive because the studies were poorly designed, were too few in number, were on animals, or had other problems such as not proving safety and effectiveness. Studies were related to asthmatic bronchitis, burn healing, cardiovascular disease, glaucoma, liver disease, and ischemic stroke. One of the outcomes of the studies was establishing the possibility of interaction between salvia and warfarin (a drug to prevent blood clotting).[60] Salvia is known to affect blood clotting and could cause hemorrhaging if a patient is taking warfarin and salvia at the same time.[60]

By reviewing the scientific studies of these Chinese herbs, we can discern that Western medical science believes Chinese herbal medicine needs much more scientific study. Just because more studies are needed does not, however, mean that these drugs are not effective, nor does it mean they are. We have to keep in mind that many of these herbal medicines have been used for hundreds of years, and there must be a good reason that practitioners would continue to make their formulas and use them for people who are ill or injured. If an herb or combination of herbs were found to achieve a desired effect, it would follow that the herb would be used again, and again, and again. To satisfy Western science, however, the future will surely bring more and better research studies of herbal medicines.

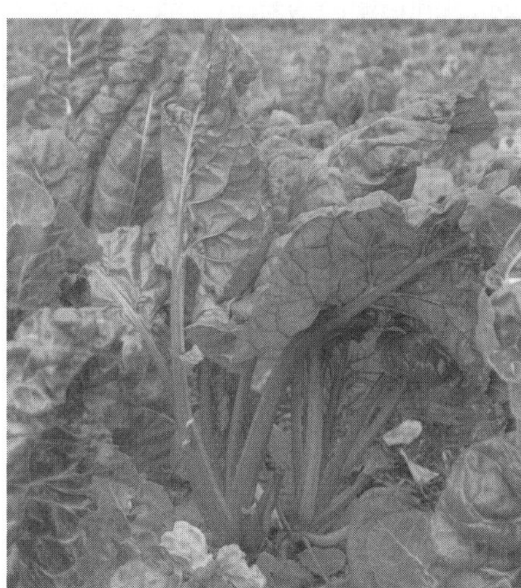

FIGURE 9.11 Rhubarb.

We have just explored two of the mainstream traditional Chinese medicine treatments, acupuncture and herbal medicines. Massage, diet, and exercise are also important Chinese treatments and are presented next.

WHAT IS CHINESE MASSAGE THERAPY?

Chinese massage or Oriental body therapy has been used in China for over 2,000 years.[61] It is a type of therapeutic bodywork called *tui na* (also spelled tuina and pronounced tway-nah), which means to "push" and "pull."[1] The focus of tuina is to stimulate or subdue qi energy in the body and bring the patient's body back into balance. A wrist pulse diagnosis aids the practitioner to find the meridians that need work. The use of hand techniques to massage soft tissue (muscles and tendons) is combined with acupressure to directly affect the flow of qi, and manipulation techniques to realign musculoskeletal and ligament relationships.

The following four styles are taught in the main schools in China:

Rolling method: The rolling method is used for joint and soft tissue problems, insomnia, migraines, and high blood pressure.

One-finger method: The one-finger method is similar to a deep tissue work massage called Shiatsu. In the one-finger method, practitioners push points (tsubo) along the meridian with the tip of the thumb or finger. It is supposed to help chronic and internal problems, pediatric patients, and gynecological problems.[1]

Nei gung method: The *nei gung* method utilizes *nei gong* qi energy exercises and specific massage methods to revitalize depleted energy systems.[61]

Bone setting method: The bone setting method specializes in joint injuries and nerve pain. Manipulative massage is used to realign the musculoskeletal and ligament relationships.

The two tuina methods most used today are the rolling and the one-finger method. The rolling method uses vigorous rolling with the knuckles and the back of the hand on body parts. Along with that could be "scrubbing" with the pinky finger side of the hand, applying elbow pressure, pulling at the back and spine with splayed fingers and interlocked thumbs, and brisk tapping with the cupped hands or edges of the palms.[62] See **BOX 9.5** for more on tuina rolling.

One-finger massage uses the index finger or thumb to stimulate tsubo points on the meridians. Dependent on the body condition, the tuina practioner will make a decision about which moves to use (pushing, pulling, nipping, strong pinching, chopping, rubbing, or kneading).[62] Sometimes walking massage is used with the aid of a steel bar frame that the practitioner hangs onto while walking on the client (legs, back). See **BOX 9.6** for tuina sensations.

Box 9.5

Tuina Rolling

"A favorite move for a client's leg now is rolling my forearm and wrist. With tui na, I can use my whole arm. The movements are more rapid and can wake the muscles up. Runners love it!"

—Erica Williams, a Western-trained massage therapist who added tuina to her practice

Source: Excerpts from Kovach V. The tui na touch: the intensity of Chinese medicine at your fingertips [Massagetherapy.com]. Available at: http://www.massagetherapy.com/articles/index.php/article_id/The-Tui-Na-Touch. Accessed August 18, 2010. Originally published in *Massage & Bodywork* magazine, April/May 2003.

Box 9.6

Tuina Sensations

"A few moments later, I'm experiencing another set of surreal sensations: the back of my neck is being kneaded and grasped with upward motions that make my whole spinal column feel like it's floating, suspended, above the table."

—Quote online from a person receiving tuina massage

Source: Excerpts from Kovach V. The tui na touch: the intensity of Chinese medicine at your fingertips [Massagetherapy.com]. Available at: http://www.massagetherapy.com/articles/index.php/article_id/The-Tui-Na-Touch. Accessed August 18, 2010. Originally published in *Massage & Bodywork* magazine, April/May 2003.

Because tuina massage focuses on specific problems, rather than being used for generalized massage, it is becoming an excellent adjunct therapy for many joint injuries and muscle strains, and is often used as a complement to traditional Western massage (e.g., Swedish-style massage).[62]

WHAT IS CHINESE DIET AND EXERCISE THERAPY?

Diet Therapy

The Chinese believe that the diet is one of the sources of qi energy, and is grounded in the five element and eight guiding principles theory.[42] Rather than emphasizing a balance of protein, carbohydrates, and fats, foods are identified as having yin and yang, warming and cooling, drying and moistening properties. According to Chinese medicine, if a person presents with a cold or damp condition, they should not eat raw fruits and vegetable (yin foods) because those would cause a further loss of body heat and fluid secretion.[1] They might be encouraged to eat ginger to help with digestion and barley to help with dampness.[63] Dampness is a by-product of eating popular foods such as cheese, yougurt, white flour, and sugar, and the person might present symptoms of sinus-type problems and loose stools or constipation.[63]

On the other hand, a person who has a hot or dry diagnosis would be advised not to eat fried, broiled, high fat, or spicy foods (yang) because they are warming foods and would generate even more heat and stimulate circulation.[1] The Chinese diet is planned to optimize digestion and aid organ function. Foods not found on the menu are cold, raw foods such as salads, iced drinks, and frozen foods because it is difficult for the body to process them.[63] The type of foods selected are built around steamed rice, cooked vegetables, and small quantities of animal protein or beans.

Exercise Therapy (Qi Gong and Tai Chi Ch'uan)

Qi Gong Exercise

Exercise in TCM includes qi gong, a practice that is supposed to optimize the flow of qi. Qi gong exercises are intended to regulate the mind and breathing; therefore, posture, movement, breathing, meditation, and visualization are all incorporated. Qi gong can be considered a psychosomatic therapy because it has a physical component but also helps to regulate and balance the mind. It is a practice that works to ease and regulate breathing while storing up energy in the body.[1] Research shows that qi gong can help premenstrual pain; head, neck, shoulder, back, and wrist pain; headaches/migraines; and the side effects of chemotherapy.[64] Two types of qi gong are practiced: internal and external. Internal qi gong is used to maintain health by regulating qi and harmonizing the internal energy of the body. Internal qi gong movement postures are the most common form of practice today. Certain movements and breath work or visualization gather and circulate qi in the body. External qi gong is used by the practitioner to transfer qi to another person for healing purposes, and is similar to other bodywork modalities in the West, such as therapeutic touch. More about qi gong may be found in Chapter 15 of this text. An example[64] of a simple qi gong arm-swing exercise follows.

Begin with feet firmly planted, shoulder-width apart. Rotate on the heels while turning left to right from the hips. Arms hang limply at the sides, swinging as the lower body turns from side to side. Lead from the hips, not from the shoulders.

Breathing: Breathe consciously, in and out through the nose. Use deep, low belly breaths from the diaphragm.

Repetition: 10–15 minutes each day, in morning and evening.

Benefits: Prevents stagnation (or pain) in shoulder, hip, knee and ankle joints, wrists, and back.

Tai Chi Ch'uan Exercise

Tai chi (simplified spelling) is another Chinese medicine exercise that is practiced by millions of Chinese each day and is growing in popularity in the United States. It originates from the martial arts, complete with self-defense applications. Young and old can learn and use it. Tai chi involves very slow movements. Those who practice it are likely to get stronger, improve balance, improve flexibility, and have less anxiety.[63] There are several forms of tai chi, some short (12 movements) and some long (55 movements). One example is the tai chi form 24 Taiji, also known as Standard 24 Form; as its name suggests, it contains 24 movements[65] (see **FIGURE 9.12**).

A video of tai chi Form 24 Taiji can be accessed at the Web site. Tai Chi instructors say that it is suitable for the young and the old because people are taught stretching and flexing joints, and it reflects Chinese traditional philosophy.[66] Tai chi is discussed further in Chapter 15 of this text.

Research on Qi Gong and Tai Chi

Researchers in Arizona, California, and North Carolina analyzed 77 studies related to tai chi and qi gong. The studies were published between 1993 and 2007 and included 6,410 participants. Their review indicated the two practices can have a positive effect on bone health, cardiorespiratory fitness, balance, accidental falls, and psychological benefits (stress reduction).[34,67] A 10-year research trial through Harvard, Emory, and Yale Universities published in the *Journal of the American Geriatrics Society*[65] found that tai chi practitioners had overall better balance and reduced their risk of falling by 47.5 percent.[65] A study by Lan, et al.[68] found that those who practice tai chi had a reduced risk of cardiovascular disease due to improved vagal nerve function. (Stimulation of the vagal nerve causes a reduction in heart rate or breathing.) A comprehensive review of randomized controlled studies to assess the health benefits of both qi gong and tai chi found a significant number of health benefits.[69]

CONCLUSION

This concludes the chapter on traditional Chinese medicine. You have been given a bird's eye view about TCM philosophy, diagnostics, and mainstream treatment methods. Please keep in mind that there is so much more to learn. We hope that you will be motivated to investigate and further explore more TCM concepts and practices.

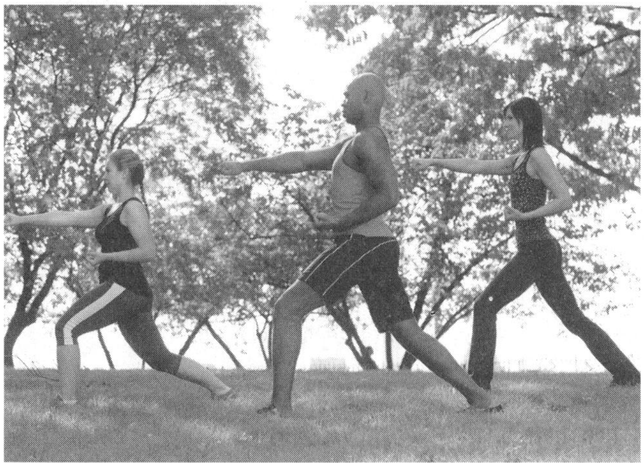

FIGURE 9.12 24 Movement Tai Chi.

Suggestions for Class Activities

1. Invite a traditional Chinese medicine doctor to class to discuss TCM philosophy and treatment modalities.
2. Research one or more of the Web sites listed for acupuncture research. Report your findings to the class.
3. Visit a Chinese pharmacy and note the types of herbals and their forms.
4. Ask a tai chi instructor to engage classmates in tai chi.
5. Invite a Chinese massage therapist to class to demonstrate tuina massage.
6. Go on a field trip to an herbal garden. Take pictures of various herbs.
7. Research the common Chinese herbs and assess if new information is revealed.
8. Research online several meridian charts including the triple heater meridian points chart.

Review Questions

1. What does TCM stand for?
2. Explain the theory of the meridians and the concept of qi.
3. What is the theory of yin and yang?
4. Name a yin organ and a yang organ.
5. What are the five elements, and how are they applied to traditional Chinese medicine?
6. What is different about the TCM observation diagnostic practice compared to traditional Western medicine practice?
7. Explain how TCM utilizes the tongue for diagnosis.
8. Compare and contrast TCM pulse diagnosis with traditional Western medicine's technique.
9. Name five different ways acupuncture may be given.
10. Compare and contrast moxibustion and cupping.
11. Which acupuncture style is used by U.S. medical doctors?

12. What does the research say about acupuncture?
13. What kind of training does a person need to have to become an acupuncturist?
14. Where in the United States can a person go for acupuncture school?
15. Name two properties of herbal medicines.
16. How may herbal plant therapy be classified?
17. What are the five taste classifications of herbal plant therapy?
18. What does the research show about the 15 most commonly used Chinese herbal medicines?
19. Describe what rolling massage and one-finger Chinese massage are.
20. What would the diet prescription be for someone who is considered cold/damp?
21. What is the purpose and function of qi gong exercise?
22. From what practice did tai chi originate?
23. How many movements are there in tai chi?
24. What advice would you give to someone considering going to a traditional Chinese medical practitioner or doctor?

Key Terms

acupuncture Procedure that increases the flow of qi energy to treat illness or provide local pain relief by the insertion of stainless steel needles at specified sites on the body.

acupuncture point injection Sterile syringes are used to inject vitamins or herbal products into the system via the trigger points.

auricular acupuncture Uses points in the ears that correspond to areas of the body and bodily symptoms.

chondritis Inflammation of a cartilage.

decoction The process of boiling a substance in water to extract its essence.

diagnosis Identification of a diseased condition.

diet therapy Prescribed to increase qi energy; it is grounded in the theories of five elements and eight guiding principles.

Doppler ultrasound A form of ultrasound that can detect and measure blood flow.

electro-acupuncture Mild electrical pulses are relayed via acupuncture needles to various trigger points in the skin.

endorphins Natural pain-killing substances produced in the human body and released by stress or trauma.

external qi gong The practice of transferring the practitioner's qi to another person for healing purposes. This form of qi gong is similar to other bodywork modalities in the West, such as therapeutic touch.

five elements (or tattwa) Earth, water, fire, air, and ether or space.

halitosis Offensive odor of the breath.

holistic A concept in medical practice upholding that all aspects of people's needs, psychological, physical, mental, emotional, and social, should be taken into account and seen as a whole.

incontinence Inability to control excretion of urine and feces.

internal qi gong Uses certain movements and breath work or visualization to gather and circulate qi in the body.

Japanese-style acupuncture Uses fewer and thinner needles with less stimulation than traditional Chinese acupuncture.

Korean acupuncture Uses points in the hand that correspond to areas of the body and bodily symptoms.

laser acupoint stimulation Uses rays or laser beams rather than acupuncture needles to facilitate the trigger point.

medial Pertaining to the middle.

medical acupuncture Acupuncture performed by a Western medical doctor.

meridians Unseen channels in the body in which qi energy circulates.

moxibustion The stimulation of an acupuncture point by burning herbs called moxa, which are placed at or near the point.

naturopathic medicine A system or method of treating disease that employs no surgery or synthetic drugs but uses special diets, herbs, vitamins, massage, and so on to assist the natural healing processes.

osteoarthritis A type of arthritis of the joints that leads to joint pain, stiffness, and swelling.

osteopathy A traditional medical system originally based on the premise that manipulation of the muscles and bones to promote structural integrity could restore or preserve health.

pathology The science or the study of the origin, nature, and course of diseases.

pharmacopoeia A pharmaceutical book that contains a list of drugs, their formulas, methods for making medicinal preparations, requirements and tests for their strength and purity, and other related information.

physiology The functions and activities of the body.

placebo A substance having no pharmacological effect but administered as a control in testing experimentally or clinically the efficacy of a biologically active preparation.

podiatrist A person qualified to diagnose and treat foot disorders.

putrid Having the odor of decaying flesh.

qi (chi) According to TCM, qi is a bodily energy that flows through unseen channels in the body called meridians. Illness is believed to occur when qi is blocked.

qi gong A type of energy therapy that uses gentle movement to access and redistribute energy surrounding and within the human body. Incorporates posture, movement, breathing, meditation, visualization, and conscious intent in order to move qi energy throughout the body.

intent in order to move qi energy throughout the body.

rancid Having a bad smell or taste. Fats and oils when stale become spoiled or rancid.

stagnate To stop developing, growing, progressing, or advancing.

tai chi A Chinese exercise system that uses slow, smooth body movements to achieve a state of relaxation of both body and mind.

tonify Gentle stimulation of an acupuncture point.

traditional Chinese herbal medicine (CHM) The study and use of plants for medicinal purposes.

tuina A type of massage to stimulate or subdue qi energy in the body and bring the patient's body back into balance.

urinary retention Holding urine in the urinary bladder.

veterinary acupuncture Acupuncture used on animals to treat a variety of conditions (e.g., arthritis and hip problems, back pain and disc disease, incontinence and urinary retention).

visceral organs Internal organs of the body, specifically those within the chest (as the heart or lungs) or abdomen.

World Health Organization The directing and coordinating authority for health within the United Nations system.

yin-yang Two energies that control different bodily systems but cannot exist without each other.

References

1. Reller P. A history of traditional Chinese medicine. 2008. Available at: http://www.acupuncturesf.com/history.html. Accessed August 3, 2010.
2. Freeman L, Lawlis G. *Mosby's complementary and alternative medicine: a research-based approach*. St. Louis: Mosby; 2001.
3. Purify Our Mind. History of traditional Chinese medicine. Available at: http://www.purifymind.com/HistoryMed.htm. Accessed August 3, 2010.
4. Burke A, Upchurch D, Dye C, Chyu L. Acupuncture use in the United States. *J Altern Complement Med*. 2006;12(7):639–648.
5. Pelletier K. *The best alternative medicine*. New York: Simon & Schuster; 2000.
6. Maciocia G. *The foundations of Chinese medicine: a comprehensive text for acupuncturists and herbalists*. Philadelphia: Churchill Livingstone; 2005.
7. Shen R. Concept of qi in traditional Oriental medicine. Available at: http://www.rotemshen.co.uk/Chinese%20Medicine.htm. Accessed August 4, 2010.
8. Compassionate Dragon Healing. Five elements table. Available at: http://www.compassionatedragon.com/astrology3.html. Accessed August 3, 2010.
9. Sacred Lotus Arts: Traditional Chinese Medicine. TCM diagnosis. Available at: http://www.sacredlotus.com/diagnosis/looking.cfm. Accessed August 4, 2010.
10. Yin Yang House. Pulse diagnosis in TCM acupuncture theory. Available at: http://www.yinyanghouse.com/theory/chinese/pulse_diagnosis#meridiancorrelations. Accessed August 5, 2010.
11. Chinese Medicine Sampler. Welcome. Available at: http://www.chinesemedicinesampler.com. Accessed August 5, 2010.
12. Acupages.com Acupuncture styles. Available at: http://www.acupages.com/Acupuncture-Center/Acupuncture-Styles.html. Accessed August 5, 2010.
13. Tiegen R. What is acupuncture? Available at: http://www.spineuniverse.com/treatments/alternative/what-acupuncture. Accessed August 8, 2010.
14. All 4 Natural Health.com. How is acupuncture done? Some methods explained. Available at: http://www.all4naturalhealth.com/how-is-acupuncture-done.html. Accessed August 10, 2010.
15. Suvow S. History of acupuncture in China. 1998. Available at: http://www.acupuncturecare.com/acupunct.htm. Accessed August 10, 2010.
16. Beck M. Decoding an ancient therapy: high-tech tools show how acupuncture works in treating arthritis, back pain, other ills. *Wall Street Journal*. March 22, 2010.
17. Xun L, Jun Hu, Wang X, Zhang H, Liu J. Moxibustion and other acupuncture point stimulation methods to treat breech presentation: a systematic review of clinical trials. *Chin Med*. 2009;4:4doi:10.1186/1749-8546-4-4
18. Russell M. Methods in acupuncture. Available at: http://ezinearticles.com/?Methods-in-Acupuncture&id=435536. Accessed August 10, 2010.
19. Fratkin J. Acupuncture styles [Acupuncture.com: Gateway to Chinese Medicine Health and Wellness Newsletter]. February 2008. Available at: http://www.acupuncture.com/newsletters/m_feb08/Acupuncture%20Styles.htm. Accessed August 14, 2010.
20. Tanaka T. Styles of acupuncture treatment. Available at: http://www.acupuncture-treatment.com/styles.html. Accessed August 14, 2010.
21. altMD. Acupuncture styles. Available at: http://www.altmd.com/Articles/Acupuncture-Styles. Accessed August 14, 2010.
22. Joswick D. What are the different styles of acupuncture? Available at: http://www.acufinder.com/Acupuncture+Information/Detail/What+are+the+different+styles+of+acupuncture+. Accessed August 14, 2010.
23. Blue Sky Natural Vet. Veterinary acupuncture. Available at: http://www.blueskynaturalvet.com/acupuncture.html. Accessed August 16, 2010.
24. Berman BM, Lao L, Langenberg P, Lee WL, Gilpin AMK, Hochberg MC. Effectiveness of acupuncture as adjunctive therapy in osteoarthritis of the knee: a randomized, controlled trial. *Ann Intern Med*. 2004;141(12):901–910.
25. Hollifield M, Sinclair-Lian N, Warner TD, Hammerschlag R. Acupuncture for posttraumatic stress disorder: a randomized controlled pilot trial. *J Nerv Ment Dis*. 2007.
26. Manheimer E, Zhang G, Udoff L, et al. Effect of acupuncture on rates of pregnancy and live birth among women undergoing in vitro fertilization: systematic review and meta-analysis. *Br Med J*. Published online February 2008.
27. Cherkin DC, Sherman KJ, Avins AL, et al. A randomized trial comparing acupuncture, simulated acupuncture, and usual care for chronic low back pain. *Arch Intern Med*. 2009;169(9):858–866.
28. Meade CS, Lukas SE, McDonald LJ, et al. A randomized trial of transcutaneous electric acupoint stimulation as adjunctive treatment for opioid detoxifiction. *J Subst Abuse Treat*. 2010;38(1):12–21.
29. Dhond RP, Yeh C, Park K, et al. Acupuncture modulates resting state connectivity in default and sensorimotor brain networks. *Pain*. 2008;136(3):407–418.
30. Linde K, Allais G, Brinkhaus B, et al. Acupuncture for tension-type headache. *Cochrane Database System Rev*. 2009;(1):CD007587.
31. Zhang RX, Li A, Liu B, et al. Electroacupuncture attenuates bone cancer-induced hyperalgesia and inhibits spinal preprodynorphin expression in a rat model. *Eur J Pain*. 2008;12(7):870–878.

32. Internet Health Library. Available at: http://www.internethealthlibrary.com/Therapies/Acupuncture.htm#top. Accessed August 17, 2010.
33. Singh S, Ernst E. *Trick or treatment: the undeniable facts about alternative medicine*. New York: Norton; 2008.
34. National Center for Complementary and Alternative Medicine. Acupuncture: an introduction. Available at: http://nccam.nih.gov/health/acupuncture/introduction.htm. Accessed August 12, 2010.
35. Accreditation Commission for Acupuncture and Oriental Medicine. ACAOM accreditation manual: structure, scope, process, eligibility requirements and standards. July 2008. Available at http://www.acaom.org/documents/file/policies_and_procedures_handbook(1).pdf. Accessed August 15, 2010.
36. American Board of Medical Acupuncture. Home page. Available at: http://www.dabma.org. Accessed August 15, 2010.
37. American Academy of Medical Acupuncture. Licensure. Available at: http://www.medicalacupuncture.org/acu_info/licensure.html. Accessed August 18, 2010.
38. Classical Chinese Herbal Therapy. History of traditional Chinese herbal medicine. Available at: http://www.traditionalchinesetherapy.com/content/history/. Accessed August 17, 2010.
39. TravelChinaGuide.com. Chinese herbal medicine. Available at: http://www.travelchinaguide.com/intro/medicine/herbal.htm. Accessed August 17, 2010.
40. Somerville R, ed. *The alternate advisor*. Alexandria, VA; Time-Life Books; 1997.
41. Dharmananda S. The lessons of Shennong: the basis of Chinese herb medicine. Available at: http://www.itmonline.org/arts/shennong.htm. Accessed August 14, 2010.
42. Traditional Chinese Medicine Information Page. Herbal therapy. Available at: http://www.tcmpage.com/herbal_therapy.html. Accessed August 14, 2010.
43. Bradford N, consultant ed. *The one-spirit encyclopedia of complementary health*. London: Octopus; 2000.
44. Dharmananda S. An introduction to Chinese herbs. Available at: http://www.itmonline.org/arts/herbintro.htm. Accessed August 14, 2010.
45. Professional Associations Chinese Herbal Medicine. Register of Chinese herbal medicine. Available at: http://www.internethealthlibrary.com/Therapies/MedicalHerbalism.htm. Accessed August 16, 2010.
46. Huang K. *The pharmacology of Chinese herbs*. 2nd ed. Boca Raton, FL: CRC Press; 1996.
47. Oriental Medicine. The properties of herbs. Available at: http://www.orientalmedicine.com/the-properties-of-herbs. Accessed August 16, 2010.
48. Huang HL, Chen CC, Yeh CY, Huang RL. Atractylodes reactive oxygen species mediation of baizhu-induced apoptosis in human leukemia cells. *J Ethnopharmacol*. 2005;97(1):21–29.
49. Zhu J, Leng E, Gui X, Chen D. Experimental study for effects of some Chinese herbals on gastrointestinal motility. Available at: http://alternativehealing.org/bai_zhu.htm#Gastrointestinal%20Motility. Accessed August 20, 2010.
50. Zhion.com. Atractylodes. February 22, 2009. Available at: http://www.zhion.com/herb/Atractylodes.html. Accessed August 20, 2010.
51. Han SB, Lee CW, Yoon YD, et al. Prevention of arthritic inflammation using an Oriental herbal combination BDX-1 isolated from *Achyranthes bidentata* and *Atractylodes japonica*. *Arch Pharm Res*. 2005;28(8):902–908.
52. Dong H, He L, Huang M, Dong Y. Anti-inflammatory components isolated from *Atractylodes macrocephala* Koidz. *Nat Prod Res*. 2008;22(16):1418–1427.
53. Mayo Clinic Health Manager. Ephedra (*Ephedra sinica*)/ma huang. Available at: http://www.mayoclinic.com/health/ephedra/NS_patient-ephedra. Accessed August 19, 2010.
54. EphedraOutlet. Available at: http://ephedraoutlet.com. Accessed August 19, 2010.
55. MedlinePlus. Ephedra (*Ephedra sinica*) ma huang. Available at: http://www.nlm.nih.gov/medlineplus/druginfo/natural/patient-ephedra.html. Accessed August 19, 2010.
56. ZhiZhong G. Clinical study of Dahuang (medicinal rhubarb)-Chishao (common peony) decoction on liver cirrhosis endotoxemia. *Chin J Info Trad Chin Med*.
57. Mantani N, Sekiya N, Sakai S, et al. Rhubarb use in patients treated with Kampo medicine—a risk for gastric cancer? *Yakugaku Zasshi*. 2002;122:403–405.
58. Zhang ZJ, Cheng WW, Yang YM. Study on low dose of processed rhubarb in preventing pregnancy induced hypertension. *Chung-Hua Fu Chan Ko Tsa Chih* [*Chin J Obstet Gynecol*]. 1994;29:463–464, 509.
59. Ding Y, Zhao L, Mei H, et al. Exploration of emodin to treat alpha-naphthylisothiocyanate-induced cholestatic hepatitis via anti-inflammatory pathway. *Eur J Pharmacol*. 2008;590(1–3):377–386.
60. Aetna InteliHealth. Danshen (*Salvia miltiorrhiza*). Available at: http://www.intelihealth.com/IH/ihtIH/W/8513/31402/351410.html?d = dmtContent. Accessed August 18, 2010.
61. Acupuncture.com. Tui na—Chinese bodywork therapy. Available at: http://www.acupuncture.com/qigong_tuina/tuinabodywork.htm. Accessed August 18, 2010.
62. Kovach, V. The tui na touch: the intensity of Chinese medicine at your fingertips [Massagetherapy.com]. Available at: http://www.massagetherapy.com/articles/index.php/article_id/60/The-Tui-Na-Touch. Accessed August 18, 2010.
63. Inner Light Wellness. The Chinese medicine diet. Available at: http://innerlight-wellness.net/articles/the-chinese-medicine-diet. Accessed August 19, 2010.
64. Marazita E. Alternative medicine: qi gong; Chinese exercise for better health. Available at: http://www.seattlepi.com/health/288318_altmed12.html. Accessed August 19, 2010.
65. Everyday Tai Chi. Tai chi form Beijing 24 teaching clips. Available at: http://www.everyday-taichi.com/tai-chi-form-beijing-24.html. Accessed August 19, 2010.
66. Garofalo, MP. Taijiquan 24 form. Available at: http://www.egreenway.com/taichichuan/short.htm. Accessed August 19, 2010.
67. Inner Idea. Tai chi: moving slow in a fast world. Available at: http://www.inneridea.com library/tai-chi-movements. Accessed August 19, 2010.
68. Lan, C., Chen, S., Lai, J., & Wong, M. (1999). The effect of Tai Chi on cardiorespiratory function in patients with coronary artery bypass surgery. *Med & Sci in Sports & Exercise*. 1999:31(5):634–638.
69. Jahnke R, Larkey LK, Rogers CE, Etnier J, Lin F. Comprehensive review of health benefits qigong and tai chi. *Sci Health Promotion*. 2010;24(6):e1–e25.

Alternative Medical Systems: Naturopathic and Homeopathic Medicine

LEARNING OBJECTIVES

As a result of reading this chapter, students will:

1. Assess the impact of naturopathy on the way health care has been conducted in the United States.
2. Explain how naturopathy functions as a medical system without using traditional medical diagnostics and treatments.
3. Compare and contrast the training of the naturopath to that of traditional allopathic physicians.
4. Analyze reasons why homeopathic substances can be effective when they are so diluted that not even a molecule of original substance is left.

WHAT IS NATUROPATHIC MEDICINE AND HOW DID IT DEVELOP?

Naturopathic medicine is a holistic, whole body health care system based on the belief that the body has the potential to heal itself and that the physician's role is to support the body's efforts.[1] Naturopathy has been defined in similar but different ways by three naturopathy pioneers[2]:

> *"Naturopathy is the perfected Science of Human Wholeness, and it includes all agencies, methods, systems, regimes, practices and ideals of natural origin and divine sanction whereby human health may be restored, 'enhanced, maintained."*
>
> —Edward E. Purinton

> *"Naturopathy is the science, art, philosophy of adjusting the framework, correcting the mental influences, and supplying the body with its needed elements."*
>
> —Dr. J.E. Cummins

> *"Naturopathy is a distinct school of healing, employing the beneficent agency of Nature's forces, of water, air, sunlight, earth power, electricity, magnetism, exercise, rest, proper diet, various kinds of mechanical treatment, and mental and moral science."*
>
> —Dr. Benedict Lust

As can be discerned from these definitions, naturopathy is viewed as a way of life, and the practice of naturopathic medicine employs multidisciplinary means of preventing and treating disease. Currently, naturopathy is considered a primary health care program that includes eclectic forms of treatment modalities.[3]

Historical Development

The philosophical roots of naturopathic medicine stem from the time of Hippocrates, the Greek father of medicine (about 400 BCE).[4] Hippocrates incorporated natural means such as diet, exercise, manipulative therapies, and hydrotherapy into his practice.[5] At that time, other physicians also studied the laws of nature and applied those principles within their medical practices. *Vis medicatrix naturae*, Latin for the healing power of nature, was their code and became the mantra for present-day naturopathic medicine. The practice of naturopathy began as a part of the European *nature cure*, which evolved during the eighteenth and nineteenth centuries.[6] Six cholera epidemics occurred during the nineteenth century in Asia, Europe, North Africa, and the Americas. Paris and London were affected especially hard, with thousands of deaths. In 1842, Chadwick submitted a *Report on the Sanitary Conditions of the Laboring Population of Great Britain* to the English Parliament.[7] In it, Chadwick wrote that the spread of cholera was due to contaminated drinking water from human sewage. His solution was to change the urban sanitation infrastructure by incorporating flushing toilets, an enclosed sewage systems, and garbage collection. Chadwick did not accept Dr. John Snow's germ theory as the cause of Cholera. He believed instead that dirt was the main cause. In 1848, Arnold Rikli added to the water cure by emphasizing the importance of fresh air and sunlight. Rather than scientific medicines, changing the environment (nature) was believed to be the *real* cure for cholera or Typhoid epidemics.

The term "naturopathy" was coined in 1892 and described a system of natural therapies.[8] The word comes from Greek and Latin and translates to "nature disease."[9] In 1902, German immigrant Benedict Lust founded the American School of Naturopathy in New York after having cured himself of tuberculosis by a natural means, hydrotherapy. Some of the courses that he taught included herbal medicine, nutrition, physiotherapy, psychology, homeopathy, and manipulation techniques.[10] In 1919, Lust founded the American Naturopathic Association, which was incorporated in 19 states.[1] In the ensuing years, however, naturopathic medicine did not become a popular discipline here in the United States. After Lust's death, there was conflict among the various schools of natural medicine (homeopathy, herbalism, physio-medicalism). Medical technology had advanced, and conventional medicine had consolidated politically and virtually "swamped natural means of medical care."[5,p99] During the 1970s and 1980s, however, a movement of health consciousness began to inspire people to move from the pharmaceutical to a more natural and holistic means of healing, and naturopathic medicine again began to gain in appeal.

WHAT ARE THE MAJOR BELIEFS OF NATUROPATHY?

The following are the five major beliefs of naturopathy:

Disease is a natural part of nature. Disease is viewed as a natural part of nature and is caused by a violation of nature's laws (e.g., sleeping poorly, eating poorly, irrational thinking patterns, irresponsible alcohol drinking behaviors, unprotected sexual conduct). When healthy functioning is disturbed, the naturopathic belief is that disease will result in humans just as it does in the plant and animal kingdoms.

Promote health and prevent disease. Prevention of disease is another major belief in naturopathy. Naturopathic practitioners or physicians work on promoting health to prevent disease.[11] They encourage patients to be responsible for their own health by living healthy lifestyles. Good health is seen as a triad: maintaining a balance among the body's structure, its biochemistry, and the emotions.

The body will heal itself. A major belief of naturopathy is that the body is its own best healer and knows what it needs to get well or heal itself.[12] Symptoms of disease are viewed as a result of the body trying to purify itself. The preferred mode is to allow the body to heal on its own by using positive strategies to strengthen the immune system (diet, fluids, rest). In naturopathy, the cause of the symptoms (problem) is investigated and diagnosed before treatment is prescribed, which would include treating the patient in a holistic, and natural, fashion.[11–13]

Germs are not the major cause of disease. Naturopaths invoke a few simplistic theories to explain the causes of disease. They don't believe that pathogens or germs are the main cause of disease. They believe that disease is caused by several other phenomena that could include the actions of "toxins" (accumulation of waste materials and bodily refuse); food allergies; dietary sugar, fat, and gluten; inadequate vitamin and mineral intake; vertebral misalignments; imbalances of qi energy; and a few others.[12,13] Acute (short-acting) diseases such as fevers, measles, childhood chicken pox, colds, and the like are believed to be the body's attempt to get rid of waste products that are interfering with the body's functioning systems. On the other hand, all the chronic (long-lasting) diseases are viewed as the result of continued suppression of the same acute diseases or from self-initiated attempts at body cleansing.[14]

First, do no harm. Finally, a naturopathic medicine belief is to "First, do no harm." Based on this belief, the naturopathic physician uses methods and substances that are as nontoxic and noninvasive as possible.[10,12,13]

WHAT ARE THE NATUROPATHIC DIAGNOSTIC METHODS?

Traditional Diagnostic Methods

Naturopathic practitioners use many of the diagnostic methods of the traditional physician, such as observing the overall look of the patient, taking the pulse and blood pressure, listening to the heart and breathing, and so forth. Naturopaths will take a detailed history and will ask questions related to lifestyle and diet. They may order standard blood and urine laboratory tests.[15,16] Naturopaths also may order radiology for diagnostic purposes although they do not use radiology for treatment purposes.

Biotypes

Besides the traditional diagnostic methods, naturopaths assess biotype or constitution to aid in diagnosis because they believe that each type has certain characteristics that are related to the risk of acquiring particular diseases. The biotypes are endomorph (soft and round), mesomorph (muscular and perhaps stocky), and ectomorph (long and lean) (see **FIGURE 10.1**).[17]

Endomorphs may have more gall bladder problems, whereas ectomorphs are more prone to rheumatoid arthritis

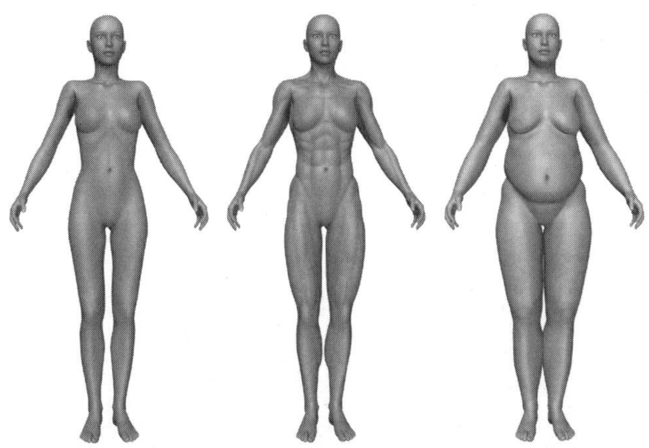

FIGURE 10.1 Biotypes: Ectomorph, Mesomorph, and Endomorph.

and mesomorphs are more inclined to suffer degenerative arthritis.[5] The naturopath may use the body type as a start in the diagnostic process.

Iridology

Iridology is the examination of the iris or colored portion of the eye for markings that supposedly reveal changing conditions of every part and organ of the body. In 1670, a physician, Phillippus Meyens, wrote a book called *Chromatica Medica* in which he wrote about the eye and the relationship of its appearance to the physical body.[18] In the middle of the nineteenth century, when still a child, Ignatz Von Peczely caught an owl, and as the owl struggled, it accidentally broke its leg. Just after, the boy saw a black line rising in the owl's eye. Later in life, Von Peczely became a physician and began to study the irises of his patients. Because he believed there was a relationship between changes in the body and iris markings, he developed an iris chart.[18,19]

Around the same time, a 14-year-old Swedish boy, Nils Liljequist, became severely ill following a vaccination. He was treated with quinine and other potent drugs, after which his iris color changed. His iris color changed again after his ribs were broken years later. He, like Von Peczely, believed there was a relationship between the iris and body injuries and disease. In 1893, Liljequist published over 258 drawings showing the iris/body relationship. His iris maps were very similar to Von Peczely's.[19] Through the years, the iris chart was continually researched and revised. Some of the most widely used maps for iridology were eventually published by Dr. Bernard Jensen in the 1950s. Dr. Jensen was a chiropractor, an entrepreneur, and the author of numerous books and articles on health and healing.

Certain areas of the iris are believed to correspond to organ and body systems and are analyzed to reveal inherent weaknesses and strengths in the organ systems. Those who study the iris (iridologists) do not claim that it will diagnose disease, but believe that the markings on the iris can indicate if an individual has overactivity or underactivity in areas of the body.[20] For example, an underactive pancreas might indicate a diabetic condition. See **FIGURE 10.2** for an iridology chart.

The theory of iridology includes the view that the iris contains four layers that indicate tissue activity: acute changes, subacute changes, chronic changes, and degenerative changes. The color of the iris is also used in assessment. See **BOX 10.1** for differentiation of blue-eyed, mixed, and brown-eyed types.[19]

The markings on the iris are designated as white, yellow-white, yellow, orange, red-brown, brown, and black. Each is thought to indicate pathology within the body (as reflected in **BOX 10.2**).

The iridologist, besides observing the layers, colors, and markings on the iris, will assess the rings and spots on the iris that supposedly indicate certain body conditions. Spots that move across the iris are said to indicate deficiencies of a particular organ or system. Several types of rings may be found on the iris, each of which is said to indicate body deficiency. See **BOX 10.3** for how iris rings relate to pathology.[19] Those illustrated represent only a few of the major rings.

Practitioner qualifications vary. One can acquire a Diploma of Holistic Iridology in person or through distance education though the International Institute of Iridology and the DaVinci College of Holistic Medicine.[21] The International College of Iridology[22] is a professional society for the study and advancement of iridology. Its Web site states that it is dedicated to the education and unification of iridologists around the world. It provides continuing education forums, support research, and clinical practice of iridology.[22]

Problems with Iridology

One of the problems associated with iridology is that this practice is not regulated or licensed by any government agency in the United States or Canada. What is more important, there seems to be no scientific evidence that iridology should be used for diagnostic purposes.[23] All double-blinded, rigorous tests of iridology have failed to find any statistical significance.[23] Usually the studies were set up so that iridologists would view photographs or slides of individuals and then be asked to diagnose disease. For example, a kidney disease and iridology study was published in the *Journal of the American Medical Association* and a gall bladder disease and iridology study was published in the *British Medical Journal*.[24] Both showed no statistical significance for using iridology as a diagnostic tool for disease. Many more studies have been attempted. Even though there have been research studies that showed iridology was a valid diagnostic tool, they have been discounted because they did not use good scientific procedures such as control groups and unmasked studies. Studies like these are biased and should not be used to promote any benefit of the use of iridology for diagnostic purposes.[16,23,25]

Mineral Analysis

Naturopaths may analyze hair for trace mineral content. Testing is performed on hair that is cut 1½ inches from the

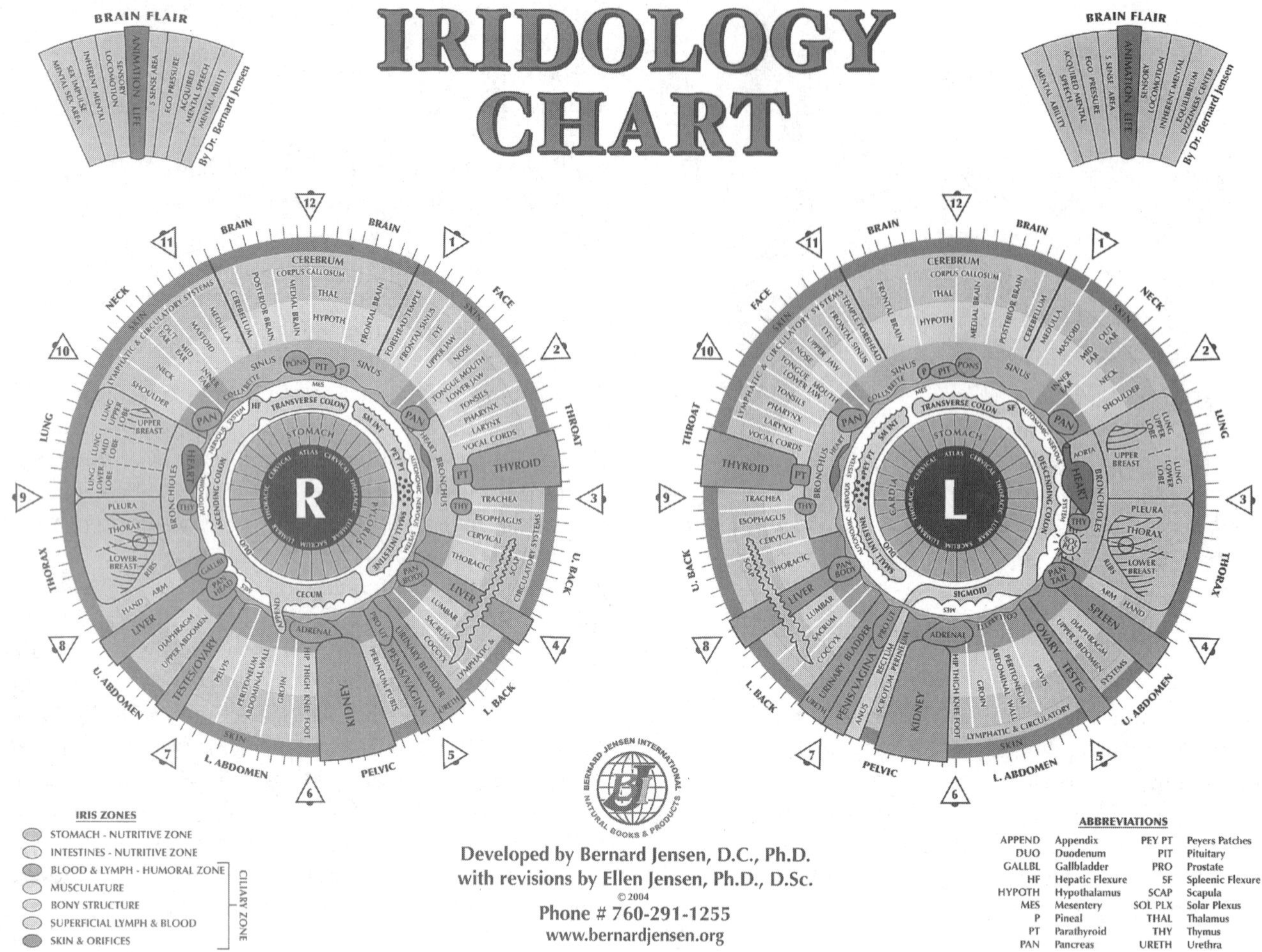

FIGURE 10.2 Iridology chart.

Box 10.1

Iris Colors Used for Diagnostic Purposes

Blue-eyed type: Supposedly have increased risk for upper respiratory, digestive tract, urogenital tract, lymphatic tissue, joint, kidney, and adrenal gland imbalances.

Mixed eye type: Has discolorations (usually light brown) on top of a blue background. Supposedly has increased risk for liver-related problems, digestive tract problems, and allergies.

Brown-eyed type: Supposedly predisposed to blood disorders and imbalances of minerals. Cautioned to pay attention to the circulatory system, liver, bone marrow, spleen, digestive system, and endocrine glands.

Box 10.2

Eye Markings and Their Relationship to Pathology

- White indicates an area of the body working hard to "maintain."
- Yellow-white indicates an area of the body losing a battle.
- Yellow indicates poor kidney function; yellow sclera (white part of the eye) suggests gallbladder disease.
- Orange indicates problems metabolizing carbohydrates and weakness in the liver and/or pancreas. Glucose levels should be checked.
- Red-brown indicates deterioration.
- Brown indicates poor liver function and "dirty blood."
- Black indicates dying tissue.

Box 10.3

Iris Rings and Their Relationship to Pathology

- Scurf Rim or Ring of Purpose is a dark band around the iris. This may indicate that the skin is not functioning properly (perhaps does not easily sweat).
- Stress Rings or Rings of Freedom look like growth rings on a tree. They may indicate neuromuscular tension and stress.
- Lipid Ring or Ring of Determination is a heavy white ring partially or completely covering the outer edge of the iris. This ring is mostly found in older people, and it may be indicative of arteriosclerosis and other cardiovascular problems. It may also indicate problems with the liver and thyroid, and an increased risk of Parkinson's disease.
- Lymphatic Rosary or Ring of Harmony looks like a tiny ring of clouds around the outer iris. People with this ring may have lymphatic congestion and swollen lymph nodes.

scalp, and the hair sample is then sent to a laboratory for analysis. Supposedly, the hair sample can reveal mineral status and toxic metal accumulation following long-term or even acute exposure. Diet, stress, medications, pollution, nutritional supplements, and inherited patterns are all factors that are believed to affect a mineral imbalance.[26] A study of six commercial U.S. laboratories, which analyze 90 percent of the hair samples in the United States, showed laboratory differences in highest and lowest reported mineral concentrations.[27] There were variations in laboratory sample preparation methods and calibration standards. The conclusion was that hair mineral analysis is unreliable and should not be used to assess individual nutritional status or exposure to environmental pollution.[27]

BioResonance Diagnosis

BioResonance is the practice of using an electronic device to measure the body's electromagnetic radiation and electric currents. The theory is that damaged organs and cancer cells emit electromagnetic oscillations that are different from healthy cells and that a BioResonance device can detect this information.[28] Thus far, there is no scientific evidence that BioResonance works.[28] BioResonance machinery was supposed to cure smoking addiction and cancer, but it was shown to be fake gadgetry.[16,23] In March of 2002, the Federal Trade Commission charged an Internet entrepreneur, David L. Walker, with making false claims about the efficacy of his supposed cancer cure, the "CWAT-Treatments: BioResonance Therapy and Molecular Enhancer.[29] Walker had advertised his products, which also included herbal and mineral mixtures, as so effective in fighting cancer that people would not need surgery, chemotherapy or other conventional cancer treatments. He also charged thousands of dollars for the treatment. The settlement with Walker and the FTC occurred in October, 2002 with Walker having to pay $229,000 in fines and was permanently prohibited from making the same or similar claims.[29]

Kirlian Photography As Diagnosis

In Kirlian photography, colorful photographs of images surrounding the body and within the body are made after applying high-frequency electrical currents to a patient's body. An object is placed in contact with a photographic plate and connected to a source of high voltage, high frequency, but low current electricity. The electricity stimulates electrons so they ionize the surrounding air. Those promoting Kirlian photography say it is photography of the aura, or electrical field, surrounding people. Those debunking Kirlian photography say it is due to natural phenomena such as pressure, electrical grounding, humidity, and temperature.[30] To date, there are no rigorous scientific studies showing the worth of Kirlian photography for use in diagnosing disease.[16,23]

Thus far, several naturopathic diagnostic tests have been discussed, but either they have not been scientifically tested or they have been tested and shown not to be effective. Naturopathic treatments are presented next.

WHAT ARE THE NATUROPATHIC TREATMENTS?

Balancing Four Major Body Systems

Naturopaths employ a system of noninvasive health care and health assessment in which neither surgery nor drugs are the first treatment of choice, although they know that there are times and certain body conditions that require them.[30] Naturopaths believe that the key to successful treatment is in balancing four major body systems: the immune system, the elimination (or detoxification) system, the nervous system, and the hormonal system.[10,31] In order to achieve this balance, naturopaths encourage patients to use natural therapies such as fresh air, sunlight, water, rest, and exercise. [10,31]

Education and Counseling

Naturopaths rely on educating and counseling clients about lifestyle and diet. In fact, at Bastyr University in Seattle, a major hub for educating naturopaths, students take counseling courses so that they can better work with clients.[32]

Nutrition

Nutrition and its relationship to diseases is a primary focus of naturopathy. Naturopaths believe that diet alone or with the use of proper supplements may improve conditions. Fasting may be prescribed for a day or more (1-, 3-, 5-, and 7-day fasts). The purpose is to give the digestive system a rest and to detoxify the body. Juice may be drunk or grapes may be eaten during days of fasting.[5]

Botanicals and Traditional Medicines

Medicines prescribed usually come from nature rather than a laboratory. Naturopaths use botanical medicine (phytotherapy) for treating disease conditions. Vitamins and homeopathic substances (e.g., tissue cell salts) may also be prescribed. Different states have laws identifying the type of traditional medicines that naturopaths may prescribe. In the state of Washington, for example, naturopaths may prescribe antibiotics, thyroid medicine, progesterone, and other drugs.[10]

Energy Work, Massage, Physical Therapy, TCM, and Bodywork

Naturopaths might use energy work, massage therapy, physical therapy, and traditional Chinese medicine modalities (such as acupuncture, herbal medicines). Naturopathic manipulation or bodywork comprises a variety of systematic movements to heal musculoskeletal and neurological conditions, very similar to osteopathic and chiropractic medicine.

Hydrotherapy

Hydrotherapy and colonic enemas (colon hydrotherapy) may be used depending on the condition. Hydrotherapy is the treatment of physical disability, injury, or illness by immersion of all or part of the body in water to facilitate movement, promote wound healing, and relieve pain. It is usually done under the supervision of a trained therapist. Hydrotherapy may include the use of hot and cold water. Alternate hot and cold is used to stimulate the blood and lymph circulation and help to remove congestion and revive the body tissues.[5] Cold compresses may also be used to boost the elimination of toxins.

As described, naturopathic treatments are usually noninvasive and medicines are natural or herbal rather than prescription drugs. Naturopaths focus on the importance of nutrition and lifestyle not only as strategies for the prevention of disease, but also as treatment modalities.

You have now learned what naturopathy is, the diagnostic methods used, and an overview of treatment modalities. Next we explain the training of the naturopathic physician.

WHAT ARE THE NATUROPATHIC CLASSIFICATIONS AND THE TRAINING OF NATUROPATHIC PHYSICIANS?

There are three main categories of naturopathic practitioners[9]:

Traditional naturopath: The traditional naturopath does not have a university undergraduate or higher education degree. He or she can obtain training through distance learning (correspondence or Internet courses). The admission requirements are not rigorous, and naturopaths trained in this fashion are not eligible for certification. They may not prescribe drugs, x-rays, or surgery. The programs are not accredited by organizations recognized for accreditation purposes by the U.S. Department of Education and are not subject to licensing.

Health care providers: The second category is composed of medical doctors, osteopathic doctors, chiropractors, and nurses who pursued additional training in naturopathic treatment modalities.[9] Their training programs also vary.

Naturopathic physician: The third category is the naturopathic physician, whose training is similar to the training of the medical doctor.[9] Prerequisites include 3 years of premedical sciences at a university with a cumulative grade point average of 3.0 on a 4-point scale. The curriculum includes courses in the basic sciences (anatomy, physiology, histology, microbiology, biochemistry, immunology, pharmacology, and pathology), clinical disciplines (diagnostic medicine practices such as physical and clinical diagnosis, laboratory diagnosis, radiology, naturopathic assessment, and orthopedics), and naturopathic courses (clinical nutrition, botanical medicine, traditional Chinese therapeutic skills and treatments, homeopathic medicine, hydrotherapy, naturopathic manipulation, and lifestyle counseling). Clinical experience includes 1,500 hours of clinical requirements and proficiency in all aspects of naturopathic medicine. Students must also pass the board Naturopathic Physicians Licensing Examination (NPLEX) after the second and fourth years. Continuing medical education (CME) credits are required on an ongoing basis after becoming a doctor of naturopathy (ND).

Four universities in the United States and two Canadian universities offer a doctor of naturopathy (ND) or doctor of naturopathic medicine degree (NMD).[33] According to the American Association of Naturopathic Physicians (AANP),[34] the 4-year, baccalaureate professional association, there are 3,000 licensed naturopathic physicians. See **BOX 10.4** for schools accredited by the Council on Naturopathic Medical Education.

Currently, the following states and territories have licensing laws for naturopathic doctors[34]:

- Alaska
- Arizona
- California
- Connecticut
- District of Columbia
- Hawaii
- Idaho

- Kansas
- Maine
- Minnesota
- Montana
- New Hampshire
- Oregon
- Utah
- Vermont
- Washington
- U.S. territories of Puerto Rico and Virgin Islands

Box 10.4

Schools Accredited by the Council on Naturopathic Medical Education (recognized by the U.S. Department of Education)

- Bastyr University, Seattle, Washington
- University of Bridgeport College of Naturopathic Medicine, Bridgeport, Connecticut
- National College of Naturopathic Medicine, Portland, Oregon
- Southwest College of Naturopathic Medicine and Health Sciences, Tempe, Arizona

WHAT IS THE LEVEL OF NATUROPATHIC USE?

According to the 2007 National Health Interview Survey, an estimated 729,000 adults and 237,000 children in the United States had used a naturopathic treatment in the previous year.[9] Some of the more common conditions that naturopaths treat are allergies, fatigue, colds, headaches, migraine headaches, shingles, genital warts (HPV), irritable bowel syndrome, gout, depression, urinary tract infections, kidney stones, constipation, arthritis, asthma, back problems, high blood pressure, menstrual problems, chronic pain, and stress.[1,10] Many individuals visit naturopathic practitioners not only for primary care, but also for prevention of disease and to support wellness.

WHAT ARE THE RESULTS OF RESEARCH ON NATUROPATHY?

Naturopaths have shown good success in treating some cancers because of the naturopathic treatments that focus on strengthening the body's immune system.[10] The National Center for Complementary and Alternative Medicine (NCCAM) is studying a naturopathic dietary approach for type 2 diabetes, naturopathic treatments for periodontal (gum) disease, and naturopathic herbal and dietary approaches to breast cancer prevention; currently, however, there are no study results. A study at the NCCAM that involved a group of 70 warehouse workers who had lower-back pain demonstrated positive results. Naturopathic care that included acupuncture, exercise, dietary advice, relaxation training, and a back-care booklet was more cost effective than the employer's usual patient education program. Both workers and employers benefited from the naturopathic approach, which was associated with less absenteeism, lower costs for treatments, and better quality of life.[9]

The NCCAM[9] has reported that both Naturopathy and traditional Chinese medicine were effective for treating temporomandibular disorders (TMD) in women. TMD is characterized by pain and tenderness when chewing and opening the mouth. Limitations of jaw opening are often accompanied by deviations in mandible path, and clicking, popping, or grating sounds from the temporomandibular joint. Researchers evaluated two alternative healing approaches, traditional Chinese medicine ($n = 50$) and naturopathic medicine ($n = 50$) to assess whether they were as effective as usual care ($n = 50$) provided by dental clinicians. Participants were females 25–55 years of age with multiple health problems.[9]

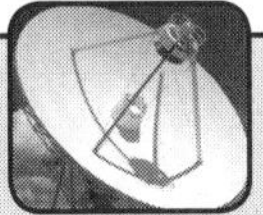

In the News

Preliminary results of a randomized trial of a whole practice model of naturopathic care for cardiovascular risk were published on the Web site of the Naturopathic Physicians Research Institute in August 2010. The study sample was Canadian postal workers at elevated cardiovascular risk. The workers' cardiovascular health improved more after being treated with naturopathic care versus those in usual care in the Framingham cardiovascular risk profile.

Also in the news was a report that two naturopathic physician principle investigators received grants from the National Institutes of Health. The first was to study integrated medicine practices versus standard oncology for breast cancer in matched cohorts. The study will take place in the Seattle area. The second award was a grant for an 18-month clinical trial of omega-3 fatty acids and alpha lipoic acid in the treatment of mild to moderate Alzheimer's disease. This study will take place in Portland, Medford, Klamath Falls, and Bend, Oregon.

Two studies published in the 1990s showed positive results for naturopathic treatment of rheumatoid arthritis using a naturopathic-controlled diet.[35,36] Many other studies cited by Pelletier[10] were published in the 1970s, 1980s, and 1990s and showed fairly positive results for naturopathic treatment. One series of studies by Hudson showed the value of naturopathic botanicals and nutritional supplements that changed abnormal pap smears to normal. Also, a pilot study conducted at Bastyr University provided herbal and nutritional therapies to HIV-infected patients, which improved their immune function. Pelletier also presented studies showing the effects of naturopathic treatment on osteoarthritis, asthma, atherosclerosis, back pain, benign prostatic hypertrophy, depression, diabetes mellitus, eczema, HIV disease, irritable bowel syndrome, migraine headaches, middle ear infections, premenstrual syndrome, upper respiratory infection, and vaginitis. Please refer to Pelletier's text,[10] *The Best Alternative Medicine: What Works? What Does Not?*, pages 184 to 194, for a closer examination of these results.

WHAT IS THE FUTURE OF NATUROPATHY?

Naturopathy is cost-effective, and because of that is being integrated into conventional medicine practices. Naturopaths have lower overhead costs and charge patients less than do medical doctors or osteopaths. The treatments are less invasive and, therefore, cost much less. In many states, naturopathy is covered by insurance. Its practitioners are becoming well educated in the sciences, nutrition, and counseling practices. The future may comprise a new vision of health care that may include naturopathy. As more scientific studies are designed and implemented that demonstrate the effectiveness of naturopathy, the practice will surely increase and be fruitful.

The executive director of the American Association of Naturopathic Physicians, Karen E. Howard, foresees that naturopathy will be a meaningful component in future health care. The AANP promotes naturopathy as a tool to change the health care system from disease management to health promotion by incorporating the principles of naturopathic medicine (presented earlier in this chapter).[37] The future of naturopathy appears to be bright.

This chapter would not be complete without presenting information on homeopathy, one of the major tools of the naturopath. This practice is discussed next.

WHAT IS THE HOMEOPATHY HEALING SYSTEM AND HOW DID IT DEVELOP?

Homeopathy is a healing system developed in 1790 by a German physician and chemist named Samuel Hahnemann.[5,38] The word *homeo* refers to similar and *pathos or pathy* refers to suffering and disease. Homeopathy is a holistic and natural system of healing that aims to prevent illness as well as treat it. Homeopathy is based on the idea that like cures like. Substances that cause specific symptoms in a healthy person are thought to be able to cure individuals who are ill displaying the same type of symptoms.

History

Hahnemann became disenchanted with the unhygienic and often brutal medical techniques such as purging, emetics, bloodletting, and the use of large doses of chemical agents such as mercury and arsenic that were used in the late 1700s. He stopped his physician's practice and became a translator. While translating a text called, *A Treatise on Materia Medica* by Scottish physician Dr. William Cullen, Hahnemann learned that quinine was supposed to cure malaria because of its astringent properties. Because he doubted that the astringent property of quinine was the reason for the cure, he began to experiment on himself. Each time he took a dose of quinine, he produced the symptoms of malaria in himself, supposedly a healthy individual.[5,38] His investigations continued as he began to experiment with small doses of substances thought to cure disease. Soon, Hahnemann began to dilute substances such as herbs, minerals, and animal extracts in an alcohol–water solution. Hahnemann found that the more he diluted substances, the less the side effects and the more he could boost the potency of the drug. As the solutions were diluted, shaking became a necessary action because this process released what Hahnemann called stores of *vital energy*.

Although Hahnemann popularized the idea of *like cures like*, Hippocrates, the Father of Medicine, and the Egyptians used the idea of similars in the fifth century BCE.[38] Over time, the more orthodox practice of curing with substances contrary to the symptoms took over. In folk medicine, however, the principle of similars persisted for hundreds of years until Hahnemann began his more scientific investigation of homeopathy.[1] The more that Hahnemann tested subjects, the more he found a "drug picture of substances" and then finally a "symptoms picture" of each patient that made his prescriptions more effective.[5] He developed three essential principles of homeopathy that remain today:

1. *The principle of similars:* Like cures like.
2. *The principle of infinitesimal dose:* The more diluted the dose, the more potent its curative effects.
3. *The principle of specificity of the individual:* If the remedy is to cure, it must match the symptom profile of the patient.[38]

A student of Hahnemann, Dr. Constantine Hering, introduced homeopathy into the United States. He opened a homeopathic medical school in 1835 in Allentown, Pennsylvania.[39] By 1900, there were 22 homeopathic medical schools, close to 100 homeopathic hospitals, and over 1,000 homeopathic pharmacies in the United States. About 15 percent of all U.S. physicians were homeopathic practitioners. During the 1930s, conventional pharmaceutical medications were being produced, and a powerful American Medical Association challenged homeopathy as a viable medical system. Consequently, the practice in the United States virtually died out.[39] Homeopathy did not, however, die out everywhere; it is still practiced worldwide. There are more than 6,000 German and 5,000 French practitioners. In Great Britain, homeopathy is a part of the medical and health care system. There are many homeopathic hospitals and outpatient clinics. The practice is also used in India, where there are over 100 homeopathic colleges.

WHAT ARE HOMEOPATHIC TREATMENTS?

Homeopathic treatments are minute (diluted) remedies made from animal, vegetable, and mineral substances.[1,38] Homeopaths believe that the energy or *vibrational* pattern from a homeopathic substance that is contained in the solution stimulates healing by activating the *vital force*, first identified by Hahnemann.

Remedies come in a variety of forms: tablets, powders, wafers, and liquids in an alcohol base. Like many traditional medicines, many homeopathic remedies are found as over-the-counter products.[1,38] This allows for self-treatment of minor conditions such as flu, sore throat, headache, and insomnia.

The process of dilution takes several weeks. Plant parts are dissolved in a mixture of alcohol and water and left to stand for 2 to 4 weeks. The mixture, called *mother of tincture*, is occasionally shaken and strained. That solution is then used to make different potencies by repeatedly diluting with water or alcohol and vigorously shaking it, a process called *succussion*.[39] A dilution to a 4X remedy is done in the following way. The mother of tincture solution is diluted by a factor of 10 (1X), then again by a factor of 10 (2X), then again by a factor of 10 (3X), and again by a factor of 10 (4X). The dilution amount is calculated at 1: 10,000. That seems very dilute, but many remedies are diluted even more. For instance, some solutions are diluted by 100 at each stage and use a C scale. A 4C solution (C = Roman numeral 100) is made in the following way. One part of the mother tincture is diluted with 99 parts of water. The dilution factor is then 100, or a 1C remedy. The solution is then repeatedly diluted by a factor of 100, leading to 2C, 3C, and 4C solutions. Many homeopathic remedies are diluted to 30C. The resulting solution is unlikely to contain even a molecule of the original solution.[23] There are even higher diluting scales used by some homeopaths: a millesimal (M) scale—1 part in 1,000 and a quintamillesimal (Q) scale—1 part to 50,000 parts. Homeopaths claim that the remedy has memory of the original solution and that is enough to influence body symptoms.

Currently, there are over 2,000 homeopathic remedies, often referred to by an abbreviated name. For instance, the abbreviation for *Argentum nitricum* is Arg-n; this is a homeopathic remedy made from silver nitrate and used for nervous complaints or anxiety. In addition, a homeopath might use tissue salts, made only from mineral sources. Tissue salts are also used in diluted solutions; in fact, they are so diluted that even if toxic substances such as snake's venom are used, there are no possible side effects.[5]

Homeopathic practitioners consult repertories and materia medicas to determine the remedy to be used that matches the patient's symptoms or profile. The compendiums were written over a period of 200 years and include thousands of tests or "provings" on healthy individuals.[39] If given to a well person, the substances are supposed to cause illness, but given in diluted doses to a sick person, the substances are thought to cure illness. Rather than treating a person who has diarrhea with substances that could cause constipation, the homeopath would prescribe a minute dose of a substance that in a stronger preparation would cause diarrhea.

HOW SAFE ARE HOMEOPATHIC REMEDIES?

According to the NCCAM, a review has found that homeopathic remedies are generally considered safe and unlikely to cause severe side effects. Even though the liquid homeopathic medicines contain alcohol, no adverse effects from alcohol levels have been found or reported to the FDA. Also, homeopathic remedies have not been found to interfere with conventional drugs, although people should let their doctors know if they are using them.

WHAT TYPES OF HEALTH CONDITIONS ARE TREATED BY HOMEOPATHY?

A full range of health conditions are treated by homeopathic remedies. These include headache, sore throat, cough, earache, digestive disorders, colic, diarrhea, fever, sleep disturbances, mumps, measles, hemorrhoids, shingles, hives, allergies, joint pain, and more. See **TABLE 10.1** for homeopathic remedies for various health conditions.[1,38]

WHAT STEPS ARE USED WHEN PRESCRIBING HOMEOPATHIC TREATMENTS?

Homeopaths use five essential steps to prescribe a remedy: note the symptoms; look up the symptoms; decide which remedy is appropriate; decide the dosage, and how often and when to repeat it; and evaluate the results. The dosage is dependent on the severity of symptoms, but the rule in homeopathy is that the minimum dosage required to initiate a healing response is first given. An important principle of homeopathy is that the whole person should be studied—their temperament, personality, and emotional and physical

Table 10.1
Homeopathic Remedies and Health Conditions Treated

HOMEOPATHIC REMEDY	TARGET AILMENTS	WHERE FOUND	HOMEOPATHIC USE
Aconite (*Aconitum nacelles*)	Angina, anxiety induced by shock, arthritis, asthma, colds, flu, fevers, headaches, sore throat, colic, diarrhea, cystitis, toothaches	Bluish violet flowers called monkshood. Found in mountainous regions of Europe, Russia, and central Asia. Juices traditionally used by hunters as an arrow poison.	For symptoms similar to being poisoned; distress or fear, thirst, and unbearable aches and pains. Illnesses for which onset is sudden and acute.
Alium cepa	Colds with sinus congestion; coughs that cause a ripping, tearing throat pain; inflamed eyes; hay fever; earaches	Red onion, a common garden vegetable. Applied to skin as a poultice. Used internally for intestinal worms.	Used for same conditions as when exposed to onion: watering eyes and burning, runny nose.
Aloe	Indigestion, diarrhea, hemorrhoids	Made from the juice of the flowering succulent plant native to Africa.	Used to treat diarrhea, hemorrhoids, and indigestion.
Antimonium tartaricum	Whooping cough, nausea, fever, chest colds	Substance found in metals, mostly sulfide stibnite.	For gradual, progressive weakness; accumulation of mucus with rattling in the chest; cold sweat; and great sleepiness.
Apis (*apis mellifica*)	Bites and stings with burning, itching, or swelling; conjunctivitis; general swelling from food allergies; hives; tonsillitis; mumps; red, swollen joints; cystitis; shingles; fever	Made from the body of the honeybee found all over the world.	For ailments with symptoms similar to a bee sting: redness and swelling, restlessness, or irritability.
Arg. N (*Argentum nitricum*)	Emotional problems, headaches, eye complaints, sore throat, digestive disorders, stomach ulcers, flatulence, diarrhea, constipation, trembling, weakness	Made from pure crystals of silver nitrate.	Used for symptoms of mental exertion and anxiety. Good for exam nerves or stage fright.
Arnica (*Arnica montana*)	Muscle aches and pain, bruises, sprains, strains	Mountain daisy found in higher elevations in Europe, northern Asia, and the United States.	Used for very active people (mountain climbers) and those who suffer some sort of accident.
Arnica (*Leopard's Bane*)	For trauma, injury, and any case of major or minor physical stress, broken bones, bruises, swollen tissue, and inflammation	Known as leopard's bane. Grows in the mountains of Europe and in Siberia.	Used as a first aid remedy, particularly to treat shock and trauma. As an application, used for bruises and swelling.
Arsenicum album	Angina, anxiety disorders and panic attacks, Crohn's disease, influenza	Dilute form of arsenic made from separation from other metals such as iron, cobalt, and nickel by baking at high temperatures.	Prescribed to treat patients with various digestive complaints accompanied by dehydration and burning pains.
Belladonna	Common cold, flu, sore throat, earache, high fever with chills but no thirst, arthritis, colic, measles, mumps, sunstroke, toothaches, painful menstrual periods	Deadly nightshade plant that grows wild across Europe. Yellow flowers in July and dark red berries in late summer.	For illnesses with symptoms of dry mouth and hot, flushed skin, nausea, convulsions, and delirium.

Table 10.1
Homeopathic Remedies and Health Conditions Treated (Continued)

HOMEOPATHIC REMEDY	TARGET AILMENTS	WHERE FOUND	HOMEOPATHIC USE
Bryonia (*Bryonia alba*)	Irritability; vertigo, headache; dry, parched lips, mouth; excessive thirst; bitter taste; sensitive epigastric discomfort; constipation; dry cough; rheumatic pains and swellings	Flowered, vine-like plant that originated in England, often growing on hedgerows.	Prescribed to patients to treat back pain, sciatica, neck pain, and other general aches and pains.
Calcarea carbonica	Lower back pain, broken bones, sprains, muscle cramps, constipation, chronic ear infections, eye inflammations, headaches, insomnia, allergies, eczema, gastritis, gallstones, menstrual problems, asthma, arthritis	Comes from chalk, coral, and limestone.	Used for conditions accompanied by symptoms of exhaustion, depression, and anxiety.
Calendula	Promotes healing; used on cuts, tears, lacerations, burns, open wounds, and hemorrhages after tooth extraction; used as a mouthwash and an eyebath	Made from the fresh flowering tops and leaves of the marigold plant.	Used for first aid; antiseptic; used to bathe and sterilize wounds and abrasions.
Cantharis	Bladder infections, sunburns, scalds	A beetle found in southern France. The beetles are boiled and diluted before being used for treatment.	Prescribed to patients whose ailments are coupled with symptoms like those of cantharis poisoning.
Chamomilla	Irritability, toothaches, painful menstrual periods, earaches	The flowering German chamomile plant common in Europe.	Prescribed to patients who are extremely sensitive to pain, irritable, and impatient. Most often given to children who work themselves into violent temper tantrums.
Ferrum phosphoricum	Tickling, hacking coughs; headaches; fevers; rheumatic joints; early menstrual periods	Mineral compound of iron and phosphorus. Derived from mixing the solution with lactose to make it nontoxic.	Prescribed to patients who suffer from conditions with low energy and anemia.
Gelsemium (*Gelsemium sempervirens*)	Anxiety, flu with aches, exhaustion, headaches	A climbing vine with trumpetlike yellow flowers, commonly found in the United States.	Prescribed in diluted forms for ailments accompanied by symptoms similar to those of gelsemium poisoning.
Hepar sulphuris, Hepar sulphuris calcareum	Swollen and painful abscesses, colds, sore throat, earache, aching joints, coughing with chest pain, hoarseness, asthma, emphysema, croup, genital herpes, constipation	The flaky inner layer of oysters yields the calcium. Mixed with sulphur and heated in an airtight container. The powder is dissolved in hydrochloric acid and combined with lactose and diluted by trituration.	For infections containing pus, mental and physical hypersensitivity, and intolerance of pain and cold.
Hypericum (*Hypericum perforatum*)	Backaches, bites and stings, cuts and wounds	Also known as St. John's wort, it grows in Europe, Asia, and the United States from June to September.	Prescribed to patients for bodily injuries because of the soothing effect it has on the nerves.

(Continues)

Table 10.1

Homeopathic Remedies and Health Conditions Treated (Continued)

HOMEOPATHIC REMEDY	TARGET AILMENTS	WHERE FOUND	HOMEOPATHIC USE
Ignatia (*Ignatia amara*)	Anxiety, dry tickling cough, sore throat with feeling of a lump, tension headaches, indigestion, irritable bowel syndrome, painful hemorrhoids	Seeds (beans) from the fruit of a small tree native to China and the Philippines. Called St. Ignatius bean.	Used for symptoms similar to poisoning symptoms: increased salivation, pounding headache, cramps, giddiness, twitching, and trembling.
Ipecac, ipecacuanha	Nausea, vomiting, motion sickness, irritating cough, flu with nausea, gastroenteritis	The ipecacuanha shrub is native to Central and South America. The shrub is said to induce vomiting, but when diluted can help with these symptoms.	Prescribed to patients for nausea and vomiting.
Kali bichromicum	Acute bronchitis, mucus discharge, sinusitis	Also called potassium bichromate. Chemical compound acquired from chromium iron ore or by processing potassium chromate with a strong acid.	Prescribed for conditions that are accompanied by pain in a specific spot.
Lachesis	Choking coughs, croup, earaches, sore throats, indigestion, throbbing headaches, insomnia, hot flashes, heart arrhythmias, hemorrhoids, sciatica	South American bushmaster snake that grows to 7 feet. Venom is lachesis. Venom extracted and diluted in large quantities of lactose.	Treats symptoms similar to venom poisoning: destruction of red blood cells and clotting impairment. Heart poisoning.
Ledum (*Ledum palustre*)	Animal bites, insect sting, bruises that have discolored, deep cuts or puncture wounds, gout, aching joints	Ledum is a plant also called marsh tea. Found in bogs across northern Europe, Canada, and the United States.	Helpful for conditions accompanied by signs of infection or inflammation.
Lycopodium (*Lycopodium clavatum*)	Backache with stiffness and soreness in lower back, bedwetting, colds with stuffy nose, cystitis, headache with throbbing pain, gout, indigestion with abdominal cramps, gas, heartburn, sciatica, eczema	Known as club moss; it grows in pastures and woodlands in Great Britain, northern Europe, and North America.	Used for complaints accompanied by symptoms of digestive upset, desire for sweets, and anxiety.
Mercurius vivus	Abscesses (dental or glandular), backaches, chickenpox, earaches, eye inflammation	Made from the chemical element mercury by diluting the element with large quantities of milk sugar.	Prescribed for conditions with symptoms of shaking, hot and cold sweats, and restlessness.
Natrum muriaticum	Backaches; cold sores; colds with sneezing, watery eyes, and runny nose; constipation; fevers; genital herpes; eczema; anemia; hay fever; migraine headaches; indigestion; depression	Natrum is salt or sodium chloride.	Given for conditions with symptoms of extreme thirst, emotional sensitivity, and a strong desire for salt.
Nux vomica	Colic and stomach cramps from overeating, colds with sneezing and stuffy nose, constipation, cystitis, headache with dizziness, fevers with chills, gas and gas pains, hangovers, indigestion, insomnia, irritable bowel syndrome, stomach flu	Known as poison nut; it is made of seeds of an evergreen tree found in India, Thailand, China, and Australia. Seeds contain strychnine.	For overindulgence of alcohol, food, or coffee.

Table 10.1
Homeopathic Remedies and Health Conditions Treated (Continued)

HOMEOPATHIC REMEDY	TARGET AILMENTS	WHERE FOUND	HOMEOPATHIC USE
Phosphorus	Bronchitis, pneumonia, coughs with congestion, visual problems resulting from eyestrain, gastritis, nosebleeds, indigestion, stomach ulcers, kidney infections, nasal polyps, hepatitis, anemia, hemorrhages, diarrhea	Found in inorganic phosphate rocks.	For conditions accompanied by symptoms of fatigue and nervousness with a tendency to bleed easily and unquenchable thirst for cold water.
Pulsatilla (*Pulsatilla nigricans*)	Bedwetting, breast infections, hay fever, aching joints, late menstrual periods, depression, urethritis in men	Plant found in the meadows of northern and central Europe.	Prescribed to patients with conditions accompanied by yellow or white discharge.
Rhus toxicodendron	Arthritis, backache with spine stiffness, bursitis, carpal tunnel syndrome, eye inflammation, itching, genital herpes, influenza, hives that itch, impetigo, poison ivy, sprains with stiffness, toothaches	Vine-like shrub known as poison ivy.	Conditions accompanied by fever, restlessness, and swollen glands.
Ruta (*Ruta graveolens*)	Carpal tunnel, eye strain, sciatica, groin strain, sprains, tennis elbow, tendon and cartilage injury	A plant native to southern Europe.	For conditions or injuries accompanied by symptoms of weakness or bruised sensation.
Sepia	Backaches, violent coughing, cold sores and fever blisters, genital herpes, hair loss, gas, headaches, sinusitis, urinary incontinence, menstrual cramps, nausea from motion sickness or pregnancy	Cuttlefish, a soft-bodied mollusk related to a squid.	For conditions with symptoms of apathy, moodiness, and weakness.
Silica	Athlete's foot, constipation, hemorrhoids	Mineral present in the human body in trace amounts but is vital to the bones, cartilage, and skin.	Minute doses prescribed to patients for excessive sweating, weakness, and sensitivity to cold.
Sulphur	Asthma accompanied by rattling mucus, cough with chest pain, diarrhea, eye inflammation, bursitis, headaches, indigestion, joint pain, itching with redness, burning vaginal discharge, eczema with itching and burning	Also called brimstone.	For conditions accompanied by irritability, intense itching, burning pains, and offensive odors.

responses—before prescribing a homeopathic remedy. A person's genetic and personal health history and body type are also considerations when prescribing a homeopathic remedy.

WHERE IS HOMEOPATHY USED AND HOW MANY ARE USING IT?

Homeopathy is used in countries around the world: Australia, New Zealand, Canada, Czech Republic, France, Great Britain, Greece, India, Netherlands, Hungary, Israel, United States, Germany, and Latin America.[38] According to the 2007 National Health Interview Survey, approximately 3.9 million adults and approximately 900,000 children used homeopathy in the previous year in the United States.[9]

WHAT HAVE CLINICAL STUDIES FOUND?

According to the NCCAM, homeopathy is difficult to study using current research methods because of the difficulty in standardizing the homeopathic remedies. They simply can't be measured using current scientific methods. Also, homeopaths take into account several considerations when prescribing the right homeopathic remedy for a headache, for example. Homeopathic clinicians have identified more than 200 symptom patterns for headaches. They would note where in the brain the headache is occurring, and the individual's temperament, constitution, emotionality, and personality. They would next select a homeopathic remedy for headache that would meet these considerations. The problem is that there is not just one homeopathic remedy for headaches, but many that could be given depending on the patient's profile.[39] It makes setting up clinical trials very difficult; consequently, very little evidence has been demonstrated that supports homeopathy as an effective treatment for any specific condition.[9]

Cucherat et al. conducted a meta-analysis of homeopathy clinical trials.[40] They found some evidence that homeopathic treatments were more effective than placebo, but discounted it because of the poor quality of the trials. Townhill analyzed available homeopathic research and found evidence that homeopathy was effective in the treatment of some musculoskeletal disorders, but also reported that some studies had flaws in quality and design.[41] Freeman and Lawlis[39] described several randomized studies conducted in the 1980s and 1990s that were to assess whether homeopathy was significantly better than placebo effect. The first two described were conducted by David Reilly, a Scottish physician. Reilly et al. conducted a pilot study and then two randomized, double blind, placebo-controlled trials on homeopathic treatment of allergies and treatment of asthmatics sensitive to house dust mites. A meta-analyis of the studies on allergies and house dust mites showed that homeopathic remedies were reported to be more effective than placebo. These studies were published in the international journal *Lancet*, a peer-reviewed publication that has editorial offices in London and New York.

Other studies to assess whether homeopathic remedies were better than placebo involved treatment of fibromyalgia, influenza, carriers of hepatitis B virus, rheumatic arthritis, and childhood diarrhea. Again, these studies reported some positive effects of homeopathy. Other studies involving homeopathic remedies, however, were not so positive and had methodological flaws. An outcome from previous research is that future studies will need to be high in quality and should be replicated for specific disease conditions.[39] Homeopaths, however, are not perplexed about the inability of past research studies to demonstrate how homeopathic remedies actually work. They say that the mechanism of many allopathic drugs, such as aspirin and some antibiotics, also is not scientifically explained.[10]

ARE HOMEOPATHS LICENSED AND CERTIFIED?

Currently, there are no uniform licensing or professional standards in the United States for homeopaths. What often occurs is that a homeopathic practitioner is licensed in one of the medical professions, such as an MD or osteopathic physician, which is the rule in Arizona, Connecticut, and Nevada. Naturopaths, chiropractors, dentists, physical therapists, nurses, and veterinary physicians are allowed to employ homeopathy within their practices in many states.

CONCLUSION

It seems that naturopathy and homeopathy are an integral part of complementary and alternative medicine. Many traditional physicians are also embracing the ideas and practices of both naturopathy and homeopathy. Perhaps a fusion of the best of our traditional and alternative practices will offer hope of a better health care system in the United States.

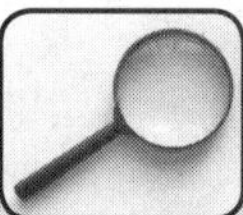

Case Study

A 22-year-old college student, Lisa, has suffered every spring for as long as she can remember with sinus headaches, sore throat, cough, and congestion. Often it would turn into a bad case of bronchitis, for which the doctor would order antibiotics. After several weeks, all of the above would happen again. A friend has told Lisa about a naturopathic physician who uses homeopathic remedies, and is encouraging her to make an appointment. Lisa should take several steps before making the first appointment. In what order should the following steps be taken?

- Check credentials of the doctor.
- Look up the definition of naturopathy and gain an understanding of the field.
- Distinguish among the different types of naturopaths and select a doctor from the type most preferred.
- Look up the definition of homeopathy and gain an understanding of the field.
- Find a list of homeopathic remedies used for allergies and sinus congestion.
- Notify family physician.

Suggestions for Class Activities

1. Invite a naturopathic physician to class. Ask about services rendered, fees for various stages of condition (from the first office visit on), academic background, philosophy of iridology, and any other questions students want to ask.
2. Visit a health food store and note the types of homeopathic remedies. Make a presentation to the class regarding your findings.
3. Demonstrate the homeopathic dilution process in class using a simple remedy. You can find these at various Web sites.

Review Questions

1. What is naturopathic medicine and how did it develop?
2. Name five major beliefs of naturopathy.
3. Explain what iridology is and how it is thought to aid in the diagnosis of body ailments.
4. Name and describe several main naturopathic treatments.
5. How do naturopaths use hydrotherapy?
6. What type of training does a naturopathic physician receive?
7. What are the three levels of training for a naturopathic physician?
8. What is the level of naturopathic use in the United States?
9. What does the research show about naturopathy?
10. What is homeopathy?
11. Who was the founder of homeopathy?
12. Define and differentiate among the three principles of homeopathy.
13. How did homeopathy evolve into a medical discipline?
14. What is mother of tincture?
15. What is the process of homeopathic dilution?
16. What types of health conditions are treated by homeopathy?
17. What do the clinical studies show regarding homeopathy?
18. How do homeopaths become licensed or certified?

Key Terms

astringent A substance or preparation that constricts tissue. It can lessen discharges such as mucus or blood.

bioresonance The practice of using an electronic device to measure the body's electromagnetic radiation and electric currents and to detect damaged body cells.

biotypes Body types or body constitutions that naturopaths use to aid a diagnosis because they believe each type has certain characteristics that are related to risk of particular diseases.

calibration To adjust instrumentation so that it will be precise.

chiropractic A discipline and profession that focuses on disorders of the musculoskeletal and nervous systems under the belief that the effects of these disorders negatively impact health.

cholera An acute, infectious disease characterized by profuse diarrhea, vomiting, and cramps.

degenerative arthritis Chronic breakdown of cartilage in the joints; the most common form of arthritis, occurring usually after middle age.

ectomorph Body type in which the appearance of the body is thin.

endemic Diseases belonging exclusively or confined to a particular place.

endomorph Body type in which the appearance of the body is round and soft. The physique presents the illusion that much of the mass has been concentrated in the abdominal area.

epidemic Diseases that affect many persons at the same time, and spread from person to person from one locale to another.

fasting To abstain from all food.

hemochromatosis A disorder wherein the body is not able to break down iron; therefore, too much is absorbed from the gastrointestinal track, causing abdominal pain and fatigue.

homeopathy The use of extremely diluted substances given to cure disease using the law of similars: *like cures like*.

hydrotherapy The treatment of physical disability, injury, or illness by immersion of all or part of the body in water to facilitate movement, promote wound healing, and relieve pain. It is usually done under the supervision of a trained therapist. May involve the use of hot, moist soaks or dry heat for pain relief and to promote healing.

infrastructure The basic, underlying framework or features of a system or organization.

iridology The examination of the iris or colored portion of the eye for markings that supposedly reveal changing conditions of every part and organ of the body.

Kirlian photography Colorful photographs of images surrounding the body and within the body that are made after applying high-frequency electrical currents to a patient's body.

mesomorph Body type in which the appearance of the body is a natural, athletic physique.

modalities The application of a therapeutic agent, usually a physical therapeutic agent.

mother of tincture The homeopathic mixture first made from plants that is diluted in alcohol and left to sit for 2 to 4 weeks.

naturopathic medicine A holistic, whole body health care system based on the belief that the body has the potential to heal itself and that the physician's role is to support the body's efforts. A system or method of treating disease that employs no surgery or synthetic drugs but uses special diets, herbs, vitamins, massage, and so on to assist the natural healing processes.

osteopathic A therapeutic system originally based on the premise that manipulation of the muscles and bones to promote structural integrity could restore or preserve health. Current osteopathic physicians use the diagnostic and therapeutic techniques of conventional medicine as well as manipulative measures.

pathogen A disease-producing agent such as a virus, bacterium, or other microorganism.

periodontitis Gum disease that begins when permeability of the mouth tissue permits pathogenic bacterial components to invade deeper periodontal connective tissues.

phytotherapy Using botanical medicine to treat disease conditions.

quinine A white, bitter, slightly water-soluble alkaloid, having needlelike crystals, obtained from cinchona bark. Used in medicine chiefly in the treatment of resistant forms of malaria.

rheumatoid arthritis A chronic autoimmune disease characterized by inflammation of the joints, frequently accompanied by marked deformities, and ordinarily associated with manifestations of a general, or systemic, affliction.

succussion Act of shaking a homeopathic mother of tincture solution during the dilution process.

temporomandibular disorder (TMD) A condition characterized by pain and tenderness of the jaw when chewing and opening the mouth.

tuberculosis An infectious disease that may affect almost any tissue of the body, but especially the lungs. It is caused by the organism *Mycobacterium tuberculosis*, and is characterized by tubercles.

References

1. Somerville R, ed. *The alternate advisor*. Alexandria, VA: Time Life Books; 1997.
2. Corinthian Naturopathic College. Naturopathy as defined by pioneers. Available at: http://www.corinthiannaturopathiccollege.com/naturopathy_as_defined_by_pioneers. Accessed September 6, 2010.
3. Smith MJ, Logan AC. Naturopathy. *Med Clin North Am*. 2002:86(1):173–184.
4. Heartland Naturopathic Clinic. The history of naturopathic medicine. Available at: http://www.heartlandnaturopathic.com/history.htm. Accessed September 6, 2010.
5. Bradford N., ed. *The one spirit encyclopedia of complementary health*. Hong Kong: Hamlyn; 2000.
6. University of Maryland Medical Center. Naturopathy. Available at: http://www.umm.edu/altmed/articles/naturopathy-000356.htm. Accessed August 26, 2011.
7. The Natural Health Perspective. A history of Western natural healing practices in Europe. Available at: http://naturalhealthperspective.com/tutorials/history.html. Accessed September 10, 2010.
8. Bastyr University. History of naturopathic medicine. Available at: http://www.bastyr.edu/education/naturopath/about/history.asp. Accessed September 10, 2010.
9. National Center for Complementary and Alternative Medicine. Naturopathy: an introduction. Available at: http://nccam.nih.gov/health/naturopathy/D372.pdf. Accessed August 26, 2011.
10. Pelletier K. *The best alternative medicine: what works? What does not?* New York: Simon & Schuster; 2000.
11. Vercillo K. 10 underlying beliefs of naturopathy. Available at: http://hubpages.com/hub/10-Underlying-Beliefs-of-Naturopathy. Accessed September 7, 2010.
12. Atwood K. Naturopathy: a critical appraisal: the naturopathic belief system. Available at: http://www.medscape.com/viewarticle/465994_3. Accessed September 7, 2010.
13. Micozzi, M. *Fundamentals of Complementary and Alternative Medicine*. 3rd ed. New York: Elsevier; 2006.
14. Oler C. Naturopathic philosophy. Available at: http://www.naturalpathhealthcenter.com/index.php/Tour-the-Center/Naturopathy/Tour-the-Center-About-Naturopathy.html. Accessed September 10, 2010.
15. Ernst E, ed. *The desktop guide to complementary and alternative medicine: an evidence-based approach*. New York: Mosby; 2001.
16. Ernst E, Pittler M, Wider B, eds. *The desktop guide to complementary and alternative medicine: an evidence-based approach*. 2nd ed. New York: Mosby Elsevier; 2006.
17. Formerfatguy.com. A solution for hardgainers and ectomorphs. Available at: http://www.formerfatguy.com/weblog/2009/05/solution-for-hardgainers-and-ectomorphs.asp. Accessed September 12, 2010.
18. Carter S. Iridology history. Available at: http://sandycarter.com/iridologynow/iridology-history.html. Accessed September 16, 2010.
19. Niebergall L, Karu A. Iridology. Available at: http://altmed.creighton.edu/Iridology/. Accessed September 16, 2010.
20. Wolfe F. Healing feats. What is iridology? Available at: http://www.healingfeats.com/whatis.htm. Accessed September 18, 2010.

21. Da Vinci College of Holistic Medicine. Available at: http://www.collegenaturalmedicine.com. Accessed September 28, 2010.
22. International College of Iridology. Available at: http://www.iridologycollege.org. Accessed September 16, 2010.
23. Singh S, Ernst E. *Trick or treatment: the undeniable facts about alternative medicine*. New York: Norton; 2008.
24. Knipschild P. Looking for gall bladder disease in the patient's iris. *BMJ*. 1988;297(6663):1578–1581.
25. Simon A, Worthen DM, Mitas JA. An evaluation of iridology. *JAMA*. 1979;242(13):1385–1389.
26. Gero G. Trace mineral analysis [Holistic Naturopathic Center]. Available at: http://www.holisticnaturopath.com/hairmineral.htm. Accessed September 25, 2010.
27. Seidel S, Kreutzer R, Smith D, McNeel S, Gilliss D. Assessment of commercial laboratories performing hair mineral analysis. *JAMA*. 2001;285:67–72.
28. Memorial Sloan-Ketting Cancer Center. BioResonance Therapy. Available at: http://www.mskcc.org/mskcc/html/69136.cfm#References. Accessed August 26, 2011.
29. Federal Trade Commission. Bogus cancer cure guru settles FTC charges. Available at: http://www.ftc.gov/opa/2002/10/walker.shtm. Accessed August 26, 2011.
30. Carroll RT. Kirlian photography [Skeptic's Dictionary]. 1994. Available at: http://www.skepdic.com/kirlian.html. Accessed August 26, 2011.
31. Great Lakes Natural Medicine. About Naturopathic medicine. Available at: http://www.greatlakesnaturalmedicine.com/wp/?page_id=2. Accessed September 22, 2011.
32. Bastyr University Naturopathic Medicine Program. Available at: http://www.naturalhealers.com/schools/bastyr/. Accessed September 27, 2010.
33. Albert DP, Martinez D. The supply of naturopathic physicians in the United States and Canada continues to increase. *Compl Health Pract Rev*. 2006;11:120–122.
34. American Association of Naturopathic Physicians. Licensed states and licensing authorities. Available at: http://www.naturopathic.org/content.asp?contentid=57. Accessed September 25, 2010.
35. Kjeldsen-Kragh J, Haugen M, Borchgrevinck CF, et al. Controlled trial of fasting and one-year vegetarian diet in rheumatoid arthritis. *Lancet*. 1991;338(8772):899–902.
36. Haugen M, Kjeldsen-Kragh J, Nordvag BY, Førre O. Diet and disease symptoms in rheumatic diseases--results of a questionnaire based survey. *Clin Rheumatol*. 1991;10(4):401–407.
37. Howard K. The future of naturopathic medicine: a message from Karen E. Howard, Executive Director of the American Association of Naturopathic Physicians. *Natural Med J*. 2010;2(1):1–2. Available at: http://naturalmedicinejournal.net/pdf/NMJ_JAN10_HP.pdf. Accessed September 20, 2010.
38. Dannheisser I, Edwards P. *Homeopathy: an illustrated guide*. Boston, MA: Element; 1998.
39. Freeman L, Lawlis F. *Mosby's complementary and alternative medicine: a research-based approach*. St. Louis: Mosby; 2001.
40. Cucherat M, Haugh MC, Gooch M, Boissel JP. Evidence of clinical efficacy of homeopathy. A meta-analysis of clinical trials. HMRAG. Homeopathic Medicines Research Advisory Group. *Eur J Clin Pharmacol*. 2000;56(1):27–33.
41. Townhill S. Homeopathy and musculoskeletal disorders—an overview and critique of available research. 2009. Available at: http://hpathy.com/homeopathy-scientific-research/homeopathy-and-musculoskeletal-disorders---an-overview-and-critique-of-available-research/. Accessed September 25, 2010.

Botanicals: A Biologically Based Therapy

LEARNING OBJECTIVES

As a result of reading this chapter, students will:

1. Describe how invested Americans are socially and economically in the use of biologically based therapies.
2. Explain ways in which botanicals could be better standardized.
3. Examine the impact of botanicals on the pharmaceutical industry.
4. Analyze the impact of biologically based therapies on U.S. health costs.

WHAT ARE BIOLOGICALLY BASED THERAPIES?

Biologically based therapies use a variety of natural techniques to maintain health and/or treat diseases. A major biologically based therapy is the use of botanicals, which are fresh or dried plants, plant parts, or chemicals extracted from the plants. Some botanicals are classified as herbs and some as spices. Some botanicals are used in cosmetics, prescription drugs, and nonprescription drugs.

Biologically based therapies also make use of minerals, vitamins, fatty acids, proteins, and probiotics (live bacteria often found in whole grains, yogurt, and functional foods). Biologically based therapies may involve orthomolecular medicine (which emphasizes supplementing diet with mega doses of vitamins, minerals, enzymes, hormones, and amino acids) and chelation therapy (use of a drug to bind with, and remove, excess or toxic amounts of metal or minerals from the blood). This chapter focuses mainly on the use of botanicals for therapeutic use.

WHAT ARE BOTANICALS?

Botanicals is a term for the use of plants or plant parts to create scents or to develop therapeutic medicinal treatments.[1] Several terms are also used synonymously: herbal medicine, "phytotherapy" (plant therapy) or medical herbalism. Botanicals may include using a mixture of different herbs or a single herb.[1] Herbal substances may come from all parts of plants such as the roots, stalks, flowers, bark, and seeds, and may include chemicals extracted from the plants. Over 1,600 botanicals and their derivatives are sold in the United States as dietary supplements. The herbs are sold as dried materials of plant origin either in bulk whole form, cut-and-sifted, or powdered.[2,3] Herbal remedies are used to restore and maintain health by relying on the curative properties of certain herbs to stimulate our body's healing system.[4] Herbs are used to alleviate disease, prevent it from recurring, detoxify the body, and support the immune system.

Nutritional Supplementation, Spices, and Other Uses

Botanicals may be used to supplement a person's normal diet with additional extracts, nutrients, herbs, and/or certain foods. They also may be used to provide fragrance (aromatherapy). Botanicals classified as spices are used to flavor foods. Spices are said to be piquant (pungent or tart in taste; spicy). Aromatic plant materials, usually tropical in origin, such as cloves, cinnamon, nutmeg, and pepper are used in seasoning food.[3]

In addition, the cosmetics industry uses over 360 botanical additives to add fragrance and enhance the looks of their products. Moreover, botanicals are used in prescription and nonprescription drugs. They may be present in crude form (whole dried plants or plant parts) or as a chemical constituent.

HOW HAVE HERBS BEEN USED HISTORICALLY?

Herbs have been used by many cultures for centuries, in fact before recorded history.[5] Herbs were used in Ayurvedic medicine as long ago as 1900 BCE and in traditional Chinese medicine from around 2700 BCE. Chinese herbalism is based on the concepts of yin and yang and qi (chi) energy. Herbs used for cooling are yin herbs and those used for stimulating are yang herbs. For more information on the use of traditional Chinese herbal medicines, please see Chapter 9; for more information on Ayurvedic herbal use, please see Chapter 8.

The use of herbs has been traced back to 5,000 years ago by the Sumerians, who wrote of well-established medicinal uses for such plants as laurel, caraway, and thyme. The ancient Egyptians (1000 BCE) relied heavily on garlic, opium, myrrh, cumin, caraway, fennel, olive oil, and licorice. Native American Indians and early Americans used plants and the bark of certain trees. The native Indians of Peru used quinine to treat malaria and limes to prevent scurvy, a vitamin C deficiency. They also used a plant called foxglove to obtain a chemical now known as digitalis to treat certain heart conditions. In 1960, the body of a Neanderthal man living 60,000 years ago was uncovered, and several herbs used to treat him were present. Eight different species of plants were found at the burial site, and seven of those eight are used for medicinal purposes today.[6]

WHAT IS AN HERBALIST?

An herbalist is a practitioner, and contributor to the field, of herbal medicine. Native healers, shamans, scientists, holistic medical doctors, nutritionists, pharmacists, naturopaths, traditional Chinese medicine doctors (TCM), and traditional Ayurvedic medicine doctors may use and promote herbal medicines. Medical herbalists combine modern scientific concepts with their knowledge of herbs. They are academically trained in examination techniques and knowledge of the human body.[4]

WHAT ARE THE DIFFERENT FORMS OF HERBS?

Herbs come in their natural state or are processed into many forms. The different forms are listed and described as follows:

- *Crude herbs:* Herbs that are collected and dried, cut, and sifted. Crude herbs may be cooked into teas.[5,7]
- *Concentrated herbal extracts:* These herbs may be in liquid or solid form and are anywhere from 2 to 100 times as concentrated as crude herbs.[5,7,8]
- *Powders:* Ground crude herbs. They may be ingested in natural form or cooked to make teas.
- *Teas:* Aqueous extractions of crude herbs or herbal powders.
- *Dried decoctions or concentrated granules:* Decoctions are concentrated brews made by simmering tougher forms or parts of herbs such as roots, barks, and woody stems.[5,7,8] Decoctions are cooked as teas and the solid residue is removed, after which the remaining liquids are dried out until only powders remain.[8] The powders are about four times as potent as the original herbs.
- *Tinctures:* Herbal concentrates or extracts made by soaking herbs in solutions, usually alcohol, glycerin, or a vinegar base.[5,7] These are designed to bring out the herbal properties.
- *Infusions:* Concentrates made by steeping 1 ounce of herb in 2 cups of water. The more delicate parts of the plant such as leaves, flowers, and light stems are used.
- *Bolus:* A suppository made from herbs that is to be inserted into the rectum or vagina. Powdered herbs mixed with cocoa butter, water, or honey can be formed into a suppository. If made with cocoa butter or honey, the preparation needs to be refrigerated or it will lose its shape. If made with water, it needs to be heated on a cookie sheet at a low temperature of 120 degrees or so until hardened. At time of insertion, a lubricant should be applied to the bolus.[7]
- *Capsules:* Powdered herbs, dried decoctions, or concentrated extracts are placed in gelatin capsules.
- *Tablets:* Powdered herbs, dried decoctions, or concentrated herbal extracts are mixed with a binding substance and then pressed into tablets.
- *Gelcaps:* Sealed gelatin capsules that hold either tinctures or concentrated liquid herbal extracts.
- *Bath:* Two to four quarts of a decoction or infusion, strained and then added to a tub of bathwater.
- *Poultice:* A preparation of a fresh, dry, ground, or powdered herb or herbal mixture that is wrapped in thin cotton or wool cloth and applied to the skin. Sometimes the poultice is applied directly to the skin.[7,8]
- *Fomentation:* A cloth is soaked in an infusion or decoction from which all the herb has been strained. The cloth is then applied to the skin.[7]
- *Liniment:* A liniment has a liquid base and is rubbed into sore muscles and joints. It is made by making a decoction or infusion and then adding ¼ to ½ part olive oil and/or rubbing alcohol.[7]

WHAT ARE THE CHEMICALS AND PROPERTIES OF HERBS?

Various plants contain chemicals, many of which are used in today's prescription medications as well as herbal medicines. Some of the chemicals found in plants and herbs include the following:

Alkaloids: Alkaloids are used in painkiller drugs, narcotics, hypotensives (to lower blood pressure), hypertensives (to increase blood pressure), bronchodilators, stimulants, antimicrobials, and anti-inflammatory herbs. Coffee bean and the plant *Ephedra sinica* contain stimulating alkaloids.[8]

Cardiac glycosides: These chemicals have a marked action on the heart, strengthening the force and speed of systolic contractions. The foxglove plant contains *Digitalis purpurea*, one of the glycosides.[8]

Carotenoid pigments: These are pigments found in yellow to red plants such as carrots, sweet potatoes, red and yellow peppers, squash, and tomatoes. Two carotenoids are beta-carotene and lycopene (red pigment found in tomatoes). They help maintain healthy epithelial tissue and mucous membranes, aid growth and repair of body tissue, and more. Carotenoid pigments transfer light energy to chlorophyll for use in photosynthesis and act as antioxidants for chlorophyll.[8,9]

Chlorophyll: This is a pigment found in dark green leafy vegetables such as spinach, parsley, kale, green beans, and leeks. Chlorophyll absorbs energy from the sun to facilitate photosynthesis (synthesis of carbohydrates from carbon dioxide and water) in plants. According to Michael T. Simonich of the Linus Pauling Institute, chlorophyll has antioxidant properties and retards cancer cell growth.[10,11] Two types of chlorophyll are found in plants and green algae, chlorophyll a and chlorophyll b.

Fixed oils: Fixed oils are referred to as vegetable, carrier, or base oils and contain nutrients such as minerals, antioxidants, and fat-soluble vitamins. They are not volatile and do not evaporate. Many fixed oils are used with essential oils for aromatherapy because they do not compete with the aroma. They may also be mixed with essential oils that are used for massage therapy.[12] Some examples of fixed oils are almond oil, avocado oil, aloe vera, castor oil, flaxseed oil, and evening primrose oil.[13]

Flavonoids: Flavonoids are a set of chemicals that include brilliant plant pigments seen in fruits and vegetables. They are thought to be potent antioxidants, and have anti-inflammatory and metal-chelating properties.[14] There are six subclasses: anthocyanidins are found in red, blue, and purple berries; red and purple grapes; and red wine. Flavanols are found in teas, chocolate, grapes, berries, apples, and red wine. Flavanones are found in citrus fruits and juices. Flavonols are found in yellow onions, scallions, kale, broccoli, apples, berries, and teas. Flavones are found in parsley, thyme, celery, and hot peppers. Isoflavones are found in soybeans, soy foods, and legumes.

Lignans: Lignans are phytoestrogens with weak estrogenic or anti-estrogenic activity. Lignans may be found in nuts, seeds, breads, vegetables, fruit, and wine. Examples of nuts and seeds are milk thistle seed, flax seed, sunflower seed, sesame seed, cashews, peanuts, and poppy seeds. Whole grain, multi-grain, rye, and wheat bread also contain lignans. Vegetables such as broccoli, cauliflower, onions, and green beans contain lignans, as do fruits such as apricots, strawberries, peaches, and pears.[15] Research studies are conflicting about the health benefits of lignans. Although a diet rich in lignans lowers cardiovascular disease risk, research is unclear as to whether the effect is due to lignans alone or to other foods in the diet. Velentzis et.al[16] conducted a meta-analysis study of publications up to September 2008 and found there was little evidence to suggest that lignans with their mild estrogenic activity are associated with increased breast cancer risk. On the other hand, for postmenopausal women, the meta-analysis found that high lignan intake was associated with a 15 percent reduction in the risk for getting breast cancer.[16]

Phytoestrogens: Phytoestrogens are estrogen-like chemicals that can act like the hormone estrogen. They come from three chemical classes: the lignans, the isoflavonoids, and the coumestans. More than 300 foods contain phytoestrogens.[17] Isoflavonoid phytoestrogens are found in the legume family (e.g., soybeans) and coumestan phytoestrogens are found in various beans, such as pinto beans and lima beans, but also in alfalfa and clover sprouts. Research studies about the use of soy products are conflicting. Half of the studies reported no increased risk of breast cancer associated with ingesting soy milk or soy products. Other studies have indicated a decrease in the risk of breast cancer among women eating soy compared to women who did not.[17]

Phytoprogesterones: Phytoprogesterones are plant chemicals that bind to progesterone receptors. Phytoestrogens are found in the lignans, the isoflavonoids, the flavonoids, and the coumestans. Examples of plant sources are flaxseed, soybeans, tofu, sesame seeds, blueberries, and almonds.[18]

Plant coumarins: Coumarin was first isolated from the tonka bean (*Dipteryx odorata*), which is in a classification known as coumarou; thus similar plants were named plant coumarins. Coumarins are mainly synthesized in the leaves of plants, but occur at the highest levels in the fruits, next highest in the roots, and at the lowest levels in the stem. Coumarin has no anticoagulant activity, but once converted to dicoumarol by fungi it becomes anticoagulant in nature. Sweet clover disease in cattle is caused by cattle eating moldy, sweet clover silage. The cattle hemorrhaged to death from the effects of the clover.[18] Coumarin is also found in sweet woodruff, vanilla grass, sweet grass, Cassia cinnamon, and red clover blossoms.

Oral anticoagulants are derived from plant coumarins. Warfarin was used as a rat killer (rodenticide) prior to its 1954 introduction into clinical medicine as an anticoagulant.[19]

Salicylates and salicins: These are aspirin-like compounds that have pain-relieving and anti-inflammatory action. Salicin is a glycoside found in willow bark. It acts as an antipyretic, antiseptic, and anti-inflammatory. It is a bitter tonic (gastric stimulant) and is useful for mild feverish colds, headaches, and rheumatic conditions.[20] Herman Kolbe synthesized salicylic acid from coal tar; it was found to be stronger than salicin.[20,21] Today, it is an active ingredient in many skin care products used to treat acne. Because salicin and salicylic acid use caused many side effects such as stomach irritation leading to nausea and vomiting and hearing problems (tinnitus), scientists synthesized acetylsalicylic acid, the main ingredient in today's aspirin products.

Saponins: Saponins are glycosides or chemicals found in plants such as oats, vegetables, and beans that cause plants placed in water to "soap up," or froth to form a lather. They are also found in several herbs: alfalfa, agave, fenugreek, and ginseng.[22] They get their name from the soapwort plant (*Saponaria*); the root of the plant was used for making soap.[23] Because of the detergent properties, saponins are used in shampoos, facial cleansers, and cosmetic creams.[24] They act on internal surfaces of membranes and blood vessels to lower surface tension. Saponins are thought to have several health benefits, including reducing blood cholesterol levels, boosting immunity, reducing cancer risk, reducing bone loss, and having antioxidant properties.[24]

Tannins: Tannins are polyphenols obtained from various parts of plants. They are found in tree bark, wood, fruit, leaves, and roots. Tannins bind with proteins and form a protective layer on the skin and mucous membranes.[25] Tannins are used in dyeing and photography, as an astringent in medicines, and for refining beer and wine.[26] Tannins can reduce diarrhea or intestinal bleeding, and are used externally to inhibit infections of the eye, mouth, vagina, and rectum.[26] Coffee, black tea, green tea, and wine contain tannins.

Volatile oils: Volatile oils are compounds of vegetable origin that evaporate at room temperature and allow us to enjoy the smell. They are made through steam distillation and expression.[27] *Steam distillation* is done by immersing the plant in a still filled with water and then boiling it. The vapors are condensed on a cold surface and the essential oils then separate. During *expression*, the process calls for an abrasive action on the surface of fruit while being washed with water. The solid waste is eliminated and essential oil is separated by centrifugation. Volatile oils have many health benefits: antiseptic properties (oil of thyme); antispasmodic properties (ginger, lemon balm, rosemary, peppermint, chamomile, fennel, caraway); perfumes (oil of rose); and flavoring (oil of lemon). They may be used in medicine as stimulants, and some exhibit antifungal and insect-repellent actions. Eucalyptus, garlic, oregano, and tea tree also contain volatile oils.[27]

HOW DO YOU USE HERBS?

Shopping for Herbs

If you are considering obtaining herbs, you may buy them in bulk or buy standardized medicinal herbs.[28] *Bulk herbs* are those harvested from an herbalist who has grown them in an herb garden or those that you have grown. You may also purchase bulk herbs at a health food store or herbal shop where you may see bins of dried bulk herbs. One problem is that you can't be sure of the level of constituents in the bulk herbs or plant material. But buying bulk herbs allows you to learn how to process and store the herbs. You can also experiment somewhat by mixing some preparations.[28]

The advantage of buying *standardized herbs* is that they have been processed, so a known minimum level of one or more of the major active ingredients is present. They may be more expensive than bulk herbs, but are still quite a bit less expensive than pharmaceuticals that treat the same conditions.[28]

Care and Storage of Herbs

If you are considering obtaining herbs, you should gather them when they are as fresh as possible. You will need to be careful to obtain them from reputable sources and should buy them in a form allowing positive identification. You should check to be sure the herbs are insect free, and you should store them in tightly closed glass containers in cool, dry places away from the sun. Empty 35 mm film containers are a good size for storing small amounts of herbs when traveling. They can be placed in glove compartments or backpacks and heat does not affect the 35 mm container.[7] Herbal brews can be kept in the refrigerator for a couple of days, but then begin to weaken in medicinal strength.

Utensils for Making Herbal Preparations

Pans that are aluminum or cast iron should not be used for brewing teas because the metals disintegrate into the herbal preparation. It is best to use stainless steel, glass, or ceramic pots and bowls. Even the stirring spoon should be stainless steel, but wooden spoons may be used. To avoid contaminating your herbs, you should keep a clean set of spoons that are used only for herbal preparation and nothing else.[7]

HOW DOES THE GOVERNMENT CONTROL HERBS?

Governmental Control of Herbs in Germany Compared with the United States

In 1976, the Federal Republic of Germany (then West Germany) developed a mechanism to assure herbal safety. The country commissioned an expert panel (German Commission E) that was composed of physicians, pharmacists, pharmacologists, toxicologists, and representatives of the pharmaceutical industry and laypersons. To determine with "reasonable certainty" the safety and efficacy of each herb being evaluated, the commission checks herbal data independently of other drugs. They assess data from clinical trials, field studies, case studies, and independent medical association members.[6] Approximately 600 to 700 different plant drugs are sold in pharmacies, health food stores, and markets. About 70 percent of German physicians prescribe registered herbal remedies, and government health insurance helps pay a significant proportion of the $1.7 billion in annual sales.

In the United States, the Food and Drug Administration (FDA) evaluates the safety and efficacy of new drugs based on data supplied by the drug manufacturer (pharmaceutical company). The process to get a new drug can take 12 years and cost over $350 million. It costs the pharmaceutical industry about $12.6 billion a year for new drug development.[29] Even though the FDA was petitioned by phytomedicine manufacturers from Europe and the United States to allow well-researched European drugs the status of old drugs so they would not have to go through new drug applications, the FDA has never responded to those petitions.[7]

In 1994, the U.S. Dietary Supplement Health and Education Act (DSHEA) allowed herbal products to be labeled with certain information such as side effects, potential safety problems, and contraindications. Nutritional support information and how the product affects the body's physiology can be included, but the label cannot make a statement that the herb is therapeutic or can treat or cure a disease condition.[7]

Herbals are defined by the DSHEA as dietary supplements.[18] They are described as a product that:

- Is intended to supplement the diet
- Contains one or more dietary ingredients (including vitamins, minerals, herbs or other botanicals,

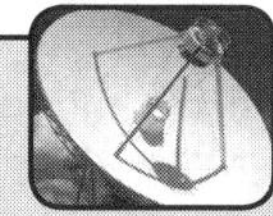

In the News

The FDA released a new release in January 2002,[30] titled, Tips for the savvy supplement user: Making informed decisions and evaluating information. Main tips are the following:

Basic points to consider: thinking about total dietary needs, checking with personal doctor before using supplements, information about prescription drug and over-the-counter medicine interactions, unwanted effects from supplements during pregnancy, adverse effects and who you should report it to, and who is responsible for ensuring safety and efficacy of dietary supplements.

Tips on searching the web for dietary supplement information: who operates the site, purpose of the site, source of the information and references, checking to be sure information is current, and reliability of the internet site.

More tips and to-do's. Asking yourself if it sounds too good to be true; thinking twice about chasing the latest headline; checking assumptions about safety of the herb such as equating the word, natural, to mean healthful and safe or safe because there is no cautionary information on the label or safe because it has not been recalled.

Contacting the manufacture if you can't tell if the product meets same standards as those in research studies you have read. Look for information about substantiating claims, tests conducted for safety or efficacy, what quality control systems are in place, and if the firm has received any adverse effects from people who have used the product.

Questions:

1. What are your thoughts about the FDA approval process?
2. How could the FDA speed up the approval process (or should it)?
3. What are your thoughts about the approval process for herbal products?
4. What main point did you learn from the FDA tips displayed in the In The News section?
5. Do you believe that the United States could learn from and adopt policies that have been developed in Germany?

amino acids, and certain other substances) or their constituents

- Is intended to be taken by mouth, in forms such as tablet, capsule, powder, softgel, gelcap, or liquid
- Is labeled as being a dietary supplement

How the FDA Approves New Drugs and Medical Devices

The FDA's drug approval process, aimed at proving the safety and effectiveness of new drugs, is an important hurdle for new companies seeking a piece of the international market. If the FDA would accept herbal supplements for the approval process, the following steps would be taken:

1. *Investigational new drug application (IND):* Researcher submits preliminary animal and lab testing data, a proposal for tests on humans, and expected findings. The FDA has 30 days to submit questions, which delays the process, or to allow the next step.[29]
2. *Clinical studies*
   a. *Phase 1:* Safety, dosage, and effects on the body are tested on 20–80 healthy volunteers (about 1 year).
   b. *Phase 2:* Effectiveness and side effects are tested on 100–300 people with the disease to be treated by the drug (about 2 years).
   c. *Phase 3:* The drug is tested on 1,000 to 3,000 people with the disease who are in clinics or hospitals. Benefits and long-term side effects are compared. Marketing information, including labels and warnings, are developed (about 3 years).
3. *New drug application (NDA):* An NDA is then submitted (usually about 100,000 pages). Researchers submit applications containing all scientific data, how the drug is processed, what it is made of, and how it would be packaged, along with samples and labeling. On receiving the NDA, the FDA starts a 180-day approval period that can be delayed at any time for questions and additional research. FDA chemists, pharmacologists, physicians, statisticians, microbiologists, and other specialists review the NDA. This approval process usually takes around 2½ years.

See **BOX 11.1** for the different types of applications required by the U.S. Food and Drug Administration.

Sometimes, the FDA will move drugs or medical devices through a streamlined process. An example of this process is exemplified by an article published in the *Healthcare Business News*.[30] It could be that some herbals already approved by the German commission or other European commissions could be streamlined through the U.S. FDA process.

Box 11.1

FDA Application Types

Animal and Veterinary

Biologics, Blood, and Vaccines

Cosmetics

Tobacco products

Drugs

Foods

Medical devices

Radiation-emitting products

All other topics

HOW SAFE ARE HERBAL SUPPLEMENTS?

Even though an herbal supplement is on the shelf of a store, the FDA is still supposed to monitor its safety. If the FDA finds a product unsafe, it could take action against the manufacturer and/or issue a warning. The product could also be removed from the market. Herbal supplements, however, do appear to have a better safety record than that of pharmaceutical drugs.[4] That does not mean that all herbals are safe or that they cannot be abused. Safety depends on many factors, including chemical makeup, how the herb works in the body, how it is prepared, dosage, and interaction with other herbs or pharmaceutical products.[31] We should be aware that many herbals contain ingredients that elicit strong effects in our bodies and could have potential side effects. Moreover, taking the products along with prescription drugs could be dangerous if the herb potentiates (adds to the effect) or negates the effect of the prescription drug. An example is the use of herbs such as ginkgo, garlic, ginseng, ginger, and St. John's wort, which increase the effect of prescription drug blood thinners and blood thinning effects of over-the-counter medicines such as nonsteroidal anti-inflammatory drugs such as ibuprofen.[32]

In addition, St. John's wort is taken to aid mild depression, but some people find it makes their skin more sensitive to the sun's ultraviolet rays and have an allergic reaction. The FDA has issued a public health advisory concerning many of these interactions. Examples follow:

- Kava kava (an antianxiety herb) has been linked to liver toxicity. Kava has been taken off the market in several countries because of this toxicity.
- Valerian (taken as a sleep aid) may have the unexpected effect of overstimulating instead of sedating.
- Garlic, ginkgo, feverfew, and ginger, among other herbs, may increase the risk of bleeding.

- Evening primrose (*Oenothera biennis*) may increase the risk of seizures in people who have seizure disorders.
- In 2007, the FDA put out a warning to consumers to avoid red yeast rice products promoted on the Internet as treatments for high cholesterol. Products put out by Swanson Healthcare Products, Inc. and manufactured by Nature's Value Inc. and Kabco Inc. contained an unauthorized ingredient called lovastatin, which is found in a prescription drug called Mevacor. The ingredient does lower cholesterol, but has side effects of adverse muscle reaction and kidney complications.[29]

In addition, some herbal supplements, especially those imported from Asian countries, may contain high levels of heavy metals, including lead, mercury, and cadmium. Talk to your health care provider for more information. Certainly, you should talk to your doctor if you are thinking about buying and using herbal supplements.

WHAT ARE HEALTH CARE PROFESSIONALS' KNOWLEDGE OF AND RECOMMENDATIONS REGARDING HERBAL SUPPLEMENTS?

Research studies have been employed to ascertain health care professionals' knowledge and attitudes regarding herbal supplement use for various conditions. The first study discussed is a review of studies[33] through March 2006 of U.S. or Canadian pharmacists' attitudes, knowledge, or professional practice behaviors regarding herbal supplements. Results show inconsistency. A majority of respondents believed that herbal supplements could be beneficial but they also believed that the majority of their colleagues do not accept herbal medicine. A majority believed that herbal medicine could increase the profit margin. Studies showed inconsistency about pharmacists' views regarding how selling herbal supplements affects the pharmacy's image. Some believed it affected the pharmacy negatively and some did not.[33]

Results of a survey study[34] of 184 board certified psychiatrists in New Jersey revealed that 62 percent did not recommend herbal products. Of the 38 percent responding who did recommend herbal remedies, 30 percent recommended St. John's wort, 25 percent recommended gingko, 13 percent recommended valerian, and 8 percent recommended other herbal products.[34]

An online survey was administered to a random sample of subscribers to the *Drug and Therapeutic Bulletin*, primarily physicians and pharmacists. Of the 164 respondents, results showed that 75.5 percent of the health care professionals said they believed that their profession was poorly informed about herbal supplements, and 86.3 percent of the respondents believed the general public was poorly informed.[35] Respondents also rated their own knowledge abut herbal supplements as *quite* (36.2 percent) or *very* (10.4 percent) poor.

HOW MUCH MONEY IS SPENT ON HERBAL SUPPLEMENTS EACH YEAR?

According to the 2007 National Center for Health Statistics (NCHS) survey,[36] out-of-pocket spending for all complementary and alternative medicine (CAM) therapies was estimated at $33.9 billion dollars. Of that amount, the cost of non-vitamin, non-mineral products was 14.8 billion dollars and 2.9 billion dollars was spent on homeopathic medicine.

WHO USES HERBALS, AND WHICH HERBALS ARE THE MOST POPULAR?

According to the same NCHS 2007 study,[36] 17.7 percent of U.S. adults had used natural products during the past 12 months.[18] The 10 natural products most commonly used by U.S. adults during the last 30 days were fish oil omega 3 (37.4 percent), glucosamine (19.9 percent), echinacea (19.8 percent), flaxseed oil/pills (15.9 percent), ginseng (14.1 percent), combination herb pills (13.0 percent), ginkgo biloba (11.3 percent), chondroitin (11.2 percent), garlic supplements (11.0 percent), and coenzyme Q-10 (8.7 percent).

There are hundreds of herbs—too many to include in one chapter of a textbook—but the following represents those more commonly used for certain disorders and disease conditions. Some have been studied scientifically, some are still being studied, and some have not been studied.

Certain precautions should be taken before buying an herb for medicinal use. The main one is to discuss your idea with your physician. If you are taking any prescription medications, talking with your physician is extremely important because of the possibility of drug interaction. A second precaution is to research the company that is producing the herbal. You might want to get a membership in Consumerlab.com, an Internet site that researches and tests herbals, minerals, and vitamins to ensure that the ingredients listed on the label are actually in the herbal preparation.

WHAT ARE COMMON HERBAL SUPPLEMENTS AND NON-PLANT BASED DIETARY SUPPLEMENTS?

The following are some of the most commonly used herbal and non-plant based dietary supplements:

Alfalfa (Medicago sativa): This versatile herb is also a folk remedy for arthritis, diabetes, asthma, and hay fever. It is said to detoxify the body, especially the liver. It contains vitamin K, which helps the body form blood clots, and should not be taken in combination with warfarin (Coumadin), an anticoagulant drug. It is possibly effective for lowering cholesterol in people with high cholesterol levels. It may also lower blood sugar. Taking alfalfa seeds may cause extra sensitivity to the sun, and taking alfalfa pills along with estrogen birth control pills may lower their effectiveness. It may mimic lupus erythematosus symptoms and should not be taken by people with lupus.[28]

Aloe vera: Known as burn plant, lily of the desert, and elephant's gall. See **FIGURE 11.1**. Aloe is used topically for skin wounds and other skin conditions. Aloe supplements can be used for peptic ulcers and for gastrointestinal health. Aloe latex (the green part of the leaf that surrounds the gel) contains a laxative compound. The FDA has banned OTC aloe laxative products because manufacturing companies did not provide necessary safety data.[18] Aloe vera contains three anti-inflammatory fatty acids helpful for the stomach, small intestine, and colon. It alkalizes digestive juices to prevent overacidity. The leaves contain a clear gel that is used as a topical ointment.

Arginine (L-arginine): Arginine is an amino acid that can raise levels of nitric oxide in the blood and body tissues, which can increase blood flow necessary for arousal. Because of the vasodilation effect, conditions such as chest pain from clogged arteries and headaches due to blood vessel swelling may be helped. Arginine has also been studied for its wound healing properties, as an aid to sperm production, and for its body building properties. It is also being studied for wasting disease in people who have AIDS and similar conditions.[38]

Arnica (Arnica montana): An extract of the bright yellow, daisy-like flower is used. It is rubbed on the skin to soothe and heal bruises and sprains, and relieve irritations from trauma, arthritis, and muscle or cartilage pain. Applied as a salve, arnica is also good for chapped lips, irritated nostrils, and acne. It has also been used as a mouthwash for swollen gums and mouth ulcers.[28,37]

Astragalus (Astragalus membranaceus, Astragalus mongholicus): Astragalus is a tonic and immune-enhancing herb that is supposed to increase natural killer (NK) cell activity. This type of plant has been used in China for nearly 4,000 years for chronic hepatitis and as an adjunct in cancer therapy. It is used by those with AIDS today. The root of the plant is used in soups, teas, extracts, and capsules.[18] The herb is presently being studied by the NCCAM. Preliminary studies indicated some effectiveness for boosting the immune system, benefits for the heart and liver, and as a useful adjunct for cancer therapy. See **FIGURE 11.2**.

Bee pollen: Bee pollen is collected from flowers by honeybees and is their main food source. It is a popular energy booster, strengthens the immune system, and enhances vitality. It is said to slow the effect of premature aging of the skin as well as act as an aid for weight control. Animal studies on mice and rats showed benefits of bee pollen, and in a study of 60 men in Wales, researchers found that pollen extract was effective as a treatment for prostate enlargement and inflammation of the prostate.[39]

Bilberry: Bilberry is a little blue berry related to cranberries and blueberries. It is said to be a powerful anti-inflammatory and antioxidant. It contains nutrients (e.g., flavonols, anthocyanosides) needed to protect eyes from eyestrain or fatigue, and can improve circulation to the eyes. It may help with night vision and/or help the eyes to adjust to changes in light.[40] Clinical studies suggest that bilberry may prevent diabetic retinopathy and improve visual acuity and retinal function. Because of the coumarins present in bilberry, an additive effect with blood thinners could result.[41]

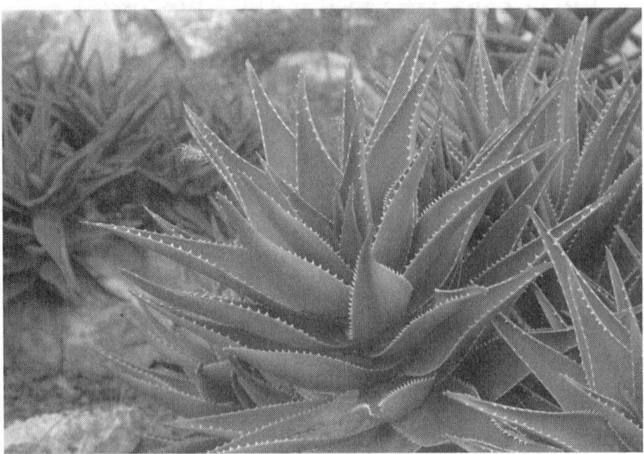

FIGURE 11.1 Aloe vera plant.

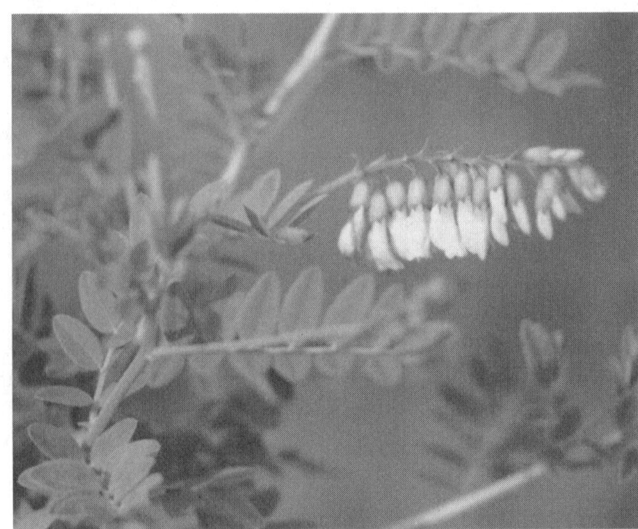

FIGURE 11.2 Astragalus.

Black cohosh: A plant native to North America that is a member of the buttercup family. (See **FIGURE 11.3**.) It has been used as a treatment for arthritis and symptoms of menopause (hot flashes, night sweats, vaginal dryness). Scientific studies have not shown effectiveness for treating menopausal symptoms, but laboratory study of mice showed promotion of bone formation.[42]

Butterbur: Also known as butter dock, bog rhubarb, and exwort. It is an herb native to Europe, Asia, and north Africa. Both the leaf and roots may be used. Herbalists use an extract from its roots, called petasins. Extracts have been used to treat allergies, bronchial asthma, headache, pain, and muscle and urinary tract spasms. Several clinical studies have demonstrated the effectiveness of butterbur for migraine headache.[43–46]

Calendula (Calendula officinalis): Calendula is grown in the United States. (See **FIGURE 11.4**.) The flower is used medicinally to prevent muscle spasms, start menstrual periods, and reduce fever. The plant is said to be antibacterial, antifungal, anti-inflammatory, and antiviral. Calendula stimulates white blood cells to engulf harmful microbes and helps speed wound healing. Commercial calendula flower ointments can be purchased and applied as needed.[28,36]

Cascara sagrada aged bark (Rhamnus purshiana): Cascara is a species of buckthorn found predominantly in the western United States. The aged bark has been used for centuries as a laxative herb because of the plant's glycosides. Only organic bark, aged at least a year, should be used; fresh bark induces vomiting and diarrhea. Cascara sagrada was a primary ingredient in many over-the-counter laxatives in the United States until the FDA banned its use along with aloe in 2002. The FDA banned the herb because of a controlled clinical study that found cascara sagrada could potentially cause liver damage with long-term usage due to the glycosides present in the plant's chemical makeup.[46,47]

Cat's claw (Uncaria tomentosa, Uncaria guianensis): Cat's claw is most commonly used to support the immune system. Cat's claw is used to help treat viral infections, Alzheimer's disease, cancer, kidney disease, and arthritis.[18] The inner bark of cat's claw is used to make liquid extracts, capsules, and teas. Small studies in humans have shown a possible benefit of cat's claw in osteoarthritis and rheumatoid arthritis, but no large trials have been done. In fact, there is not enough scientific evidence to determine whether cat's claw works for any health condition. The National Institute on Aging has funded a study to look at how cat's claw may affect the brain. Findings may point to new avenues for research in Alzheimer's disease treatment. Few side effects have been reported for cat's claw when taken at recommended dosages. Women who are pregnant or trying to become pregnant should avoid using cat's claw because of its past use for preventing and aborting pregnancy.[18]

Cayenne pepper (Capsicum anuum): Also known as chili pepper, Cayenne is not cooked or used raw (undried) because of its irritant effect on the gastrointestinal system. It is intended to be used in a dry, usually powdered form to heal bleeding ulcers in the digestive system.[7] Excessive ingestion may cause gastroenteritis or liver or kidney damage. The chemical that causes

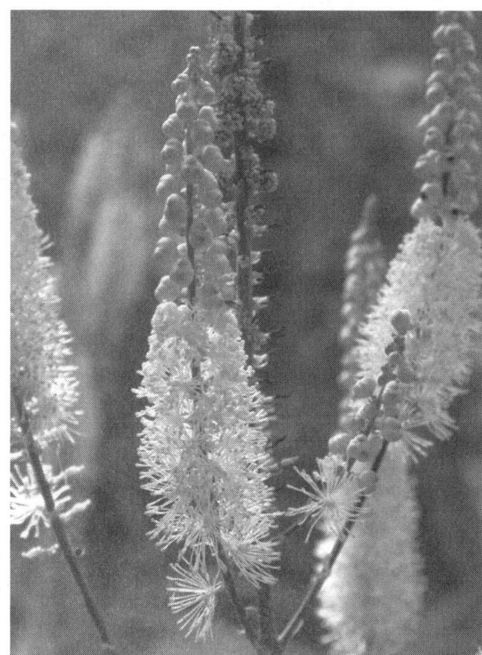

FIGURE 11.3 Black cohosh.

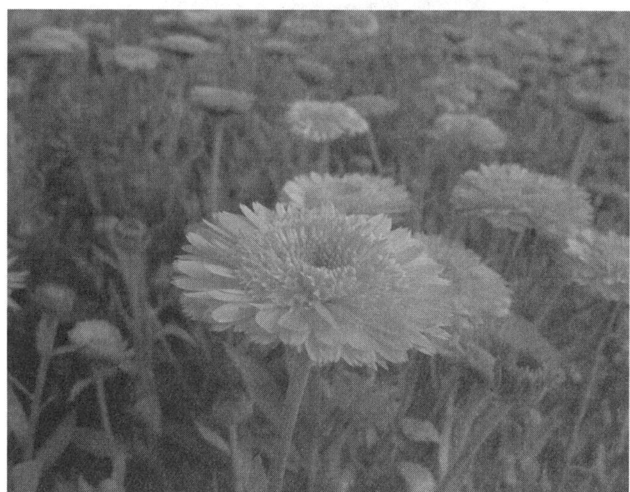

FIGURE 11.4 Calendula.

the hotness is capsaicin. Cayenne has antioxidant properties. Regular consumption of cayenne increases the resistance of blood lipids to oxidation and may slightly decrease insulin levels after a meal. Cayenne is reported to possibly interfere with MAO inhibitors and antihypertensive therapy, and may increase hepatic metabolism of drugs.[48]

Celery seed: Celery seed is used primarily as a diuretic (increasing urine output to help the body get rid of excess water). Celery seed is also suggested for treating arthritis and gout, and to help reduce muscle spasms, calm the nerves, and reduce inflammation. However, there are no scientific studies in humans that show whether celery seed is effective for these conditions or any others. Studies do show that celery seeds act as a mosquito repellent. Pregnant women should not use celery seed because it may lead to uterine bleeding and muscle contractions in the uterus, which could cause miscarriage.[5]

Chaste tree extract (chasteberry): Chasteberry is the fruit of the chaste tree, a small shrub-like tree native to Central Asia and the Mediterranean region. (See **FIGURE 11.5**.) It has been used for menstrual problems, such as premenstrual syndrome, as well as for symptoms of menopause, some types of infertility, and acne. The chasteberry is dried when ripe and used to prepare liquid extracts or solid extracts that are put into capsules and tablets. Some studies show chasteberry improves premenstrual syndrome, breast pain, and some types of infertility, but many of the studies were not well designed and/or not scientifically reliable enough to determine whether chasteberry has any effect on these conditions. It can cause gastrointestinal problems, acne-like rashes, and dizziness.[8,18,28]

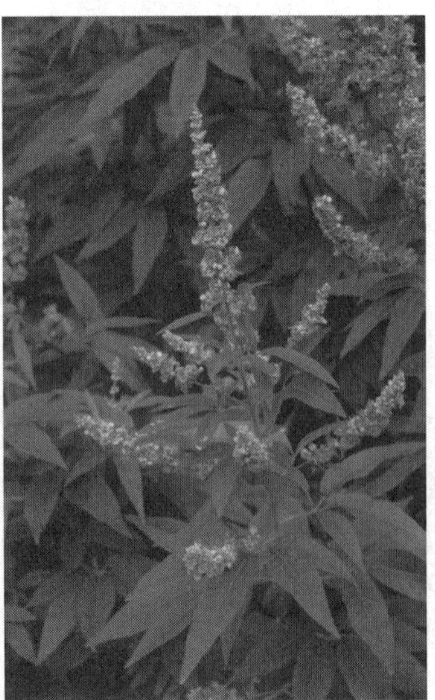

FIGURE 11.5 Chasteberry.

Cranberry fruit (Vaccinium macrocarpon): Historically, cranberry fruits and leaves were used for a variety of health conditions such as wounds, urinary disorders, diarrhea, diabetes, stomach ailments, and liver problems. Many people take cranberry juice or the fruit for preventing or treating urinary tract infections (UTIs). Research shows that components found in cranberry may prevent bacteria, such as *E. coli*, from clinging to the cells along the walls of the urinary tract and causing infection. There is no evidence, however, that cranberry can treat urinary tract infections.[18] Cranberry has been reported to have antioxidant and anticancer activity. Cranberry may be found in the form of fruit, fruit juice, extracts, capsules, or tablets.[18]

Creatine: Although not a plant herb, creatine is a dietary supplement used by athletes and we wanted to include information about it. Creatine is naturally synthesized in the human body and during the 1800s was found to be an organic constituent present in meat. It began to be used by athletes as a "natural" way to enhance athletic performance and build lean body mass. Adolescent athletes have been found to take doses that are not consistent with scientific evidence, and to frequently exceed recommended loading and maintenance doses. The National Collegiate Athletic Association has now banned the use of school funds to buy and supply creatine for athletes, although the athletes may buy creatine for themselves and consume it.[49]

Dong quai root (Angelica sinensis): Dong quai is an herb in the celery family native to China, Japan, and Korea. (See **FIGURE 11.6**.) The root is medicinally active, and different parts of the dong quai root are believed to have different actions. The head of the root has anticoagulant activity; the main part of the root is a tonic; and the end of the root eliminates blood stagnation. It is considered the "female ginseng" because of its balancing effect on the female hormonal system. However, studies have not found dong quai to have strong hormone-like effects.[49] Dong quai should not be used by people with bleeding disorders, excessive menstrual bleeding, diarrhea, or abdominal bloating, or during infections such as colds and flu. Dong quai may contain weak estrogen-like compounds and should not be taken by pregnant or nursing women, children, or people with breast cancer.[50]

Echinacea: There are nine known species of echinacea, all of which are native to the United States and southern Canada. Echinacea is believed to stimulate the immune system to help fight infections and has been used to treat or prevent colds, flu, and other infec-

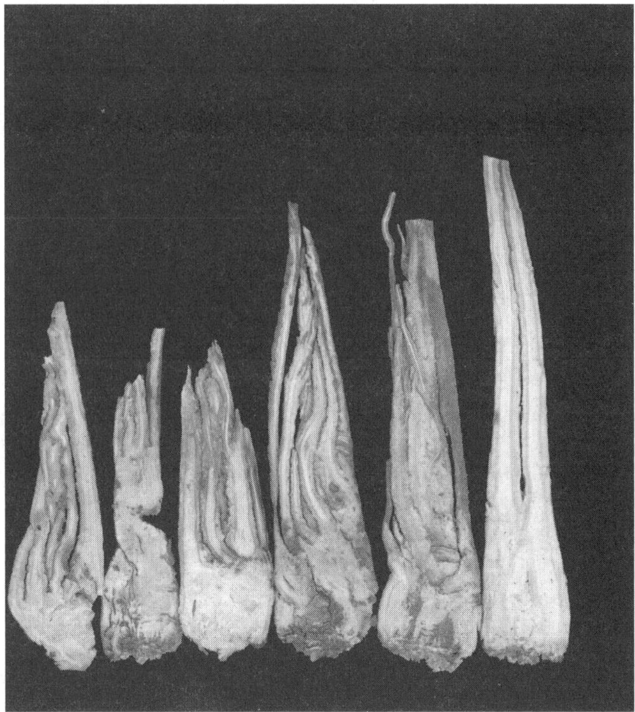

FIGURE 11.6 Dong quai root.

tions. The above-ground parts of the plant and its roots are used fresh or dried to make teas, squeezed (expressed) juice, extracts, or preparations for external use. Two NCCAM-funded studies did not find a benefit from echinacea, either as a fresh-pressed juice for treating colds in children or as an unrefined mixture of two strains of echinacea. However, other studies have shown that echinacea may be beneficial in treating upper respiratory infections. NCCAM is continuing to support the study of echinacea for the treatment of upper respiratory infections and for its potential effects on the immune system.[8,18,28]

Ephedra or ephedrine: Ephedra is an evergreen shrub-like plant native to Central Asia and Mongolia. The principal active ingredient, ephedrine, is a compound that can powerfully stimulate the nervous system and heart. Ephedra has been used for more than 5,000 years in China and India to treat conditions such as colds, fever, flu, headaches, asthma, wheezing, and nasal congestion. It has also been an ingredient in many dietary supplements used for weight loss, increased energy, and enhanced athletic performance. The dried stems and leaves of the plant are used to create capsules, tablets, extracts, tinctures, and teas. In 2004, the FDA banned the U.S. sale of dietary supplements containing ephedra after finding that the supplements had an adverse health risk (namely, cardiovascular complications). The ban does not apply to traditional Chinese herbal remedies or to products such as herbal teas regulated as conventional foods.[8,18]

Evening primrose (Oenothera biennis): Evening primrose is a plant native to North America, but it grows in Europe and parts of the Southern hemisphere as well. It has yellow flowers that bloom in the evening. Evening primrose oil has been used since the 1930s for skin disorders such as eczema (inflamed, itchy, or scaly skin). It is also used for inflammation, such as rheumatoid arthritis, and for breast pain associated with the menstrual cycle, menopausal symptoms, and premenstrual syndrome (PMS).[8,18,28]

Feverfew (Tanacetum parthenium): Feverfew was originally found in the Balkan mountains of Eastern Europe. It now grows throughout Europe, North America, and South America. It is a short bush with daisy-like flowers (see **FIGURE 11.7**) and has been used for centuries for many conditions such as fevers, headaches, stomachaches, toothaches, insect bites, infertility, problems with menstruation, and with labor during childbirth. Some research suggests that feverfew may be helpful in preventing migraine headaches; however, results have been mixed, and more evidence is needed from well-designed studies. Feverfew may be helpful in treating mild rheumatoid arthritis symptoms.[8,18,28]

Flax (Linum usitatissimum): The flax plant is believed to have originated in Egypt, but grows throughout Canada and the northwestern United States. Flaxseed is used for many conditions: as a laxative, for hot flashes, and for breast pain. Studies of flaxseed preparations to lower cholesterol levels report mixed results, some positive and some not. There is not enough reliable information to determine whether flaxseed is effective for heart conditions.[18]

Garlic (Allium sativum): Garlic is the edible bulb from a plant in the lily family. It is used to treat high cholesterol, heart disease, and high blood pressure. Garlic

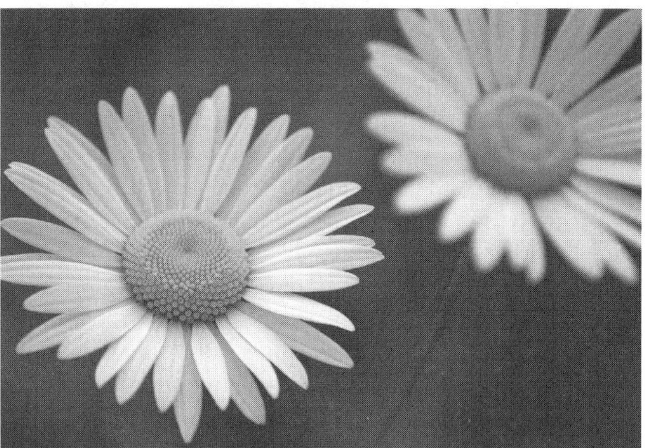

FIGURE 11.7 Feverfew.

is also used to prevent certain types of cancer, including stomach and colon cancers. Some evidence indicates that taking garlic can slightly lower blood cholesterol levels; studies have shown positive effects for short-term use (1 to 3 months). However, an NCCAM-funded study on the safety and effectiveness of three garlic preparations (fresh garlic, dried powdered garlic tablets, and aged garlic extract tablets) for lowering blood cholesterol levels found no effect. Preliminary research suggests that taking garlic may slow the development of atherosclerosis (hardening of the arteries), a condition that can lead to heart disease or stroke. Garlic may also slightly lower blood pressure and it may lower the risk of certain cancers. However, no clinical trials have examined this. A clinical trial on the long-term use of garlic supplements to prevent stomach cancer found no effect.[18]

Ginger root (Zingiber officinale): Ginger is a tropical plant that has green-purple flowers and an aromatic underground stem (called a rhizome). Ginger is used in Asian medicine to treat gastrointestinal conditions such as stomachaches, nausea, diarrhea, and nausea from motion, chemotherapy, and pregnancy. Ginger has been used for rheumatoid arthritis, osteoarthritis, and joint and muscle pain. Studies suggest that the short-term use of ginger can safely relieve pregnancy-related nausea and vomiting. Studies are mixed on whether ginger is effective for nausea caused by motion, chemotherapy, or surgery. It is unclear whether ginger is effective in treating rheumatoid arthritis, osteoarthritis, or joint and muscle pain.[7,28]

Ginkgo biloba: Ginkgo comes from the leaves of the ginkgo biloba tree. Ginkgo leaf extract has been used to treat a variety of ailments and conditions, including asthma, bronchitis, fatigue, and tinnitus (ringing or roaring sounds in the ears). The NCCAM funded a study of the well-characterized ginkgo product EGb-761[18] In a clinical trial, known as the Ginkgo Evaluation of Memory study, researchers recruited more than 3,000 volunteers age 75 or older who took 240 mg of ginkgo daily. They were followed for an average of approximately 6 years. Results of the study found that EGb-761 was ineffective in lowering the overall incidence of dementia and Alzheimer's disease in the elderly and ineffective in slowing cognitive decline, lowering blood pressure, or reducing the incidence of hypertension. Side effects of ginkgo may include headache, nausea, gastrointestinal upset, diarrhea, dizziness, or allergic skin reactions. More severe allergic reactions have occasionally been reported.[18,28]

Ginseng (Panax ginseng): Although Asian ginseng has been widely studied for a variety of uses, research results to date do not conclusively support health claims associated with the herb. Traditional and modern uses of ginseng include improving the health of people recovering from illness, increasing a sense of well-being and stamina, improving both mental and physical performance, and treating erectile dysfunction, hepatitis C, and symptoms related to menopause. Some studies have shown that Asian ginseng may lower blood glucose levels. Other studies indicate possible beneficial effects on immune function. Of all the studies, only a few large, high-quality clinical trials have been conducted.[18,28] (See **FIGURE 11.8**.)

Glucosamine and chondroitin: Glucosamine and chondroitin are not plant herbs, but are dietary supplements used by many today. Glucosamine is a natural compound found in healthy cartilage. Available evidence from randomized controlled trials supports the use of glucosamine sulfate in the treatment of osteoarthritis, particularly of the knee. Glucosamine is commonly taken in combination with chondroitin, a glycosaminoglycan derived from articular cartilage.[38]

Goldenseal (Hydrastis canadensis): Goldenseal is a plant that grows wild in parts of the United States but has become endangered by overharvesting. Goldenseal is used for colds and other respiratory tract infections, infectious diarrhea, eye infections, and vaginitis (inflammation or infection of the vagina). It is also applied to wounds and canker sores, and is used as a mouthwash for sore gums, mouth, and throat. The NCCAM is funding research on goldenseal, including studies of antibacterial mechanisms and potential cholesterol-lowering effects. Few studies have been published on goldenseal's safety and effectiveness, and there is little scientific evidence to support using it for any health problem. Goldenseal is considered safe for short-term use in adults at recommended dosages.[18,28]

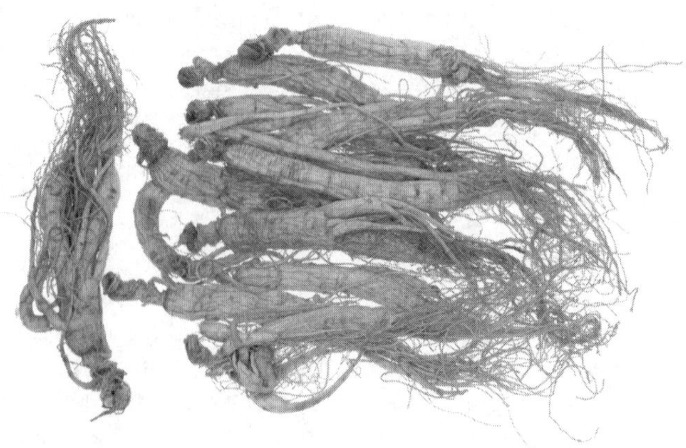

FIGURE 11.8 Ginseng.

Gotu kola (Centella asiatic): A perennial plant native to India, Japan, China, Indonesia, South Africa, Sri Lanka, and the South Pacific. It has been used to treat leprosy, bronchitis, asthma, and syphilis. It also has been used in Ayurvedic medicine for wound healing. Gotu kola is used most often to treat chronic venous insufficiency (a condition where blood pools in the legs). People with liver disease should not take gotu kola because it has been shown in clinical trials to affect the liver.[5]

Grape seed extract (Vitis vinifera): Grape seed extract is used for heart and blood vessel conditions such as atherosclerosis (hardening of the arteries), high blood pressure, high cholesterol, and poor circulation. Grape seed extract has also been used for complications related to diabetes, such as nerve and eye damage; vision problems, such as macular degeneration (which can cause blindness); and swelling after an injury or surgery. It has been used for cancer prevention and wound healing. Even though small randomized trials have found beneficial effects, larger clinical trials are needed to determine the efficacy of grape seed extract for diabetic retinopathy and for vascular fragility.[18,28]

Green tea (Camellia sinensis): Fresh leaves from the *Camellia sinensis* plant are steamed, producing green tea. Green tea and green tea extracts have been used to prevent and treat a variety of cancers, including breast, stomach, and skin cancers. Green tea and green tea extracts have also been used for improving mental alertness, aiding in weight loss, lowering cholesterol levels, and protecting skin from sun damage. Even though laboratory studies suggest that green tea may help protect against or slow the growth of certain cancers, studies in people have shown mixed results. Green tea does contain some caffeine, giving a sense of mental alertness. There is not enough evidence to show whether green tea supports weight loss.[18,28]

Hawthorn (Crataegus laevigata): Hawthorn is a spiny, flowering shrub or small tree of the rose family. Hawthorn is used for problems associated with heart disease, digestion, and kidney problems. The hawthorn leaf and flower are used to make liquid extracts, usually with water and alcohol. Dry extracts can be put into capsules and tablets. There is scientific evidence that hawthorn leaf and flower may be safe and effective for milder forms of heart failure, but study results are conflicting. There is not enough scientific evidence to determine whether hawthorn works for other heart problems.[18,28]

Hoodia (Hoodia gordonii): Hoodia is a flowering, cactus-like plant native to the Kalahari desert in southern Africa. (See **FIGURE 11.9**.) Hoodia currently is used as an appetite suppressant. Dried extracts of hoodia stems and roots are used to make capsules, powders, and chewable tablets. Hoodia can also be used in liquid extracts and teas. The safety of hoodia is still unknown.[18]

Kava (Piper methysticum): Kava is used primarily for anxiety, insomnia, and menopausal symptoms. The FDA has issued a warning that using kava supplements has been linked to a risk of severe liver damage and has been associated with several cases of dystonia (abnormal muscle spasm or involuntary muscle movements). Kava can interact with drugs used for Parkinson's disease and cause scaly, yellowed skin when used over a long period of time.[18]

Kudzu (Pueraria lobata): Kudzu is a coiling, climbing, and trailing vine native to southern Japan and southeast China. It now grows in the Southeastern part of the United States. It has been used in China to treat alcoholism, diabetes, gastroenteritis, and deafness. A 2005 study found that an extract of the root reduces alcohol drinking by heavy drinkers.[51] More research needs to be done on the herb and its possible effects before drawing any conclusions.

Lavender (Lavandula angustifolia): The name "lavender" comes from the Latin root *lavare*, which means "to wash." Lavender is native to the mountainous zones of the Mediterranean region. It also flourishes in the southern United States. Essential oil is extracted from the blue-violet flowers (see **FIGURE 11.10**), and when diluted, may be applied to the skin. It is used for conditions such as anxiety, restlessness, insomnia, and depression. Lavender is also used for headache, upset stomach, and hair loss. Dried lavender flowers can be used to make teas or liquid extracts that can be taken by mouth. There is little scientific evidence of lavender's effectiveness for most health uses. Small studies on lavender for anxiety showed mixed results.[18]

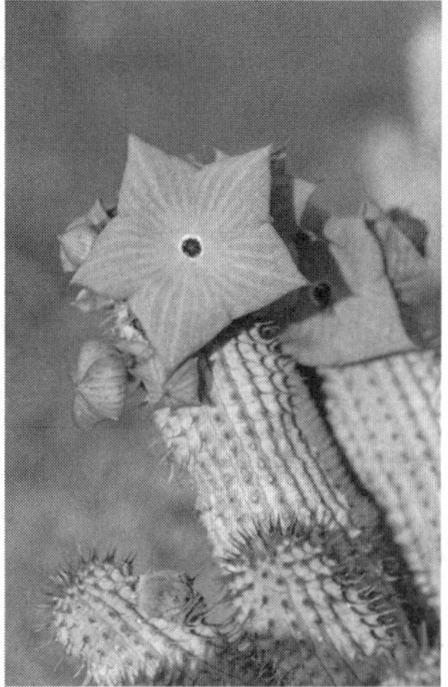

FIGURE 11.9 Hoodia.

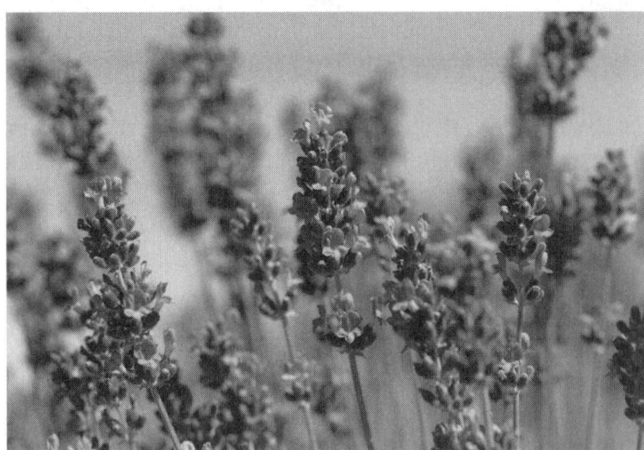

FIGURE 11.10 Lavender.

Melatonin: Melatonin may be found in animals, plants and microbes. It is not considered a plant herb like most of the others in this section, but it is another dietary supplement used by many. Melatonin is a hormone normally secreted by the pineal gland and was first promoted as a cure for jet lag and then as a sleep aid. Some clinical research has found that melatonin may help elderly people with insomnia who are tapering off or stopping benzodiazepines. It may help with sleep problems associated with menopause. Positive studies have shown that melatonin can help with complications during chemotherapy for breast cancer and it may also be linked positively with prostate cancer; however, more research is needed to study both of these areas. Melatonin should not be taken if pregnant or nursing because not enough research has been conducted to demonstrate that it is safe for the developing fetus or the infant after birth.[5]

Milk thistle seed (Silymarin, Silybum marianum): The milk thistle seed plant is native to the Mediterranean and grows wild throughout Europe, North America, and Australia. It is a potent anti-inflammatory and antioxidant. The plant's small, hard fruits have been shown to protect the liver against a variety of toxins. It alters liver cell membrane structure, blocking the absorption of toxins into the cells. It is used to treat liver cirrhosis, chronic hepatitis (liver inflammation), and gallbladder disorders. Results from clinical trials of milk thistle for liver diseases have been mixed, and most studies have not been rigorously designed. The National Cancer Institute is studying the effectiveness of silymarin for patients with leukemia who experience chemotherapy-related liver damage.[18]

Nettle (Stinging nettle, Urtica dioica): A perennial flowering plant, native to North America and the Mediterranean region. Reports say that nettle can provide relief from painful muscles and joints, arthritic pain, and gout. Extracts also can be used to treat anemia, hay fever, kidney problems, and pain by inactivating inflammatory cytokines. It is used in Europe for benign prostatic hyperplasia. The potency and effectiveness of nettle are still being assessed.[5,52]

Peppermint (Mentha piperita): Peppermint is a cross between two types of mint (water mint and spearmint), and it grows throughout Europe and North America. It is used for a variety of health conditions, including nausea, indigestion, and cold symptoms. Peppermint oil is also used for headaches and muscle and nerve pain. Although some studies have shown no effects, several suggest that peppermint oil may improve symptoms of irritable bowel syndrome.[5,18]

Pomegranate juice: Pomegranate juice contains antioxidants at higher levels than do other fruit juices. Research has not yet proven that drinking pomegranate juice can help lower cholesterol or assist with any other health issue. If you choose to drink pomegranate juice, be sure that it is 100 percent pure pomegranate juice. Dr. Dean Ornish maintains that blood flow to the heart improved 17 percent in men and women with coronary heart disease who drank 8.5 ounces a day for 3 months. Research findings from Israeli studies showed that it can lower blood pressure and help shrink plaque buildup in the neck arteries.[5]

Probiotics: Probiotics are not a plant herb but are live bacteria similar to beneficial microorganisms found in the human gut. They are also called "friendly bacteria" or "good bacteria." Probiotics are used by many as a dietary supplement. Probiotics are thought to prevent and treat certain illnesses and support general wellness. The largest group is lactic acid bacteria, the type found in yogurt (*Lactobacillus acidophilus*). Research suggests that probiotics are useful to treat diarrhea, irritable bowel syndrome, and urinary tract infection; shorten intestinal tract infections; reduce recurrence of bladder cancer; and prevent and manage atopic dermatitis.[18,53]

Red clover (Trifolium pratense): Red clover is used for relieving coughing and skin problems, and for preventing symptoms caused by menopause. It has also been used for cancer and respiratory problems such as whooping cough. The primary side effects reported were nausea and upset stomach. Several small studies assessed the effects of red clover on menopausal symptoms, but the results were inconclusive. Further research needs to be conducted on this herb in order to determine whether it is effective.[18,37]

Sage (Salvia officinalis, Salvia lavandulaefolia, Salvia lavandulifolia): Sage is used for mouth and throat inflammation, indigestion, and excessive sweating.

Sage is also used as an ingredient in some dietary supplements for mouth, throat, and gastrointestinal problems. Some people may use sage to improve mood, or boost memory or mental performance. Sage is available as dried leaves, liquid extracts and sprays, and essential oils. It may be gargled, applied topically, or drunk as a tea. Two small studies suggest that sage may improve mood and mental performance in healthy young people and memory and attention in older adults.[18]

Saw palmetto berry (Serenoa repens): Saw palmetto is a small palm tree native to the eastern United States. Its fruit was used medicinally by the Seminole tribe of Florida. It is mainly used for urinary symptoms associated with an enlarged prostate gland. It is also used for chronic pelvic pain, bladder disorders, decreased sex drive, hair loss, hormone imbalances, and prostate cancer. Some research shows that saw palmetto might work as well for benign enlarged prostate gland as do some prescription medications such as finasteride (Proscar) and tamsulosin (Flomax). But other research shows that taking saw palmetto might have little or no benefit for some men. There currently is not enough scientific evidence to prove that saw palmetto is effective.[18,36]

St. John's wort (Hypericum perforatum): St. John's wort is a plant with yellow flowers (see **FIGURE 11.11**) whose medicinal uses were first recorded in ancient Greece. St. John's wort has been used for centuries to treat mental disorders and nerve pain. It has also been used as a sedative and a treatment for malaria, as well as a balm for wounds, burns, and insect bites. St. John's wort is most commonly used today for depression, anxiety, and sleep disorders. There is scientific evidence that St. John's wort may be useful for short-term treatment of mild to moderate depression. Although some studies have reported benefits for more severe depression, others have not. St. John's wort has significant interactions with some other medications. More research is being conducted by the NCCAM on this topic.[18,36]

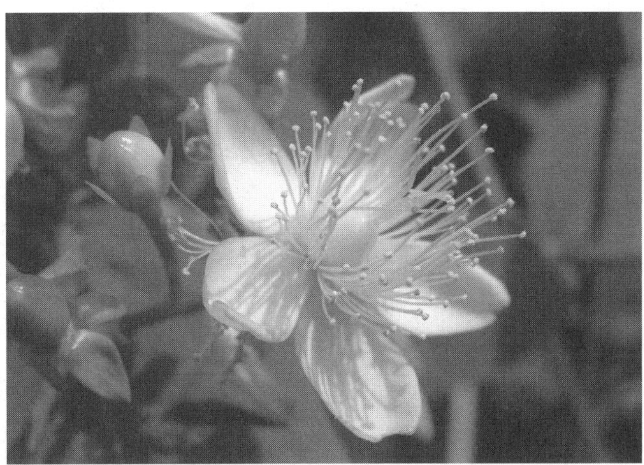

FIGURE 11.11 St. John's wort.

Valerian (Valeriana officinalis): Valerian is a perennial plant native to Europe and Asia and is now grown in North America. The plant has an odor that is offensive. It was used by Hippocrates and Galen for insomnia, nervousness, headaches, and even heart palpitations. Valerian currently is used for sleep disorders and anxiety. Research suggests that valerian may be beneficial to sleep disorders; however, there is not enough evidence at this time to confirm this or any of the other use of valerian.[18,53]

White willow bark: White willow bark is used today for the treatment of pain, headache, and inflammatory conditions such as bursitis and tendinitis. Researchers believe that the chemical salicin, found in willow bark, is responsible for these effects. However, studies have identified several other components of willow bark that have antioxidant, fever-reducing, antiseptic, and immune-boosting properties. Some studies have shown white willow bark is as effective as aspirin for reducing pain and inflammation (but not fever), and at a much lower dose.[36,52]

Wild yam: Wild yam is a plant that contains a chemical, diosgenin, that can be made into steroids such as estrogen and dehydroepiandrosterone (DHEA). It is used to treat menstrual cramps, nausea, and morning sickness associated with pregnancy; inflammation; osteoporosis; menopausal symptoms; and other health conditions. Several studies have found that wild yam has no effect at all on these conditions because by itself, wild yam does not contain progesterone.[5,36]

Yarrow (Achillea millefolium): Yarrow has been used for thousands of years for medicinal purposes. It is thought to have anti-inflammatory properties and has the ability to staunch blood flow from slow healing wounds. It is used by modern herbalists to treat wounds. Yarrow has also been used to make tea[54] and to flavor beer, wine, and soft drinks. The leaves and flowers are used as seasoning. Young leaves may be used in salads or boiled as greens. Yarrow has been found to have an anti-inflammatory and anti-edema effect. It is used for stomach upset and for liver and gallbladder problems.[55]

Yohimbe: Yohimbe comes from the bark of the yohimbe tree (see **FIGURE 11.12**), which is found in Zaire, Cameroon, and Gabon. It is used to treat erectile dysfunction in males and also to increase weight loss. Studies are conflicting as to whether the herb is effective in

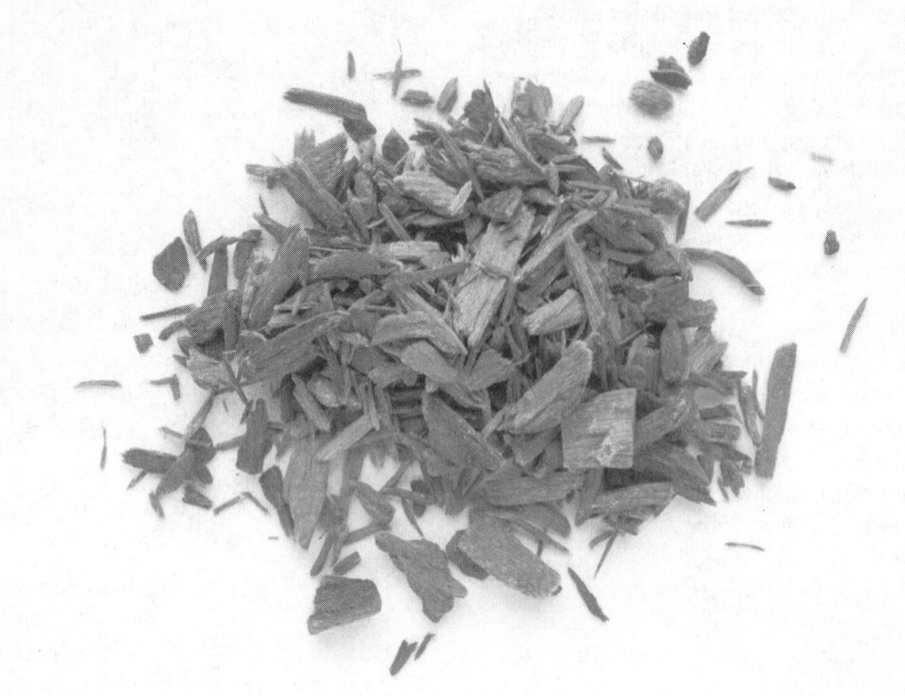

FIGURE 11.12 Yohimbe tree and bark.

increasing weight loss. An overdose can cause serious problems such as weakness and nervous stimulation, followed by paralysis, fatigue, stomach disorders, and ultimately death.[52,56]

CONCLUSION

In sum, there are a myriad of herbs available but you should be diligent about the ones you use. Valid and reliable herbal information is available from the NCCAM,[18] MedlinePlus,[36] Mayo Clinic,[38] University of Maryland Medical Center,[5] and similar Web sites. The *Physician's Desk Reference for Herbal Medicines*[55] also is a great resource. There are many herbals that can be safely used, but you need to take personal responsibility when selecting them for your bodily conditions or just as a preventive method for staying well.

Suggestions for Class Activities

1. Invite an herbalist to class to discuss the properties of various herbs and how to grow them.

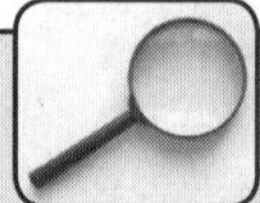

Case Study

Robert is a 55-year-old man who has been experiencing urinary frequency during the night and sometimes during the day. He has been feeling fatigued at work because he has not been getting a good night's sleep. His wife, Sandy, has been urging him to see a urologist (genitourinary specialist). While playing golf, Robert revealed his problem to one of his friends. The friend told Robert that he had been having similar symptoms. He recommended an herb called saw palmetto because he was taking it and his urinary frequency problem had lessened.

Questions:

1. What steps should Robert follow before obtaining this herb?
2. How important is it that Robert see a physician?
3. If Robert did decide to purchase the herb, where should he get it?
4. What other precautions should Robert take?

2. Visit an herbal garden and take photos. Bring the photos to class and let classmates guess the herbs. You can make a game of this by dividing the class into two teams.
3. Research the benefits and side effects of selected herbs. Present your findings to the class.
4. Start your own herbal garden using three common herbs. Report to the class the care required for the herbal garden.

Review Questions

1. What are biologically based therapies?
2. What are two examples of biologically based therapies?
3. What is the definition of phytotherapy?
4. Give two examples of nutritional supplements.
5. What is the definition of an herbalist?
6. Distinguish among crude herbs, decoctions, and herbal extracts.
7. Name and explain four chemicals and properties of herbs.
8. What are phytoestrogens?
9. What is the difference between bulk and standardized herbs?
10. How should herbs be cared for and stored?
11. What is the difference between the United States and Germany regarding the assessment of the safety and efficacy of herbs?
12. What is the definition of herbals according to the DSHEA?
13. If an herb is found to be unsafe, what action can the FDA take?
14. How much money is spent on herbals each year, and what percentage of U.S. adults use them?
15. Name and discuss five herbals and the conditions/diseases they are used for.

Key Terms

alkaloids A group of chemicals made by plants and are alkaloid in nature. Examples of alkaloids include cocaine, nicotine, and caffeine.

biologically based therapies Use of natural techniques to maintain health and/or treat diseases.

cardiac glycosides These chemicals have a marked action on the heart, strengthening the force and speed of systolic contractions.

carotenoid pigments Pigments found in yellow to red plants such as carrots, sweet potatoes, red and yellow peppers, squash, and tomatoes.

chelation therapy Use of a drug to bind with, and remove, excess or toxic amounts of metal or minerals from the blood.

chlorophyll Pigment found in green plants and dark leafy green vegetables such as spinach, parsley, kale, green beans, and leeks.

fixed oils Referred to as vegetable, carrier; or base oils; they contain nutrients such as minerals, antioxidants, and fat-soluble vitamins.

flavonoids A set of chemicals that include brilliant plant pigments seen in fruits and vegetables.

herbalist A practitioner of, and contributor to the field of, herbal medicine.

lignans Phytoestrogens with weak estrogenic or anti-estrogenic activity.

nutritional supplements Also called dietary supplements. Nutritional supplements are preparations that provide additional nutrients and may include vitamins, minerals or herbals.

orthomolecular medicine Emphasizes supplementing the diet with mega doses of vitamins, minerals, enzymes, hormones, and amino acids.

phytoestrogen Estrogen-like chemicals that can act like the hormone estrogen.

phytotherapy Plant therapy. Using botanical medicine to treat disease conditions.

plant coumarins Oral anticoagulants. Coumarin was isolated from the tonka bean (Dipteryx odorata), which is in a classification known as coumarou; thus, similar plants were named plant coumarins.

salicylates and salicins Aspirin-like compounds that have pain-relieving and anti-inflammatory action.

saponins Glycosides or chemicals found in plants such as oats, vegetables, and beans that cause plants placed in water to "soap up," or froth to form a lather.

tannins Polyphenols obtained from various parts of plants. Found in tree bark, wood, fruit, leaves, and roots.

volatile oils Compounds of vegetable origin that evaporate at room temperature and allow us to enjoy the smell.

References

1. National Center for Complementary and Alternative Medicine. Available at: http://nccam.nih.gov/health/whatiscam/#natural. Accessed August 27, 2011.
2. MedlinePlus. Herbal medicine. Available at: http://www.nlm.nih.gov/medlineplus/herbalmedicine.html. Accessed October 2, 2010.
3. Answers.com. Botanical. Available at: http://www.answers.com/topic/botanical#ixzz1BsZLWhqI. Accessed October 2, 2010.
4. Bradford N, ed. *The one spirit encyclopedia of complementary health*. London: Hamlyn; 1996.

5. University of Maryland Medical Center. Herbal medicine. Available at: http://www.umm.edu/altmed/articles/herbal-medicine-000351.htm. Accessed October 2, 2010.
6. Freeman L, Lawlis GF. *Mosby's complementary and alternative medicine: a research-based approach*. St. Louis: Mosby; 2001.
7. Thomas L. *10 essential herbs*. Prescott, AZ: Hohm Press; 1996.
8. Boon H, Smith M. *The complete natural medicine guide to the 50 most common medicinal herbs*. 2nd ed. Canada: Robert Rose Inc.; 2004.
9. Science Encyclopedia. Plant Pigment—Carotenoids. Available at: http://science.jrank.org/pages/5303/Plant-Pigment-Carotenoids.html. Accessed October 5, 2010.
10. Simonich MT. Cancer prevention by chlorophylls. *Research Newsletter*. Fall/Winter 2006. Linus Pauling Institute at Oregon State University. Available at: http://lpi.oregonstate.edu/fw06/chlorophylls.html. Accessed October 5, 2010.
11. Anderson E. Chlorophyll can help treat cancer. Available at: http://www.naturalnews.com/023422_chlorophyll_cancer_carcinogen.html#ixzz1BuQ3jfYP. Accessed October 6, 2010.
12. Squidoo. Essential oils versus fixed oils. Available at: http://www.squidoo.com/essential-oils-versus-fixed-oils. Accessed October 6, 2010.
13. Fixed Oils.Com. Fixed oils. Available at: http://www.fixedoils.com/oils/index.html. Accessed October 6, 2010.
14. Linus Pauling Institute. Flavonoids. Available at: http://lpi.oregonstate.edu/infocenter/phytochemicals/flavonoids/#disease_prevention. Accessed October 6, 2010.
15. Dietary Fiber Food. Lignans: foods high in lignans. Available at: http://www.dietaryfiberfood.com/lignan.php. Accessed October 6, 2010.
16. Velentzis LS, Cantwell MM, Cardwell C, Keshtgar MR, Leathem AJ, Woodside JV. Lignans and breast cancer risk in pre-and post-menopausal women: meta-analyses of observational studies. Br J Cancer 2009;100(9):1492-8 Epub 2009 Mar 31. Available at: http://www.ncbi.nlm.nih.gov/pubmed/19337250?dopt=Citation. Accessed August 27, 2011.
17. Cornell University. Phytoestrogens and breast cancer. 2001. Available at: http://envirocancer.cornell.edu/FactSheet/Diet/fs1.phyto.cfm. Accessed October 7, 2010.
18. National Center for Complementary and Alternative Medicine. Health information. Available at: http://nccam.nih.gov/health/. Accessed October 3, 2010.
19. Thangavelu A, Irizarry L. Plant poisoning, glycosides—coumarin. Available at: http://emedicine.medscape.com/article/816897-overview. Accessed October 6, 2010.
20. Schror K. *Acetylsalicylic acid*. Weinheim, Germany: Wiley-Blackwell; 2009.
21. Singh AP. Salicin—a natural analgesic. Available at: http://www.ethnoleaflets.com/leaflets/salicin.htm. Accessed October 8, 2010.
22. Sahelian R. Saponin in plants benefit and side effects. Available at: http://www.raysahelian.com/saponin.html. Accessed October 11, 2010.
23. Cornell University Department of Animal Science. Saponins. Available at: http://www.ansci.cornell.edu/plants/toxicagents/saponin.html. Accessed October 11, 2010.
24. Phytochemicals. What is saponins? Available at: http://www.phytochemicals.info/phytochemicals/saponins.php. Accessed October 11, 2010.
25. Goode J. Tannins. Available at: http://www.wineanorak.com/tannins.htm. Accessed October 11, 2010.
26. Herbs 2000. Tannins. Available at: http://www.herbs2000.com/h_menu/tannins.htm. Accessed October 11, 2010.
27. Volatile oils [Powerpoint slides]. No author listed. Available at: www.fantastic-flavour.com. Second online reference is www.fantastic-flavour.com/yahoo_site.../volatile_oils.240183302.ppt Accessed October 11, 2010 and August 27, 2011.
28. Duke J. *The green pharmacy*. Emmaus, PA: Rodale Press; 1997.
29. U.S. Food and Drug Administration. How drugs are developed and approved. Available at: http://www.fda.gov/drugs/developmentapprovalprocess/howdrugsaredevelopedandapproved/default.htm. Accessed October 13, 2010.
30. Daly R. FDA moves to speed device approval process. Healthcare Business News. Available at http://www.modernhealthcare.com/article/20110119/NEWS/301199967/#. Accessed March 10, 2011 and August 27, 2011.
31. Office of Dietary Supplements, National Institutes of Health. Background information: botanical dietary supplements. Available at: http://ods.od.nih.gov/factsheets/BotanicalBackground/#h5. Accessed October 14, 2010.
32. Corwin A, Zahorik L, Hurlbutt M. Herbal supplements: health-care implications and considerations. *CDHA Journal*. Winter 2009,24(2): 7–14.
33. Kwan D, Hirschkorn K., Boon H. U.S. and Canadian pharmacists' attitudes, knowledge, and professional practice behaviors toward dietary supplements: a systematic review. *BMC Comp and Alternat Medi*, 2006,6(31). Available online at: http://www.biomedcentral.com/1472-6882/6/31. Accessed August 27, 2011.
34. Scimone A, Scimone AA. Recommendation of herbal remedies by psychiatrists. Available at: http://www.orthomolecular.org/library/jom/2001/articles/2001-v16n03-p155.shtml. Accessed August 27, 2011.
35. Drugs and Therapeutic Bulletin. DTB survey on herbal medicines. BMJIJournals. Available at: http://dtb.bmj.com/site/about/DTB_survey_on_herbal_medicines.pdf. Accessed August 27, 2011.
36. Barnes P, Bloom B, Nahin R. Complementary and alternative medicine use among adults and children: United States, 2007. National Health Statistics Reports; no 12. National Center for Health Statistics. 2008. Available at: http://www.cdc.gov/nchs/data/nhsr/nhsr012.pdf. Accessed August 27, 2011.
37. MedlinePlus. Alfalfa. Available at: http://www.nlm.nih.gov/medlineplus/druginfo/natural/19.html. Accessed October 18, 2010.
38. Mayo Clinic. Arginine (L-arginine). Available at: http://www.mayoclinic.com/health/l-arginine/NS_patient-arginine. Accessed October 18, 2010.
39. Broadhurst C. What's the buzz? Medicine from the bee hive. Available at: http://www.bee-pollen-health.com/bee-pollen-research.html. Accessed October 18, 2010.
40. Gibb J. The health benefits of bilberry [Ezine Articles]. Available at: http://ezinearticles.com/?The-Health-Benefits-of-Bilberry&id=386416. Accessed October 18, 2010.
41. Memorial Sloan-Kettering Cancer Center. Bilberry fruit. Available at: http://www.mskcc.org/mskcc/html/69134.cfm#Clinical Summary. Accessed October 18, 2010.
42. Geller SE, Shulman LP, van Breemen RB, et al. Safety and efficacy of black cohosh and red clover for the management of vasomotor symptoms: a randomized controlled trial. *Menopause*. 2009;16(6):1156–1166.
43. Diener HC, Rahlfs VW, Danesch U. The first placebo-controlled trial of a special butterbur root extract for the prevention of migraine: reanalysis of efficacy criteria. *Eur Neurol*. 2004;51(2):89–97.
44. Grossman W, Schmidramsl H. An extract of *Petasites hybridus* is effective in the prophylaxis of migraine. *Altern Med Rev*. 2001;6(3):303–310.
45. Lipton RB, Gobel H, Einhaupl KM, et al. *Petasites hybridus* root (butterbur) is an effective preventive treatment for migraine. *Neurology*. 2004;63(12):2240–2244.
46. Agosti R, Duke RK, Chrubasik JE, Chrubasik S. Effectiveness of *Petasites hybridus* preparations in the prophylaxis of migraine: a systematic review. *Phytomedicine*. 2006;13(9–10):743–746.
47. Pravel D. Cascara sagrada: a safe laxative herb or not? June 17, 2010. Available at: http://www.suite101.com/content/

cascara-sagrada-a-safe-laxative-herb-or-not-a250496. Accessed October 19, 2010.

48. Sahelian R. Cayenne pepper supplement health benefit and use in medicine. Available at: http://www.raysahelian.com/cayenne.html. Accessed October 19, 2010.
49. WebMD. Find a vitamin or supplement: Creatine. Available at: http://www.webmd.com/vitamins-supplements/ingredientmono-873-CREATINE.aspx?activeIngredientId = 873&activeIngredientName = CREATINE. Accessed November 3, 2011.
50. Wong C. Dong quai. Available at: http://altmedicine.about.com/od/herbsupplementguide/a/DongQuai.htm. Accessed October 19, 2010.
51. Lukas SE, Penetar D, Berko J, et al. An extract of the Chinese herbal root kudzu reduces alcohol drinking by heavy drinkers in a naturalistic setting. *Alcohol Clin Exp Res*. 2005;29(5):756–762.
52. Livestrong. Explore dietary supplements. Available at: http://www.livestrong.com/dietary-supplements/. Accessed September 23, 2011.
53. National Institutes of Health, Office of Dietary Supplements. Valerian. Available at: http://ods.od.nih.gov/factsheets/valerian/
54. Kroeger H. *Healing with herbs A-Z*. Carlsbad, CA: Hay House. 1998.
55. Gruenwald J, Brendler T, Jaenicke C, eds. *PDR for Herbal Medicines*, 2nd ed. Montvale, NJ: Medical Economics. 2000.
56. WebMD. Yohimbe. Available at: http://www.webmd.com/vitamins-supplements/ingredientmono-759-YOHIMBE.aspx?activeIngredientId = 759&act. Accessed October 20, 2010.

Aromatherapy and *Bach® Original Flower Remedies*

LEARNING OBJECTIVES

As a result of reading this chapter, students will:

1. Define aromatherapy and describe several historical examples of the use of aromatherapy.
2. Explain how aromatherapy has become a complement to traditional medical health care.
3. Examine ways in which nurses, health educators, and other health professionals could incorporate aromatherapy within their practices.
4. Analyze how Western medicine can learn from, and build upon, alternative methodologies, such as aromatherapy to improve health and change behaviors.
5. Explain the history and philosophy of the *Bach® Original Flower Remedies.*
6. Name the three *Bach® Original Flower Remedies* groups.

WHAT IS AROMATHERAPY?

Aromatherapy is an ancient therapy that has gained in popularity in recent years. The word *aromatherapy* means "treatment using scents."[1] Aromatherapy is the use of concentrated plant oils (essential oils) to help improve general health and well-being.[2] It is a branch of herbal medicine, but unlike herbal medicine, essential oils are typically not taken internally, although some naturopaths and doctors in France and even here is the United States use internal essential oil preparations. More commonly here in the United States, aromatherapy preparations are inhaled or applied to the skin. Aromatherapy is a holistic practice that considers the mind, body, spirit, and emotions during the healing process. It helps to reduce stress, enhance relaxation, relieve anxiety, and alleviate some emotion-related disorders.[2,3]

WHAT ARE THE MOST COMMON WAYS TO USE AROMATHERAPY?

Aromatherapy is most often used in one of three ways. The first is inhalation or breathing in the scent of essential oils. Approximately 6–12 drops of essential oil may be added to a bowl of steaming water and then inhaled. Eucalyptus, pine, lavender, black pepper, lemon, or peppermint oils are helpful for coughs, colds, and sinus problems.[2] A diffuser also may be used. Diffusers can be electrical, burners that use candles, or a simple ceramic ring that is warmed by a light bulb. For this, one to six drops of oil are heated to release molecules into the air. Lemon and rosemary are stimulating oils that could be used in the workplace; relaxing oils such as lavender or chamomile could be used in the bedroom. Drops of essential oils may be placed near the person receiving aromatherapy so that the scent is inhaled, or one to two drops may be placed in a handkerchief and inhaled.

The second way is to apply a diluted form of essential oil directly to the skin, such as when receiving massage (five drops of essential oil added to a light base massage oil). When bathing, five to eight drops of essential oil may be placed in the bathwater. Lemon, cypress, eucalyptus, and lavender are good for chills. Some essential oils are added to perfumes and lotions. Even hot/cold compresses can be made by soaking a cloth in a water solution of one or two drops of essential oil (e.g., lavender) in a bowl of water.[2,3] Some essential oils may be applied directly from the bottle to the skin, usually only a drop or two. The drops may be applied to any area on the body but many are applied to the soles of the feet.

The third method of using aromatherapy is not commonly used but is a legitimate methodology. It involves ingesting pills, capsules, or drops of essential oils. This method should not be used without consulting a physician or a trained expert in aromatherapy.

WHAT IS THE HISTORICAL RECORD REGARDING AROMATHERAPY USE?

Plant oils have been used as a therapeutic aid for thousands of years. The earliest written record was that of Tisserand who wrote a book, *The Art of Aroma Therapy*, in 2650 BCE.[2] Historical Chinese, Ayurvedic, and Arabic medical texts document the use of aromatic oils for spirituality and health. Roman soldiers bathed in water that contained scented oils and received massages with plant oils. In ancient Greece, Hippocrates recommended regular aromatherapy baths and scented massage.[2] One of the first aromatic practices was fumigation. Plant oils were burned, creating a great deal of smoke that engulfed sickrooms, supposedly combating evil spirits and getting rid of them from patients' bodies.[3] Hippocrates used aromatic oils as fumigation to rid Athens of plague.[1] A Greek perfumer by the name of Megallus created a perfume called Megaleion. Megaleion included myrrh in a fatty-oil base that was used to produce a pleasing aroma, had anti-inflammatory properties towards the skin and was used to heal wounds.

The Egyptians were the experts, however, in the use of essential oils. Approximately 6,000 years ago, the Egyptian physician Imhotep recommended scented oils for massage and bathing.[2] In Egypt, the essential oils were prepared by placing plants in a stone trough along with fatty oils. The plants would be crushed until the base oil was saturated with the essential oils. Priests in Egypt administered scented ointments to worshipers during rituals. Incense was burned three times a day in the city of Heliopolis and was always burned at the opening of a shrine, at the coronation of a pharaoh, and at all national celebrations. One recipe that was supposedly a perfume for the gods was named Kyphi, a cocktail of essential oils that contained peppermint, saffron, juniper, acacia, and henna.[2] These were combined with wine and honey, resin, myrrh and raisins; made into a paste; and solidified. The solidified mixture was then burned as an offering to the gods. This passion for incense nearly wiped out the cedar forests of Lebanon because of the military campaigns that were mounted to ensure a large supply of the prized cedar.

Because the Egyptians believed in an afterlife, they went to great lengths to ensure a comfortable journey into the next world. Alabaster jars and ebony coffers contained ointments the Egyptians believed would make the skin of the deceased supple after he or she arrived in the new world.[2] During the embalming process, bodies were washed with salt and body cavities were filled with myrrh and oakmoss, imported from Greece. Oakmoss has an exquisite, sweet scent and contains usnic acid, an antibiotic that helped with the mummification process. Pine resin also had antimicrobial properties and was used for mummification.[3] See **FIGURE 12.1**.

In daily lives, the Egyptians used heavy mascara on their eyelids and lashes to help protect their eyes from the sun. They also used many creams and lotions as anti-aging remedies. The Egyptians extracted oils from plants by a method of infusion for use as cosmetics. Their cosmetics contained scents from lily, bitter almond, mint, frankincense, and myrrh. Later, people from all around the world traveled to Egypt to learn the secrets of aromatherapy because they finally understood that the Egyptians' aromatherapy practices were therapeutic for the skin and body.[1] At the time of the Crusades, the art of aromatherapy was carried to the West.

A Persian-born physician, Avicenna (980–1037 CE), developed the distillation method for oils that is still used today. Some argue that distillation had been used for many centuries and maintain that Avicenna merely refined the process. For example, within the 12th century, an abbess in Germany named Hildegard grew and distilled lavender for its medicinal properties. Avicenna, however, devised a coiled cooling pipe to condense steam and collect the evaporated essence.

The methods of distilling oils were imported to northern Europe in the Middle Ages (14th century). Documents exist that show herbal oils were used to fight diseases such as the Black Death. At the end of the 15th century, Paracelsus, an army surgeon and alchemist, used aromatherapy to treat leprosy. Records also show that it was used during the 16th

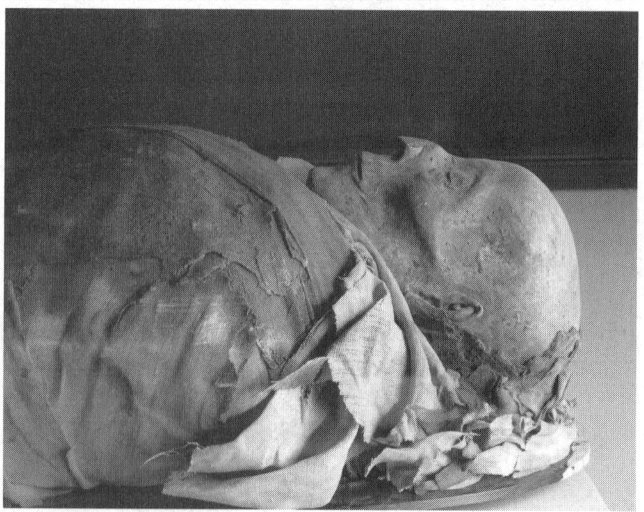

FIGURE 12.1 Mummification.

and 17th centuries by European herbalists to treat several diseases.[1]

In the late 1930s, impressive research was conducted by Rene-Maurice Gattefosse, a French chemist who sparked interest in aromatherapy. In fact, it was Gattefosse who originated the term *aromatherapy* and defined the use of essential oils as a discipline. His research began after he burned his hand in a laboratory experiment and quickly plunged it into a pot of the closest liquid, which happened to be lavender oil.[2] His hand healed with no infection or scarring. That event spurred him to do a great deal of research about aromatherapy's healing power. Dr. Jean Valnet, a French army surgeon, expanded the works of Gattefosse by using essential oils as antiseptics during World War II. In 1977, Valnet wrote a book called *The Practice of Aromatherapy*.

Another key player in the establishment of modern aromatherapy was Marguerite Maury, an Austrian biochemist and two-time winner of an international prize for exceptional scientific contributions to cosmetic research. Maury introduced the concept of prescribing oils for people, and she developed a way to apply essential oils in massage.[2] Micheline Arcier studied under Maury and opened clinics, now famous in Great Britain, using aromatherapy as a holistic health system.[3]

In the 1980s, California practitioners began to use essential oils in treatment. Today, one can find a wide selection of books about aromatherapy and can find many essential oils in local health food stores, although many are not considered pure essential oils. Aromatherapy products are also easily accessible through the Internet. Most practicing aromatherapists in the United States are trained as massage therapists, psychologists, or chiropractors who incorporate the use of essential oils into their practices.

IS AROMATHERAPY SAFE?

Aromatherapy is safe for the young to the elderly, although some preparations are strong and instructions need to be followed very carefully. Adverse reactions are rare, but it is important to remember that essential oils are medicines; taken in the wrong doses they could be toxic to the body. Most undiluted essential oils should not be applied directly to the skin or mucous membranes because they are too strong and could cause skin irritation or allergic reaction,[3] but some may be applied if only using a drop or two. For example, lavender and tea tree oil can usually be used undiluted; however, severe sensitivity has been noted by some people. It is a good idea to perform a patch test to assess if you could be allergic to a particular oil. You could apply a couple drops of the essential oil mixed in with some sort of carrier oil (e.g., olive oil or sweet almond oil) to the inside of your forearm. If there is no reaction, the essential oil should be safe to use.

Women who are pregnant should consult with their physician before obtaining aromatherapy.[2] People with high blood pressure, asthma, epilepsy, or other health problems should also either avoid essential oils or consult with their doctors before using them because they may be taking medications that the aromatherapy oil may interact with.

Aromatherapy may be used on babies during baby massage. It is purported to speed the development of the nervous system and brain, help balance the baby's developing systems, and encourage growth.[3] Aromatherapy massage on babies should be done gently using a firm hand and special aromatic baby oils. Baby formulas should not contain more than two drops of essential oil per 1¾ fluid ounces of carrier oil.[3] Generally accepted essential oils for babies are lavender, rose, and chamomile.

To be very safe, if you are considering the purchase of essential oils, you should check for an expiration date. Be sure to store your essential oils away from children. Always remember that less is more. If one drop will get the job done, don't use two drops. You should never take essential oils internally based on your own judgment. Someone highly trained in aromatherapy, such as a naturopathic doctor or medical doctor, could prescribe internal use, but you should

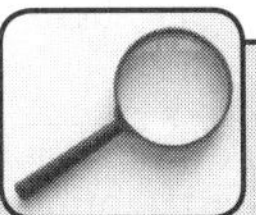

Case Study

Cathy has epilepsy and is taking medication for it. She also has insomnia many nights. She went to a spa and was impressed with an aromatherapy treatment she was given in conjunction with her massage. The aromatherapy scent made her remember smells associated with pleasant childhood memories, and now Cathy is very interested in obtaining her own essential oils for home use. She found an online source and bought several, one of which was lavender, thought to be good for insomnia because of its sedative effect. That night, Cathy placed some drops of lavender essential oil in a diffuser, took her epilepsy medication (primidone [Mysoline]), and went to bed.

Questions:

1. What should Cathy have done before using lavender essential oil in her diffuser?
2. Research the potential interactive effects of lavender and medications for epilepsy. What did you find?

not do this on your own. Finally, a very important safety tip is to keep essential oils away from fire hazards because they are quite flammable.[3]

WHO CAN USE AROMATHERAPY ESSENTIAL OILS AND FOR WHAT PURPOSES?

An aromatherapist can use essential oils because they are trained in their use, but the oils are available for anyone to use. That means you could buy your own supply of essential oils for personal use.

The purposes for using aromatherapy vary. Some traditional physicians and naturopaths learn about the biochemistry of the oils and their action on our bodies, so their purpose is medicinal. They may use aromatherapy to treat the physical body or they may use it to treat emotional or psychological disorders.[3] Prescriptions may be for internal or external essential oil treatment.[3] Practitioners may use essential oils as a part of beauty treatments or in cosmetics. Certainly, massage therapists use essential oils in massage oil preparations. The main purpose of aromatherapy, however, is to maintain health by boosting the body's immune system via the senses of touch and smell.

WHAT ARE AROMATHERAPY TERMS?

The following are some common terms used in aromatherapy:

- *Absolute:* Plant extraction obtained by using chemical solvents.
- *CO_2:* Plant oil extracted by the carbon dioxide method.
- *Hydrosol:* Floral water or distillate water that remains after distilling an essential oil.
- *Carrier oil:* Base or vegetable oil derived from the fatty portion of plants such as the seeds, kernels or the nuts. They are used to dilute CO_2s and absolutes before applying them to skin. Examples are olive oil, sweet almond oil, avocado oil, sesame oil, sunflower oil and peanut oil.
- *Essential oil:* Distilled liquid from the leaves, stems, flowers, bark, roots, or other elements of a plant.
- *Infused oil:* A carrier oil that has been mixed with one or more herbs.
- *Resin:* A thick sticky substance produced by trees.

Although some sources differentiate plant extracts into essential oils, absolutes, hydrosols, and CO_2s, *essential oils* is used as a blanket term to include all natural, aromatic, and volatile plant oils, including CO_2s and absolutes.[4]

WHAT ARE THE VARIOUS PROCESSES FOR MAKING ESSENTIAL OILS?

Just as with herbals (see Chapter 11), essential oils also are extracted from the bark, roots, leaves, stalks, flowers, berries, and sap of trees and plants. Essential oils are very concentrated. For example, it takes about 220 pounds of lavender flowers to make about 1 pound of essential oil. Essential oils are very volatile, evaporating quickly when exposed to the air.

Steam distillation is the most common method used to extract the oils. The plant parts are heated and then the plant molecules evaporate and are carried in the steam along a pipe, where they are cooled and condensed into a liquid. Finally, the molecules separate, the water is drawn off the oil, and the result is a pure, natural essential oil.[3]

Soaking or macerating is another method employed when the aromatic components of the plant could be ruined with high heat. Maceration involves soaking aromatic plants in animal fats or vegetable oils. Plates loaded with animal fat or vegetable oil are laid on wooden frames. Flower petals are then placed on the plates to soak. Every few days, new petals are placed on the plates so that the fat is soaked with scent. Later, the fat is washed with pure grain alcohol, which serves to dissolve the essential oil compounds while the fat is left behind. Vacuum distillation is used to remove the alcohol, and what is left behind is the floral absolute. This method is costly and labor intensive, so it is rarely used anymore.[3]

Expression is a method to extract essential oils from the rinds of citrus fruit. Again, no heat source is used. First, the fruit is removed and the rinds and pith are soaked in water, then they are removed and turned upside down. The cells containing the oils break apart, and the oil drips out and soaks into nearby sponges. When the sponges become saturated, they are squeezed into containers.[2,3]

Cold-pressed extraction is also used to extract essential oils from citrus fruit, as well as nuts and seeds. It is similar to expression except this process involves high mechanical pressure to force the oils out. The oils contain water, which will eventually evaporate. Cold-pressed oils spoil more quickly than oils extracted from other processes, so you should purchase only small quantities at a time.[5]

Solvent extraction is used for plants such as jasmine and linden blossom that cannot survive the distillation process. Blossoms are laid on perforated trays and washed with a solvent such as hexane. The solvent dissolves the non-aromatic waxes, pigments, and volatile aromatic molecules. The solution is filtered and the filtered material goes through a low pressure distillation process. A waxy mass called the concrete remains, which can contain as much as 55 percent of the volatile oil. The concentrated concrete is then processed to remove the waxy materials. The waxy concrete is warmed and stirred with alcohol, which breaks up the concrete into minute globules. The volatile oil separates, as does some of the wax. The solution is agitated and frozen to precipitate out the wax. The absolutes are left.[5,6]

Carbon dioxide (CO_2) extraction gives a richer, more intense scent because more of the aromatic chemicals are released. High pressure is placed on the CO_2, which turns it into a liquid and a solvent that can extract aromatic molecules in an extraction process similar to the solvent extraction process. The advantage to the CO_2 process is that no solvent residue remains because the CO_2 reverts back to a gas and evaporates.[5,6]

Florasols/phytols extraction is a process that uses other types of gaseous solvents. Dr. Peter Wilde used the solvent Florasol (R134a) in the late 1980s to extract aromatic oils and biologically active components from plant materials for use in the perfume industry as well as in food and aromatherapy. Because the extraction occurs at, or below, the outside (ambient) air temperature, there is no heat breakdown of the plant products used. A free-flowing clear oil free of waxes is obtained.[6]

HOW DO YOU CARE FOR AND STORE ESSENTIAL OILS?

Ultraviolet rays can decrease the storage life of essential oils. They should be stored in dark amber, cobalt blue, or violet glass bottles. In addition, they should be kept in a cool, dark place away from direct sunlight, heater vents, and registers. Heat and water are major spoilers of essential oils. They should never be left in the car, especially in the summer. If keeping essential oils in the bathroom, the tops should be shut tightly to keep out moisture. The bottles should not be left in sun or in a window because the light will enter the bottle and warm up the oil. Heat will speed the oxidation process and make the oil prematurely age.[7]

The size of the bottle is also important. Smaller bottles expose the oil to less oxygen, which will keep the oil intact longer. With care, the shelf life can be greatly extended. The shelf life of most oils varies from 6 months to several years, but keep in mind that citrus oils have the shortest shelf life and should be stored carefully.

WHAT ARE CARRIER OILS?

Carrier oils are vegetable oils derived from the fatty part of a plant, usually from the seeds, kernels, or nuts.[8] The oils are used to dilute essential oils prior to application. They carry the essential oil onto the skin. Some carrier oils are odorless, but many have a sweet, nutty aroma. If the scent is strong and bitter, the oil has probably become rancid. Some examples of vegetable oils that are used as a carrier in aromatherapy are sweet almond oil, apricot kernel oil, avocado oil, borage seed oil, camellia seed oil (tea oil), cranberry seed oil, evening primrose oil, grape seed oil, hazelnut oil, hemp seed oil, jojoba, macadamia nut oil, olive oil, peanut oil, pecan oil, pomegranate seed oil, rose hip oil, sesame oil, sunflower oil, and watermelon seed oil.[8]

Carrier oils are best if they have been cold pressed. The oil is pressed from the fatty portion of the botanical without the use of added heat. Cold expeller–pressed carrier oils are also acceptable. These oils have been processed under conditions that keep the heat to a minimum. If carrier oils are not processed with low heat, the nutrients in the oils are damaged.[8]

If you are attempting to select carrier oils for purchase, you should consider other factors than the processing methods. Some nutrients and essential fatty acids are contained within carrier oils. For example, some contain fat-soluble vitamins and minerals and act as antioxidants, helpful to the skin. Carrier oils that contain fatty acids are also nourishing to the skin, but may cause the oil to become rancid much faster.[8] You should select a carrier oil that has an aroma that won't conflict with the scent of the essential oil and a color that you will be satisfied with when mixed with your essential oil. Certainly price is a consideration. For example, organic carrier oils are more costly than conventional oils. You should not purchase mineral oil or petroleum jelly for aromatherapy use. Mineral oil and petroleum jelly can clog pores and prevent the skin from breathing naturally.

To keep carrier oils for a longer period of time, they should be stored in dark glass bottles with tight fitting tops and in a cool, dark location. Carrier oils may, however, be stored in plastic, unlike essential oils, which should always be stored in glassware. To prolong the lifespan of some fragile carrier oils, they should be stored in the refrigerator. Usually the producer of the carrier oil will affix specific storage instructions on the carrier oil bottle. Some oils, such as avocado oil, should never be stored in the refrigerator, so read the labels carefully.

WHAT DO THE CLINICAL STUDIES SHOW?

There are completed and ongoing aromatherapy studies. Some of the studies have not been well designed and some are inconclusive. Cook and Ernst conducted a systematic review of the literature using Medline, Embase, British Nursing Index, CISCOM, and AMED to analyze randomized controlled trials of aromatherapy.[9] The researchers found 12 trials: 6 had no replication and 6 found relaxing effects of aromatherapy combined with massage. The authors concluded that the effects of aromatherapy were not strong enough to be considered a treatment for anxiety, but that aromatherapy has a mild, transient anxiolytic (relaxing) effect.[9]

In a clinical study of the effects of lemon and lavender, the findings revealed that lemon appeared to enhance mood, but lavender had no effect on mood. Neither lemon (considered a stimulant) nor lavender affected participants' heart rate, blood pressure, wound healing, pain ratings, or levels of interleukin-6 or interleukin-10. The findings did show that blood levels of norepinephrine (stress hormone) remained elevated following participants' immersion in ice water after inhaling lemon scent. After smelling lavender, participants' levels of norepinephrine declined to prestressor levels.[10]

A controlled research pilot study to examine the effects of aromatherapy using clary sage and lavender showed positive results in decreasing stress and relieving anxiety in 14 ICU nurses over 42 nursing shifts.[11] The sample, however, was small and the authors conclude that the study should be replicated.

Aromatherapy seems to promote relaxation in people with cancer and sleep disorders. Some of the oils or natural plants have been reported as useful when treating a wide variety of conditions such as burns, infections, depression, insomnia, agitation in Alzheimer's patients, and high blood pressure. The problem, however, is that there is very little clinical evidence to support claims that aromatherapy can prevent or cure diseases.[12] As reported on the WebMD site, some studies have shown that lavender and tea tree oils have been found to have some estrogenic (female hormone-like) effects. The site also reports that lavender and tea tree oils may block or decrease the effect of androgens (male sex hormones). An example the site gives is that when lavender and tea tree oils were applied to the skin of prepubertal boys over a long period of time, there was a relationship to breast enlargement. If lavender and tea tree oil are indeed estrogenic, they may not be safe for women who have a high risk for estrogenic receptive breast cancer.[13]

WHAT ARE SOME COMMON AROMATHERAPY ESSENTIAL OILS?

The following are common aromatherapy essential oils.[3,4,14] Even though they are presented as having benefits, keep in mind that most have not been scientifically tested here in the United States.

Bergamot Oil (*Citrus bergamia*)

Source: Comes from the pear-shaped yellow fruit of the bergamot tree (see **FIGURE 12.2**) that Christopher Columbus discovered in the Canary Islands and then introduced to Italy and Spain. The rind of the fruit is used. It takes peels from approximately 1000 bergamot fruits to make 30 ounces of oil.

Benefits: Cooling and refreshing action to help nervous emotions and frustration. Benefits the gastrointestinal tract, aid for oily skin and acne, and used to soothe breathing difficulties.

Uses: Is a component in perfumes and is the main aromatic taste of Earl Grey tea. Used as a skin tonic and has a deodorizing action.

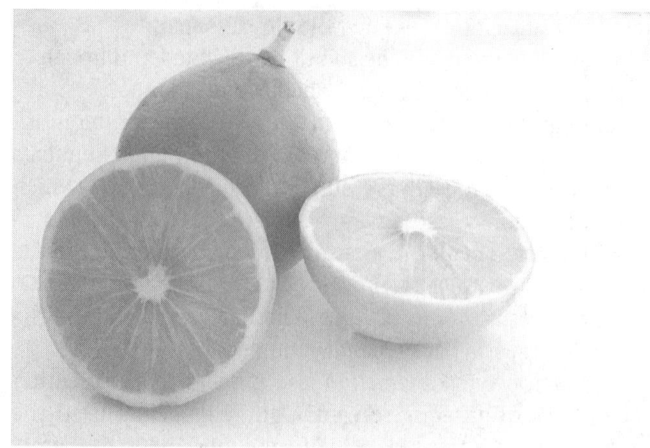

FIGURE 12.2 Bergamot.

Cedarwood Oil (*Juniperus virginiana*)

Source: Flower from the cedarwood tree. It has the faint smell of sandalwood. Pale yellow to light orange in color.

Action: Helps calm and balance energy. Clears the respiratory system of excess phlegm. Aids urinary tract infections. Improves oily skin and dandruff. It should not be used on infants or women who are pregnant.

Uses: Egyptians used the oil in the mummification process, in cosmetics, and as an insect repellant.

Chamomile Oil (Roman chamomile, *Anthemis nobilis*, and German chamomile, *Matricaria chamomilla*)

Source: Flowers of the chamomile plant (see **FIGURE 12.3**). The word *chamomile* comes from the Greek word meaning *earth apple*.

Action: The Roman chamomile is said to promote relaxation whereas the German chamomile is reported to be a powerful anti-inflammatory. Benefit the gastrointestinal tract, and relieves allergies, PMS, psychological problems, abdominal pain, gall bladder upsets, and ear and throat infections. Safe for use on children and pregnant women.

Uses: Used in teas, massage oils, as a poultice for wounds, in burners, and in steam baths.

Clary Sage Oil (*Salvia sclarea*)

Source: Clary sage plant. Gives a sweet, nutty, and floral aroma.

Action: Acts as anticonvulsant, antidepressant, antiseptic, antispasmodic, deodorant, sedative, and tonic. Helps with aging skin, diffuses hot flashes during menopause, relieves cramps, and reduces tension and stress.

Uses: Used in skin tonics, potpourri, poultice, massage oil, and baths.

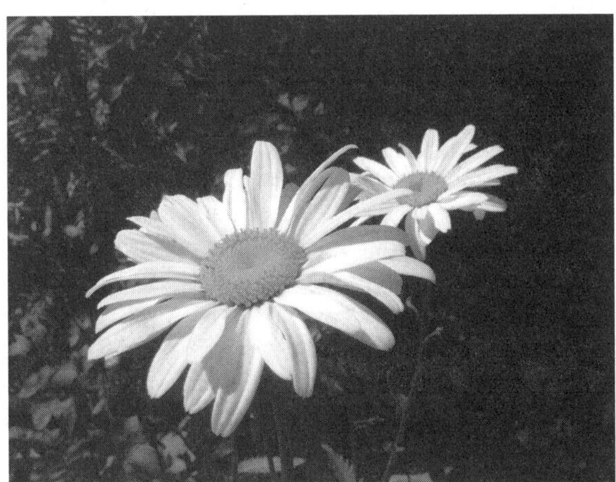

FIGURE 12.3 Chamomile.

Clove Oil (*Eugenia caryophyllata*)

Source: Evergreen tree native to Indonesia and the Malacca Islands. It has bright green leaves and nail-shaped rose-peach flower buds that turn deep red-brown when dried. Oil is extracted from the leaves, stems, and buds.

Action: Analgesic, antiseptic, antispasmodic, antineuralgic, carminative, antimicrobial, disinfectant, insecticide, and tonic.

Uses: Perfumes, mulled wines and liqueurs, dental products (toothache), pomade, insect repellant, lotions, creams, massage oil, burners and vaporizers, and as a mouthwash.

Eucalyptus Oil (*Eucalyptus radiata*)

Source: Eucalyptus plant native to Australia. South Africa, Portugal, Spain, Brazil, and Chile also grow eucalyptus (see **FIGURE 12.4**). The leaves are steam distilled to obtain the oil.

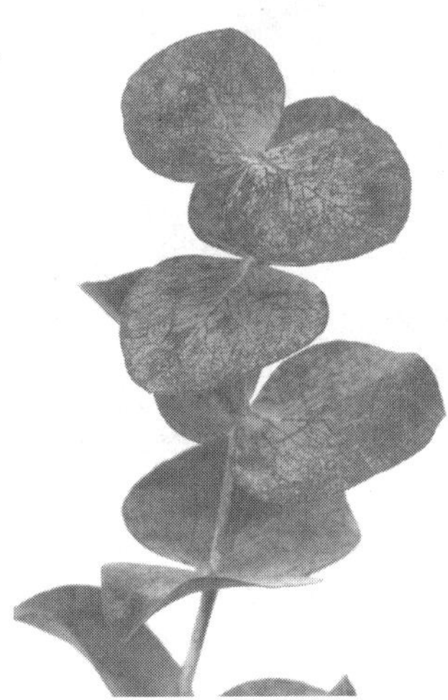

FIGURE 12.4 Eucalyptus.

Actions: Stimulant, decongestant, antimicrobial, anti-inflammatory and breathing enhancer. Used to treat asthma, kidney infection, and sore muscles.

Uses: Steam inhalations, compresses, poultices, and massage.

Jasmine Oil (*Jasminum grandiflorum*)

Source: Evergreen, climbing shrub that can grow 33 feet high. Has dark green leaves and small white star-shaped flowers (see **FIGURE 12.5**). Originally from China and Northern India and then brought to Spain, France, Italy, Egypt, Morocco, Japan, and Turkey. Floral fragrance; rich sweet scent.

Action: Promotes feeling of optimism and well-being (antidepressant), helps muscular spasm, soothes irritating coughs and laryngitis, helps with labor and painful periods, and relieves anxiety and nervousness. Helps promote the flow of breast milk and reduces stretch marks.

Uses: Massage oils, baths, lotions, burners, and vaporizers.

Juniper Oil (*Juniperus communis*)

Source: Evergreen shrub. Oil is extracted by steam distillation from the berries, needles, and wood. Has a clear, slightly woody aroma and is a pale oil.

Action: Antiseptic, antirheumatic, antispasmodic, astringent, diuretic, stimulating, and tonic effect. Should not be used during pregnancy or by people with kidney problems. Helps with the digestive system and has a tonic effect on the liver. Effective for acne, eczema, oily skin, and dandruff.

Uses: Burners and vaporizers, massage oils, baths, lotions, creams, and compresses.

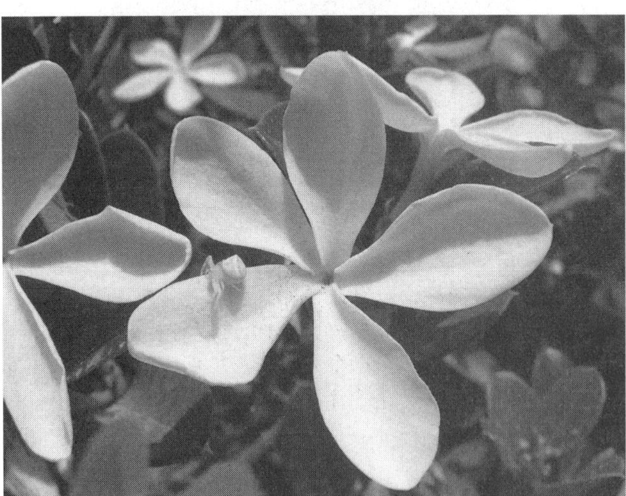

FIGURE 12.5 Jasmine.

Lavender Oil (*Lavandula angustifolia*)

Source: Evergreen shrub with pale green leaves and violet flowers (see **FIGURE 12.6**). Comes from the Latin word *lavare*, which means *to wash*. Has a delicate floral fragrance. Oil is steam distilled from flowering tops.

Action: Disinfectant, pain relief (chronic muscle aches, back discomfort, menstrual pain, arthritic and rheumatic pain), and sedative. Helps to treat insomnia, anxiety, high blood pressure, burns, wounds, respiratory problems, and digestion disorders. Is used in skin care and hair care, stimulates urine production, and helps ease discomfort of insect bites. Should not be used by women who are pregnant or who are breastfeeding.

Uses: Cold compresses, massage oils, lotions, soaps, baths.

Lemon Oil (genus *Citrus* of the *Rutaceae* family of plants)

Source: Citrus lemon tree that grows to 15 feet high. Produces highly scented lemon fruit and white blossoms year-round. Early forms originated in China and then were grown in Italy and the Mediterranean area. Columbus brought the lemon tree to the new world in 1493. Extraction by cold pressing the peel.

Action: Antiseptic, astringent, and detoxifying. Good for skin conditions, insomnia, fever, stomach disorders, weight loss, asthma, and hair care. Immune system booster.

Uses: Cleaner for cleansing the body and metal surfaces, perfumes, soaps, cosmetics, and drinks. Used in baths, massage, and inhalation.

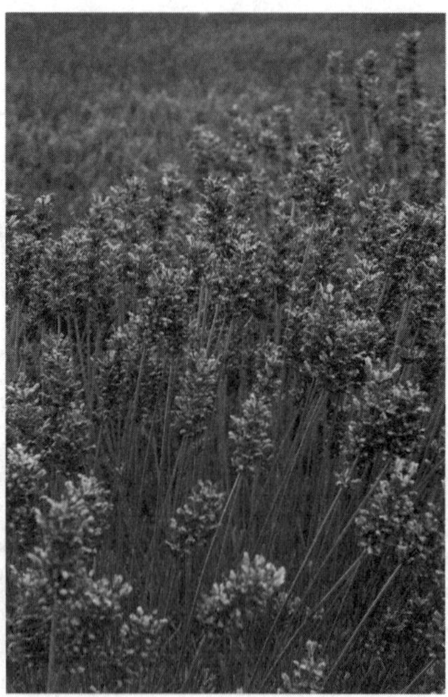

FIGURE 12.6 Lavender.

Orange Oil (*Citrus sinensis*)

Source: Orange tree. Extraction is from peels of orange by expression or cold compression.

Action: Anti-inflammatory, antidepressant, antispasmodic, sedative, aphrodisiac, antiseptic, and carminative. Good for indigestion, dental care, respiratory problems, irritable bowel syndrome, urinary tract infections, hair care, and skin care. Can be used as a diuretic and tonic. Is a detoxifier.

Uses: Adds orange flavor to beverages and desserts. Used in soaps, lotions, creams, cosmetics, room fresheners, deodorants, and bakery items.

Peppermint Oil

Source: Cross between watermint and spearmint plants. Native to Europe. Known as the world's oldest medicine. Strong spicy mint flavor. May be safely ingested (see **FIGURE 12.7**).

Action: Reduces pain of headache, digestive disorders, nausea, fever, stomach and bowel spasms, sore throats, muscle aches, and toothaches. Can be used as a skin cleanser and breath sweetener.

Uses: Soap, shampoo, toothpaste, chewing gum, tea, perfume, and ice cream. Enemas, pills, cold rubs, tonics, massage, steam baths, and burners.

Rose Oil (*Rosa centifolia/Rosa damascena*)

Source: Flower. Deep floral, rich, sweet scent. It takes 30 roses to make a single drop of oil, and 60,000 roses to produce just 1 ounce of rose oil. It is also known as rose otto (attar of roses) or rose absolute. Rose ottos are

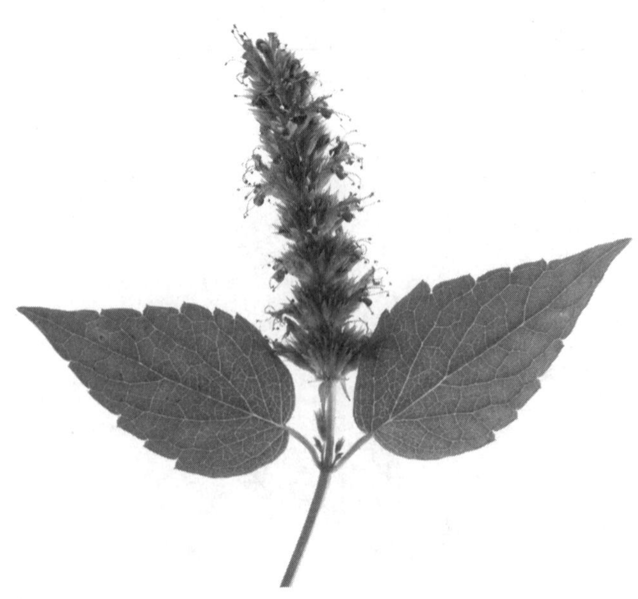

FIGURE 12.7 Peppermint.

extracted by steam distillation while rose absolutes are made by solvent or carbon dioxide extraction.

Action: Antidepressant, antiseptic, antispasmodic, antiviral, aphrodisiac, astringent, laxative. Speeds up clotting for people suffering from hemorrhage. Good for liver health and as a tonic for the nerves. Soothes the stomach, helps the uterus function better, provides menstrual pain relief, and in mild concentrations is good for headaches.

Uses: Skin tonics, massage, baths, infused in the air.

Tea Tree Oil (*Melaleuca alternifolia*)

Source: Extracted by steam distillation of twigs and leaves of the tea tree (see **FIGURE 12.8**).

Action: Antibacterial, antimicrobial, antiseptic, antiviral, expectorant, fungicidal, and insecticidal. Stimulates wound healing, circulation, and hormone secretions; boosts immunity; rids the body of toxins; and gives muscular pain relief.

Uses: Diluted doses for wounds, sores, or acne. A couple drops mixed with vodka can be given as a douche to treat yeast infections. Applied to toenails to treat fungus infections. Not recommended for baths because it can irritate sensitive areas.

Ylang Ylang Oil (*Cananga odorata*)

Source: Flowers of the ylang ylang tree, which is found in the rain forests of Asia-Pacific Islands such as Indonesia, Philippines, Java, Sumatra, Comoro and Polynesia. Ylang ylang means *flower of flowers* (see **FIGURE 12.9**). Extracted by steam distillation of fresh flowers of the tree.

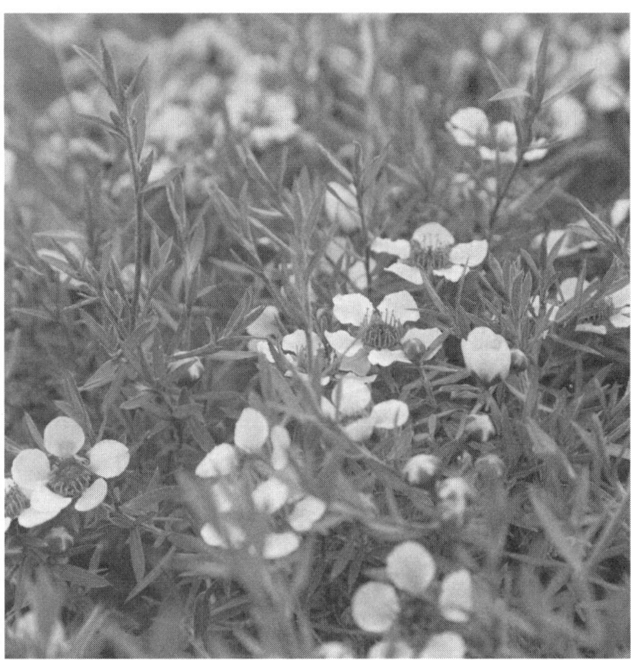

FIGURE 12.8 Tea tree leaves and flowers.

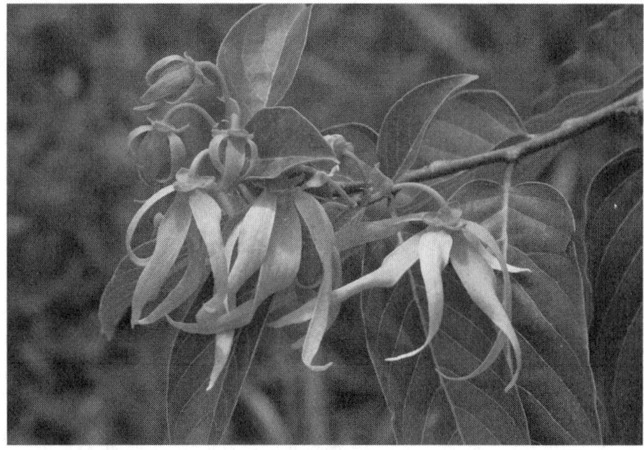

FIGURE 12.9 Ylang-ylang flowers.

Action: Antidepressant, antiseborrheic, antiseptic, aphrodisiac, lowers blood pressure, nerve booster, sedative, sleep enhancer, and anti-infective. Effective in maintaining moisture and oil balance of the skin.

Uses: Massage, baths, infused in the air.

The essential oils listed and discussed in the previous section are the more common ones, but the list is certainly not exhaustive. If you are interested in learning about more essential oils, check the reference list at the end of this chapter.

As you can see, there is a lot to learn about essential oils. For fun, see In the News for an article found online that explains how to make aromatherapy candles.

Note: Please see Appendix 12.A at the end of this chapter for simple aromatherapy recipes.

Now that you have learned basic aromatherapy information, the next topic in this chapter is Bach Flower Remedies, a field related to homeopathy, herbals, and aromatherapy.

WHAT ARE *BACH® ORIGINAL FLOWER REMEDIES* AND WHAT IS THEIR HISTORY?

There are 38 bottles of tincture on the shelves of many health food stores and pharmacies that are known as the *Bach® Original Flower Remedies*. Dr. Edward Bach (pronounced Batch) was a renowned English physician and bacteriologist who had worked for years trying to find treatments that were less toxic than those he had available in the late 1920s and early 1930s. Dr. Bach (see **FIGURE 12.10**) began to perceive that healing lay in nature rather than in the laboratory. In 1930, Bach gave up his practice and left London. He developed a holistic practice in which he talked to patients and comforted them.[2,16] Bach believed that disease was a manifestation of negative thoughts (fear,

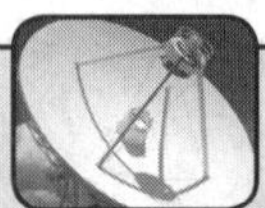

In the News

The following information is paraphrased and condensed from an online article from eHow.com.[15]

The first thing to do is gather your aromatherapy soy candle-making supplies (see **BOX 12.1**):

Box 12.1
Aromatherapy soy candle-making supplies.

- Soy wax flakes, chips or blocks (flakes or chips melt faster). There are approximately 20 ounces (oz) of volume per pound of wax. If your jars are 8 oz. and you want to make 8 jars, you will need 240 total ounces. 240 divided by 20 equals 12 pounds of wax.
- Essential oils (5–10 drops per pound of wax)
- Wicks. Enough for one per jar. They should be trimmed to about 1 inch longer than the jar.
- Jars 8 or 16 oz in size. Mason jars are good for soy candles. Number and size of jars will depend on the amount of wax you use.
- Newspapers
- Glue dots
- Double boiler pan
- Thermometer to measure the temperature of the wax (candy thermometer may be used)
- Pouring pot (aluminum)
- Candle dye is optional. May use liquid dyes or dye blocks.

Lay the newspaper on a flat surface and place all your materials on it. Put the glue dots in the center of your jars so that you can secure the wicks, and then place the wicks on top of the glue dots. Next, heat water in the bottom pan of your double boiler. (If you don't have a double boiler, you can use two pans, placing two inches of water in the larger of the two.) Melt your wax in the top pan. Stir often to keep it from sticking to the bottom of the pan. Remove the top pan that contains the melted wax and add your dye (if using) in small increments. Stir so that the color is evenly distributed. Now it is time to put in a few drops of essential oils (5 to 10 per pound of wax). Mix them in quickly before the wax hardens. By this time, the wax should have begun to harden a little and using your pouring container, you can pour the wax into your jars. You will need to hold the wicks so that they don't fall over in the jars. After the wax has been poured in and hardened, you will need to trim the wicks to about an inch from the top. If you want to make your jars attractive, tie ribbons around the mouth of the jars. Viola! You now have candles to keep or to give away as gifts. Caution people, however, to remove the ribbons when lighting the candles so that the ribbons will not catch on fire.

anxiety, jealousy, grief, frustration, despair), and the way to help and cure them was to address those negative thoughts. Bach had been trained in homeopathy, and while working at the London Homeopathic Hospital developed the seven Bach nosodes, still used today. Nosodes are made from the discharges of diseases, but diluted so that only minute quantities or reminiscences of molecules are retained in the homeopathic solution.[2] Dr. Bach, however, wanted to develop medicines even less toxic than the nosodes.

Historical accounts relate how Dr. Bach began to use flowers as remedies for emotional disorders. One day Dr. Bach strolled through the English countryside and stopped in front of several different flowers. As he was standing in front of a particular flower (such as a rose), he would feel a strong emotion, but after tasting the dew drop from the flower, the emotion would subside. He would move on to other flowers, experiencing different emotions that would subside after tasting the flower. Because of this, Dr. Bach conceived the idea that he could make liquid tinctures prepared from flowers. Over years of trial and error, Bach developed his 38 Flower Remedies to support every negative state of mind possibly conceived. Dr. Bach believed that if he could help rebalance his patients' emotions, then no matter what the disease condition, it would improve.

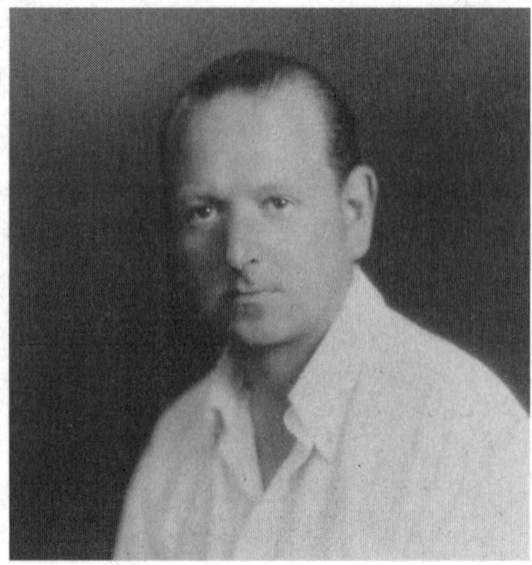

FIGURE 12.10 Dr. Edward Bach.

Dr. Bach died in 1936 at the age of 50. He had been diagnosed with cancer some 20 years previously and finally succumbed to the disease. Before his death, Bach gave instruction that no more remedies should be formulated. Today, the *Bach® Original Flower Remedies* are used alone, or as a supplement to homeopathy, herbalism, and aromatherapy, and the Bach Centre still thrives today in the house where he lived, Mount Vernon, in Brighwell-cum-Sotwell, England.

The Remedies

The *Bach® Original Flower Remedies* are unique in that they are used to treat negative emotional states, not diseases, although the intent is to aid healing by treating the emotional disorder. The Bach Remedies were at one time classified into three groups: the *Twelve Healers*, the *Seven Helpers*, and the *Second 19*. Currently, the remedies are classified into seven groups according to emotions (see **BOX 12.2**).

The following lists all the *Bach® Original Flower Remedies*; pictures of Remedies in the Twelve Healers and Seven Helpers classifications are featured. The use of each is paraphrased from the Bach Centre Web site,[16] wherein most of the explanations were developed by Dr. Bach.

Agrimony: (*Twelve Healers*) Used for people who keep their troubles and unhappiness hidden. They may use alcohol or other drugs to stay happy and like to be around friends, parties, and bright lights. See **FIGURE 12.11**.

Aspen: (*Second Nineteen*) Remedy for feeling of fear when one doesn't know what is causing the fear.

Beech: (*Second Nineteen*) Flowers from the tree. In Dr. Bach's words, "Remedy for people who feel the need to see more good and beauty in all that surrounds them."

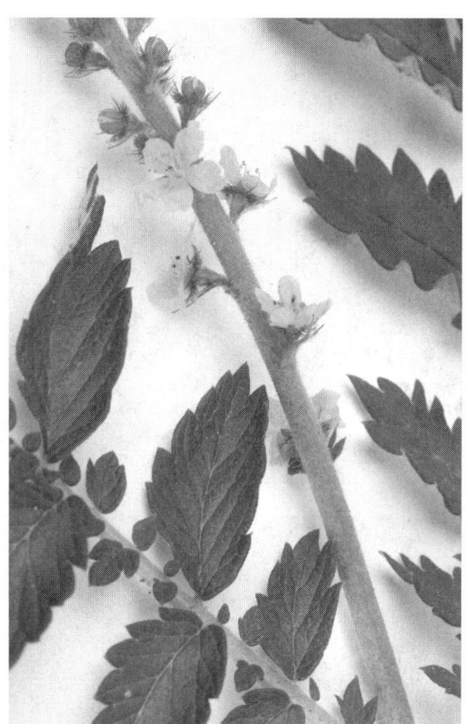

FIGURE 12.11 Agrimony.

Centaury: (*Twelve Healers*) For people who find it difficult to say no. They are usually kind, gentle people who are overanxious to serve others. See **FIGURE 12.12**.

Cerato: (Twelve Healers) Remedy for people who make decisions, then question themselves or doubt if they have made the right decision. See **FIGURE 12.13**.

Box 12.2

The *Bach® Original Flower Remedies* Classified According to Emotions

FEAR	UNCERTAINTY	INSUFFICIENT INTEREST IN PRESENT CIRCUMSTANCES	OVER-CARE FOR WELFARE OF OTHERS	OVER-SENSITIVE TO INFLUENCES AND IDEAS	LONELINESS	DESPONDENCY OR DESPAIR
Aspen	Cerato	Chestnut Bud	Beech	Agrimony	Heather	Crab Apple
Cherry Plum	Gentian	Clematis	Chicory	Centaury	Impatiens	Elm
Mimulus	Gorse	Honeysuckle	Rock Water	Holly	Water Violet	Larch
Red Chestnut	Hornbeam	Mustard	Vervain	Walnut		Oak
Rock Rose	Scleranthus	Olive	Vine			Pine
	Wild Oat	White Chestnut				Star of Bethlehem
		Wild Rose				Sweet Chestnut
						Willow

Source: Courtesy of The Bach Centre.

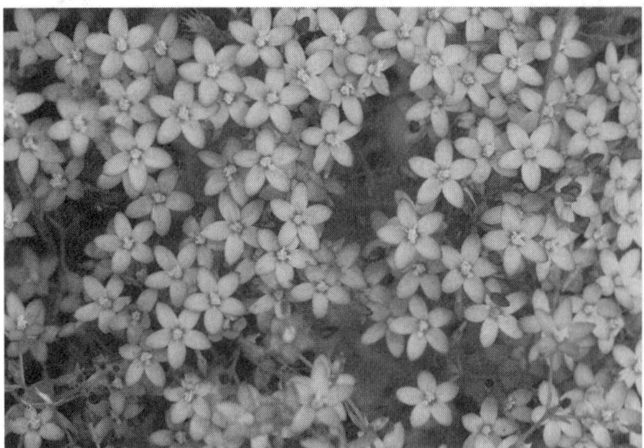

FIGURE 12.12 Centaury.

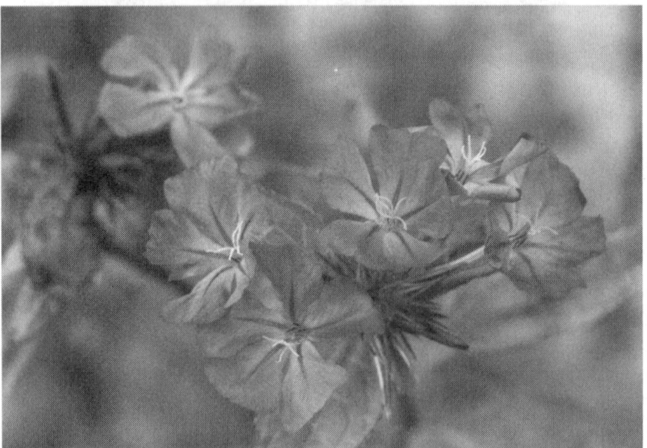

FIGURE 12.13 Cerato.

Cherry plum: (Second Nineteen) Flowers from the tree. Also a remedy for fear, but it is fear of losing control of oneself and doing something crazy. Cherry plum is an ingredient in Dr. Bach's Rescue Remedy or crisis formula.

Chestnut bud: (*Second Nineteen*) Tree buds. For people who make the same mistake over and over because they have not learned the lessons of life.

Chicory: (*Twelve Healers*) An aid to help someone love unconditionally rather than expecting to receive love and attention from someone after giving it. These people feel slighted and hurt if they don't get all they expect. See **FIGURE 12.14**.

Clematis: (*Twelve Healers*) Remedy for those who live in daydreams or whose minds drift away from reality into fantasies of the future. See **FIGURE 12.15**.

Crab apple: (*Second Nineteen*) Flowers from the tree. It is known as the cleansing remedy and is in the cream version of the Rescue Remedy. It is supposed to help people who have poor self-concept or self-esteem. They may not like their own personality or bodies.

Elm: (*Second Nineteen*) Flowers from the tree. Remedy for people who have lost confidence in themselves or who have taken on a huge responsibility and don't feel they can handle it.

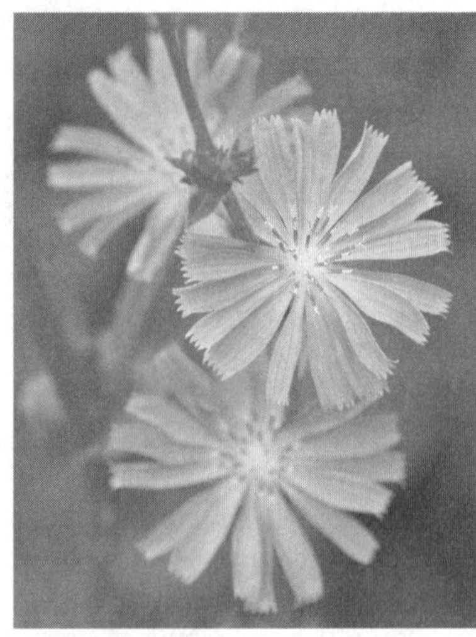

FIGURE 12.14 Chicory.

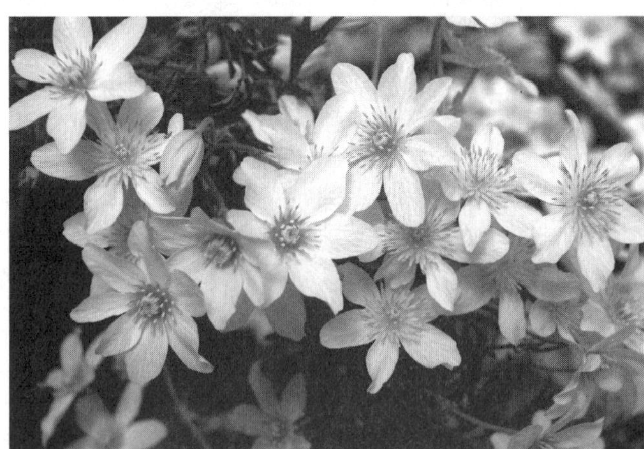

FIGURE 12.15 Clematis.

Gentian: (*Twelve Healers*) Remedy for those times when people are feeling down. These people are easily discouraged, and small life delays cause doubts and the blues. See **FIGURE 12.16**.

Gorse: (*Seven Helpers*) Remedy for people who have given up belief and hope. Remedy for uncertainty; these people need to see things in a different light to move forward. See **FIGURE 12.17**.

Heather: (*Seven Helpers*) For people who do not like to be alone even though they are obsessed with themselves. Because of their need to talk about themselves, people avoid them and then they are alone, the one thing they don't like to be. See **FIGURE 12.18**.

Holly: (*Second Nineteen*) Remedy for negative, aggressive feelings towards others. They may feel hatred, suspicion, envy, and have an absence of love. The remedy is supposed to encourage openness and better feelings towards others.

Honeysuckle: (*Second Nineteen*) Remedy for those who live in the past when they felt happy. These people believe their best days were those they lived in the past.

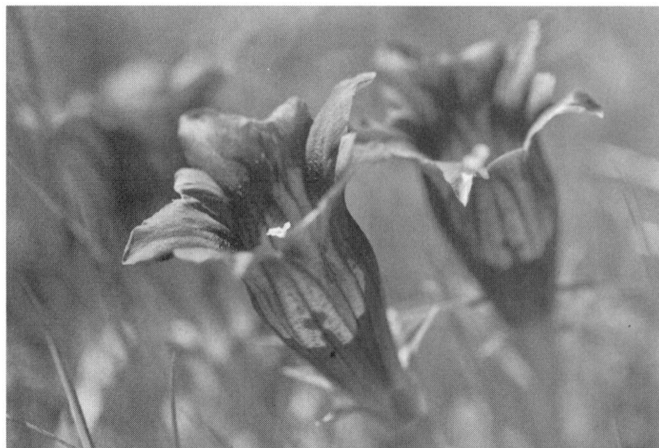

FIGURE 12.16 Gentian.

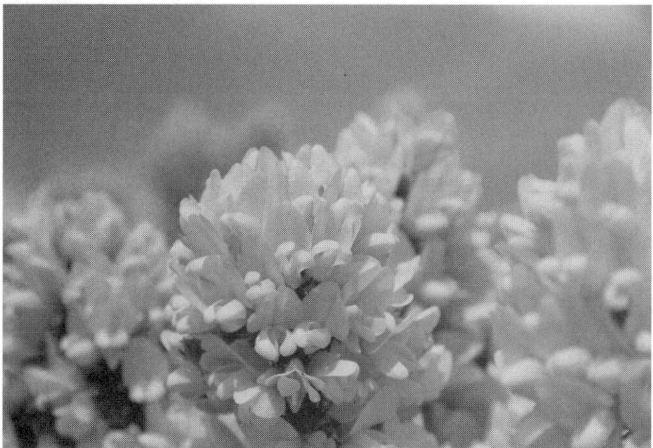

FIGURE 12.17 Gorse.

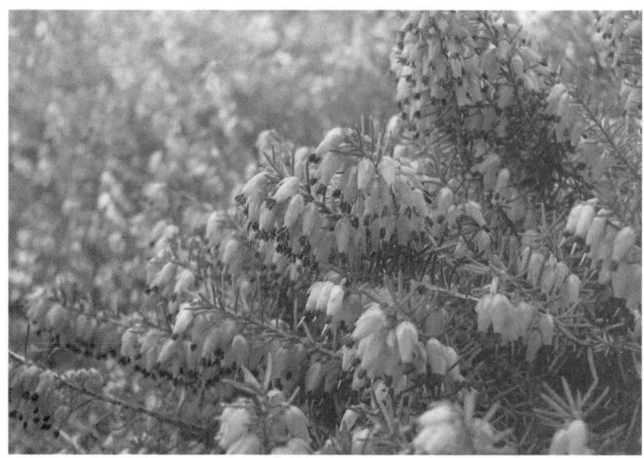

FIGURE 12.18 Heather.

Hornbeam: (*Second Nineteen*) Flowers from the tree. Remedy for those who feel they can't take care of the burdens of life or daily affairs. Used to help those who feel exhausted and tired just thinking about what they have to do.

Impatiens: (*Twelve Healers*) Remedy for those who are impatient and who feel frustrated and irritable. They may live life in a rush, rather than in a methodical way, and they are impatient with people who are slow. See **FIGURE 12.19**.

Larch: (*Second Nineteen*) Cones from the tree. Remedy for people with a lack of confidence in themselves. They don't consider themselves as good as others around them, and they may expect failure.

Mimulus: (*Twelve Healers*) Remedy for known fears such as fear of public speaking, getting sick, having an accident, being poor, being alone, and other misfortunes. See **FIGURE 12.20**.

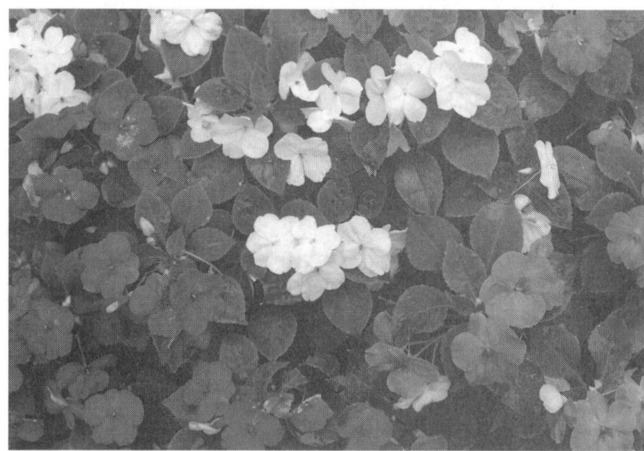

FIGURE 12.19 Impatiens.

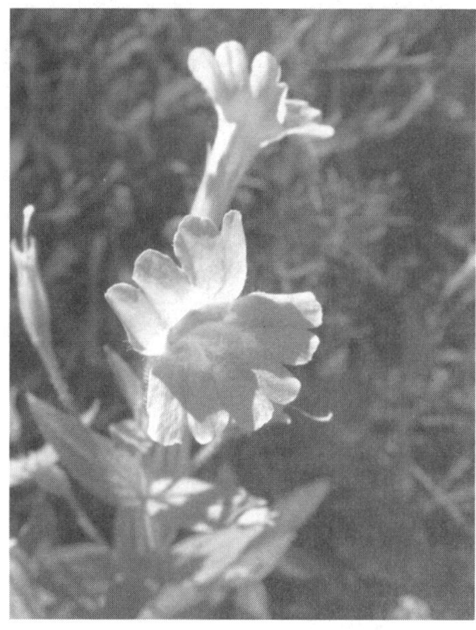

FIGURE 12.20 Mimulus.

Mustard: (*Second Nineteen*) Remedy for people who experience deep gloom or despair. They may be able to state all the reasons they have to be happy, but still experience this gloom.

Oak: (*Seven Helpers*) Remedy for people who are strong and steady and don't give up even when life hands them adversity. That seems very positive, but the negative side is that they don't rest or let others help them. See **FIGURE 12.21**.

Olive: (*Seven Helpers*) Remedy for those who have had severe mental or physical exhaustion after an illness or other tiring event. They may feel they have no strength left and no pleasure in their daily lives. See **FIGURE 12.22**.

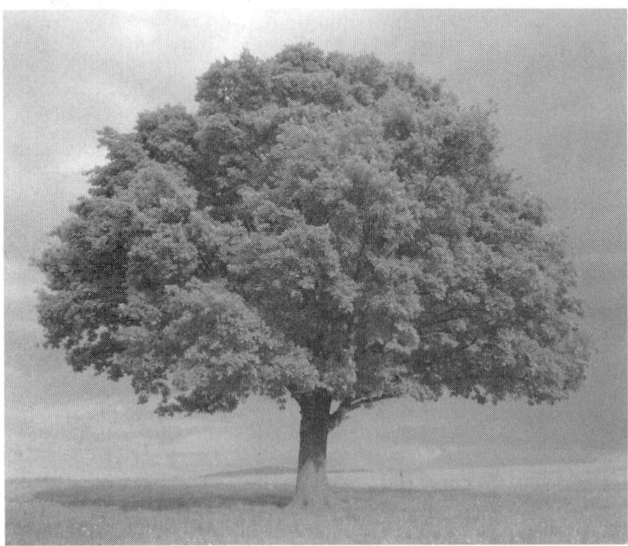

FIGURE 12.21 Oak.

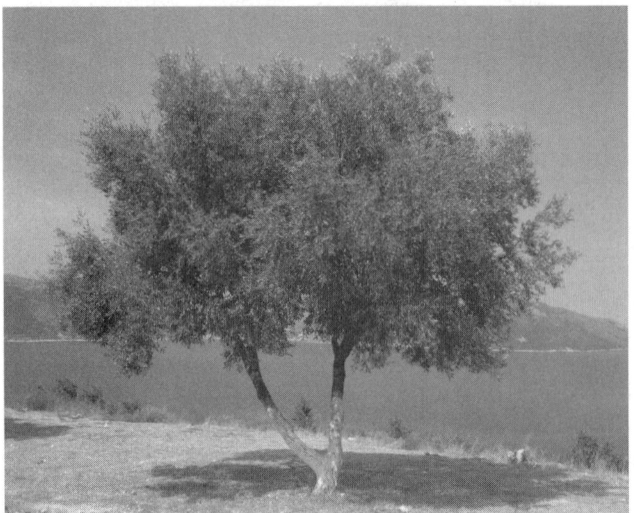

FIGURE 12.22 Olive tree.

Pine: (*Second Nineteen*) Remedy for people who blame themselves for an event or who may even blame themselves for mistakes made by others. They may be often asking for forgiveness even when they are not responsible.

Red chestnut: (*Second Nineteen*) Remedy for those who experience fear because they are concerned or anxious about others. It can be a negative effect on the people who they are concerned about.

Rock rose: (*Twelve Healers*) Remedy to help feelings of terror. It is an ingredient in the Rescue Remedy or crisis formula. This is a panicky and terror type of fear. The remedy is to help provide calm and courage. See **FIGURE 12.23**.

Rock water: (*Seven Helpers*) Remedy for those who deny themselves the joys and pleasures of life because it might interfere with their work. They take this self-denial to extremes and try to perfect themselves. The remedy is supposed to help people become kinder to themselves. See **FIGURE 12.24**.

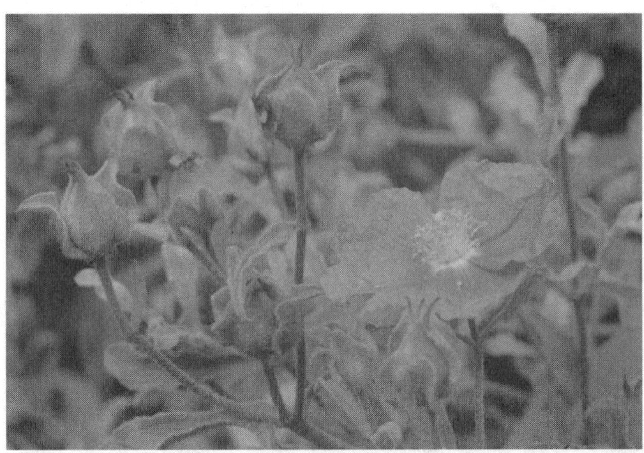

FIGURE 12.23 Rock rose.

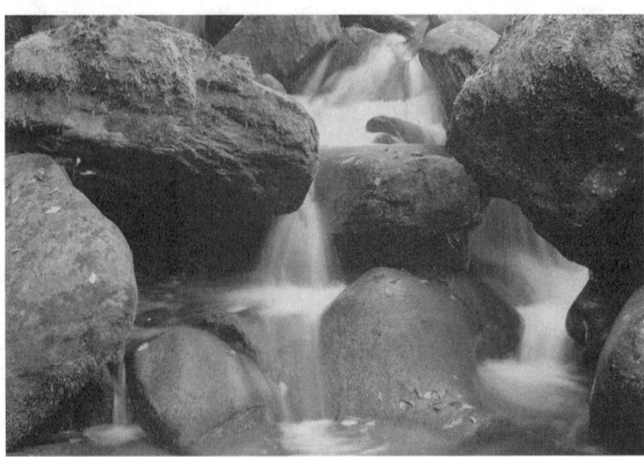

FIGURE 12.24 Rock water.

Scleranthus: (*Twelve Healers*) Remedy for people who don't seem to be able to make up their minds or make a decision. They may end up with mood swings. The remedy is supposed to help people clarify what they want. See **FIGURE 12.25**.

Star of Bethlehem: (*Second Nineteen*) Included in the Rescue Remedy or crisis formula. Remedy for the after effects of shock that may have been caused by bad news (loss of family member or friend, car crash, etc.).

Sweet chestnut: (*Second Nineteen*) Remedy for times of anguish so strong that people don't know if they can face it. This is final despair for them. The remedy is supposed to help people remain masters of their own lives and help them to renew hope and strength.

Vervain: (*Twelve Healers*) Remedy for people who have rigid ideas and principles about life. They are perfectionists who try to persuade others to align their views with them. They are in danger, however, of becoming fanatics. The remedy encourages the wisdom to enjoy life, to calm themselves, and to listen to alternative views. See **FIGURE 12.26**.

Vine: (*Seven Helpers*) Remedy for people who know their own minds and who think they know best for others. They may try to dominate others, as tyrannical fathers or overbearing bosses. They may have a positive side from which they have the ability to make wise, gentle, and loving suggestions for others; the remedy encourages this disposition. See **FIGURE 12.27**.

Walnut: (*Second Nineteen*) Remedy to help protect against those times when others attempt to lead them away from their own ideas and convictions. The remedy helps protect them from outside influences.

Water violet: Remedy for quiet and dignified people who are talented and capable but who seem proud and disdainful of others. The remedy is needed when a barrier appears between them and others and leaves them lonely. See **FIGURE 12.28**.

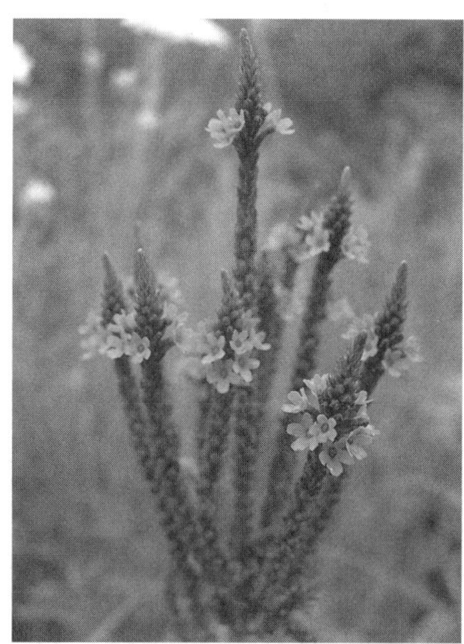

FIGURE 12.26 Vervain.

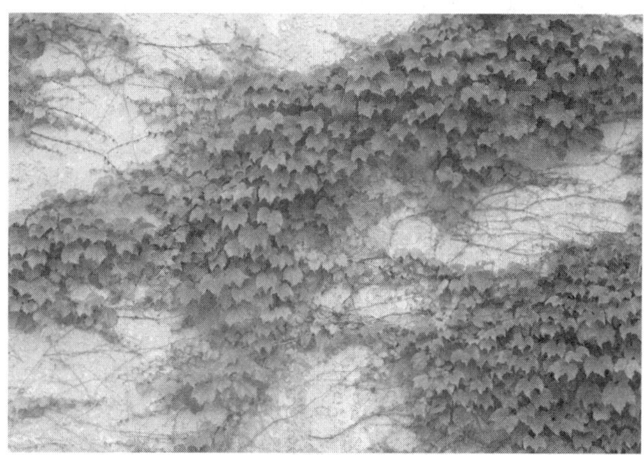

FIGURE 12.27 Vine.

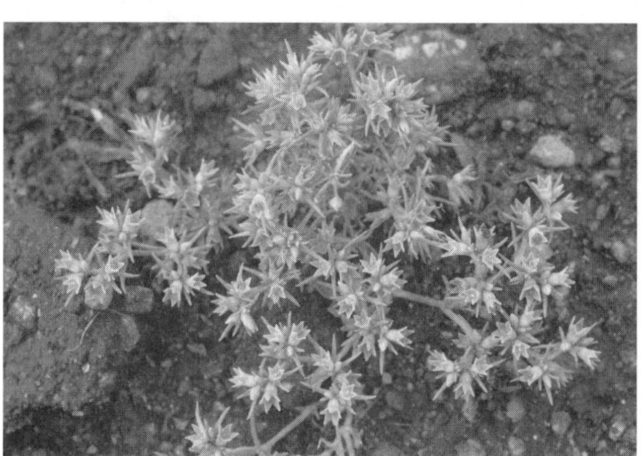

FIGURE 12.25 Scleranthus.

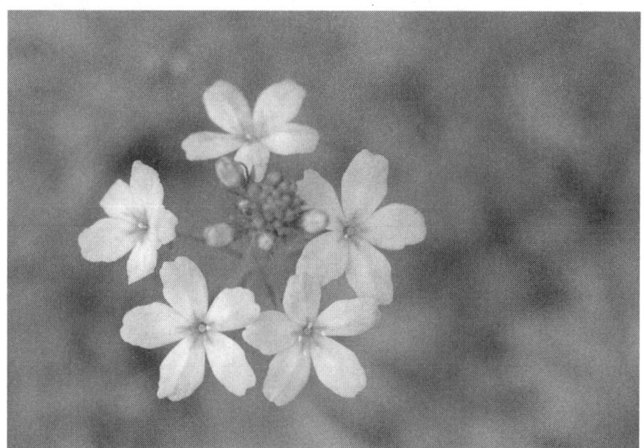

FIGURE 12.28 Water violet.

White chestnut: Remedy for unwanted thoughts and mental arguments that cause a person to stop concentrating on other issues. The remedy helps them think more calmly and rationally.

Wild oat: Remedy for people who have the ambition to do something worthwhile but don't know how to go about doing it. The remedy is supposed to help these people get in touch with their sense of purpose. See **FIGURE 12.29**.

Wild rose: Remedy for those who become resigned to life and don't make the effort to improve their lives or find joy. The remedy is supposed to help them reawaken their interest in life

Willow: Remedy for those who have suffered adversity and who feel resentful and bitter about their lives. They may begrudge others their success. The remedy encourages them to once again experience optimism and faith and to feel more generous about others.

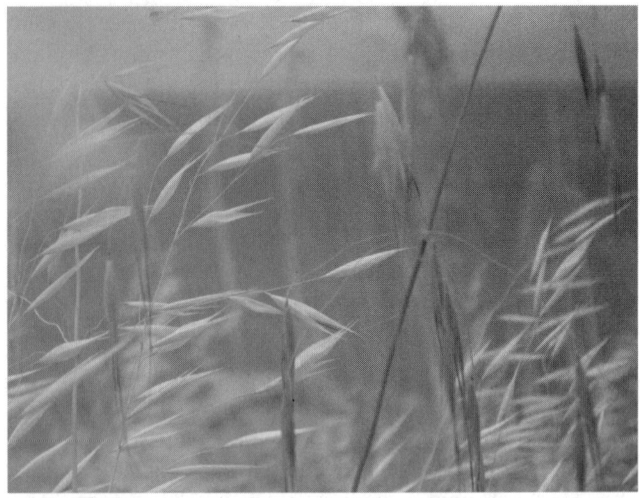

FIGURE 12.29 Wild oat.

Special Use of *Bach® Original Flower Remedies*

Rescue Remedy (also known as crisis formula) is a unique combination of five *Bach® Original Flower Remedies*.[3,16] The five flowers are rock rose, for terror; impatiens, for impatience; clematis, for dreaminess or lack of interest in the present; star of Bethlehem, for the after-effects of shock; and cherry plum, for fear of the mind giving way. Rescue Remedy is purported to help people cope with everyday situations such as taking an exam or driving test, the after-effects of a bitter argument, wedding-day nerves, going to the dentist, working toward a tight deadline, coping with bereavement, going for a job interview, speaking at an important meeting, fear of flying, receiving bad news, being stuck in a traffic jam, and coping with the kids. What do you think? Do you believe that one remedy can help all those emotions?

Another application of Bach Rescue Remedy is a cream called Bach Rescue Cream.[16] It is a general skin salve to soothe and restore and is supposed to help a wide range of skin conditions, such as rough, flaking, or chapped skin. Bach Rescue Cream contains the same combination as Bach Rescue Remedy, but also contains crab apple, a cleansing remedy.

Choosing the *Bach® Original Flower Remedies* for Personal Use

Recognizing exactly how we are feeling is very important when it comes to choosing the most appropriate *Bach® Original Flower Remedies* for personal use. Certainly we should carefully research all the remedies. Just as an exercise, let's talk about what you would have to do to choose a Bach Flower Remedy. First, you will have to pinpoint exactly how you are feeling at the moment or have been feeling during the past few weeks. Then you would need to match the mood you're in with the appropriate Bach Flower Remedy. It can be difficult to admit to ourselves some of our negative emotions—few of us want to be seen as jealous or overprotective. But, once we have admitted how we feel, we are halfway towards treating that emotion. If you find it too difficult to work out your feelings, why not ask someone

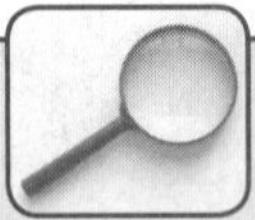

Case Study

Michael is a college student who began feeling a lack of self-confidence that he could make it through nursing school. He has begun counseling and is learning a lot about himself. He learned that he is a worrier and is extremely fearful that he would make a nursing medical error. He also seems to need other people's permission to do and be what he wants. His mother was fine with his choice of profession, but his father wanted him to get a business degree. Michael has a quiet and sensitive nature. He has a part-time job, but his studies are getting more intense and soon he will need to do his clinical nursing practices. He could not make a decision about whether to keep his part-time job or to quit and take out more school loans. Michael's worries have led him to get irritable bowel syndrome and other stress-related conditions (e.g., his hair is thinning).

Questions:

1. List and describe all the emotions you identified when reading this case study.
2. For each emotion, which Bach Flower Remedy might be appropriate to help Michael?

who knows you well (your partner, a member of your family, or a work colleague) to describe you. With their help, you should be able to make an intelligent choice.

CONCLUSION

This chapter has introduced you to aromatherapy and the *Bach® Original Flower Remedies*. If you are considering using them, please confer with your physician to be sure that the remedy or remedies will not interact with any prescription or over-the-counter drugs that you may be taking.

Suggestions for Class Activities

1. Invite an aromatherapist to class to explain how he or she uses aromatherapy as a healing process.
2. Research the amount of money it would cost to acquire 10 aromatherapy essential oils.
3. Make the aromatherapy candles in class or on your own at home. If you make them on your own, bring some samples in to show the class.
4. Make an aromatherapy treatment using a simple aromatherapy recipe found in the appendix at the end of this chapter.
5. Invite a Bach Flower Remedies practitioner to class to discuss treatment procedures and costs.
6. If a Bach Flower Remedies practitioner does not live in your area of the state, research treatment procedures and costs and report back to class.

Review Questions

1. What does the term *aromatherapy* mean?
2. What are essential oils?
3. What are the three ways to use aromatherapy?
4. Who wrote the earliest written record of the therapeutic use of plant oils and in what year?
5. Why did early Greeks use aromatherapy for fumigation?
6. Which civilization was considered the experts in the use of essential oils?
7. What aromatherapy plants were used in mummification?
8. Identify the French chemist who originated the term *aromatherapy* and defined the use of essential oils as a discipline.
9. What are some side effects of the use of aromatherapy?
10. Name three essential oils that may be safely used on babies.
11. Name and describe four of the seven ways to make essential oils.
12. From which of the methods of making essential oils are concretes formed?
13. What are four tips in the care and storage of essential oils?
14. What are carrier oils? Give three examples.
15. Overall, what does the research show about the effects of aromatherapy?
16. What are four examples of aromatherapy oils? Please give a source, a benefit, and a use when answering.
17. How many Bach Flower Remedies are there?
18. How many flowers are in the Bach Flower Rescue Remedy formula?

Key Terms

absolutes Plant extractions that are obtained by using chemical solvents.

aromatherapist A person trained in the use of essential oils.

aromatherapy Means "treatment using scents"; the use of concentrated plant oils.

Bach® Original Flower Remedies Tinctures made from flowers to treat emotions rather than disease.

carrier oils Base or vegetable oils used to dilute CO_2s and absolutes before applying them to skin.

CO_2s Plant oils extracted by the carbon dioxide method.

cold-pressed extraction Process involving mechanical pressure to force the oils out of citrus fruit, nuts, and seeds.

concrete Waxy mass that remains after solvent extraction. The waxy concrete is then processed to remove the waxy materials.

essential oils Distilled liquid from the leaves, stems, flowers, bark, roots, or other elements of a plant.

expression A method to extract essential oils from the rinds of citrus fruit without using heat. Requires squeezing by hand and collecting oils with a sponge.

florasols/phytols extraction method A process that uses gaseous solvents to extract essential oils.

fumigation Burning of plant oils to create a great deal of smoke.

hydrosol Floral water or distillate water that remains after distilling an essential oil.

infused oil Carrier oil that has been mixed with one or more herbs.

maceration Soaking aromatic plants in animal fats or vegetable oils to prepare for vacuum distillation.

Rescue Remedy Five Bach Remedy flowers that make up a formula to treat a crisis.

solvent extraction Process of washing blossoms with a solvent such as hexane to dissolve the nonaromatic waxes, pigments, and volatile aromatic molecules.

vacuum distillation A process to remove the alcohol and what is left behind to make the floral absolute.

References

1. Shealy CN. *The illustrated encyclopedia of natural remedies*. Boston, MA: Element; 1998.
2. Bradford N., ed. *The one spirit encyclopedia of complementary health*. London: Hamlyn; 1996.
3. Goldstein N. *Essential energy: a guide to aromatherapy and essential oils*. China: Time Warner; 1997.
4. Worwood V. *The complete book of essential oils and aromatherapy*. San Rafael, CA: New World Library; 1991.
5. West Coast Institute of Aromatherapy. Essential oil extraction: expression. Available at: http://www.esscentually.com/blog/essential-oil-information/essential-oil-extraction-expression29/. Accessed October 27, 2010.
6. White Lotus Aromatics. Methods of extracting essential oils. Available at: http://www.naturesgift.com/extraction.htm. Accessed October 27, 2010.
7. Gritman Essential Oils. Care and storage of essential oils. Available at: http://www.gritman.com/EO_Papers/Care_and_Storage_of_Essential_Oils.html. Accessed October 28, 2010.
8. AromaWeb. What are carrier oils? Available at: http://www.aromaweb.com/articles/whatcarr.asp. Accessed October 28, 2010.
9. Cook B, Ernst E. Aromatherapy: a systematic review. *Brit J Gen Pract*. 2000;59:493–496.
10. National Center for Complementary and Alternative Medicine. Summary of journal article. Kiecolt-Glaser JK, Graham JE, Malarkey WB, et al. Olfactory influences on mood and autonomic, endocrine, and immune function. *Psychoneuroendocrinology*. 2008;33(3):328–339.
11. Pemberton E, Turpin P. The effect of essential oils on work-related stress in intensive care unit nurses. *Holistic Nursing Pract*. 2008;22(2):97–102.
12. WebMD. Aromatherapy (essential oils therapy)—topic overview. Available at: http://www.webmd.com/balance/stress-management/tc/aromatherapy-essential-oils-therapy-topic-overview. Accessed November 1, 2010.
13. WebMD. Public information from the National Cancer Institute. Aromatherapy and essential oils—questions and answers about aromatherapy. Available at: http://www.webmd.com/cancer/tc/ncicdr0000458089-questions-and-answers-about-aromatherapy. Accessed November 1, 2010.
14. Organic Facts. Health benefits of essential oils. Available at: http://www.organicfacts.net/organic-oils/natural-essential-oils/health-benefits-of-essential oils.html. Accessed November 2, 2010.
15. Lambert E. How to make aromatherapy candles [eHow Home & Garden and Lifestyles]. Available at: http://www.ehow.com/how_4796468_make-aromatherapy-candles.html. Accessed November 15, 2010.
16. The Bach Centre. Our founder, Dr Edward Bach. Available at: http://www.bachcentre.com/centre/drbach.htm. Accessed November 15, 2010.
17. Kroeger H. *Healing with herbs A-Z*. Carlsbad, CA: Hay House; 1998.
18. Gillerman H, Arnold J. *The essential oils deck: Simple blends for health and beauty*. San Francisco: Chronicle Books; 2009.

APPENDIX 12.A

Aromatherapy Recipes[17,18]

Remember to do a patch test before placing any of the essential oils on your body. Apply a few drops to the inside of your elbow and sole of your foot. If any irritation occurs, immediately clean it off and do not use. Some descriptions of oils in the following recipes were not described in this chapter and, therefore, are given.

DIGESTIVE AID RECIPE

Makes 1 ounce (30 ml) of abdominal massage oil.

- 7–8 drops sweet marjoram (steam distilled from an aromatic plant grown in the mediterranean and central European and North African countries)
- 22–25 drops tangerine
- 15 drops sweet fennel (steam distilled from crushed seeds of fennel plant)
- 7–8 drops peppermint
- 1 tablespoon (15 ml) olive oil
- 1 tablespoon (15 ml) grape seed oil
- 1 teaspoon (5 ml) sesame oil

Combine 30 drops of the essential oil mixture with 2 tablespoons (30 ml) of carrier oil in a 1-ounce amber glass bottle.

IMMUNE SUPPORT FOOT RUB

Makes 1 ounce (30 ml) of massage oil for feet after the morning shower.

- 7–8 drops geranium
- 15 drops Atlas cedar
- 22–25 drops hyssop decumbens (steam distilled from Hyssop herb)
- 1 tablespoon (15 ml) sesame oil

MUSCULOSKELETAL INJURIES MASSAGE OIL

Makes 1 ounce (30 ml).

- 7–8 drops chamomile
- 1/4 teaspoon plus 22 drops litsea (steam distilled from litsea cubeba fruit)
- 22–25 drops vetiver
- 1 tablespoon (15 ml) arnica
- 1 tablespoon (15 ml) St. John's wort

Combine 30 drops of the essential oil mixture with 2 tablespoons (30 ml) carrier oil in a 1-ounce amber bottle.

MOODS AND EMOTIONS RECIPE

Makes 1 ounce (30 ml) of mood-balancing anointing oil.

- 1/4 teaspoon plus 15–18 drops palmarosa (steam distilled from grass leaves of wild herbaceous plant)
- 1/4 teaspoon plus 15–18 drops petitgrain (steam distilled from bitter orange plant)
- 2 drops rose

Put a drop on your finger and anoint the center of your chest and pulse points.

RESPIRATION RECIPE

This is an inhalation-diffusing blend recipe. Makes 1/2 ounce. Do not use if you are have asthma.

- 22–25 drops eucalyptus citriodora
- 22–25 drops pine
- 22–25 drops spruce
- 1/4 teaspoon plus 8 drops ravensara (steam distilled from plant grown in Madagascar)

Put 2–3 drops of the blend into a bowl of steaming hot water. Close eyes tightly, place towel over your head, and inhale the steam (good for colds and congestion).

For sinus congestion, place a drop inside nostrils or on the center of your chest.

You could also inhale any of the oils from their bottle or from a blend of the oils.

SKIN CARE OIL

Makes 2 ounces of everyday body oil.

Combine 1 1/2 teaspoons essential oil blend with 2 tablespoons Vitamin E and 7 ounces hydrating carrier oil. Choose kukui nut, safflower, or sunflower oil.

- 1/4 teaspoon plus 8 drops rosewood
- 7–8 drops sandalwood
- 2 drops lemon
- 1 tablespoon safflower, sunflower, or apricot kernel oil
- 1/2 teaspoon avocado oil
- 1/2 teaspoon vitamin E

SKIN CARE FOR THE FACE

Combine 20 drops of the essential oil blend with 2 tablespoons of a carrier blend. After washing your face, leave skin damp. Apply 2–3 drops to your fingers and rub them together.

- To regenerate mature skin: Stroke skin in upward movement with Rose hip seed oil blend.
- For oily skin: Jojoba. Pat on skin.
- For dry skin: Avocado or olive oil. Use your fingers to spread the oil with upward strokes.
- For hormone balancing and smoothing transitions of puberty or menopause: Massage lightly with Evening primrose oil.
- For sunburn: Rub gently with Aloe vera gel.

Manipulative and Body-Based Therapies: Chiropractic Medicine, Massage, and Reflexology

LEARNING OBJECTIVES

As a result of reading this chapter, students will:

1. Explain what chiropractic medicine is and trace the practice from its origins to its present day place within the healthcare field.
2. Explain how internal philosophical conflicts within the various camps of chiropractors have impacted the entire chiropractic medicine field of study.
3. List and describe several reasons that bodywork therapies such as massage and reflexology benefit the physical, emotional, mental, and social domains of health.
4. Predict the future of chiropractic, massage, and reflexology as healing professions.

WHAT IS CHIROPRACTIC MEDICINE?

Chiropractic medicine is a method of treatment based on the belief that the nervous system (spinal column, nerves), skeletal system (bones, joints), and muscular system (muscles, ligaments, tendons) interact, and if that interaction is blocked, disease and/or pain will occur.[1] The chiropractic belief is that the body has an inherent ability to heal itself if nerve impulses can travel freely between the brain and the rest of the body. The chiropractic method of treatment is to relieve the blockage by using spinal manipulation or by manipulating joints throughout the body. Chiropractic doctors generally treat people who present with neuromusculoskeletal disorders.[2] The word *chiropractic* is derived from the Greek words *cheir*, meaning hand, and *praktikos*, meaning done for.[3–5]

A major focus of chiropractic is to adjust the spinal vertebrae that surround the spinal cord to release pressure on the spine and spinal nerves that connect to, and innervate, the rest of the body. The term *subluxation* refers to one or more bones of the spine that have moved out of position and cause pressure on or irritate spinal nerves.[1] The chiropractic *adjustment* is a process of manipulating misaligned vertebrae or other joints in the body (e.g., wrist bones and joints) back into place.

The Origins of Chiropractic

Chiropractic care (spinal manipulation) can be traced back to between 2700 and 1500 BCE in writings from China and Greece. Other ancient cultures, including Japan, Polynesia, India, Egypt, and Tibet, also shared the concepts of basic manipulation. A variety of native North and South American cultures also practiced therapeutic manipulation, including the Aztec, Toltec, Tarascan, Inca, Maya, Sioux, and Winnebago. Even Hippocrates (460–379 BCE), the father of medicine, practiced manipulation and devoted two chapters of his text, *Corpus Hippocrateum*, to the use of manipulative procedures.[3] Later, the physician Galen (130–202 AD), who was influenced by the writings of Hippocrates, used manipulation within his practice. He was said to have used cervical manipulation to heal the paralysis of the right hand of a prominent Roman scholar, Eudemas.[3]

A form of chiropractic was practiced by people called bonesetters who set the broken bones of people without conducting surgery. During the Middle Ages, bonesetting was practiced in Europe, North Africa, and Asia, where practitioners were apprenticed into the trade. Western folk medicine contains many references to "bonesetters," said to be early chiropractors, and those references contain many tales of bonesetters curing patients after doctors had failed.[4,6] Two

English bonesetters, Sarah Mapp (an 18th-century bonesetter) and Sir Herbert Barker (1869–1950) became famous for their bonesetting skills.[3] Even today, in some countries such as England and Ireland, bonesetters still practice their bonesetting techniques.

Here in the United States, Daniel D. Palmer (1845–1913) founded the concept of chiropractic medicine in 1895 in Davenport, Iowa (see **FIGURE 13.1**). Palmer had been a schoolteacher, a farmer, and a grocer before turning to magnetic healing, which he stayed with until chiropractic. He was a self-taught student of anatomy and physiology, at a time when many physicians had no formal medical education. One day, in a building where his office was located, he met a janitor who told Palmer he had been deaf for 17 years, ever since an occasion when he strained his back while in a small, cramped spot in a stooped position. After examining the man, Palmer found a prominent, painful, misaligned vertebra in the upper spine and convinced the man that he could help him. He used the spinous process of the vertebra as a lever, and "racked" (gave a sharp thrust) the vertebra back into place.[3] The man could immediately hear again.

Not only did Palmer have success on this one occasion, but some time later, he met a woman who had heart trouble that was not improving. After examining her spine, Palmer found a displaced vertebra that was pressing on the nerves that innervated the heart. After adjusting her vertebra, she had immediate relief from her heart symptoms. Palmer became confident that spinal manipulation could heal about 95 percent of all diseases.[7]

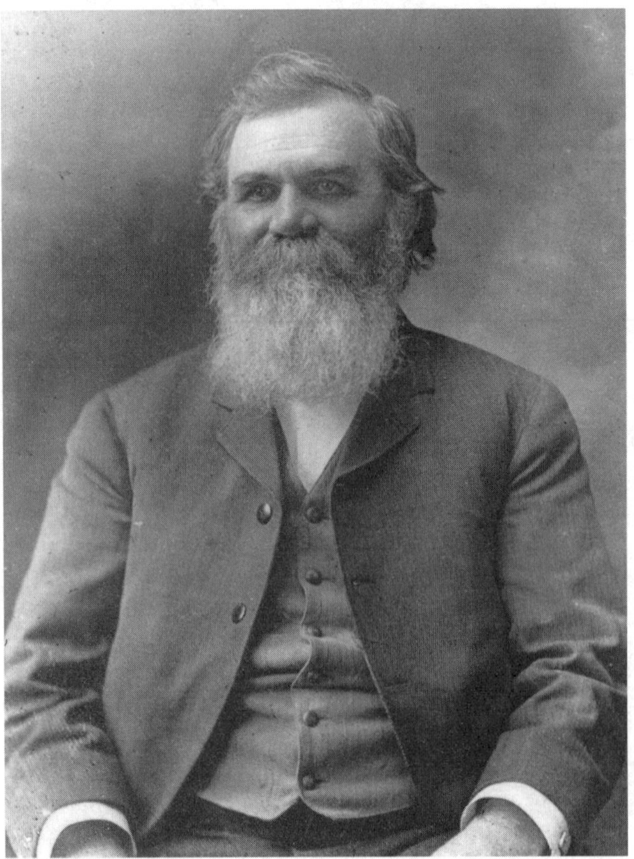

FIGURE 13.1 Daniel D. Palmer.

Many believe that Palmer learned manipulation from A.T. Still, the founder of osteopathy. Palmer had traveled from Davenport to observe Still's practice and had other things in common such as magnetic healing. Palmer, however, disputed that he was influenced by Still, and claimed that he learned his techniques from a person who lived in Davenport. In 1898, Palmer opened the Palmer School of Chiropractic in Davenport; 4 years later the school graduated four students, one of whom was his son, B.J.

Palmer had many problems as a founding chiropractor. In 1906, he was jailed for a short time (until he paid a fine) for treating people without a license. Soon after that, he sold his business to his son, B.J., who is credited with developing chiropractic medicine. B.J. widely advertised the school, set up a correspondence program, and published two magazines. He also bought an x-ray machine and offered a course leading to a special diploma in x-ray technology. The school boasted 1,000 students by 1920.[3] During the ensuing years, chiropractic has developed and changed.

Chiropractic Philosophy

Chiropractors believe that good health is determined by a healthy nervous system, particularly a healthy spinal column. The primary belief is in using natural and conservative methods of health care and to allow the body to heal itself without the use of surgery or medication.[2]

Tedd Koren, D.C., wrote an article presenting a philosophical view of chiropractic and contrasted it with allopathic medicine.[8] His article stems from the philosophical roots of healing from the early writings of Hippocrates to the present. Even then, there were two conflicting views about healing. One camp was known as the Empiricists or Vitalists, and the other camp was known as the Rationalists or Mechanists. Koren believes that chiropractic medicine is similar to the views of the Vitalists. The following quotes provide some of his philosophical comments. If you are interested in the full "debate," refer to the online article at http://www.chiro.org/LINKS/ABSTRACTS/Medical_Philosophy.shtml.[8]

> "Living creatures are fundamentally different from nonliving creatures," they say. "The laws of physics, chemistry, mechanics, and mathematics cannot give us a complete knowledge or understanding of biological systems because the whole body is greater than the sum of its parts." Vitalists learn how the body works by studying the living body, not isolated chemicals in a test tube or by making up theories.
>
> "The body is intelligent and reacts to the environment. Symptoms are its response to environmental stress, a sign that the body is fighting to return to its homeostatic balance. Symptoms must be permitted to express them-

selves so the body may cleanse and heal and return to normal balance."

"More important than diagnosing and treating disease, the individual's innate power of resistance needs to be strengthened so it may heal."

People are chemically, emotionally, and structurally unique. When caring for a sick person, we should try to learn why that one person is sick in his or her own unique way, and we should not generalize to other people. 100 people with cancer are, if you look closely enough, really expressing 100 unique conditions that have some things in common but many things unique to their situation. The more their care is tailored to their unique needs, the more successful the results.

The body is essentially unknowable. It has billions of parts, each doing its own thing at a fantastic rate. The body is constantly reacting to its environment and changing moment by moment. How can anyone know what is happening at any one time to all those parts? And doesn't the very act of observing alter our results?[8]

Chiropractic philosophy differs depending on views about chiropractic treatment. Chiropractic is rooted in mystical concepts, leading to internal conflict between two camps, called straights and mixers, which continues to this day. Even though there are two distinct camps of chiropractic, both believe in subluxations and the use of spinal manipulation,[9] and each of those two camps have off-shoots.

Philosophy of Straights

There are two straight camps: objective straights and traditional straights. *Objective straights* focus solely on the correction of chiropractic vertebral subluxations, whereas *traditional straights* claim that chiropractic adjustments are a plausible treatment for a wide range of diseases.[10] Traditional straights believe in the concept of innate intelligence, which has been called a faith-based, unscientific belief, and which has led to criticism for chiropractors.[5,10,11] The traditional straights strictly adhere to chiropractic origins, limiting the scope of their practice to manual manipulations of the spine. They follow Palmer's doctrine that vertebral subluxations can either cause or contribute to most diseases and disorders. Traditional straights do not claim to be able to diagnose diseases but only that they can detect and cure subluxations. They recognize the Palmer School of Chiropractic in Davenport and two other schools having similar views about the use of chiropractic for treatment of disorders and also diseases. Rather than using treatment adjuncts such as heat and electricity, traditional straights use only spinal manipulation or joint manipulation to treat every sort of disease. Members see pinched nerves as the cause of dizziness, eye and ear problems, high or low blood pressure, skin disorders, hay fever, congestion, asthma, and other diseases. About 15 percent of all chiropractors are identified as straights.[11] The International Chiropractic Association, based in Davenport, supports the views of the straights.

Philosophy of Mixers

Mixers believe that disease can be caused by pathogens such as bacteria, viruses, fungi, and the like.[5,11] However, they believe that subluxations can lower resistance to disease or cause a neurological imbalance within the body, thus lowering resistance to disease. They use adjustments to treat back pain, neck pain, and other musculoskeletal disorders. Mixers comprise the majority of practitioners,[11] and are supported by the American Chiropractic Association (ACA) based in Arlington, Virginia. Members offer consultation, education, and various treatment modalities. Besides spinal manipulation and adjustments, mixers may use heat, light, water, electricity, vitamins, colonic irrigation, and other physical and mechanical adjuncts.

Philosophy of Reform Chiropractic

An offshoot of the mixers are a group called reform chiropractors. They reject traditional Palmer philosophy and tend not to use alternative medicine methods. Reform chiropractors promote scientific studies and practices and are considered the most biomedical of the groups.[12] They recommend chiropractic care only for musculoskeletal disorders and do not believe that spinal joint dysfunction is the cause of disease; therefore, they do not focus on subluxations only.[13] The association they developed is the National Association for Chiropractic Medicine (NACM), an association of chiropractors working for reform.[14]

Chiropractic Philosophy Regarding Vaccination and Fluoridation

Chiropractors have historically been opposed to vaccination and water fluoridation based on their belief that all diseases were traceable to causes in the spine, and therefore could not be affected by vaccines. Some chiropractors continue to be opposed to vaccination, but others are beginning to accept the practice.[15] Fluoridation, however, remains controversial. Many countries in Europe are rejecting water fluoridation because they believe drinking water is not the appropriate vehicle for delivering medication. Many believe that ingesting fluoride is less effective than topical application.

Now that chiropractic philosophy has been presented, it is important to gain an understanding of the techniques employed by chiropractors. How do chiropractors adjust or align spinal vertebrae? Are there side effects from adjustments? Do people die from having adjustments? What does the research show? Answers to these questions follow.

The Process of Chiropractic

Occasionally vertebrae become misaligned and place pressure on the nerves exiting the spinal cord. The misalignment of a vertebra is called a subluxation. When subluxations occur, chiropractors use specific techniques to return the vertebrae into their proper positions or mobilize them so they can move freely. These techniques are called spinal manipulations or adjustments. During an adjustment, the vertebra is freed from the misaligned position and returned to the proper position in the spinal column. Once performed, chiropractors believe the adjustment allows the body to heal and maintain homeostasis.

Chiropractic Diagnosis

X-ray studies are a major diagnostic tool for chiropractors and are often used during the initial evaluation. In addition, a physical examination of the injured area is completed and a history is taken. Based upon the diagnosis, the chiropractor will formulate a treatment plan.

Chiropractic Techniques

There are a variety of chiropractic techniques. The most common technique is the chiropractic adjustment, which includes a wide variety of manual and mechanical procedures usually directed at specific joints. The adjustment may be delivered in many ways using the following basic techniques: high or low velocity speed, short or long lever (direct application of force to spinous processes), high or low force, and with or without recoil.[3] The combination most used is high velocity, short lever, and low force.[3]

A direct or indirect thrust technique may be used. Different parts of the hand may be used to direct the thrust. If the neck is to be adjusted, the middle or base of the index finger may be used. If the lumbar spine is adjusted, the chiropractor may use the wrist bone to direct the thrust. If a direct thrust would be too painful, the chiropractor could use an indirect thrust by gently stretching the joint over a pad or wedge-shaped block.

The Thompson chiropractic technique involves analyzing the length of the legs and uses a drop table for adjustment. A gentle thrust is applied to the joints, which sets the drop table into motion. After the leg check analysis, the chiropractor adjusts the legs using a combination of multiple thrusts.[16]

The Gonstead chiropractic technique is the application of different levels of pressure to address all misaligned joints (subluxations). It is used to increase muscle and joint mobility.[16]

The Cox Flexion/Distraction chiropractic technique is thought to restore range of motion in joints and muscles. It is performed on a special table that flexes and bends various muscles and joints to restore herniated discs, reduce headaches, and improve posture.[16]

One mechanical aid to chiropractic adjustment is the activator, a small tool that delivers a light and measured force to correct a misalignment. It gently and painlessly moves the vertebrae.[17]

Often, before the adjustment is done, soft-tissue techniques may be used to relax joints or muscle tension. This could include massage therapy, which also serves to increase blood circulation, reduce swelling, and aid in recovery and range of motion. One type of massage therapy is a technique called active release technique (ART). It is designed to treat scar tissue adhesions that can cause symptoms such as pain, weakness, and restricted range of motion. It is also used to treat overused muscles that may have small tears or that are not getting enough oxygen. ART uses motion and hands-on muscle manipulation of the affected part. Exercises and stretches would be taught to the patients as an adjunct to this therapy.[18]

Other adjuncts that chiropractors use include the following:

- *Hydrotherapy and heat therapy:* Use of hot, moist soaks or dry heat for pain relief and to promote healing. Many chiropractors use heat to loosen back muscles before giving adjustments.[1]
- *Cold therapy:* Use of ice packs to decrease swelling and relieve pain.[1]
- *Immobilization therapies:* Use of splints, casts, wraps, and traction to immobilize body parts so that the injured part may heal.[1]
- *Electrotherapy:* Use of several techniques to provide deep tissue stimulation and improve circulation.
  - *Galvanic stimulation:* High-voltage pulsed galvanic stimulation using direct current to stimulate deep tissue without producing tissue damage.
  - *Radio frequency rhizotomy:* Application of heated radio frequency waves to the joints' nerves.
  - *Transcutaneous electrical nerve stimulation (TENS):* Delivery of alternate current electrical stimulation through small electrodes placed inside an elastic-type belt. Usually applied to tissue by the spine before spinal adjustments by chiropractors.
  - *Interferential current (IFC):* A kind of TENS therapy in which high-frequency alternate current electrical impulses are introduced into the tissue near the pain center.
- *Ultrasound:* Use of deep heat by sound waves. Used to treat muscle pain and spasms and to reduce swelling and inflammation.[1]
- *Diet and nutrition counseling:* Chiropractors may educate people about their nutrition and lifestyle. They may give modification counseling regarding exercise, smoking, mental stress, poor posture, improper lifting, and more.[19]

Contraindications and Adverse Effects of Chiropractic

Contraindications to having chiropractic adjustment include advanced osteoporosis, bleeding abnormalities or being on anticoagulants, or having spinal malignancy or other spinal inflammatory disease. Chiropractic side effects could include temporary headaches, tiredness, or local discomfort,[20] which is fairly common in about 50 percent of all patients. Serious adverse effects are reportedly rare. A 2007 study by

Thiel and others[21] of 19,722 patients in the United Kingdom concluded that minor side effects such as local tenderness or soreness were fairly common, but serious adverse events were low to very low immediately or even up to 7 days post-treatment.

Although rare, some serious side effects have occurred. Upper spinal manipulation could cause arterial dissection and stroke; lower spinal manipulation could cause cauda equina syndrome. The cauda equina are a bundle of spinal nerve roots that arise from the lower end of the spinal cord. The syndrome is characterized by dull pain in the lower back and upper buttocks and lack of feeling in the buttocks, genitalia, and thigh, together with disturbances of bowel and bladder function.

A study by Cassidy et al.[22] reinforced findings that stroke is not associated with chiropractic manipulation. The authors concluded that the increased risks of vertebral artery (VBA) stroke associated with chiropractic and primary care physicians was likely due to patients with headache and neck pain from VBA dissection seeking care before their stroke. The researchers found no evidence of excess risk of VBA stroke associated with chiropractic care as compared to primary care.

Training of the Chiropractic Doctor (DC)

According to the American Chiropractic Association, the proper title for doctors of chiropractic (DC) is "doctor" because they are considered physicians under Medicare and in an overwhelming majority of states. They are often referred to as chiropractic physicians as well.

Doctors of Chiropractic must complete 4 to 5 years at a chiropractic college accredited by the Council on Chiropractic Education (CCE), which is certified by the U.S. Department of Education.[14] Students must have 90 hours of undergraduate courses with a major emphasis on science courses. The curriculum includes a minimum of 4,200 hours of classroom, laboratory, and clinical experience and 555 hours devoted to learning about adjustive techniques and spinal analysis. A major focus is on the structure and function of the human body in health and disease. The educational program includes training in the basic medical sciences, including anatomy with human dissection, physiology, and biochemistry. The curriculum also includes differential diagnosis, radiology, and therapeutic techniques.

After their course of study, candidates must pass the national board exam and any exams required by the state in which they want to practice. In addition, they must meet all individual state licensing requirements. Doctors of chiropractic can both diagnose and treat patients, which separates them from nonphysician status providers, like physical therapists.[2] Specializations require an additional 3 years of study. Some of the postgraduate programs available include family practice, clinical neurology, orthopedics, sports injuries, pediatrics, and nutrition.[3]

The Critics' Thoughts on Chiropractic

There are those who remain critical of chiropractic. Ernst[6] conducted a narrative review of selected articles from chiropractic literature and came to the conclusion that the core concepts of subluxation and spinal manipulation are not based on sound science. He says chiropractic therapeutic value has not been demonstrated beyond reasonable doubt. During the 1960s, the American Medical Association (AMA) began a campaign to discredit the chiropractic profession, but in 1976 their efforts backfired. A source called "Sore Throat" leaked materials that revealed the AMA's tactics, prompting a Chicago chiropractor to file an antitrust lawsuit against the AMA. After a decade, the lawsuit ended. The judge on the case agreed that the AMA had acted unfairly against chiropractors. The AMA then took the case to the Supreme Court, but the appeal failed in 1990.[7] Thereafter the AMA could not make the same claims nor discourage patients from seeing chiropractors.

Research on Chiropractic

Freeman and Lawless[3] reviewed and presented in their text several published studies from the 1980s and 1990s comparing chiropractic adjustments for treating various conditions to therapies that included heat, bed rest, soft tissue massage, hospital outpatient treatment, and physical therapy. Please refer to the Freeman and Lawless text for more details (*Mosby's Complementary and Alternative Medicine: A Research-Based Approach*). In some of the studies, chiropractic was more effective during the first 2 weeks.[23,24] In two studies, there was no difference between chiropractic and physical therapy results in the treatment of neck pain[25] or lower back and neck pain.[26]

The NCCAM-supported research[20] includes funding to Palmer College of Chiropractic on spinal manipulation for hypertension (FY 2009) and temporomandibular disorders (FY 2009); however, as of August 2011, results of those studies have not yet been published.

Bronfort et al.[27] published a study in 2010 that indicated positive results for some conditions and inconclusive or negative results for others. The study consisted of systematic reviews of randomized clinical trials using U.K. and U.S. evidence-based guidelines. The authors concluded that spinal manipulation/mobilization is effective in adults for acute, subacute, and chronic lower back pain; for migraine and cervicogenic dizziness; and for several extremity joint conditions. They also concluded that thoracic manipulation/mobilization is effective for acute/subacute neck pain and that massage is effective in adults for chronic lower back pain and chronic neck pain. They found, on the other hand, that the evidence was inconclusive that chiropractic adjustment alone was effective for neck pain and mid-back pain for any duration, tension headaches, sciatica, temporomandibular joint disorders, fibromyalgia, and other conditions such as asthma and dysmenorrhea. They found the evidence was inconclusive regarding the effects of chiropractic care to help children who had middle ear infections (otitis media) and bedwetting (enuresis).

The Pros and Cons of Chiropractic

The pros of chiropractic care are that it has been shown to be effective for back and neck pain, can help decrease frequency of headaches,[1] and provides benefits for several other conditions. Chiropractic does not require drugs and is considered a natural treatment. Because of the nature of chiropractic, many doctors develop close relationships with patients and they stress educating patients about their backs and healthy lifestyles.

The cons of chiropractic care stem from those chiropractors who adhere to a philosophy that they can treat disease. It is not scientifically proven and could deter people from seeking medical advice. Even though they have learned a lot about the neuromusculoskeletal system, chiropractors do not have the training, knowledge, or experience to recognize, identify, or differentiate human pathology or disease processes.

In conclusion, we feel that chiropractic definitely has its place in the healing professions. It is a relatively safe and effective practice for many conditions and offers a complement or an alternative to traditional medical or physical therapy.

One of the adjuncts to chiropractic is massage, and we present that topic next.

WHAT IS MASSAGE?

Massage therapy is a system of manipulating soft tissue and muscles using a variety of physical methods including applying fixed or moveable pressure, holding, vibrating, rocking, applying friction, kneading and compressing, and/or causing movement to the body. Therapists mainly use their hands, but some use their feet, forearms, and elbows. The definition of massage excludes some other kinds of bodywork such as craniosacral therapy, and Feldenkrais and Traeger therapies. Even though those are sometimes identified as massage, manipulation of soft tissue is not their main focus.[28] The definition also excludes energy therapies such as healing touch (therapeutic touch) and Reiki as well as acupressure and reflexology.

Massage uses touch, a sense that most of us are especially responsive to. As an infant, a time when we are most dependent on safe handling, we rely on touch. Perhaps as adults, when we are touched, as in massage therapy, the experience may cause a memory or feeling about the touch we experienced as infants.[29]

The Origins of Massage

Massage is another therapy that has been used since ancient times. The word *massage* may come from the Arabic verb *mass*, meaning to touch, or from the Greek word *massein*, meaning to knead.[30] Massage was an important part of movement therapy and gymnastics before it was adopted by the medical community.[28] Massage was used for the treatment of fatigue, illness, and injury. Hippocrates reported that the act of rubbing up (*anatripsis*) during massage was more effective than rubbing down.[29] Greek centers for health, called gymnasiums, had massage schools. Massage also has been practiced continually since ancient times in Eastern cultures. In the Far East, performers in dance and music used massage as an aid to their artistic development. In the Chinese book, *The Yellow Emperor's Classic of Internal Medicine*, written in 2700 BCE, massage of the skin and flesh was recommended.[31] In the traditional Indian system of medicine, Ayurveda, great emphasis was placed on the therapeutic benefits of massage.[31] Egyptian tomb paintings depict people being massaged. In Europe, massage was an important practice of the Roman Empire. In the sixteenth century, doctors in France praised massage as a treatment for many ailments. In the nineteenth century, Swedish massage was developed by Per Henrik Ling (1776–1839), a Swedish doctor, poet, and educator. His massage therapy techniques were based on the techniques of China, Egypt, Greece, and Rome; physiotherapy was originally based on Ling's manual methods.[31,32]

Beginning in the 1970s until the present, there has been a movement to establish massage as a treatment for stress and a way to maintain health outside of the medical practice; however, it has yet to receive a uniform definition by the various U.S. states. Many states, in fact, after providing an explanation of what massage is and the modalities it can include (e.g., oil, ice, hot and cold packs, tub, shower, steam or dry heat, or cabinet baths) will also emphasize that massage does not encompass diagnosis, prescribing of drugs, spinal or joint manipulation, or any other service for which a license to practice medicine is required.[30]

Types of Massage

There are two main categories of massage: Western and Oriental (Eastern).[29] Western massage methods tend to be more soothing and calming whereas Oriental massage uses direct and focused pressure and is more stimulating. Eastern methods incorporate the concept of chi (qi) energy; massage is used to help chi flow through the body better.[29] Most types of massage therapy use varying massage oils, soothing music, and aromatherapy.

Western Massage

Western massage methods include Swedish massage, Esalen, and holistic massage.

- *Swedish massage* uses firm but gentle pressure to promote relaxation, ease muscle tension, and create other types of health benefits (e.g., stress relief, improvement of blood circulation).[33] Swedish massage may include deeper pressure on specific areas of muscle tension. This is called deep tissue massage.
- *Esalen massage* was developed in California at the Esalen Institute. Its staff has trained massage practitioners in the Esalen techniques and they practice all over the world. The Esalen Institute is located at Big Sur and massage was conducted with the view and sound of waves breaking. Massages were done near the cliffside natural hot springs. Esalen massage incorporates the sound of waves in the background and if not close to water, uses recordings of waves breaking onto a beach or rocks. The rationale is that the ocean provides a slow-moving rhythm said to be similar to the internal rhythm of our bodies. Long, slow strokes are given to awaken awareness and then the contact deepens and muscles are kneaded. It is said to be a wellness/stress management type of massage.[34]
- *Holistic massage* therapy claims to deal with the person as a whole. The massage therapist doesn't just focus on symptoms, but will attempt to address the underlying cause of the symptoms. At first consultation, the client completes a detailed health history including what they've eaten and what they've eliminated. The massage combines kneading strokes on tight muscles with strokes to aid lymphatic drainage.[29,35]

Eastern Massage Therapy

Eastern massage includes Ayurvedic (India), tuina (China), lomi-lomi (Hawaii), and shiatsu (Japan).

- *Ayurvedic massage* does not use a massage table, but rather a massage mat, usually made of reeds, that is placed on an Indian-style futon or cotton mattress. Massage chairs may also be used. These massages are said to provide relaxation, help circulation, and rid the body of toxins. Ayurvedic traditional Indian massage techniques are based on the Ayurvedic doshas and marmas (pressure points). They may also include Muslim massage techniques with pressure points called *Muqame Makhssos*. Massages are always given using Ayurvedic massage oils. Specific Ayurvedic massage techniques are practiced for certain disease conditions under the supervision of an Ayurvedic doctor.[36]
- *Tuina* is a bodywork therapy that has been used in China for over 2,000 years and uses the theory of the flow of chi through the meridians. Through the application of massage, chi flow is increased and allows the body to heal itself. The therapist uses hand techniques that massage soft tissues, muscles, and tendons, and uses acupressure to directly move the flow of chi. External herbal poultices, compresses, liniments, and salves may also be used.[37]
- *Lomi lomi* Hawaiian massage therapy also uses massage to increase energy flow in the body. The words *lomi lomi* mean massage. It is a unique healing massage derived from ancient Polynesians and master healers of Hawaii. The Hawaiian healing philosophy is called *Huna*, and it holds the assumption that everything seeks harmony and love. Massage is related to that philosophy through gently, yet deeply, working the muscles with loving hands. It uses continuous, long flowing strokes and relaxes the entire being. The therapist may use the forearms as well as the hands so that people who experience it say it feels like gentle waves moving over the body. The massage therapist may work on more than one part at a time (e.g., massaging a shoulder with one hand while massaging a hip with the other).[38]
- *Shiatsu massage* is a holistic type of body work and is a method to gain relaxation. In earlier days it was mainly used within families. In this century, Japanese therapists like Namikoshi and Masunaga developed shiatsu into a professional therapy and introduced it in Europe. Shiatsu uses acupressure techniques applied with hands, thumbs, elbows, and knees. Acupressure is used to unblock meridian points where chi energy is blocked so that health and energy will be restored. The basic acupressure techniques focus on specific acupuncture points called *Tsubo*, which are located on the 12 meridians. Pressure is applied slowly and softly, but deeply, and it may feel uncomfortable. The client has to change positions during the massage, lying on the back, the stomach, and both sides.[39] Watsu is a form of shiatsu massage given in a therapeutic pool of water. It involves focusing on deep breathing while the massage therapist moves the client through the warm water. The therapist maneuvers the client into gentle stretches and will rock their client's body into cradle position. The therapist will then apply acupressure to the upper and lower body while continually supporting the spine.[40]

Massage Techniques

Massage is given in a flowing sequence so that one stroke blends into the next one. The first four described in the following list are used in Swedish massage, although they also may be used in other massage forms. Just enough massage oil is used to decrease friction on the skin, but not so much that the massage cannot be given deeply.

Effleurage is a stroke that can blend all strokes (see **FIGURE 13.2**). In effleurage, the hands are placed across the body with fingers together and thumbs slightly stretched. The stroke should be smooth, initially without

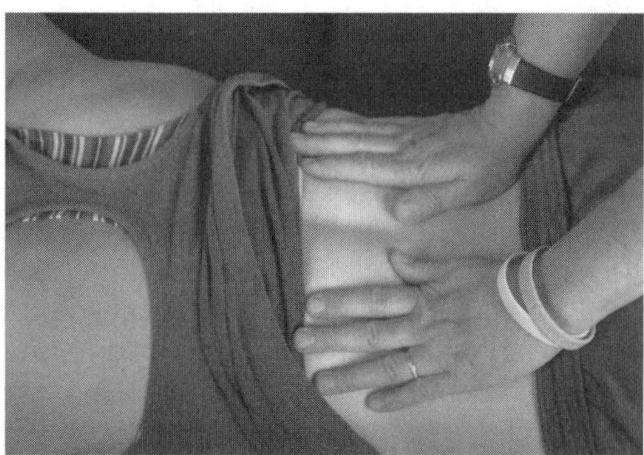

FIGURE 13.2 Effleurage.

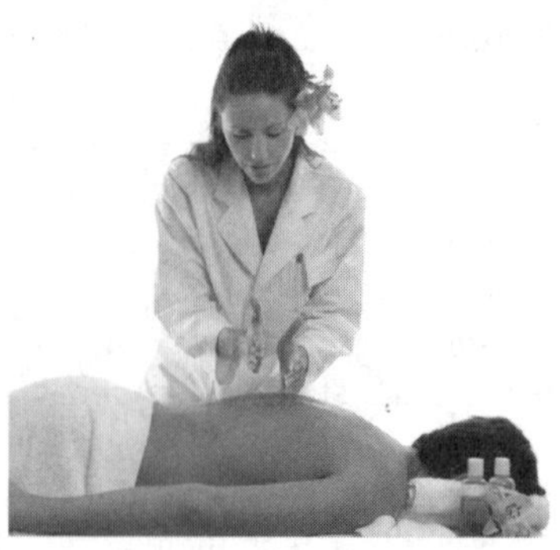

FIGURE 13.4 Tapotement.

pressure. The contours of the body should be followed and the skin should be smoothed towards the heart.

Petrissage is the act of kneading using the whole hand, with fingers together and thumbs outstretched so that the rounder contours of the body are squeezed (**FIGURE 13.3**).

Percussion is lightly striking the body using different parts of the hands, keeping the wrists loose. This stroke should begin slowly and increase to moderate speed, then build to a crescendo and stop abruptly.[35]

Tapotement is a superficial form of percussion that can be carried out with great speed. It is given by tapping the body or face. It may be done by cupping, hacking, and pinching (**FIGURE 13.4**). It makes a great end to a facial massage.

Deep sustained pressure up the full length of the sausage-shaped muscles on either side of the spine may be given during massage. The pressure is eased, however, at the cervical neck area.

Fan stroking is done by placing hands palm-side down and smoothly sliding upwards by leaning into it with a straight back. The fingers are then fanned out on both sides, slowly releasing pressure.

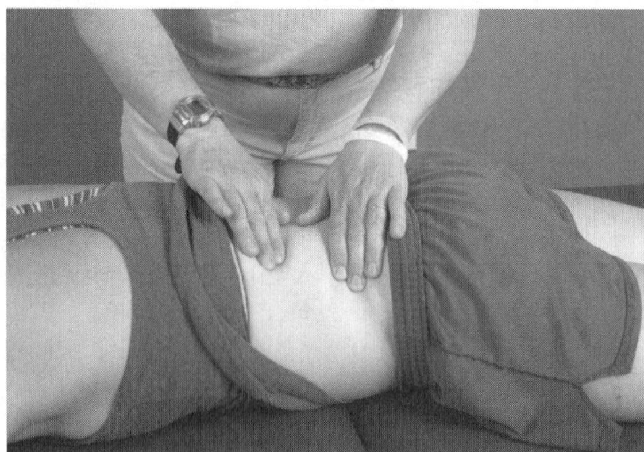

FIGURE 13.3 Petrissage.

Circular stroking is a variation of fan stroking. Both hands work on the same side at once. One hand completes a full circle motion, while the other applies a half circle. It is good for large areas like the back.

Thumb stroking is used by stroking firmly upward and out using the left thumb.[41] The stroke should be repeated higher using the right thumb.

Basic kneading is done flat and smooth, just as in kneading dough. It is good for fleshy areas and for the front of the thighs.[35]

Circular pressure is applying light pressure with the thumbs in a circular motion while gradually increasing the pressure.

Static pressure is good for releasing tension in the neck, shoulders, back, and feet. The thumbs are placed on the skin and the therapist leans into them, increasing the pressure. It is to be held for 10 seconds and then moved to another pressure point.

Cat stroking is simply placing hands at the top of the area that is being massaged and, with very light pressure, gliding the hands down the body (like petting a cat).

Knuckling is using the knuckles of the hand against the skin. The knuckles should rotate in a rippling movement in small circles on the shoulders, chest, palms, and feet.[41]

Some therapist rock, jostle, vibrate, and/or shake their clients. Some roll, rake, and pummel the skin. Some use passive stretching. Some use aromatherapy oils or light aromatherapy candles. Some use hot stones along the muscles of the spine and some use hot or cold compresses. As you can see, massage therapists are taught many techniques, which are selectively used depending on their clients and their clients' conditions.

Training of the Massage Therapist

We have discussed many types of massage, but there are many more that we have not presented. Massage therapists can specialize in more than 80 different types of massage. Education programs vary by state, but can require 500 hours or more of study to complete. A high school degree or equivalent is a prerequisite to massage therapy school.

The course of study includes anatomy and physiology, kinesiology (study of movement), and clinical massage techniques. Many states regulate massage therapy programs, and students in those states need to attend state-approved programs that may be accredited by independent agencies. After graduating, workers in states with massage therapy regulations must obtain a license prior to practicing massage therapy. They may be required to take only a state exam or one of two nationally recognized tests: the National Certification Examination for Therapeutic Massage and Bodywork (NCETMB) and the Massage and Bodywork Licensing Examination (MBLEx). A fee and periodic renewal of licensure also may be required.[42]

Benefits of Massage

Massage has physiological and psychological benefits.[35] Massage may eliminate waste products such as lactic acid from overworked muscles. Symptoms of overworked muscles are soreness, stiffness, and muscle spasms. Massage can improve circulation, bringing fresh oxygen to body tissues. It can stimulate the lymph system to rid the body of toxins. Massage can enhance a sense of well-being and reduce stress, and it can improve mood and sleep patterns.[30,32] The following case study shows one example of how massage can benefit a client.

Research on Massage

Much research has taken place to show the effects of massage therapy as a healing technique, but many studies have methodological limitations that included small sample size, inadequate control groups, lack of follow-up studies, and samples that included special patient populations. Massage is thought to be beneficial for chronic lower back pain,[43–47] as a treatment for anxiety and stress[48] and premenstrual symptoms,[49] and for pregnant women.[50] Several studies reported some benefits for a number of other conditions and problems, including anorexia nervosa,[51] autism,[52] bulimia,[53] anxiety,[54,55] diabetes,[56] eczema,[57] fibromyalgia,[58] migraine headaches,[59] and quitting smoking.[60]

A study of 598 infants by a team of researchers at the University of Warwick Medical School and Institute of Education found that massage may help infants age 6 months or younger sleep better, cry less, and be less stressed. Techniques used on infants are individualized depending on whether the infant muscles need to be relaxed or stimulated. A vegetable or plant oil such as grape seed or sweet almond oil is used because these are readily absorbed, and if the infant sucks a thumb with the oil on it, it will not be harmful. On the other hand, mineral oils are not used because they are not readily absorbed and may even be harmful.[61] A study by Livingston et al.[62] demonstrated the feasibility and safety of massage for infants with complex medical conditions. Massage was also found to create satisfaction among the caregivers, the massage instructors, and the nurses in neonatal intensive care units.

Massage has been found to be beneficial during pregnancy, but has to be conducted by someone trained in pregnancy massage to avoid pressure points that could cause uterine contractions. Massage is beneficial for relaxing anxiety during pregnancy, relieving back pain associated with muscle tension, relieving edema by stimulating circulation throughout the body, and helping promote sleep.[50] Aromatherapy oils may be used, but some are contraindicated during pregnancy, including arnica, clary sage, fennel, jasmine, and juniper.[63] Some of those that are beneficial are tangerine, lemon, tea tree, ylang-ylang, and mandarin.

Older people also benefit from massage therapy. Many who have age-related illnesses such as Parkinson's disease, arthritis, diabetes, and heart disease gain benefits due to improved circulation of lymphatic fluid and blood.

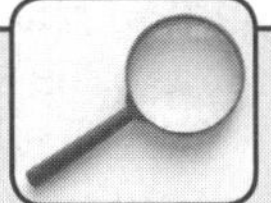

Case Study

Amy is a 54-year-old woman who has been experiencing a great deal of shoulder and neck tension. She is a computer analyst whose job requires sitting in front of a computer for long periods of time. In addition, Amy is worried about losing her job. A friend recommended that Amy should see a massage therapist, but Amy was skeptical that it could help. She felt that her problem was a pinched nerve in her neck. Eventually, Amy decided to try massage therapy.

The massage therapist took a careful history and then examined Amy's neck and shoulder. The therapist found many knots along the shoulder line and tightness in the back muscles. Simple Swedish massage and static pressure on shoulder knots was given on this first visit. Amy was instructed to do some neck and back exercises every 2 hours while sitting at the computer. Amy did feel some relief. On her next visit, the therapist began to more aggressively work out the shoulder knots. This caused Amy some discomfort but in a "good pain" way. During the third visit, the massage therapist continued to work on the shoulder knots and back muscles. Amy was feeling much better. She was trying to help herself by continuing to do her neck and back exercises and scheduled herself for regular massage therapy treatments.

Questions:

1. Have you ever received a massage? If yes, why did you go? If no, why not?

In addition, the psychological impact of loving touch may help with feelings of isolation, depression, and loneliness.[29] Usually, geriatric massage is given in 30-minute sessions, and passive stretching of shoulders, legs, and feet is given along with massage. Geriatric massage improves mobility and reduces age-related stiffness.[64]

Massage is recommended for some medically fragile individuals to improve relaxation and circulation. Techniques need to be suited to the individual so that the medically fragile person will not feel worse after the massage. The massage time may need to be shortened and the pressure may need to be light.[65] The hallmark thought is "less is better." Providing comfort for the patient is the ultimate goal. To do this, the hands of the massage therapist must be gentle, soothing, nurturing, comforting, calming, restful, simple, slow, nonjudgmental, and spacious.[65]

Several studies were reported at the National Center for Complementary and Alternative Medicine (NCCAM) Web site. A review by the Agency for Healthcare Research and Quality on CAM practices for back and neck pain showed that massage significantly reduced the intensity of acute or subacute lower back pain compared with a placebo, but did not show a difference for chronic (long-term) back pain.[66] A study of a single session of Swedish massage on hypothalamic-pituitary-adrenal and immune function produced measurable biologic effects and may have implications for managing inflammatory and autoimmune conditions.[67]

A randomized study to assess therapeutic massage benefits for chronic neck pain found that subjects receiving massage had a reduction in neck pain compared with a control group receiving a self-care book.[68] Massage therapy compared with simple touch therapy was more effective in reducing pain and improving mood in patients with advanced cancer.[69]

It seems that several studies have shown efficacy of massage for select conditions, but most of the research scientists recommend continuing research.

The next section describes a practice known as reflexology, which physical therapists as well as massage therapists use. The most skilled practitioner, however, is known as a reflexologist.

WHAT IS REFLEXOLOGY?

Reflexology is a form of massage that involves applying pressure to points on the feet, hands, and ears. The theory of reflexology is that the body is divided into 10 energy loops that start at, and then return to the hands and feet. By stimulating the origins of these loops in the feet or hands, reflexologists believe that the pressure will cause a response in any of the organs or systems found within that particular loop. It is a holistic and relaxing therapy that is thought to balance homeostasis within the body and to boost the immune system.

The body is believed to be mirrored in the shape of the feet, so if you are lying down with your feet together, heels resting on the floor and toes pointed toward the ceiling, the shape of your feet would match the outline of your body. Pressure on certain points of the feet, hands, and ears are thought to heal parts of the body that correspond to the pressure points.

The Origins of Reflexology

Reflexology techniques can be traced back 5,000 years to ancient Egypt, India, and China. During the time of the Egyptian Sixth Dynasty (2323 to 2150 BCE) a high-ranking official, Ankhmahor, was buried in the ancient burial ground at Saqqara. Pictographs display multiple scenes of people undergoing medical treatment and work on the hands and feet. Another Egyptian pictograph was found in the temple of Amon at Karnak, which was built during Ramses II's reign (1279 to 1213 BCE), and depicts a "healer tending to the feet of foot soldiers at the battle of Qadesh."[71]

In 1900, William Fitzgerald, a medical physician, introduced zone therapy to the United States. In zone therapy, the body is divided into 10 vertical zones, running from the tips of the toes to the top of the head. He wrote and published a book called *Zone Therapy*. Fitzgerald shared his knowledge with Dr. Joe Riley, a chiropractor, who began to apply pressure to his patients' feet and hands to relieve pain in other parts of their bodies. Through Riley, Dr. Eunice Ingham, a physiotherapist, began to use zone therapy on her patients (see **FIGURE 13.5**). Dr. Ingham noticed her

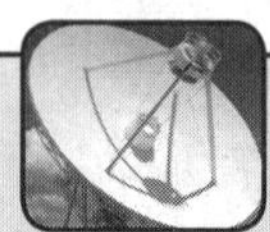

In the News

September 23, 2010. The American Massage Therapy Association (AMTA)[70] released results of a consumer survey at the AMTA National convention in Minneapolis. Results showed that the use of massage among men has decreased from 18% in 2009 to 10% in 2010. During the last year, more men also have not scheduled health care appointments for regular checkups, vaccinations or screenings. One of the reasons given was the drop in the economy. Massage use among women, however, only dropped from 26% to 25%.

Question: What do you believe might be some reasons for a greater percentage of women getting massages than the percentage of men during poor economic times?

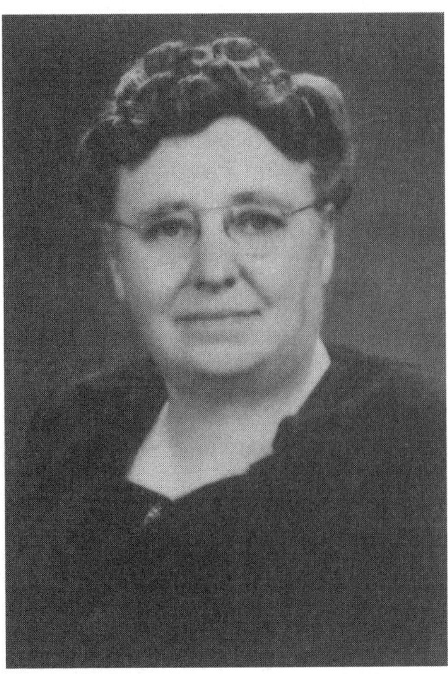

FIGURE 13.5 Dr. Eunice Ingham.

patients' healing time improved and developed the theories into a manual therapy.

Ingham renamed zone therapy as "reflexology," and mapped out the feet's reflex zones into charts that are still used today (see **FIGURE 13.6**). Ingham also discovered that applying pressure to reflex points could have a much wider effect on the body than just pain relief.[71,72,73] In 1938, Ingham published her findings in her first book, *Stories the Feet Can Tell*, and in 1951, she wrote *Stories the Feet Have Told*.

Reflexology Techniques

Reflexology is a gentle, noninvasive technique with no known side effects and is complementary to other medical therapies such as chiropractic, acupuncture, and massage. It can be an avenue to increasing human touch, which is a basic human need. No special equipment is needed, and it can be performed anywhere.

The practitioner applies pressure to the hands or feet, moving them back and forth and stretching them (see **FIGURE 13.7**). The typical session will last about 30 to 60 minutes. If practicing on the feet, only the shoes and socks need

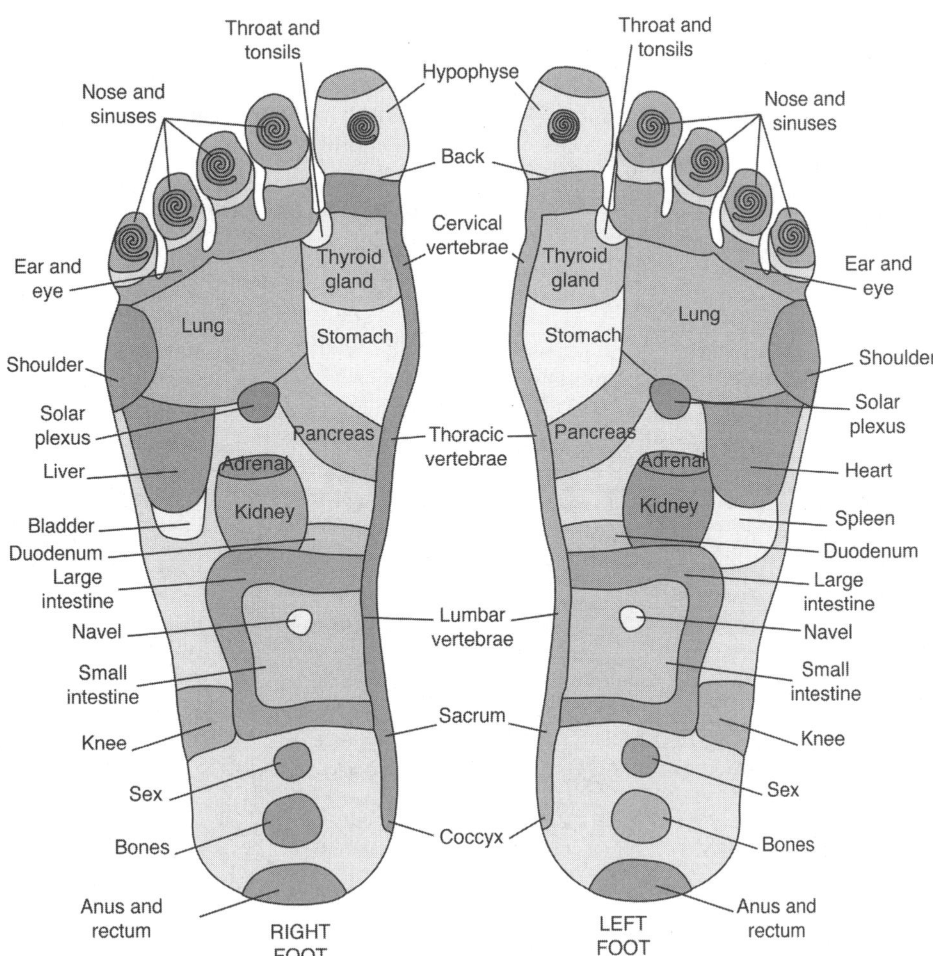

FIGURE 13.6 Foot reflexology chart.

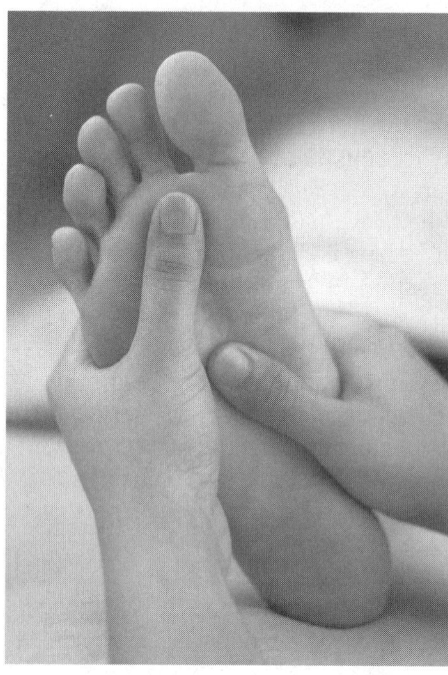

FIGURE 13.7 Reflexology therapy.

to be removed. Using the foot reflexology as an example, the basic technique uses the following steps:[74]

1. The client sits down with feet resting on a support.
2. The feet are bathed before the treatment. Rose water is often used because it helps to soothe the feet, and clients feel they are being pampered when their feet are bathed.
3. The reflexologist positions the feet close to each other and imagines looking at a map of the body.
4. Various points on the feet are pressed to stimulate the circulation.
5. Pressure is applied from the big toe down the foot, moving from side to side.

The reflexologist will hold the foot firmly and steadily. Sometimes clients feel uncomfortable or they may feel ticklish.

Oil is not used for reflexology because the fingers may slip and cause extra pressure or pain. Instead, a light dusting of talcum powder is used on the foot. Sometimes the reflexologist may feel tiny crystals under the skin and will record those on a piece of paper. To the reflexologist, it means that a particular area of the body may need special attention.

Training of the Reflexologist

Massage therapists receive some reflexology training, and many use it in their practices. Physical therapists also use reflexology. There are no licensing laws requiring special reflexology training, but it may allow a practitioner to be more effective. A national education standard has been set by the American Reflexology Certification Board (ARCB).[71] The ARCB provides a written and practical examination for certification. The training course for it consists of 110 hours of hands-on training: 40 hours in reflexology history and theory, 55 hours of anatomy and physiology, 5 hours of business ethics and standards, and 10 hours of supervised practicum. Upon graduating from such a course, an additional 90 hours of postgraduate sessions are required, bringing the total number of hours to 200 for national certification.[71]

Research on Reflexology

Reflexology has been shown effective on anxiety and pain in 23 patients with breast and lung cancer.[75] The majority of the sample were female, white, and age 65 or older. Following foot reflexology, those with breast and lung cancer experienced a significant decrease in anxiety, and patients with breast cancer showed a decrease in pain levels. Ear, hand,

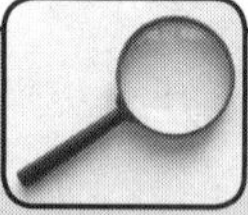

Case Study

Susan is 45 years old, divorced, has two children, and works two part time jobs to make it financially. During the last year, Susan has been suffering with migraine headaches. A friend said that her migraine headaches had been helped after she started getting reflexology treatments. Since Susan had been trying conventional medical treatments that had not helped, she made an appointment to see a reflexologist. At the initial consultation, Susan revealed that she had a history of migraine headaches. They had stopped during pregnancy with her second child 10 years ago, but had returned approximately a year ago. During the past few months she was getting them more often. After three months of a series of reflexology treatments on both her hands and feet, Susan was no longer experiencing migraine headaches.

Questions:

1. What do you think might be some reasons for the return of Susan's migraine headaches?
2. How could reflexology help Susan's migraine headaches?
3. What other reasons could explain her apparent recovery?

and foot reflexology were shown to be effective in a randomized controlled study of 35 women with premenstrual symptoms.[76] Compared to women with placebo treatment, there was a significantly greater decrease in premenstrual symptoms for women given true reflexology treatment.

Two fairly recent studies did not support reflexology as a treatment for either lower back pain or irritable bowel syndrome (IBS). In a randomized controlled study for the management of chronic lower back pain, 243 patients were assigned to one of three groups: reflexology, relaxation, or usual care. No significant differences were found among the groups on pre- and post-test lower back pain measures.[77] In the second study, reflexology was not shown effective in a single blind trial for 34 patients diagnosed with IBS.[78] Some patients were assigned to a reflexology massage and some were assigned to a nonreflexology massage. Abdominal pain, constipation/diarrhea, and abdominal distention were monitored. There was no significant difference between the reflexology group and the control group.[78]

The Future of Reflexology

The effects of reflexology in some of the clinical studies are encouraging. Some medical staff have taken up reflexology training to use as a complementary therapy. The practice is favorably received among physical therapists, massage therapists, and the nursing profession. More people are seeking out reflexologists to help with their pain conditions and body disorders. Because of these reasons, it seems that the future of reflexology is promising.

CONCLUSION

We hope this chapter has given you a better understanding of the manipulative-based therapies of chiropractic, massage, and reflexology. If you are considering a treatment using one or more of these modalities, be sure to select a practitioner who has been trained well and who is licensed or certified for their field of study.

Suggestions for Class Activities

1. Invite a chiropractor to class. Ask questions of the chiropractor about his or her philosophical beliefs and what chiropractic "camp" they belong to. Also ask about their educational background, the cost of treatments, and whether they use any adjuncts to chiropractic.
2. Invite a massage therapist to class. Ask the therapist to show class participants some simple massage techniques. Practice on each other.
3. Invite a reflexologist to class. Ask the therapist to show class participants some reflexology movements. Practice on each other.

Review Questions

1. What was the origin of chiropractic medicine?
2. Define the terms "subluxation" and "adjustment."
3. Who was the founder of chiropractic in the United States?
4. What is the difference between chiropractic and osteopathic medicine?
5. What is the overall chiropractic philosophy?
6. What is the difference in chiropractic philosophy among the straights, the mixers, and the reform group?
7. What are the Thompson, Gonstead, and Cox Flexion/Distraction chiropractic techniques?
8. What is the active release technique (ART)?
9. Name three contraindications to chiropractic adjustment.
10. What is the training of a chiropractic doctor?
11. What do the critics say about chiropractic?
12. For which conditions does research show that chiropractic is effective and for which has research shown it to be ineffective?
13. What does the word massaged mean?
14. Name several physical methods used during massage.
15. What are the two major categories of massage, and what are their philosophical differences?
16. Describe Swedish, Esalen, and holistic massage.
17. Name the four Eastern massage therapies and their countries of origin.
18. Describe tuina and lomi lomi massage therapy.
19. How does a practitioner perform shiatsu?
20. What is effleurage, petrissage, and tapotement?
21. What is the origin of reflexology, and what individuals are responsible for its development as a therapy today?
22. What professions use reflexology?

Key Terms

activator A small tool that delivers a light and measured force to correct a misalignment.

active release technique (ART) Technique designed to treat scar tissue adhesions, which can cause symptoms such as pain, weakness, and restricted range of motion. It is also used to treat overused muscles that may have small tears or are not getting enough oxygen.

adjustment A process of manipulating misaligned vertebrae or other joints in the body (e.g., wrist bones and joints) back into place.

anatripsis The act of rubbing up during massage.

bonesetters People who set the broken bones of people without conducting surgery.

chiropractic medicine A method of treatment based on the belief that the nervous system, skeletal system, and muscular system interact and if that interaction is blocked, disease and/or pain will occur.

chiropractic mixers Believe that subluxations can lower resistance to disease or cause a neurological imbalance within the body, thus lowering resistance to disease. They would use adjustments to treat back pain, neck pain, and other musculoskeletal disorders.

chiropractic objective straights Focus only on the correction of chiropractic vertebral subluxations.

chiropractic reformers Reform chiropractors promote scientific studies and practices and are considered the most biomedical of the groups. Recommend chiropractic care only for musculoskeletal disorders.

chiropractic traditional straights Claim that chiropractic adjustments are a plausible treatment for a wide range of diseases.

effleurage Massage using contours of the body; uses a smooth stroke.

galvanic stimulation High-voltage pulsed galvanic stimulation using direct current to stimulate deep tissue without producing tissue damage.

hydrotherapy and heat therapy Use of hot, moist soaks or dry heat for pain relief and to promote healing.

immobilization therapies Use of splints, casts, wraps, and traction to immobilize body parts so that the injured part may heal.

interferential current (IFC) A kind of TENS therapy in which high-frequency alternate current electrical impulses are introduced into the tissue near the pain center.

marmas Ayurvedic massage pressure points.

massage May come from the Arabic verb *mass*, meaning to touch, or from the Greek word *massein*, meaning to knead. It is manipulating soft tissue and muscles using a variety of physical methods including applying fixed or moveable pressure, holding, vibrating, rocking, applying friction, kneading and compressing and/or causing movement to the body.

muqame makhssos Muslim massage pressure points.

petrissage The act of kneading using the whole hand, with fingers together and thumbs outstretched so that the rounder contours of the body are squeezed.

radio frequency rhizotomy Application of heated radio frequency waves to the joints' nerves.

reflexology A form of massage that involves applying pressure to points on the feet, hands, and ears.

subluxation Refers to one or more bones of the spine that have moved out of position and are causing pressure on or irritating spinal nerves.

tapotement Massage that is given by tapping the body or face. It may be done by cupping, hacking, and pinching.

transcutaneous electrical nerve stimulation (TENS) Delivery of electrical stimulation through small electrodes placed inside an elastic-type belt. Usually applied to tissue by the spine before spinal adjustments by chiropractors.

ultrasound Use of deep heat by sound waves to treat muscle pain and spasms and to reduce swelling and inflammation.

References

1. Pelletier K. *The best alternative medicine: what works? What does not?* New York: Simon & Schuster; 2000.
2. American Chiropractic Association. History of chiropractic care. Available at: http://www.amerchiro.org/media/whatis/history_chiro.shtml. Accessed November 24, 2010.
3. Freeman L, Lawlis GF. *Mosby's complementary and alternative medicine: a research-based approach*. St. Louis: Mosby; 2001.
4. Bradford N, ed. *The one spirit encyclopedia of complementary health*. London: Hamlyn; 1996.
5. Somerville R, ed. *The alternative advisor*. Alexandria, VA: Time Life Books; 1997.
6. Ernst E. *The desktop guide to complementary and alternative medicine: an evidence-based approach*. New York: Mosby; 2001.
7. Singh S, Ernst E. *Trick or treatment: the undeniable facts about alternative medicine*. New York: Norton; 2008.
8. Koren T. Medical philosophy vs. chiropractic philosophy. Available at: http://www.chiro.org/LINKS/ABSTRACTS/Medical_Philosophy.shtml. Accessed November 26, 2010.
9. Ernst E. Chiropractic: a critical evaluation. *J Pain Symptom Manage*. 2008;35(5):544–562.
10. Foundation for the Advancement of Chiropractic Education. Objective straight chiropractic. Position paper. Available at: http://www.f-a-c-e.com/positionpaper1.htm. Accessed November 26, 2010.
11. Holistic online.com. Chiropractic: Two schools of chiropractors. Available at: http://www.holisticonline.com/Chiropractic/chiro_straight-and-mixers.htm. Accessed November 26, 2010.
12. Chiropractors.org. What is reform chiropractic care? Available at: http://www.chiropractors.org/resources/chiropractic-specializations/what-reform-chiropractic-care.htm. Accessed November 27, 2010.
13. The Chiropractors Directory. Types of chiropractors. Available at: http://chiropractors.healthprofs.com/cam/content/chiropractic_types.html. Accessed November 24, 2010.
14. National Association for Chiropractic Medicine. Available at: http://web.archive.org/web/20080530051351/http://www.chiromed.org/index. html. Accessed November 24, 2010.
15. Campbell JB, Busse JW, Injeyan HS. Chiropractors and vaccination: a historical perspective. *Pediatrics*. 2000;105(4):e43. doi:10.1542/peds.105.4.e43. PMID 10742364.

16. ChiropractorGuide.com. Understanding chiropractic technique. Available at: http://www.chiropractorguide.com/alternatives/understanding-chiropractic-techniques. Accessed November 24, 2010.
17. Farr G. Chiropractic techniques—an explanation. Available at: http://www.becomehealthynow.com/article/chirotechniques/663/. Accessed November 27, 2010.
18. Active Release Website. What is active release treatments (ART) to individuals, athletes, and patients? Available at: http://www.activerelease.com/what_patients.asp. Accessed November 27, 2010.
19. Grassi R, Walsh MC. Chiropractic therapies. Available at: http://www.spineuniverse.com/treatments/chiropractic/chiropractic-therapies. Accessed November 26, 2010.
20. National Center for Complementary and Alternative Medicine. Chiropractic. Available at: http://nccam.nih.gov/health/chiropractic/. Accessed November 24, 2010.
21. Thiel H, Bolton J, Docherty S, Portlock J. Safety of chiropractic manipulation of the cervical spine: a prospective national survey. *Spine*. 2007;32(21):2375–2378.
22. Cassidy J, Boyle E, Cote P, Hogg-Johnson S, Silver F, Bondy S. Risk of vertebrobasilar stroke and chiropractic care: results of a population-based case-control and case crossover study. *Spine*. 2008;33(4):176–183
23. Mathews J, Mills S, Jenkins V, Grimes S, Morkel M, Mathews W, Scott C, Sittampalam Y. Back pain and sciatica: controlled trials of manipulation, traction, sclerosant and epidural injections. *Br J Rheumatol*. 1987;26:416–423.
24. Andersson, G, Lucente T, Davis A, Kappler R, Lipton J, Leurgans, S. A comparison of osteopathic spinal manipulation with standard care for patients with low back pain. The N Engl J Med 1999;341z;1426–1431. Available online at: http://www.nejm.org/doi/full/10.1056/NEJM199911043411903. Accessed September 4, 2011.
25. Jordan A, Bendix T, Nielsen H, Hansen F, Host D, Winkel A. Intensive training, physiotherapy, or manipulation for patients with chronic neck pain. *Spine*. 1998;23(3):311–318.
26. Skargren E, Oberg B, Carlsson P, Gade M. Cost and effectiveness analysis of chiropractic and physiotherapy treatment for low back pain: six month followup. *Spine*. 1997;22(18):2167–2177.
27. Bronfort G, Haas M, Evans R, Leininger B, Triano J. Effectiveness of manual therapies: the UK evidence report. *Chiropr Osteopath*. 2010;18:3. doi:10.1186/1746-1340-18-3. Available e-version at: http://chiromt.com/content/18/1/3. Accessed November 28, 2010.
28. University of Minnesota. Massage therapy. Available at: http://www.takingcharge.csh.umn.edu/explore-healing-practices/massage-therapy. Accessed December 1, 2010.
29. Mitchell S. *The complete illustrated guide to massage: a step-by-step approach to the healing art of touch*. Boston: Element; 1997.
30. Calvert R. *The history of massage: an illustrated survey from around the world*. Rochester, VT: Healing Arts Press; 2002.
31. Holistic Online.com. History of massage. Available at: http://www.holistic-online.com/massage/mas_history.htm. Accessed December 2, 2010.
32. Carlson S. History of massage. Available at: http://www.suite101.com/content/historyofmassage-a36. Accessed December 2, 2010.
33. Brown A. Swedish massage: enjoying the most popular Western massage. Available at: http://spas.about.com/od/swedishmassage/a/Swedish.htm. Accessed December 2, 2010.
34. Esalen Massage & Bodywork Association. What is Esalen massage? Available at: http://www.esalen.org/sites/emba/html/what_is_esalen_massage_.html. Accessed December 2, 2010.
35. Michel E. What is holistic massage therapy? Available at: http://www.worldwidehealth.com/health-article-What-is-Holistic-Massage-Therapy.html. Accessed December 4, 2010.
36. Sanatansociety.org. Ayurvedic massage techniques. Available at: http://www.sanatansociety.org/ayurvedic_massage/ayurvedic_massage_techniques.htm. Accessed December 4, 2010.
37. TCM Health-Info. Tui Na (tuina)—Chinese bodywork massage therapy. Available at: http://tcm.health-info.org/tuina/tcm-tuina-massage.htm. Accessed December 4, 2010.
38. Lakainapali T. Hawaiian lomi lomi massage. Available at: http://www.huna.org/html/lomilomi.html. Accessed December 5, 2010.
39. Shiatsu Massage Guide. Shiatsu theory. Available at: http://www.topshiatsumassage.com/shiatsu-theory. Accessed December 5, 2010.
40. Massage Therapy 101. Watsu. Available at: http://www.massagetherapy101.com/massage-techniques/watsu.aspx. Accessed December 5, 2010.
41. Cardinale K. Massage techniques [Encyclomedia]. Available at: http://www.encyclomedia.com/massage_techniques.html. Accessed December 5, 2010.
42. U.S. Department of Labor, Bureau of Labor Statistics. *Occupational outlook handbook*, 2010–11 ed. Massage therapists. Available at: http://www.bls.gov/oco/ocos295.htm. Accessed December 7, 2010.
43. Ernst E. Massage therapy for low back pain: a systematic review. *J Pain Symptom Manage*. 1999;17(1):65–69.
44. Cherkin DC, Sherman KJ, Deyo RA, Shekelle PG. A review of the evidence for the effectiveness, safety, and cost of acupuncture, massage therapy, and spinal manipulation for back pain. *Ann Intern Med*. 2003;138:898–906.
45. Furlan AD, Brosseau L, Imamura M, Irvin E. Massage for low back pain. *Cochrane Database Syst Rev*. 2002;(2):CD001929.
46. Hernandez-Reif M, Field T, Krasnegor J, Theakston H. Lower back pain is reduced and range of motion increased after massage therapy. *Int J Neurosci*. 2001;106(3–4):131–145.
47. Preyde M. Effectiveness of massage therapy for subacute low-back pain: a randomized controlled trial. *Can Med Assoc J*. 2000;162(13):1815–1820.
48. Ferrell-Torry A, Glick O. The use of therapeutic massage as a nursing intervention to modify anxiety and the perception of cancer pain. *Cancer Nurs*. 1993;16(2):93–101.
49. Hernandez-Reif M., Martinez A, Field T, Quintero O, Hart S, Burman I. Premenstrual symptoms are relieved by massage therapy. *J Psychosom Obstet Gynaecol*. 2000;21(1):9–15.
50. Field T, Hernandez-Reif M, Hart S, Theakston H, Schanberg S, Kuhn C. Pregnant women benefit from massage therapy. *J Psychosom Obstet Gynaecol*. 1999;20(1):31–38.
51. Hart S, Field T, Hernandez-Reif M, Nearing G, Shaw S, Schanberg S, Kuhn C. Anorexia nervosa symptoms are reduced by massage therapy. *Eating Disord*. 2001;9:217–228.
52. Field T, Quintino O, Hernandez-Reif M, Koslovsky G. Massage therapy benefits adolescents with attention deficit/hyperactivity disorder (ADHD). *Adolescence*. 1998;33:103–108.
53. Field T, Schanberg S, Kuhn C, Fierro K, Henteleff T, Mueller C, Yando R, Burman I. Bulimic adolescents benefit from massage therapy. *Adolescence*. 1998;33:555–563.
54. Field T, Morrow C, Valdeon C, Larson S, Kuhn C, Schanberg S. Massage reduces anxiety in child and adolescent psychiatric patients. *Am Acad Child Adolesc Psychiatry*. 1992;31(1):125–131.
55. Sherman K, Ludman E, Cook A, Hawkes R, Roy-Byrne P, Bentley Sm Brooks M, Cherkin D. Effectiveness of therapeutic massage for generalized anxiety disorder: a randomized controlled trial. *Depress Anxiety*. 2010;27(5):441.
56. Field T, Hernandez-Reif M, LaGreca A, Shaw K, Schanberg S, Kuhn C. Massage therapy lowers blood glucose levels in children with diabetes mellitus. *Diabetes Spectrum*. 1997;10:237–239.
57. Schachner L, Field T, Hernandez-Reif M, Duarte A, Krasnegor J. Atopic dermatitis symptoms decreased in children following massage therapy. *Pediatr Dermatol*. 1998;15:390–395.

58. Sunshine W, Field T, Quintino O, Fierro K, Kuhn C, Burman I, Schanberg S.Fibromyalgia benefits from massage therapy and transcutaneous electrical stimulation. *J Clin Rheumatol.* 1996;2:18–22.
59. Hernandez-Reif M, Deiter J, Field T, Dieter J, Swerdlow B, Diego M. Migraine headaches are reduced by massage therapy. *Int J Neurosci.* 1998;96:1–11.
60. Hernandez-Reif M, Feld T, Hart S. Smoking cravings are reduced by self-massage. *Prev Med.* 1999;28:28–32.
61. Sinclair A. Infant massage [Childbirth Solutions]. Available at: http://www.childbirthsolutions.com/articles/postpartum/infantmassage/index.php. Accessed December 8, 2010.
62. Livingston K, Beider S, Kant A, Gallardo C, Joseph M, Gold J. Touch and massage for medically fragile infants. *Evid Based Compl Altern Med.* 2007;6(4):473–482.
63. Women's Healthcare Topics. Massage during pregnancy. Available at: http://www.womenshealthcaretopics.com/preg_massage.htm. Accessed December 9, 2010.
64. Cadena C. Geriatric massage: The next advancement in massage therapy. Available at: http://www.associatedcontent.com/article/269103/geriatric_massage_the_next_advancement.html?cat=68. Accessed December 9, 2010.
65. MacDonald G. *Massage for the hospital patient and medically frail client.* Philadelphia: Lippincott Williams & Wilkins; 2004.
66. Furlan A, Yazdi F, Tsertsvadze A, Gross A, Van Tulder M, Santaguida L, Cherkin D, Gagnier J, Ammendolia C, Ansari M, Ostermann T, Dryden T, Doucette S, Skidmore B, Daniel R, Tsouros S, Weeks L, Galipeau J. Complementary and alternative therapies for back pain II. AHRQ Pub No. 10(11)E007. Rockville, MD: Agency for Healthcare Research and Quality; 2010. Available online at: http://www.ncbi.nlm.nih.gov/books/NBK56295/. Accessed December 12, 2010.
67. Rapaport MH, Schettler P, Bresee C. A preliminary study of the effects of a single session of Swedish massage on hypothalamic-pituitary-adrenal and immune function in normal individuals. *J Altern Compl Med.* 2010;16(10):1–10.
68. Sherman K, Cherkin D, Hawkes R, Miglioretti D, Deyo R. Randomized trial of therapeutic massage for chronic neck pain. *Clin J Pain.* 2009;25(3):233–238.
69. Kutner J, Smith M, Corbin S, Hemphill L, Benton K, Mellis K, Beaty B, Felton S, Yamashita T, Bryant L, Fairclough D. Massage therapy versus simple touch to improve pain and mood in patients with advanced cancer: a randomized trial. *Ann Intern Med.* 2008;149(6):369–379.
70. American Massage Therapy Association. AMTA consumer survey shows men neglecting massage therapy in past year. Available at: http://www.amtamassage.org/articles/2/PressRelease/detail/2219. Accessed September 3, 2011.
71. Kreydin A. The history of reflexology. Available at: http://www.suite101.com/content/the-history-of-reflexology-a73343. Accessed December 15, 2010.
72. Young J. About reflexology. Available at: http://www.janineyoungreflexology.com/phdi/p1.nsf/supppages/1860?opendocument&part=2. Accessed December 15, 2010.
73. Wright J. *Reflexology and acupressure: pressure points for healing.* 2001, 2003. Summertown, Tennessee: Hamlyn and Healthy Living Publications and London, England: Octopus Publishing Group Unlimited.
74. Jerome L. Five minute foot reflexology technique. 2007. Available at: http://socyberty.com/lifestyle-choices/five-minute-foot-reflexology-technique/. Accessed December 17, 2010.
75. Stephenson N, Weinrich S, Tavakoli A. The effects of foot reflexology on anxiety and pain in patients with breast and lung cancer. *Oncol Nurs Forum.* 2000;27(1). Available at: http://www.anatomyfacts.com/Muscle/..%5CResearch%5CThe%20Effects%20of%20Foot%20Reflexology%20on%20Anxiety%20and%20Pain.pdf. Accessed December 17, 2010.
76. Oleson T, Flocco W. Randomized controlled study of premenstrual symptoms treated with ear, hand, and foot reflexology. *Obstet Gynecol.* 1993;82(6):906–911.
77. Poole H, Glenn S, Murphy P. A randomised controlled study of reflexology for the management of chronic low back pain. *Eur J Pain.* 2007;11(8):878–887.
78. Tovey P. A single-blind trial of reflexology for irritable bowel syndrome. *Br J Gen Pract.* 2002;52(474):19–23.

CHAPTER 14 Mind–Body Intervention: Meditation, Yoga, Hypnosis, Alexander Technique, Biofeedback, Prayer, and Faith Healing

LEARNING OBJECTIVES

As a result of reading this chapter, students will:

1. Assess the impact of mind–body interventions on health care in the United States.
2. Distinguish among six types of meditation and describe each one's intended effect.
3. Analyze several positive or negative effects of the use of mind–body interventions and the reason for each.
4. Explain why yoga and the Alexander Technique are considered mind–body interventions.
5. Identify the function and several benefits of yoga.
6. Explain how hypnosis is used as a therapeutic technique.
7. Analyze whether prayer and faith healing are beneficial as healing techniques.

WHAT ARE MIND–BODY INTERVENTIONS?

Mind–body interventions focus on a communication system between the mind and body.[1] This includes the mental, emotional, spiritual, social, sexual, and physical domains of health. Both Western and Eastern medical practitioners and physicians have come to the realization that this communication system is powerful, and many believe it promotes self-healing and overall health. Mind–body medicine encompasses the idea that healing does not always mean the cessation of physical symptoms, but it indicates the power to "make whole."[2]

Mind–body interventions are considered to be complementary medicine therapies, with many of the practices originating out of Chinese or Ayurvedic medicine. Some examples of mind–body interventions include meditation, hypnosis, biofeedback, Alexander Technique, yoga, faith healing, aromatherapy, autogenic and visual imagery training, progressive muscle relaxation, and tai chi. Dance movement, art therapy, and music therapy may also be included as mind–body interventions.

Several mind–body interventions result in measurable physiological responses such as lowered heart rate, blood pressure, and respirations. Stress hormones such as norepinephrine, epinephrine, and cortisol are kept in check, and blood glucose levels are decreased. One explanation for the relaxation state is that mind–body interventions may cause a placebo effect that tends to modify cognitive and body responses in a positive way by changing physiology. These positive responses are thought to boost the body's immune system.[3]

According to Pelletier,[2] there are six basic principles of mind–body interventions.

- The mind, body, and spirit are connected with one another and environmental influences.
- Stress and depression contribute to the development of, and hinder recovery from, chronic diseases because they create measurable hormonal imbalances.
- Psychoneuroimmunology explains how mental functioning provokes physical and biochemical changes that weaken immunity, lowering resistance to disease.
- Overall health improves when people are optimistic and have a positive outlook on life. Health and wellness are harmed by anger, depression, and chronic stress.
- The placebo effect—improved health and favorable physical changes in response to inactive medication

such as a sugar pill—confirms the importance of mind–body medicine and is a valuable intervention.

- Social support from family, friends, coworkers, classmates, or organized self-help groups boosts the effectiveness of traditional and CAM therapies.

This chapter is intended to introduce you to a few of the previously identified mind–body interventions. These are meditation, hypnosis, Alexander Technique, biofeedback, yoga, and faith healing.

WHAT IS MEDITATION AND HOW DOES IT WORK?

Most people think of the person who meditates as someone sitting on a cushion, legs folded in lotus position, eyes closed, and in a deep meditative trance. People, however, can meditate sitting on chairs, walking, and even dancing.

Meditation has been practiced by many cultures throughout the world. Most forms of meditation practiced today come from ancient Eastern or other religious traditions, including Buddhism and Christianity. Sakyong Mipham says that learning how to meditate is like learning how to ride a horse while staying balanced, and that we can learn how to balance our lives through meditation.[4] This introduction to meditation will explain what meditation is and how it works as a healing and "balancing" methodology.

What Meditation Is

According to Jon Kabat-Zinn,[5] a well-known mindfulness awareness meditation instructor, researcher, and author of meditation books, meditation is not a collection of techniques but is *a way of being, a way of seeing and even a way of loving*. Kabat-Zinn is the founder of the Mindfulness-Based Stress Reduction program at the University of Massachusetts Medical Center. He says that even though there are hundreds of meditation techniques and methods, those who are learning to meditate can get so caught up in learning specific techniques that it may impede their understanding of the full richness of meditation practice and what it has to offer.[5] Meditation may be considered a state in which the body is consciously relaxed, the mind is allowed to become calm and focused, and deep feelings of well-being are experienced. Meditation also may stimulate people to become aware of many feelings such as mental anguish, boredom, impatience, frustration, or body tension. Even experiencing those feelings is thought to result in a healing effect because they allow an opportunity for insight and learning.[4] According to Sogyal Rinpoche,[6] meditation brings our mind home. It is "abiding by the recognition of our true nature." It is not *out there* but *here within*. Additionally, the meditator is not required to stop thinking. Further, Rinpoche explains that meditation is a spiritual journey, and that we need to persevere along the path. We may find one day good and the next day, not so good.[6] As Allan Wallace[7] writes in *Tibetan Buddhism: From the Ground Up*:

> The point of Buddhist meditation is not to stop thinking, for ... cultivation of insight clearly requires intelligent use of thought and discrimination. What needs to be stopped is conceptualization that is compulsive, mechanical and unintelligent, that is, activity that is always fatiguing, usually pointless, and at times seriously harmful.

Meditation is intended to facilitate growth in three main areas.[8] The first is "getting to know the mind" so that a person can carefully study his or her feelings, thoughts, emotions, and various mental states. The second is "training the mind." This is the process of developing awareness, concentration, and serenity, all necessary for mental well-being. The third area of growth involves "freeing the mind," a process that is not easy but is necessary to diminish negative tendencies that decrease a sense of inner peace and harmony within oneself and the world.

Forms of Meditation

Even though there are many forms of meditation, several are acknowledged worldwide, including Vipassana meditation, Transcendental meditation, Zen meditation, Taoist meditation, Buddhist meditation, and mindfulness meditation.

Vipassana meditation is one of India's most ancient techniques and was later rediscovered by Gotama Buddha more than 2,500 years ago.[9] The word *Vipassana* may be defined in several ways: "to see things clearly," "deep insight," "to come and see," or "to come inward and see." That is why Vipassana meditation is also known as insight meditation. The Buddha believed that the cause of suffering could be erased if people could see their true nature.[10] This form of meditation is said to be a rational method for purifying the mind of all those thoughts that cause stress and pain. To exercise the technique and benefit at a maximum level, we are encouraged to take instruction from a person who is highly trained and competent to teach. During Vipassana meditation, mindfulness is employed. Mindfulness is meditating by being in the present moment. For example, we would be instructed to practice nonbiased attention, awareness, and acceptance of whatever is occurring in the present moment. Further, we would be asked to observe our own body and our mind in a nonjudgmental and unbiased way.[10] During Vipassana meditation, the most important aspect is to be watchful of our breath as it comes and goes.[11] We are not supposed to attempt to control the breath. If the breath is deep, we are supposed to let it be, and if it is shallow, the same is true. Vipassana is said to be a simple, gentle technique that is suitable for men and women of any age or race and is said to be the easiest meditation technique of all time.

Transcendental meditation (TM) was founded and introduced to the western world in 1958 by a guru (one regarded as having great knowledge) named Maharishi Mahesh Yogi.[12] TM helps people to see or transcend beyond their thoughts and to experience the source of their thoughts. This process is identified as transcendental consciousness of our most inner self, a supposedly very peaceful place and state of mind. If this state of "restful alertness" is achieved, our brain is supposed to function with significantly greater coherence and our body would gain deep rest.[13] Contrary to many other forms of meditation, TM does not require a person to concentrate (focus on something) or contemplate (think about something).[12] TM is a practical form of meditation that may be used by everyone, particularly those who lead especially hectic lives. Many forms of meditation may call for an hour or more to practice, whereas to practice TM, you just need 15–20 minutes twice daily, sitting comfortably with the eyes closed. You could do this on the bus or train, during lunch hour, or anyplace that is safe and comfortable where you could sit with eyes closed for those 15–20 minutes.

Zen Buddhist meditation, also called zazen, is practiced by way of sitting in preparation for calming the body and mind. Zazen means the "study of self." Zen Buddhism is a way to see clearly who we are, and the meditation process is supposed to help us discover insight into the nature of our being. The technique of Zen meditation gradually takes us to the state of absolute stillness and emptiness. When we think of the mind, the body, and the breath, we see them separately, but in Zen meditation, they come together as one.[14] The position used to practice Zen meditation is the pyramid structure, similar to the seated Buddha.[14] The meditation technique requires that we sit to close our mind to thought and images. Following a period of fixed concentration, our heart rate will begin to slow down and breathing will become shallow. We would then let go of past and future thoughts, and focus and react to what is being experienced in the now.[15] (Please see Appendix 14.A at the end of this chapter for a basic Zen Buddhist exercise.)

Taoist meditation is said to be much more practical than those forms requiring deeper contemplation. The fundamental principle in this form of meditation is to generate and circulate internal energy. When this particular flow of energy or force is achieved, it is known as "deh-chee," which then may be used to promote better health and longevity.[16] The first primary guideline in Taoist meditation is that we should be quiet, still, and calm. The second guideline is that we should concentrate and focus. The purpose of stillness, both mental and physical, is so that we can turn our attention inwards and cut off external sensory stimuli.[16] Within that silent stillness, we should focus attention on our breath so that we can develop intuitive insights. Taoist meditation involves breathing with the nostrils and expanding and contracting the abdomen. This form of meditation is a method that enhances self-awareness and insight.

Buddhist meditation is intended to bring our mind, body, and soul to a natural and tranquil balance. It is a method for transforming our view of reality or for getting in touch with ourselves. In Buddhist meditation, we are to become detached and objective about our thoughts, which aids us to think more clearly. Buddhist meditation is supposed to help us focus our minds and attention on a single point (*ekaggata* or one-pointedness). As stated by Francis Story, author of *Buddhist Meditation*, "The mind is hard to tame; it roams here and there restlessly as the wind, or like an untamed horse, but when it is fully under control, it is the most powerful instrument in the whole universe."[17] Buddhist meditation is a disciplined practice and must become habit to benefit our minds, bodies, and souls effectively. Through consistent practice, we should become aware of many noticeable changes such as becoming free from fear and anxiety.

Mindfulness meditation involves our focusing on the present, to be aware of our present thoughts and actions in a nonjudgmental way. There is universal agreement that at the heart of most forms of meditation lies the concept of mindfulness, or as Kabat-Zinn describes it, "Mindfulness is none other than the capacity we all already have to know what is actually happening as it is happening."[5,p.109] Kabat-Zinn has further defined mindfulness in the following way[5,p108]:

> Mindfulness can be thought of as moment-to-moment, nonjudgmental awareness cultivated by paying attention in a specific way, that is, in the present moment, and as non-reactively, as non-judgmentally, and as openheartedly as possible. It means paying attention in a particular way; on purpose, in the present moment, and non-judgmentally.

Mindfulness meditation means that we need to become aware of our physical, emotional, and mental activities in the present, meaning the here and now. This is ultimately the goal of all meditation—to awaken us to the present. Kabat-Zinn explains that the concept of mindfulness involves purposely paying attention to our experience during meditation, whether it is our breathing or our emotions. This includes deliberately noticing sensations and our response to those sensations.[5] When meditating, it is not about trying to get anywhere else, but allowing ourselves to be in the moment. Once we have learned to stay with the experience, we can then purposefully direct awareness towards some anchor to decrease the effect on our lives. In so doing, meditation can help us shape our minds.

Further, Kabat-Zinn points out that any state of mind can be a meditative state (anger, sadness, enthusiasm, delight) and is much more valuable than a blank mind or one that is out of touch.[5] Being aware of these emotions is an opportunity to learn more about ourselves. If we practiced this form of meditation, we would focus on what's happening in and around us at that very moment and become aware of all our thoughts and feelings that might be taking our energy from moment to moment. We would start by watching our breath, and then move our attention to the thoughts going through our minds, to the feelings in our bodies, and even to the sounds and sights around us. Most importantly, we would not judge or analyze ourselves.

If you are considering starting meditation, you should select a form that seems to be in keeping with your philosophy and life values. The next section describes some meditation positions that allow for individual preference and comfort.

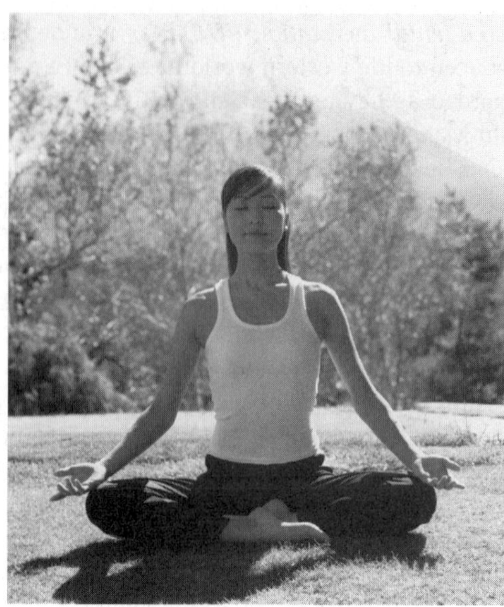

FIGURE 14.1 Burmese position.

Meditation Positions

Even though meditation may be practiced while walking, moving, or even dancing, we will explain the sitting positions first.

Seated Positions

The point of the seated positions is to allow us to be still and quiet while meditating.

The first seated position, the *Burmese position*, is likened to the pyramid structure of the seated Buddha, as reflected in **FIGURE 14.1**. You would sit on the floor and use a zafu (small pillow) to raise your hips just a little, so that your knees could touch the ground. Sitting on the pillow with two knees touching the ground forms a tripod base that gives 360-degree stability. There are other versions of Burmese. In one, the legs may be crossed and both feet placed flat on the floor or one leg may be crossed and the other extended.

The *half lotus position* is also used when meditating. In this position, the left foot is placed up onto the right thigh and the right leg is tucked under. The position is somewhat asymmetrical, and the upper body may need support to stay straight. The *full lotus position* is very stable and symmetrical.[14] In this position, both legs are placed on the opposite thigh, as reflected in **FIGURE 14.2**.

An alternative to the seated floor positions is to sit on a chair or kneel on the floor.

Movement Positions

The movement meditation positions are quite interesting. Some people and cultures like to meditate while walking, doing martial arts, or even dancing.[16] Walking while meditating has been formalized as a Zen meditation practice and is called *Kinhin*. Walking meditation focuses on awareness of self, the process of walking, and the environment. It may be practiced inside or outside. The point of walking meditation is to be in the present moment. While walking, you would first pay attention to the movement of your legs, your breathing, and your body. You would then feel your feet contacting the ground. If your mind wanders, you would refocus on the process of walking and breathing. Meditating outside can be difficult because of the distractions, but if you choose to do this outside, find a quiet place with level ground.

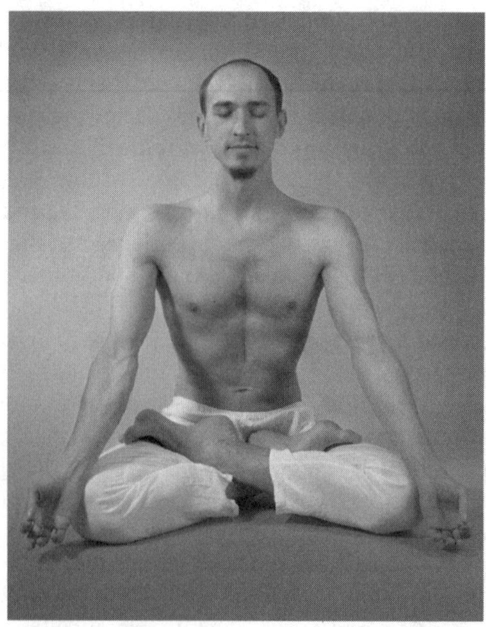

FIGURE 14.2 Full lotus position.

Some martial arts practices include Zen archery[18] (see **FIGURE 14.3**), tai chi, and qi gong. All encompass understanding the relationship of the power of breath, the life force (chi energy), the mind, and the concept of oneness.

Dance is said to be a great method to build awareness, get rid of negative feelings, and get into the present moment. Many examples of dance meditation follow.

Sufi dancing is said to be the dance of universal peace. It originated in the Islamic world and has been practiced for centuries, but not by all orders of Sufi. Sufi dancing is a part of Sama, a ritual practice developed in the mid 9th century that uses music, poetry recital, singing, and dance. The dances were first performed by religious men. All practices are intended to bring participants to a mystical experience.[19] The individual responsible for making the Sama dance a focus of Sufi doctrine is Jalaluddin Rumi, a spiritual master and a genius at poetry making who was also known as Mevlana. He was born in Iran but eventually settled in the city of Konya. Rumi established his Sufi order. He taught his followers how to use the Sama dance to guide followers to a spiritual uplifting to the Immortal one.[19]

Sufi whirling is a version of Sufi dance. In this movement, dancers whirl by themselves with arms in various positions, such as reaching out and reaching to the heavens. Sufi whirling may also be danced with a partner and is known in the West as the dance of the "whirling dervishes."[20] It is performed under strict and controlled conditions and is led by a Sufi master. The steps and motions symbolically depict the "cosmos in motion." The dance is supposed to cultivate inner peace and harmony. The dances are simple circle dances wherein dancers move around a dance floor from partner to partner (see **FIGURE 14.4**).[20] They are to let their thoughts fall away and connect on a spiritual level with other dancers. As they dance, they are to focus on the chants and songs while they connect with one another.[21]

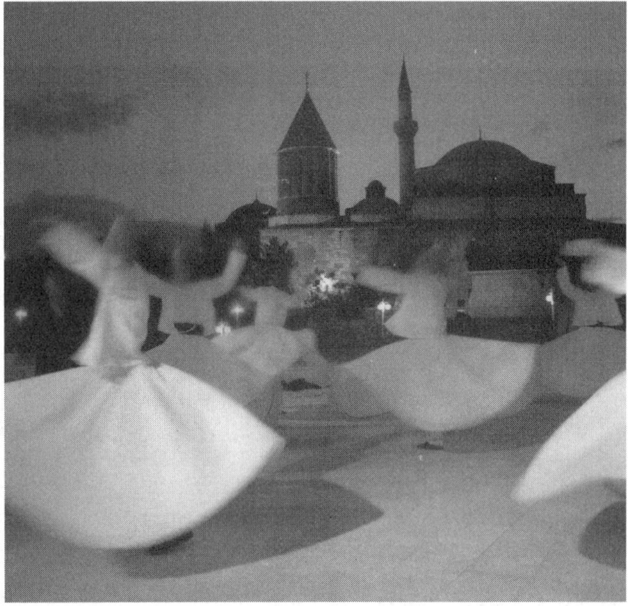

FIGURE 14.4 Sufi dancing.

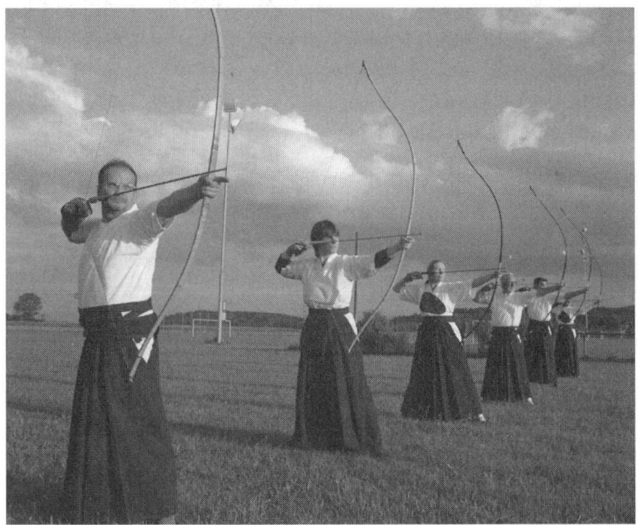

FIGURE 14.3 Zen archer.

Another form of Sufi dance is Dervish dancing by Turkish dancers, who dress in a particular style. The Dervish dancers can be said to dance to the rhythm of the cosmos or the universe as they seem to represent the solar system and the planets that revolve around the sun. During the dance, they seem to yield the body to the earth's movement. They let their bodies sway to the changing tempos of the music. As they are doing this, their consciousness also changes. They seem to be in a trance-like state as they begin to understand the possibility of the eternity of the soul. They are said to have given away the body to the earth and that the mind and soul can now concentrate on the fully transcendental.[22]

A very different dance meditation is that of Master George Ivanovich Gurdjieff. The Gurdjieff Sacred Dances use well-defined movements in which different parts of the body seem not to be related with each other.[23] The dancer is expected to coordinate different rhythms at the same time. The movements and the dance are very energetic, sometimes strange, and sometimes depict ancient rituals. The purpose of the dance is to train the dancers to be in the present moment with no thoughts of the past or future. They are to accept themselves and to be playful and relaxed (see **FIGURE 14.5**).

Again, if you are considering meditation, find the meditation form that fits your lifestyle, and find the position (sitting, walking, dancing, etc.) in which you will feel most comfortable. Next is a discussion of meditation techniques.

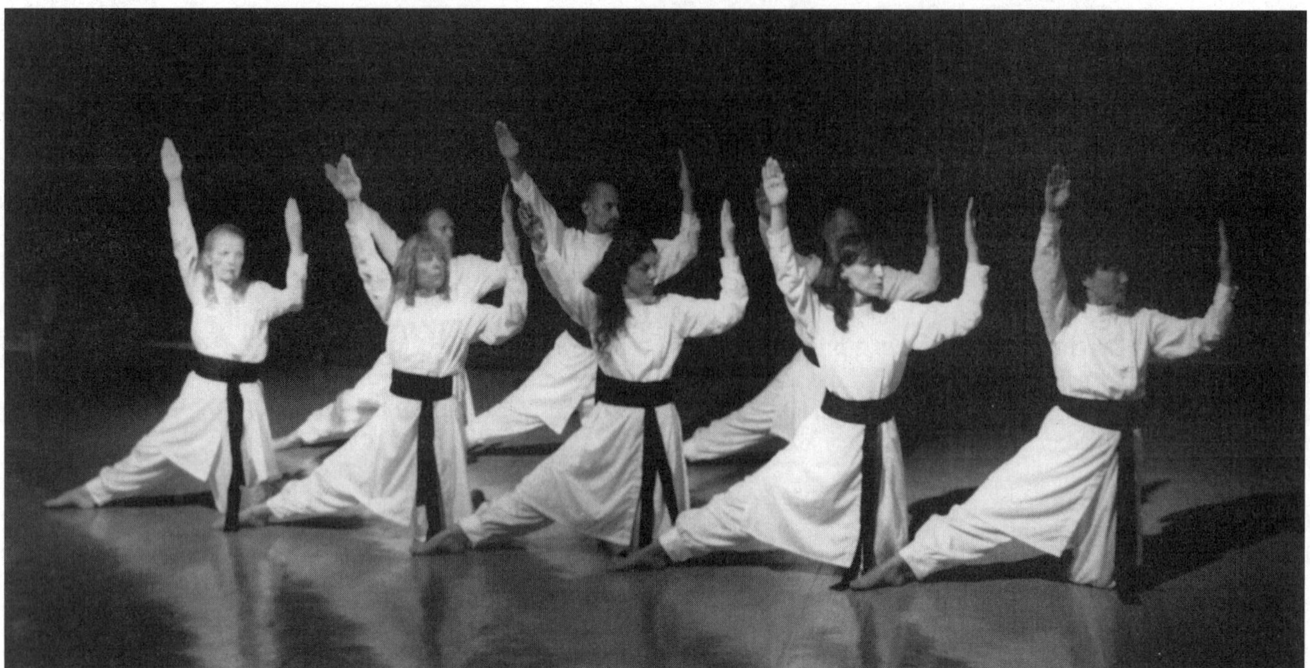

FIGURE 14.5 Gurdjieff dancers.

Meditation Techniques

There are numerous types of meditation techniques. The following presents several meditation techniques that are common to most forms of meditation, whether it is Vipassana, Transcendental, Taoist, Zen, Buddhist, mindfulness, or others.

Concentration and Visualization Techniques

To achieve concentration and visualization, you need to learn to be aware of your breath; this may occur using Zen breathing (zazen) or Vipassana breathing methods.[24] Both methods involve awareness and concentration during the breathing process to help build or shape your mind and to feel the mind and body as one. You would practice watching your breath and relax in whatever position works best. Close your eyes and start to pay attention to your breathing. Take in air through your nose and take a deep, slow breath. If your mind wanders from your breath, refocus attention to the air going in and out of your nose. As this is practiced, it is supposed to become easier to do.

Vipassana breathing entails extending awareness from the breath to the body and the sensations that rise and fall within it, and it requires being watchful of our breath as it comes and goes. Self-observation is intended to give insight into the workings of the mind.[11] Vipassana may be practiced anytime and anywhere, although when people are first practicing this form of meditation, they are encouraged to set aside a time and quiet place to meditate in a comfortable position. More experienced practitioners practice Vipassana breathing while reading, playing, swimming, and the like.

Concentration may involve focusing on an external object.[24] You could focus on anything from a point on the ceiling, to a flower, to a candle flame, to external sounds in the environment. Concentration meditations are thought to help develop focus, concentration, self-knowledge, and calmness, and to become aware of our consciousness. It allows for greater awareness and clarity to emerge.[24] After you become skilled at concentrating, you can stop concentrating on the focus point (ceiling, flower, etc.) and begin to concentrate on your mind and body as one.

Visualization techniques can range from simply moving awareness to various areas of the body, to visualizing internal flows of light, to imagining places. You could visualize images of God or places of power or peace. You could imagine that you are in a place that you love to visit and experience (see **BOX 14.1**).

Box 14.1

Imagery as a Visualization Technique

Take a moment to feel the warm sand between your toes. Look at the gentle, crystal blue water. Listen to the gentle sounds of the waves as they come in while smelling the fresh, clean air. Taste the freshness of this air. Try to totally submerge yourself into the picture you have created within your mind to ultimately create a place of total relaxation.

Insight Techniques

Techniques to acquire insight about ourselves are the WHO AM I, Koan, contemplation, silent mind, and empty mind techniques.

The *WHO AM I* technique was popularized by Shri Ramana Maharishi (see **FIGURE 14.6**).[25] It focuses on negating our false self so that we can realize our true nature or enlightenment. In the Maharishi's words:

> The moment you start looking for the self and go deeper and deeper, the real Self is waiting there to take you in. Then whatever is done is done by something else and you have no hand in it. In this process, all doubts and discussions are automatically given up just as one who sleeps forgets, for the time being, all his cares.[25]

The Koan meditation technique comes from the Zen School of Buddhism and is designed to break down an ordinary pattern of thinking. It often includes a story, question, or statement that can't be understood by rational thinking but can be solved through intuition. An example is,

"Two hands clap and there is a sound; what is the sound of one hand?"

Contemplation meditative techniques use introspection, self-study, and reflection. Contemplative meditation is supposed to help us gain a deeper understanding of some aspect of reality. The Buddhists have a technique called "meditation on the corpse," which involves imagining our own death, the burial of our body, and then our body's decomposition. It also includes instructing us to see worms feeding on our flesh and finally watching our body return to the earth.[26] Meditation on the corpse is an example of an exercise in helping us to face reality. These meditations have their roots in many Western religions and are also a part of Eastern philosophies.

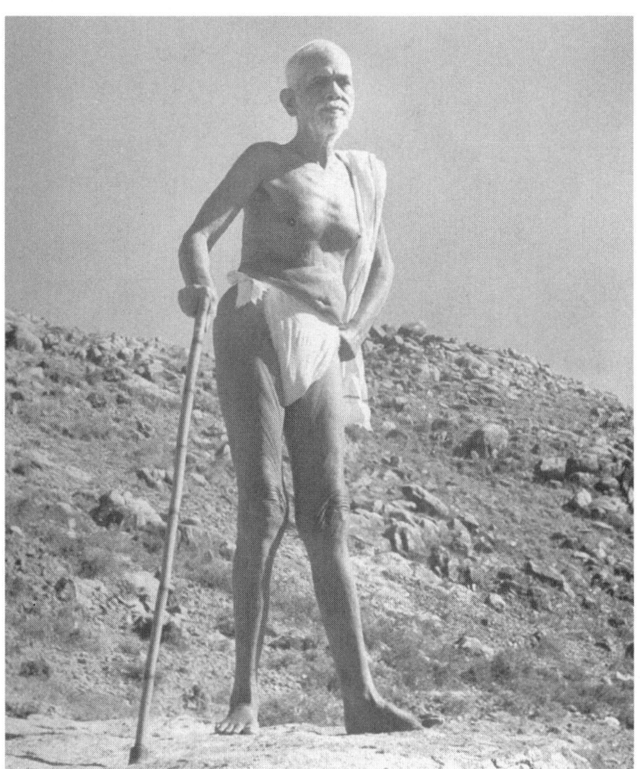

FIGURE 14.6 Shri Ramana Maharishi.

The silent mind meditation technique involves directly perceiving and feeling the world around us by focusing on how we are thinking. These meditations are an extension of the teachings of Jiddu Krishnamurti (1895–1986), who was born in India and died in California.[24] Krishnamurti was a writer and speaker on philosophical and spiritual issues. The silent mind technique is described as being sensitive of the senses, the movement of the mind, the emotions, and to others. Further, it involves being sensitive to the present. A part of the task is to develop moment-to-moment sensitivity of our physical, mental, and emotional dimensions.

The empty mind meditation technique is one that creates a kind of "awareness without object," an emptying of all thoughts from your mind.[24] The techniques for doing this involve sitting still, often in a full lotus or cross-legged position, and letting our mind go silent on its own. It is said to be difficult, because any effort seems to just cause more business in the mind.

Sound, Thought, Feeling, and Emotion Techniques

Sound (mantra) and thought meditation techniques are thought to enlighten people, and to improve their health, wealth, happiness, and so forth.[27] Sound and thought vibrations as well as music are used to purify the heart and mind. While meditating, many of us find it difficult to keep our mind from wandering, and it seems to help if we concentrate on something specific. A mantra can help. This is a word or phrase that is repeated during meditation. It may be chosen by us or by an experienced master in some traditions. The mantra may be either repeated aloud or silently as meditation progresses. Mantras supposedly help people tune into their energy field. (Please see Appendix 14.B at the end of this chapter for an example of a sound meditation exercise.)

A combination of rhythm, chanting, music, and breath are sometimes used during meditation to achieve a desired state of calmness. Others, such as many religious denominations, achieve the meditative state through song. Some meditations use positive thinking, self-hypnosis, power of intention (strong thought), and even laughter to achieve the meditative state.[27]

Often, feeling and emotion techniques are used independently, but they also can be combined with other types of meditations. Bhagwan Shree Rajneesh used laughter, crying, and silence as meditative techniques.[28] He was known as Osho, and was born in 1931 in central India (see **FIGURE 14.7**). Osho obtained a master's degree in philosophy and later founded his own spiritual movement, based on

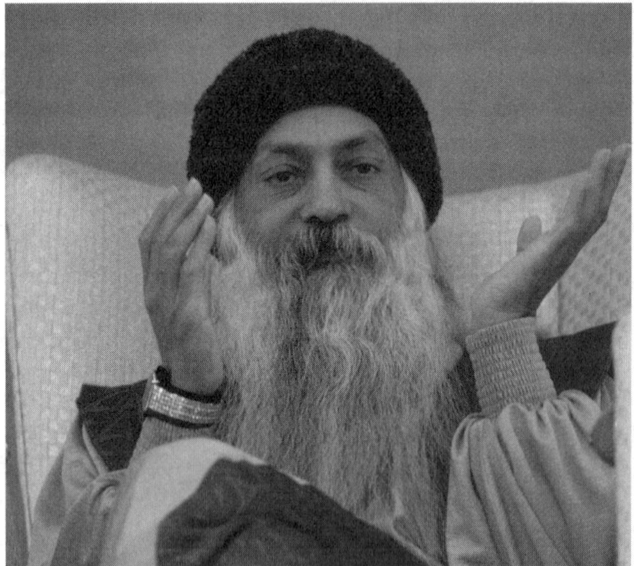

FIGURE 14.7 Osho.

an eclectic mixture of religion and philosophy.[29] Osho, like the Maharishi, was also considered a guru (one regarded as having great knowledge). Osho developed a new type of meditation that advocated letting go of all attachments to the past, future, and ego. To achieve this, Osho recommended laughter and tears, the human emotions. In letting go of attachments, Osho believed that people would become enlightened.[28]

> You will see it yourself; if you can laugh without any reason, you will see something repressed within you … . From your very childhood you have been told not to laugh—"Be serious!" You have to come out of that repressive conditioning.
>
> The second step is tears. Tears have been repressed even more deeply. It has been told to us that tears are a symptom of weakness—they are not. Tears can cleanse not only your eyes, but your heart too. They soften you; it is a biological strategy to keep you clean, to keep you unburdened. It is now a well-known fact that less women go mad than men. And the reason has been found to be that women can cry and weep more easily than men. Even to the small child it is said, "Be a man, don't cry like a woman!"
>
> But if you look at the physiology of your body, you have the same glands full of tears whether you are man or woman. It has been found that fewer women commit suicide than men. And of course, no woman in history has been the cause of founding violent religions, wars, massacres. If the whole world can learn to cry and weep again it will be a tremendous transformation, a metamorphosis.
>
> The third step is silence. I have called it "The Watcher on the Hills." Become as silent as if you are alone on the top of a Himalayan peak, utterly silent and alone, just watching, listening … sensitive, but still.

The Use of Mandalas as an Aid for Meditation

The word *mandala* comes from the classical Indian language of Sanskrit and means completion or circle. In both Hindu and Buddhist religious traditions, mandalas have a spiritual and ritual significance. The circle is a symbol found in many cultures.[30,31] They are seen in halos, prayer wheels, and other religious symbols.

Mandalas are complex designs with a circular pattern or motif. They might be incorporated into a square or rectangle, but the design retains a circular focal point and symmetry.[30,31] Sometimes line drawings of mandalas can be filled in with color, as reflected in **FIGURE 14.8**. There are several ways to color or make mandalas, including by using paint, pencils, crayons, pastels, and even colored sand. One can also buy pictures of mandalas, like the one shown in **FIGURE 14.9**.

Mandalas are said to appear in all aspects of life, such as the earth, sun, and moon. They could also represent circles of friends, family, and community.

Their use in meditation is to aid us to focus attention and to progressively move into deeper levels of the unconscious. Ultimately, mandalas are used to help us experience a mystical sense of oneness with the cosmos. We would eventually extract some sort of meaning from the mandala as we

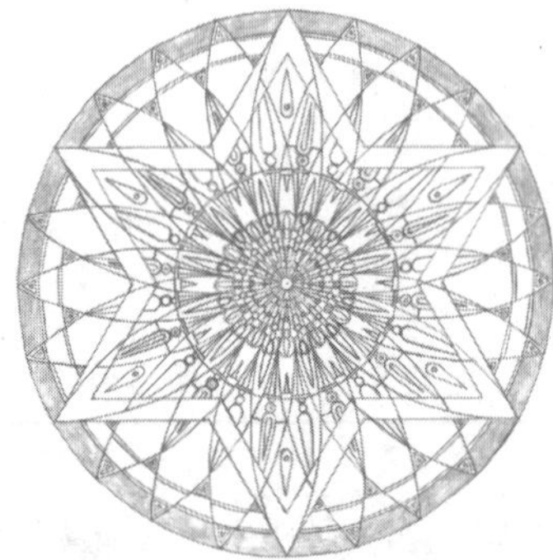

FIGURE 14.8 Mandala 1.

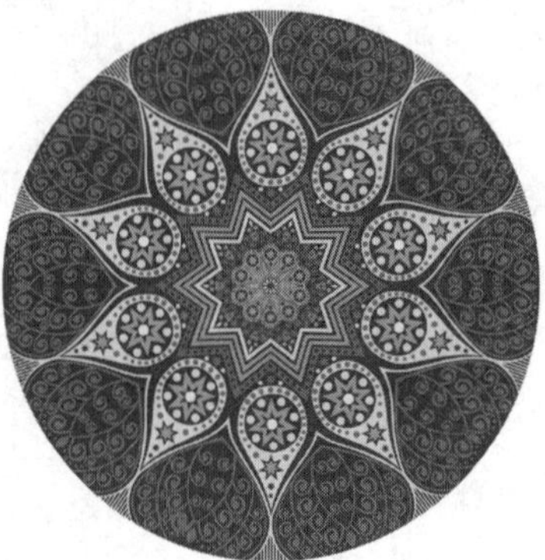

FIGURE 14.9 Mandala 2.

practiced meditation. The main purpose is to help us enter into the mandala and receive a sense of being blessed.[30,31]

Thus far, we have defined what meditation is and discussed various forms and techniques, but what does the research say about the benefits of meditation?

Benefits of Meditation

There seem to be many benefits for people who practice meditation. Some of the physiological benefits include the following[32,33]:

- Deep rest, as measured by decreased metabolic rate, lower heart rate, and reduced workload of the heart.
- Lower levels of blood lactates and, thus, reduced anxiety.
- Lower levels of cortisol and lactate, two chemicals associated with stress.
- Reduction of free radicals—unstable oxygen molecules that can cause tissue damage.
- Increased serotonin, which influences moods and behavior. Low levels of serotonin are associated with depression, headaches, and insomnia.
- Improved blood pressure.
- Higher skin resistance to wrinkles from stress related conditions. Low skin resistance (more wrinkles) is correlated with higher stress and anxiety levels.
- Drop in cholesterol levels. High cholesterol is associated with cardiovascular disease.
- Improved flow of air to the lungs, resulting in easier breathing. This has been very helpful to asthma patients.
- Slowed aging process (through increased blood flow).
- Maintenance of normal blood pressure.
- Reduced symptoms of premenstrual tension (PMT).
- Reduction of heart disease.
- Increased weight loss.

Psychological benefits of meditation include the following[32,33]:

- Increased brain wave coherence
- Greater creativity
- Decreased anxiety
- Decreased depression
- Decreased irritability and moodiness
- Improved learning ability and memory
- Increased self-actualization
- Increased feelings of vitality and rejuvenation
- Increased happiness
- Increased emotional stability
- Increased self-confidence
- Enhanced energy, strength, and vigor
- A state of deep relaxation and general feeling of well-being

Besides the physiological and psychological benefits, there are spiritual benefits. The longer an individual practices meditation, the greater the likelihood that his or her goals and efforts will shift toward personal and spiritual growth. Many individuals who initially learn meditation for its self-regulatory aspects find that as their practice deepens they are drawn more closely into the realm of the "spiritual." In her work with many cancer and AIDS patients, Borysenko observed that people who meditated became more attuned to the spiritual dimension of life. Borysenko reported that many die "healed," in a state of compassionate self-awareness and self-acceptance.[34]

Meditation Research

A 2007 nationwide U.S. survey conducted by the Centers for Disease Control and Prevention regarding CAM use found that 9.4 percent of a sample of 23,393 U.S. adults had used meditation in the past 12 months. Reasons for using meditation were to help with anxiety, pain, depression, stress, insomnia, and physical or emotional symptoms associated with chronic illnesses such as HIV/AIDS, heart disease, and cancer.[35]

Research has shown that meditation does induce changes in the body. The sympathetic nervous system is responsible for the "fight-or-flight" response produced during times of stress. Symptoms of stress include an increased heart rate, increased respirations, and a narrowing of blood vessels causing blood flow to be restricted.[36] Meditation reduces activity of the sympathetic nervous system and increases activity of the parasympathetic nervous system, which is responsible for causing heart rate and breathing to slow down, blood vessels to dilate, and digestive juices to increase.[36] Research also is focusing on meditation's effects on psychological feelings of anxiety, depression, and coping.

A 2009 study by Nidich and others[37] (funded in part by the National Center for Complementary and Alternative Medicine [NCCAM]) found that transcendental meditation (TM) showed positive effects by helping young adults cope with stress. The researchers studied 298 students from American University and other schools in the Washington, D.C., area and randomly assigned students to a TM group or a control group. The TM group had significant improvement in feelings of psychological distress, anxiety, depression, anger/hostility, and coping ability.

The NCCAM also funded a review of the scientific literature and found evidence that meditation has *potential* beneficial effects.[35] Some of the research studies reviewed were on the following topics: impact on chronic illness, alterations in brain and immune function produced by mindfulness meditation, meditation and relaxation, meditation and attention, meditation and cancer therapy, and the neural basis of the complex mental task of meditation. The researchers, however, concluded that future research needs to be more vigorous before confirming that meditation results in health benefits.

Other NCCAM-supported studies[35] include investigating meditation benefits for relieving stress in caregivers for elderly patients with dementia, reducing the frequency and intensity of hot flashes in menopausal women, relieving symptoms of chronic back pain, improving attention-related abilities, and relieving asthma symptoms. The results of those studies have not yet been reported.

Davidson, Kabat-Zinn, and others[38] recorded the brain waves of stressed-out employees of a high-tech firm in Madison, Wisconsin. The subjects were split randomly into two groups—25 people were asked to learn meditation over 8 weeks, and the remaining 16 were left alone as a control group. All participants had their brain waves scanned three times during the study: at the beginning of the experiment, when meditation lessons were completed 8 weeks later, and 4 months after that. The researchers found that participants who had meditated showed a pronounced shift in activity to the left frontal lobe, a pattern previously associated with positive effect (calmer and less stressed).[38]

Meditation is considered a safe practice, although there have been rare reports of worsening symptoms in people with certain psychiatric problems.[35] Advice on the NCCAM Web site to people who are thinking about using meditation practices includes:

- Do not use meditation as a replacement for conventional care or as a reason to postpone seeing a doctor about a medical problem.
- Ask about the training and experience of the meditation instructor you are considering.
- Look for published research studies on meditation for the health condition in which you are interested.
- Tell all your health care providers about any complementary and alternative practices you use. Give them a full picture of what you do to manage your health. This will help ensure coordinated and safe care.

Meditation is practiced by many and is one of the most important mind–body interventions of all. It is safe, and has been proven to alter body physiology in a positive way.

WHAT IS YOGA?

The yoga of today stems from a wide variety of people, practices, and time periods. The word *yoga* comes from the Sanskrit word meaning *union*.[39] Yoga dates back thousands of years in the Indian tradition. Because yoga supposedly began before the written word (prehistoric period), people learned the concepts and practices of yoga from a guru or teacher in an intimate, one-on-one, personal manner. The major purpose was to attain the highest spiritual goals: self-realization, enlightenment, and the liberation of the soul. From 7000 BCE to 1500 AD, the teachings were written down in several pieces of classical literature related to yoga and in the Vedas, four volumes written in Sanskrit: *Rig-Veda*, *Yajur-Veda*, *Sama-Veda*, and *Atharva-Veda*.[40,41]

In those years, yoga was a way of life, a culture, and a lifestyle that was more than specific yoga techniques. It included eating and bathing habits, prayer, work, and social interaction. From 1500 AD onward, yoga teachers began to focus more on the practices of Hatha Yoga, which include *asanas* (postures), *pranayama* (breath control), and *dhyana*

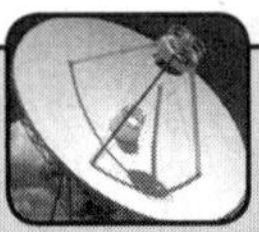

In the News

Meditation a Hit for Pain Management by Allison Aubrey—Audio version played by National Public Radio on August 19, 2011.[39]

Previously in this chapter, under Buddhist Meditation, I wrote much about the philosophy of Jon Kabat-Zinn who uses mindfulness meditation, which Kabat-Zinn says is the heart of Buddhist meditation. In an article published in 2007, Allison Aubrey interviewed Jon Kabat-Zinn and a man with shoulder and neck pain. On August 19, 2011, National Public Radio played the entire audio of this interview. A summary[39] is as follows:

> Back in 1979, Jon Kabat-Zinn was a biologist at the University of Massachusetts. Because he was trained in Vipassana tradition of Buddhist mediation, he believed that the technique could help patients at the university's medical center. His clinic was in an underground office in a medical building and had no windows. Physicians and pain specialists at the university referred patients to Kabat-Zinn and he began teaching people his mindfulness technique. Subsequently, mindfulness classes were set up in other areas of the country and they were modeled on Kabat-Zinn's teachings. Bill Mies, a man with shoulder and neck pain, learned mindfulness meditation to help him cope with his discomfort. He had received injections by doctors and had learned some exercises from physical therapists but nothing had helped until he began to learn mindfulness techniques. Mies also participated in one of the class techniques called the body scan. The instructor walked him and others in the class through a sort of mental tour of the body so that they could bring awareness into specific areas of their bodies. The techniques did not cure the pain but he and the others reported they felt better. Mies says it is a struggle because his mind would wander as he attempted to focus on body parts. He admits that it is difficult to stay "in the moment" and that it takes a lot of practice.

Questions:

1. Before you read this summary, did you ever consider that meditation could be an aid to coping with pain?
2. Please discuss with classmates how meditation may have aided Bill Mies and others.

(meditation).[42] The higher spiritual aims began to be overlooked.

In 1893, Swami Vivekananda (1863–1902) from Calcutta, India, made a historic address to the World Parliament of Religions in Chicago, where he introduced the religious practice of Hinduism. Because yoga is a major part of Hinduism, this event has often been said to be the beginning of the modern era of yoga.

In the century since then, yoga has increased in popularity and has moved a long way away from its historical foundations. Physical fitness, enhanced sexuality, and personal achievement have become the primary goals. People who practice yoga say it helps them relax and stay centered. Yoga is believed to increase the body's store of *prana*, or vital energy and, due to better posture, facilitate energy flow.[41] Today the practice of yoga has become a multi-billion-dollar industry. Various types of yogawear are a part of fashionable clothing lines, prepackaged snacks and supplements are sold as yoga food, yoga mats are sold, and yoga images of athletic people are on the covers of glossy magazines.

Function and Benefits of Yoga

Kabat-Zinn calls yoga a profound meditation practice, especially when mindfulness is incorporated. He believes that yoga develops strength, balance, and flexibility of the mind.[5] Kabat-Zinn explains that his patients in the Stress Reduction Clinic have found yoga to be a powerful form of mindfulness practice.

Yoga is believed to be helpful for a myriad of health disorders and diseases[9,43,44] ranging from back pain to pain management, respiratory problems, arthritis, weight management, stress, depression, mental performance, heart disorders, and hypertension. Studies have shown that yoga lowers blood pressure, heart rate, and body temperature and that people who practice yoga are more resistant to stress and have reduced anxiety, lower blood pressure, better respiratory function, and improved physical and sexual fitness.[9] There are claims that yoga even has anti-aging properties.

Benefits of yoga include increasing flexibility, strength, and posture. The yoga poses are called asanas, and they work by safely stretching muscles. The stretches are thought to release lactic acid from the muscles, resulting in decreased feelings of stiffness, tension, pain, and fatigue. Yoga is thought to increase joint range of motion and lubrication. Muscle tone is improved in most forms of yoga, especially the ashtanga and power yogas. Even less vigorous forms of yoga, however, are thought to increase muscle tone. Upper body strength is increased after mastering poses such as Downward Dog, Upward Dog, and Plank. Poses that strengthen the lower back include Upward Dog and Chair pose.[44] The *Halasana* position is known as the Plough position (see **FIGURE 14.10**) because *Hala* refers to plough. This position is good for stretching the neck and lower back muscles. The *Shirshasana* position is a headstand position (see **FIGURE 14.11**). It is supposed to be the king of the asanas because it has many benefits. It increases circulation to the brain and aids nervousness, tension, and fatigue. The Shirshasana position is also thought to aid correct spinal alignment.

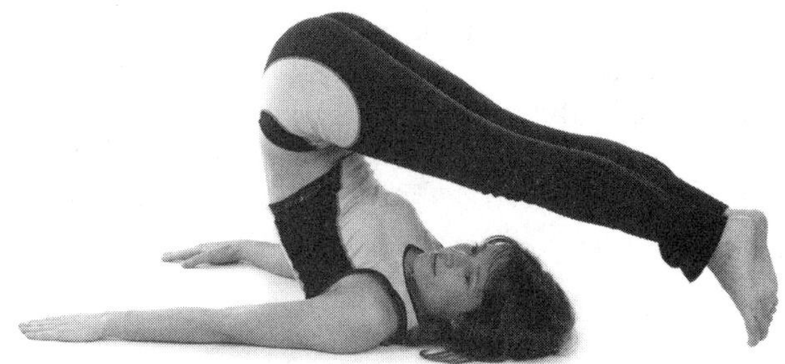

FIGURE 14.10 Halasana or Plough pose.

Posture is improved when strength and flexibility are increased. A stronger core allows a person to sit and stand "tall."[45] Full awareness of posture and movements are common in all types of physical yoga. Moreover, attention is focused on the breath during all movements, which is supposed to help open up the energy channels.

Even though yoga has been deemed safe for all ages, critics of yoga are concerned that beginners will injure themselves by trying to do the more advanced yoga positions. For example, the upside-down headstands could be dangerous for people with hypertension.[9] Critics are also concerned that people will use yoga as an alternative, rather than a complementary therapy to their prescribed, traditional

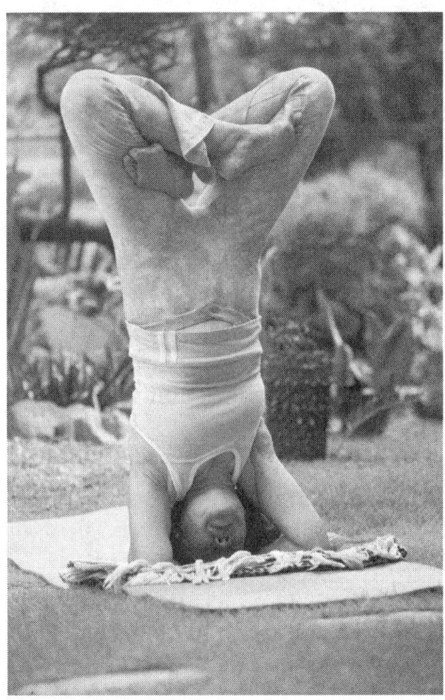

FIGURE 14.11 Shirshasana pose.

course of treatment for some specific disease or disorder.[42] Yoga experts are aware of these problems and encourage people to talk with their doctors before beginning yoga and to start with easier poses until their bodies are conditioned for the more advanced ones.[9] The secret of yoga is to be gentle to reduce the likelihood of over-stretching or straining muscles.[5]

How Yoga Works

Yoga works by promoting harmony of body, mind, and spirit, which requires correct breathing, posture, and meditation. The first thing you need to learn in doing yoga is to breathe correctly so that you make full use of your lungs, increase your circulation, and improve your energy and vitality.[42]

Power of the Breath

Breathing during meditation (or yoga) is not just the process of taking air into the lungs and breathing it out. Those are only the first and last stages of breathing (prana).[46] After air is taken in, the second form of energy occurs. This is known as *samana*, wherein the oxygen is transported to your cells. Samana is supposed to be the balancing energy, the digestive breath. The third form of prana is called *vyana*, an energy that governs the circulatory system and makes sure that oxygen reaches all cells in our bodies. This energy is supposed to awaken us emotionally. A cleansing breath is called *apana*. It eliminates stale air from our lungs each time we breathe out. The energies we have taken in are returned to the external environment.[46] The last form is called *udana*, which means "air that flies upward." This is energy that starts in our solar plexus and gains strength as it rises upwards towards the throat and mouth. Udana is energy that is said to govern our physical make-up, our ability to stand and move, our enthusiasm, and our voice.[46]

Asana Poses

After mastering the breath, you would learn yoga poses (asanas) appropriate for a beginner so that you could exercise your body muscles to improve strength and tone. The asanas are performed in a particular sequence so that all the muscle groups are exercised and toxins are flushed out. As you improve, you can move to more advanced positions. During the process of becoming more skilled with breathing and poses, you become more relaxed and gain the ability to meditate.

Yoga should be performed no less than 2 hours after eating so that food has been digested. The lessons may take from 1 to 2 hours, and you should wear loose-fitting clothing that allows movement (such as a leotard or sweat suit). Usually people go barefoot or wear a light slipper and exercise on a mat. The first 10 minutes of the class usually focus on breathing control followed by 15–20 minutes of warm-up. You would then be asked to perform the first position while concentrating on your breathing. All positions should be obtained slowly and smoothly and should be held only for as long as you are comfortable. After approximately 25 minutes of performing asanas, you would engage in about 20 minutes of relaxation exercises.

Clinical Studies

The NCCAM helped to support a study by Kiecolt-Glasser and others[47] and featured the study results on its Web site. Long-term female yoga practitioners had lower blood levels of a stress-related compound thought to play a role in cardiovascular disease and type II diabetes. In addition, the long-term practitioners had five times lower levels of C-reactive protein, which serves as a marker for inflammation.[47]

Many other studies support yoga as an adjunct for various conditions. The studies were reviews and assessments of existing literature, and several showed positive results. A review of five randomized controlled trials on depression indicated that yoga gave relief.[48] A systematic review of research by Kirkwood[49] and others indicated that yoga gave anxiety relief, but that there were methodological problems with the research.[50] Another study found that yoga was significantly better for bronchial asthma than the usual drug therapy used by a control group. A review of literature by Raub[51] found that Hatha yoga had significant psychophysiologic effects on healthy people and those compromised by musculoskeletal and cardiopulmonary disease.

Thus far, we have explained how meditation and yoga function as mind–body interventions. The next intervention discussed is hypnosis, a seemingly mysterious practice, and one people seem to fear because they feel that they will lose control over their minds and bodies. Do we?

WHAT IS HYPNOSIS?

Hypnosis is a mind–body technique that focuses on awareness and attention to internal stimuli, much like what is learned during meditation. The word *hypnosis* comes from the Greek word *hypnos*, meaning sleep. Hypnosis often, but not always, produces a trancelike state wherein the participant is highly responsive to suggestion.[2] When under hypnosis, people feel calm and relaxed, which allows them to concentrate more closely on a specific thought, memory, feeling, or sensation.[52]

Therapeutic hypnosis is used to promote health and is different from entertainment-type, stage hypnosis. Free will remains intact, and people do not lose control over their behaviors. Instead, hypnosis can help people learn to master their own states of awareness. A myth is that hypnosis causes people to lose consciousness and to lose memory of what happened during the hypnotic state (amnesia). A very small percentage might fit this description, but most people remember everything that occurs during the experience.[53]

History

Hypnosis has been used for centuries, even before the written language.[36] Trance states were used as a part of mystical and shamanic traditions since the beginning of humankind. Shamanic customs teach that the true shaman travels between many states of consciousness. In so doing, the shaman can heal people, prophesize the future, retrieve lost souls, and gain the ability to use any energies encountered.[36] It was not until the eighteenth century, however, that it was used clinically by a German physician, Dr. Franz Anton Mesmer, who created and defined a discipline using hypnotism that he called "animal magnetism."[2,36] The term *mesmerize* comes from Mesmer's hypnotism practice. During the twentieth century, Milton Erickson, a psychiatrist, began to scientifically study hypnotism as a part of his treatment process. Erickson focused his research on the process, the state, and the effects of hypnosis.[36]

Philosophies Regarding How Hypnosis Functions

Two main philosophies are used to explain hypnotic effects. The first is the neo-dissociation model, which suggests that hypnosis activates a subsystem of both psychological and physiologic parts. This activation results in an altered state of consciousness. The second is the social psychological model, which suggests that an altered state of consciousness does not occur during hypnosis; instead, hypnosis is explained by suggestibility, positive attitudes, and expectations.[36]

Researchers are at odds as to whether hypnosis affects the brain from the posterior part to the anterior or whether it affects the left and right hemispheres of the brain. Also undetermined are the types of brain waves affected—beta, alpha, theta, and delta—although most research seems to point to theta waves.[36] Theta waves are thought to be associated with mental imagery, meditation, rapid eye movement during sleep, problem solving, focused attention, and cessation of a pleasurable activity. Theta waves are also most related to hypnotic susceptibility during hypnotic states.

There are several stages of hypnosis. As a participant is being hypnotized, he or she will become very relaxed. At this stage, the participant will gain the capacity to deeply contemplate a selected theme or focal point (absorption). Absorption helps the person to become deeply engaged in the words or images that the hypnotherapist presents. The next stage is dissociation, in which the participant can let go of critical thoughts and gain the capacity to compartmentalize his or her experience. The stage of responding to or complying with a hypnotherapist's suggestion occurs next. The last stage is when the participant returns to usual awareness and reflects on the experience.

Hypnosis as Therapeutic Treatment

Hypnosis (hypnotherapy) is currently used to gain access to the deeper levels of the mind so that a change in thinking and behavior will occur. During a first visit, the therapist will ask about your medical history, the reason for coming in, and what you want to address. The hypnotherapist then will explain what hypnosis is and how it works. He or she may teach several relaxation techniques and ask you to practice them at home. The sessions last about an hour, and usually you would begin to see results within 4 to 10 sessions.[54]

Hypnotherapy is used to modify feelings of pain, fear, and anxiety and may be used as an adjunct to other conventional treatments such as analgesia in surgery, to help reduce stress, and to control allergies.[2] Research has demonstrated the effectiveness of hypnosis in treating cancer and cancer pain,[54–57] burn pain,[58,59] fibromyalgia pain,[60] and gastrointestinal disorders such as duodenal ulcers and irritable bowel syndrome.[61] Hypnosis has been helpful in treating nausea and vomiting during cancer chemotherapy,[62] pregnancy-induced nausea, and asthma, and has been used to help people who are obese lose weight. The power of suggestion from hypnosis has been used to cure warts, a condition caused by a virus. There are many published studies[63,64] of the use of hypnosis to cure warts, with a cure rate between 27 and 55 percent. Interestingly, once cured by hypnosis, the warts reportedly do not return, as they often do after traditional medical therapy.

Risks of Hypnosis

Hypnosis is considered safe when conducted under the care of a trained therapist. Adverse reactions might occur but they are rare; they could include headache, dizziness, nausea, anxiety, panic, and even the creation of false memories.[52]

How to Find a Hypnotherapist

Most hypnotherapists are physicians, registered nurses, social workers, family counselors, psychiatrists, or psychologists who have received additional training in hypnotism.[54] The National Board for Certified Clinical Hypnotherapists and the American Association of Professional Hypnotherapists[65] maintain Web sites where people can access a list of board-certified hypnotherapists in their state or area of the state. The U.S. Department of Health and Human Services' Healthfinder site offers a link to find a licensed (not certified) hypnotherapist. The sponsoring agency is the American Society of Clinical Hypnosis.

Hypnosis is a valid complementary and alternative therapy and is used by traditional and alternative health care professionals. It is a safe mind–body intervention that allows for introspection and reflection.

The next mind–body intervention to be explored is the Alexander Technique, an intervention that allows people to use their brains (mind power) to control their body posture and function.

WHAT IS THE ALEXANDER TECHNIQUE?

The Alexander Technique is a process in which people can learn to release muscular tension. Over time, our muscles become habitually overtightened, which causes our bodies to become distorted, unbalanced, and compressed.[66] Some say that we have learned walking and postural habits that cause us bodily problems and that we can learn to retrain ourselves. Proponents of the Alexander Technique say that the technique will help us learn how to monitor the way we coordinate ourselves in activities so that the activities can be carried out with a minimum of strain. Performers who sing, act, or dance often acquire this type of muscle imbalance and turn to the Alexander Technique for aid. The area in which people feel this strain is in the muscles of the back and neck, causing a stiffening of the head on the neck. Alexander Technique helps people re-educate the mind and body. It is supposed to help people discover a new balance in the body by releasing unnecessary tension.[66]

History

Frederick Matthias Alexander (1869–1955), an Australian actor, began to experience chronic laryngitis while performing, and doctors were not able to help him.[66] After he realized that his personal stress and resultant tension in his neck and body were causing his physical problems, he began to find ways to speak and move more easily. Alexander learned to how to change his breathing technique.[67] Eventually, Alexander began to teach others his technique. As people came to him for vocal training, many who had respiratory difficulties began to improve. As a result of this, medical doctors began referring their patients with respiratory ailments to Alexander (see **FIGURE 14.12**).

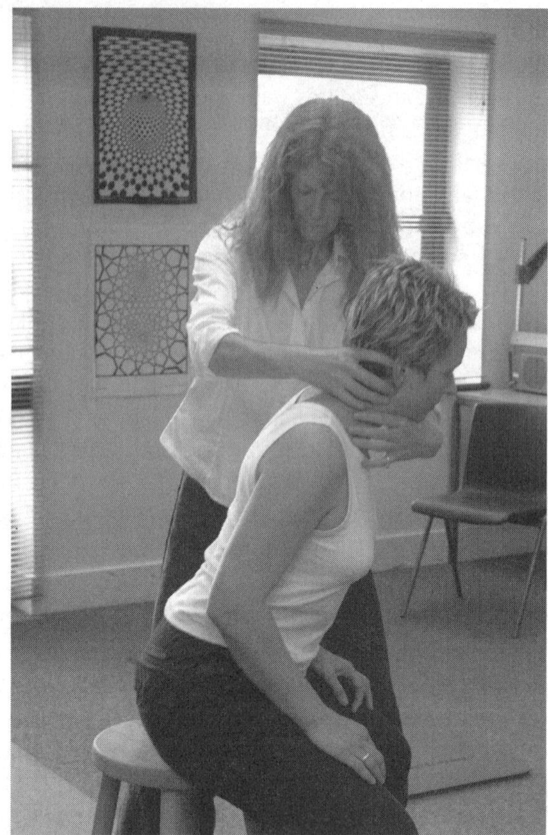

FIGURE 14.12 Alexander technique.

The Technique

The Alexander Technique can be applied when a person is sitting, lying down, standing, walking, lifting, and/or conducting other daily activities. The technique does not involve exercises, medical therapy or treatment, psychotherapy, or spiritual healing techniques.[67] It is a technique that helps people achieve core stability without specific muscle strengthening exercises. A lesson in Alexander Technique may last 30–45 minutes, and learning it appropriately will probably take a few lessons. A lot depends on how fast the participant learns new skills.[66] Many people come for several months, taking 20–40 lessons, and later come back for refresher lessons.

During the lesson, you would not need to remove your clothes or wear special clothing, although women feel more comfortable wearing pants or jeans rather than a skirt. You would be asked to walk and move around while the teacher observes your posture and movement patterns. The teacher might gently place his or her hands on your neck, shoulders, back, and hips while you are moving or sitting in a chair. This helps the teacher get more information about your patterns of breathing and moving.[68] At the same time, you would learn to think about your own movement and breathing techniques and, hopefully, be motivated to effectively change habits.

From *The F.M. Alexander Technique* by Marian Goldberg[67]

> Try this technique: Try to breathe from high up in your chest or from low down in your abdomen. Try walking or moving your arms while you breathe in one of these ways. Do you walk or move your arms differently when you change your breathing? Or make a conscious effort to change the way you walk or the way you hold your neck, or try clenching your arms: Do these efforts affect your breathing or your voice? What if these were habitual efforts—efforts which you made all the time but you were unaware that you were making them? We do make habitual excessive efforts most of the time, but we are generally unaware of making them. Excessive stress in one part of the body is usually part of a larger pattern of habitual malcoordination.

The Benefits

The benefits of the Alexander Technique are many.[67] The technique supposedly results in freer and more comfortable movement, relief from muscle strain and chronic tension, better posture, easier and healthier breathing, increased strength, and increased vitality.

Training of the Teachers

The training period to become a teacher of the Alexander Technique is quite long. Instructors in the Alexander Technique are members of a professional teaching society in the country in which they reside, and the society requires successful completion of a 3-year full-time study program at an accredited teacher training site. Student trainees are required to take 1,500–1,600 hours of instruction and attend classes four to five times each week during that time.[67] Alexander teachers may move from a focus on the postural aspects of the physical body to a focus on healing. This is commonly called "direction," in which the intent of the teacher is to allow his or her life force to be available to the life force within the student. To practice direction, the teacher will be quite still and allow his or her hands to sense what might come. The teacher might let the hands rest lightly on the student's body at whatever locations they are guided to intuitively, but does not physically manipulate the student, although the teacher might use some sort of guided movement. During lessons the hands of the teacher may become very hot or vibrate, and students often experience releases of emotions.[69]

Research Studies

Several recent studies have shown benefits of the Alexander Technique. One was a randomized study in which 579 participants with chronic or recurrent lower back pain were divided into treatment groups: 147 to massage, 144 to six Alexander Technique lessons, and 144 to twenty-four Alexander Technique lessons. In addition, half of each of these groups was randomized to exercise prescription. The exercise and Alexander Technique groups remained effective in lowering lower back pain level after 1 year, but the massage groups did not.[70] Another study by Austin and Ausubel[71] found enhanced ease of breathing in participants who learned Alexander Technique compared to a control group. A 2010 study conducted at the Cincinnati Children's Hospital found that Alexander Technique training resulted in significant improvement in posture and trunk and shoulder endurance from pre- to post-Alexander training in four pediatric urology fellows and three urology residents. The study involved assessing endurance and posture discomfort when performing basic laparoscopic skills. Another investigation was a case study of a 49-year-old woman with a 25-year history of left-sided, idiopathic (unknown cause), lumbar-sacral back pain. The Alexander Technique improved her postural coordination, and after the treatment period, she had decreased lower back pain.[72]

It seems that there are many benefits of the Alexander Technique that involve using one's own mind power to control posture and body function, including pain. It is a noninvasive and gentle technique that results in long-lasting bodily changes.

Next is a discussion of biofeedback, a mind–body intervention used by a wide variety of health and medical professionals.

WHAT IS BIOFEEDBACK?

Biofeedback is a mind–body intervention used by many professions to train people to improve their health by using their own body's electrical signals from the muscles or brain. Physical therapists use it to help stroke victims regain movement in paralyzed muscles. Health educators use biofeedback when teaching stress management. Psychologists use it to help tense and anxious clients learn to relax. Many health and medical specialists use biofeedback to help their patients cope with pain.

Origins of Biofeedback

In the 1960s, scientists were hopeful that they could train research subjects to alter brain activity, blood pressure, heart rate, and other bodily functions. They thought that biofeedback could make it possible to decrease the amount of, or could stop the need for, medications in patients with high blood pressure or other serious conditions. The research showed that we do have more control over involuntary body functions than we thought possible, but it also showed the limitations of mind over body functions.[73]

How It Works

When something frightens us or when we get angry, the stressful event produces a body response that is controlled by our sympathetic nervous system, a network of nerve tissues that help our bodies prepare to meet emergencies as in the "fight-or-flight" response. Hormones (epinephrine, norepinephrine, and cortisol) are secreted from the adrenal gland. Our pupils dilate to let in more light, and we begin to sweat. Our blood vessels contract near the skin and our gastrointestinal tract slows down. Our heart beats faster, and our blood pressure rises. When the event is over, we begin to relax again and our body responses return to normal. Scientists have used this knowledge to teach people how to relax.

The biofeedback practitioner will initiate a visual or auditory signal to stimulate stress responses. Several kinds of devices are used to monitor a variety of responses: brain wave activity (electroencephalography or EEG), skin temperature, muscle tension (electromyography or EMG), galvanic skin resistance (GSR), electrodermal resistance (EDR), blood pressure, respiratory rate, and blood flow.[73] Some of these are handheld portable devices, whereas others connect to a computer. Sensors attached to the skin send information to a monitoring box or a computer that translates the measurements into an audio tone and/or a visual meter that varies in brightness. Patients see the displayed responses and are then taught to consciously control their own body responses (e.g., respirations and heart rate). The aim is for the patient to control the stress response when not connected to the machine. The exact mechanism for how this is possible is unknown, but scientists believe that the mind–body interaction acts on the limbic system and affects the hypothalamus-pituitary axis and autonomic control.[43]

Effectiveness of Biofeedback

Biofeedback seems to be effective for a range of health and medical problems. For example, biofeedback helps treat urinary incontinence[74] and may also help people with fecal incontinence.[75,76] Thermal biofeedback has been found to ease the symptoms of Raynaud's disease (a condition that causes reduced blood flow to fingers, toes, nose, or ears), and EMG biofeedback has been shown to help people with fibromyalgia.[63] Biofeedback has also been used effectively in children. For example, EEG biofeedback revealed significant reduction in cortical stimulation in children with attention deficit disorder.[77] Thermal biofeedback helped relieve migraine and chronic tension headaches among children and teens as well.[74]

Finding a Qualified Practitioner

Psychiatrists, psychologists, nurses, dentists, physicians, physical therapists, exercise scientists, and health educators may provide biofeedback training. The Association for Applied Psychology and Biofeedback is a good resource for finding qualified biofeedback practitioners,[74] and the U.S. Department of Health and Human Services Web site, Healthfinder.gov,[78] contains a link to a site that explains how to find a biofeedback practitioner. The sponsoring agency is the Biofeedback Certification Institute of America.

The next two mind–body interventions explored in this chapter are prayer and faith healing. Can prayer work? Can people really heal others through touch? If so, how? Is healing based on faith? These are questions that perhaps won't be answered definitively, but many people offer possible explanations.

ARE PRAYER AND FAITH OR SPIRITUAL HEALING POWERFUL MIND–BODY INTERVENTIONS?

Prayer for Healing

All religions believe in prayer for healing, although people of different faiths may pray in different styles and ways.[9] In times of illness especially, religious people look toward their God or their figure of authority to help them get well.

Even people who may not believe in a particular religion hold spiritual beliefs that help them get through times of sickness, and those spiritual beliefs are said to be powerful enough to help them regain a sense of well-being.[9] Spirituality is a term that could be synonymous with religiosity, but often it is not. It may be considered an inner sense of believing that something is greater than oneself or some sense that there is a meaning to existence that is higher than oneself. As an example, Alcoholics Anonymous and other similar groups use the concept of a "higher power" to help people overcome addictions.

Questions remain about whether religion, spirituality, or prayer can be effective to help people in the healing process. To answer these questions, scientists have been inspired to use modern scientific tools and methods to test the power of prayer to cure others. Formally, studies of the mind and health healing are considered noetic science. "Noetic" means the power of inner knowing, and is a branch of metaphysics.[79] Skeptics believe it is a waste of money to validate the supernatural. On the other hand, proponents say the research is valuable because so many people believe in the power of faith and prayer to heal themselves or others.

Distant healing is perhaps the most controversial healing method. It involves people praying for and healing others at great distances away (sometimes without the ill person knowing it). It is also known as *intercessory* prayer. In a 1988 study, a San Francisco cardiologist, Randolph Byrd, asked born-again Christians to pray for 192 people who had heart disease and who were hospitalized. He compared those individuals with 201 people not targeted for prayer and who had heart disease. No one was told which group they were in, but those who were prayed for seemed to need fewer drugs and needed less help breathing. In 1998, Sicher, Targ, and others[80] published a study reporting the results of a double-blind randomized trial of distant healing in 40 patients with AIDS. Treatment subjects acquired significantly fewer new AIDS-related illnesses, had lower illness severity, required significantly fewer doctor visits, had fewer hospitalizations, and had a more positive mood compared with controls who did not receive distant healing. A randomized, controlled, double-blind study published in 1999 by William Harris and colleagues[81] involved almost a thousand heart patients, and about half of them were prayed for without their knowledge. The prayer group had lower coronary care unit scores that were derived from a chart review (scored from 1 to 6 on specific coronary needs).[81] Critics, however, say the studies were flawed because they were analyzed in the most positive ways and were due to chance, not real science. Further, a behavioral scientist at Columbia University says there is nothing that could account for how the prayers of someone in Washington, D.C., could influence the health of a group of people in Iowa.

The study of intercessory prayer and healing continues. A study led by Dr. Mitch Krucoff[82] in 2001 at Duke University Medical Center studied the effects of intercessory prayer on cardiac patients. Those who received intercessory prayer in addition to having stents placed in their diseased coronary arteries had better clinical outcomes than those not receiving prayer. Another study published in 2004 looked at how a belief in intercessory prayer affected patients.[83] Even though patients didn't know they were being prayed for, those who were prayed for did better. A study published in *Research on Social Work Practice* in 2007 found that a meta-analysis of intercessory prayer among social workers indicated a small, but significant healing effect.[83]

Does this research mean that intercessory prayer is the main reason the people who participated in these studies gained better health? The answer is no. Even most of the authors agree that there are problems in their research: short time periods of study, other uncontrolled and unknown confounding reasons, small samples, statistical methodology, and so forth. Most, however, are promoting the value of and need for future studies.

Faith or Spiritual Energy Healing

In Chapter 7 of this text, we wrote about the practices of shamans, healers among Native American people, and provided a review of healers from other cultures around the world. Spiritual energy healing has occurred since earliest times among all cultures, religions, and medicinal practices. Healers have used various healing techniques such as chants and prayer, touching, or hands placed close to the body within the energy fields that surround the body. Popular current methods used for energy healing include Reiki therapy, therapeutic touch, qi gong healing, and crystal healing. These are discussed in Chapter 15 of this book.

Examples of Faith Healing Throughout History

Many examples of faith healing have been recorded throughout history, and are presented in the following paragraphs.

By 1000 BCE, the Egyptian, Imhotep, had become a famous healer—so much so that on his death, he was deified as the Egyptian god of healing. A symbol of healing showing snakes entwined around a staff originated from the temples of Imhotep,[84,85] and reoccurred in the Greek and Roman Aesculapius caducei (see **FIGURE 14.13**).

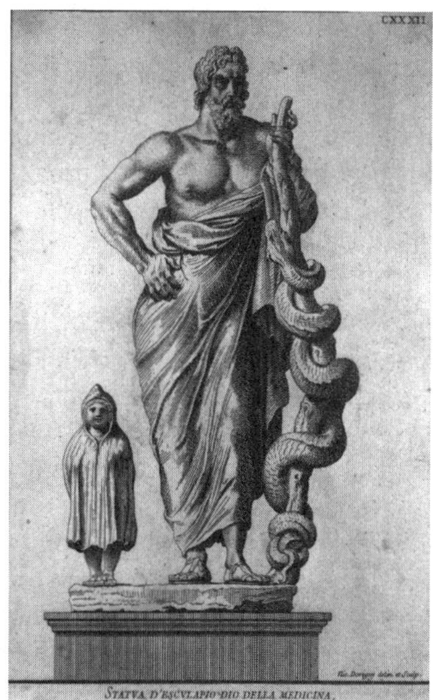

FIGURE 14.13 Caduceus of healing.

Many references to healing can be found in the Bible in both the Old and New Testaments. In the New Testament, Jesus was recorded as having cured both physical and spiritual illnesses after touching people with diseases and disorders such as blindness, lameness, deafness, and insanity.

In 1858, a 14-year-old peasant girl visited a grotto on the edge of Lourdes, a town in France. The girl was Bernadette Soubirous, who was said to have seen visions of the Blessed Mother on 18 difference occasions. During one of those incidents, Bernadette was told to dig in the grotto soil and drink the water that would be released. A natural spring was found below the grotto, and the water was thought to have curative powers. This event led to thousands of sick and injured people coming to the spring in hopes of getting cured. They prayed at the spot and bathed in the waters. The healing Grotto of Bernadette was constructed on the site, and people from all around the world have visited. Claims of being cured of cancer, blindness, and other conditions through the ensuing years has led to Lourdes being one of the busiest tourist spots in France.[86]

Mary Baker Eddy (see **FIGURE 14.14**) established the first Christian Science church in 1879. She was a notable faith healer who believed she was the recipient of cures

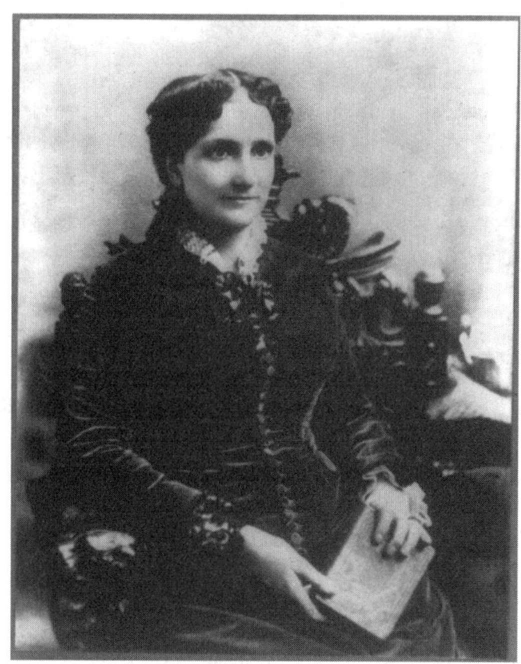

FIGURE 14.14 Mary Baker Eddy.

after professing to the "truth in Christ." Mary Baker Eddy believed that the basis of all disease was psychosomatic. She wrote that disease was an illusion and could be erased by mind control. Her philosophy became imbedded in the philosophy of the Christian Science church, which holds that the real person is spiritual and reflects God whereas the material body is unreal. Christian Scientists therefore believe that the proper treatment for illness is prayer.[87,88]

Agnes Sanford (1891–1982), an Episcopalian, is viewed as an important twentieth-century healer. In her first book, *The Healing Light*, she outlined her experiences with the healing power of God. In it, she described healing a child's knee. After having touched the knee, the child called to Agnes to take away her hand because "it's hot." Sanford told the child that it was God's electricity and power working in her knee.[89]

Edgar Cayce (1877–1945) is said to be one of the most famous, if not the most famous, healer of the modern era. He was a psychic healer and psychic trance channeller who claimed that he was a devout Christian, though others say he was the founder of the New Age movement. Cayce was most famous for channeling answers to questions concerning the health problems of distant patients. He was known as the Sleeping Prophet because he would lie down, enter a trance state, and then give his readings. It is reported that he gave about 20,000 readings in his lifetime.[90]

Barbara Brennan is a famous healer who runs the Barbara Brennan Healing School. Brennan teaches her students about the human energy field or aura and how to heal it. She is a scientist, healer, author, and trainer. One of her most popular healing books is *Hands of Light: A Guide to Healing Through the Human Energy Field*.[91] In her book, she cites medically verified case studies of a variety of people with diverse illnesses being healed by healers.

Historical and present day spiritual healers hold some common beliefs. Healers believe that the mind, body, and spirit are one interdependent unit and that all three must work in harmony.[42] They believe that all of us have an energy force around our physical bodies, our minds, and our spirits. Healers believe that the energy force gets disrupted from adverse factors such as stress, negative attitudes, poor dietary habits, and lack of exercise, and when that occurs, our own power to heal gets blocked. They believe that illness begins in the mind or the spirit and affects the body. When healers lay their hands on people, they believe they can channel or direct energy from some unknown spiritual source via themselves into their patients or clients. Healers also believe that they can help people die more peacefully.

Case Study

The following is a synopsis of a case study publicized on a Web site.[91] A man who had been addicted to alcohol for 17 years attended a meeting in March 1999 held by two seekers of the Spiritual Science Research Foundation (SSRF). They explained the science of Spirituality in brief and explained its influence on various aspects of people's daily lives. They talked about how to begin spiritual practices and explained scientifically how specific spiritual remedies helped in overcoming many of the otherwise insurmountable difficulties in life. One of the examples they gave was an explanation about addictions and their belief that they were caused by spiritual factors such as negative energies. The man attended a second meeting that was led by another spiritual advisor. He began to feel optimistic that by applying the science of Spirituality he could overcome his drinking habit. The advice the spiritual advisors offered was that he should begin chanting the name of God as per his religion of birth and that he should chant the Name of Lord Datta, which is a specific remedy to overcome difficulties due to ancestral problems. He was also instructed to pray to God.

The following response is in his own words:

> I started chanting the name of my family deity on the spot. Over the next few days, I slowly started experiencing a change within me. My restlessness and anxiety decreased. I could attend to my job better and I actually started enjoying it. Previously, I would find it stressful to complete obligations at work but now I found that I could meet all the deadlines and still find enough time, energy and enthusiasm to participate in the preparations for the public discourse. I found myself looking forward to the evenings, when I would meet with the seekers of SSRF and work till late into the night with the preparations. The need for alcohol that ordinarily would have been at the top of my mind took a backseat without my knowledge or conscious effort. Soon I found that I did not need it to sustain my day. In one and a half months, my drinking habit of 15 years was gone. Since then for the last 6 years, I have been totally abstinent.

Questions:

1. After reading the case study, what explanations could you give for the man's apparent recovery from alcohol addiction?
2. Why does he believe that chanting aided his recovery?
3. Do you think it is possible that prayer and chanting could be a healing methodology?

CONCLUSION

You have now been introduced to many mind–body interventions, some of which have valid scientific studies that indicate they are effective. Some need much more study before reaching that conclusion. Our hope is that the contents of this chapter will motivate you to explore and experience some of these practices so that you can assess for yourself whether they are healing techniques that you could use when needed.

Suggestions for Class Activities

1. Invite a person skilled in meditation to class and practice a simple meditation technique. Write a reflection paragraph about how you felt practicing meditation. If a meditation instructor is not available, practice a walking meditation routine.
2. Invite a yoga instructor to class. Be sure that you can obtain a room in your building suitable for practicing some simple yoga techniques. Write a reflection paragraph about how you felt practicing yoga.
3. Invite a hypnotist into class to talk about their techniques when using hypnotism for healing.
4. Obtain a biofeedback machine or computerized biofeedback DVD. Practice biofeedback in class.

Review Questions

1. What are mind–body interventions?
2. Define meditation and discuss three overall benefits.
3. Name five forms of meditation.
4. Who was the founder of transcendental meditation, and how is it used?
5. What is Vipassana meditation, and how is it practiced?
6. What is zazen meditation, and how is it practiced?
7. Which of the forms of meditation focus on generating and circulating internal body energy?
8. How would you describe mindfulness meditation?
9. Name four meditation positions.
10. Name and explain four meditation techniques.
11. What are five physiological and five psychological benefits of meditation?
12. How can meditation aid spiritual growth?
13. What does the research on the effects of meditation indicate?
14. What is the history and origin of yoga?
15. What are six health benefits of yoga?
16. Why is posture important when practicing yoga?
17. What does "the power of breath" mean?
18. Name three asanas.
19. What does the research indicate about the benefits of yoga?
20. How would you define hypnosis?
21. What is the history of hypnosis?
22. Name and discuss two philosophies explaining hypnotic effects.
23. What are the four stages of hypnosis, and what occurs at each stage?
24. How is hypnosis used as a therapeutic treatment?
25. How could you find a qualified hypnotist?
26. What is the Alexander Technique process?
27. What are three benefits of the Alexander Technique?
28. What is the history of the Alexander Technique?
29. Describe a typical Alexander Technique session.
30. How are Alexander Technique teachers trained?
31. What does the research indicate regarding the benefits of Alexander Technique?
32. What is biofeedback and what are its origins?
33. How does biofeedback work as a mind–body intervention?
34. Explain the biofeedback process.
35. What does the research indicate regarding the benefits of biofeedback?
36. How could you find a qualified biofeedback practitioner?
37. What does the research indicate about the effects of prayer and faith or spiritual healing?
38. What is noetic science?
39. What is intercessory prayer?
40. Name and explain three examples of faith or spiritual healing through the ages.
41. Who was Mary Baker Eddy, and what was her contribution to faith healing?

Key Terms

Alexander technique A process in which people can learn to release muscular tension and habitually overtightened muscles that cause our bodies to become distorted, unbalanced, and compressed.

asanas Another name for Yoga poses.

biofeedback A mind–body intervention that helps train people to improve their health by using their own body's electrical signals from the muscles or brain.

blood lactate A chemical associated with stress.

Buddhism A religion that originated in India by Buddha (Gautama) and later spread to China, Burma, Japan, Tibet, and parts of southeast Asia. It holds life is full of suffering caused by desire, and the way to end this suffering is through enlightenment that enables one to halt the endless sequence of births and deaths to which one is otherwise subject.

Burmese position Sitting on the floor and using a zafu—a small pillow—to raise the hips just a little, so the knees can touch the ground. Sitting on the pillow with two knees touching the ground forms a tripod base that gives 360-degree stability.

concentration technique Involves concentrating on an external object as a focus point for the mind.

contemplation meditative techniques Use introspection, self-study, and reflection. Contemplative meditation is supposed to help people gain a deeper understanding of some aspect of reality.

cortisol A chemical associated with stress.

dervish dancers Turkish dancers who dress in a particular style and seem to dance to the rhythm of the cosmos or the universe.

distant healing Involves people praying for and healing others at great distances away (sometimes without the ill person knowing it). Also known as intercessory prayer.

empty mind meditation Involves sitting still, often in a full lotus or cross-legged position, and letting the mind go silent on its own.

faith or spiritual energy healing Spiritual energy healing has occurred since earliest times among all cultures, religions, and medicinal practices. Various healing techniques are used (including chants and prayer, touching, or placing the hands close to the body within the energy fields that surround the body). Popular current methods used for energy healing include Reiki therapy, therapeutic touch, qi gong healing, and crystal healing.

feeling and emotion meditation techniques These may be used independently but also may be combined with other types of meditation practices.

free radicals Unstable oxygen molecules that can cause tissue damage.

full lotus position A seated position in which each leg is placed on the opposite thigh.

Gurdjieff Sacred Dances A technique wherein the movements are very defined and different parts of the body seem not to be related to each other.

guru One who is regarded as having great knowledge, wisdom, and authority in a certain area and who uses it to guide others.

half lotus position A seated position in which the left foot is placed onto the right thigh and the right leg is tucked under the left thigh.

hypnosis A mind–body technique that focuses on awareness and attention to internal stimuli, much like what is learned while doing meditation. The word "hypnosis" comes from the Greek word *hypnos*, meaning sleep. It was first termed "animal magnetism."

hypnotherapy Therapy using hypnosis to gain access to the deeper levels of the mind so that a change in thinking and behavior will occur.

intercessory prayer Involves people praying for and healing others at great distances away (sometimes without the ill person knowing it). Also known as distant healing.

Koan meditation technique Meditations from the Zen School of Buddhism that are designed to break down an ordinary pattern of thinking.

mandala Means completion or circle. A word coming from one of the languages of India called Sanskrit.

mantra meditation A word or phrase repeated during meditation.

martial arts Encompass understanding the relationship of the power of breath, the life force (qi energy), the mind, and the concept of oneness.

meditation A way of being, a way of seeing, and even a way of loving.

menopause The period of permanent cessation of menstruation, usually occurring between the ages of 45 and 55.

mesmerize Term stemming from Dr. Franz Anton Mesmer, who defined the discipline of hypnotism.

metabolic rate The amount of energy liberated or expended in a given unit of time.

mindfulness meditation To become aware of your physical, emotional, and mental activities in the here and now.

neo-dissociation model A model that suggests hypnosis activates a subsystem of both psychological and physiologic parts.

noetic science The study of the mind and health healing. Noetic means the power of inner knowing, and is a branch of metaphysics.

parasympathetic nervous system Responsible for causing heart rate and breathing to slow down, blood vessels to dilate, and digestive juices to increase.

rhythm and song methods of meditation A combination of rhythm, chanting, music, and breath used during meditation to achieve a desired state of calmness.

Sama A ritual practice developed in the mid 9th century that uses music, poetry recital, singing and dance.

Sanskrit Is one of 22 languages spoken in India and is the liturgical (church language) of Hinduism and Buddhism. The language originated about 1500 B.C.E.

serotonin Levels of this chemical influence moods and behavior; low levels are associated with depression, headaches, and insomnia.

silent mind meditation Technique involving directly perceiving and feeling the world around us by focusing on how we are thinking.

social psychological model A model that suggests during hypnosis, an altered state of consciousness does not occur; instead, hypnosis is explained by suggestibility, positive attitudes, and expectations

Sufi dancing Said to be the dance of universal peace and is supposed to bring participants to a mystical experience and cultivate inner peace and harmony. The dance involves whirling by oneself or with partners. Dancers whirl with arms in various positions, such as reaching out and reaching to the heavens.

sympathetic nervous system Responsible for the "fight-or-flight" response produced during times of stress.

thought and laughter methods of meditation Using positive thinking, self-hypnosis, power of intention (strong thought), and even laughter to achieve the meditative state.

Vipassana Is known as insight meditation. Mindfulness is employed during meditation. Requires being watchful of your breath during inhalation and exhalation.

visualization techniques Used to achieve a meditative state.

walking meditation Focuses on awareness of self, the process of walking, and the environment.

WHO AM I Focuses on negating the false self in order to realize one's true nature or enlightenment.

yoga Requires full awareness of posture and movements. Attention is focused on the breath during all movements and helps open up the energy channels. Thought to be a powerful meditation technique.

zazen The breathing technique of Zen meditation, also known as the meditation of the Buddha. This involves awareness and concentration during the breathing process to help build or shape the mind and to free oneself from dualistic thinking (separation of mind and body).

References

1. Rice B. Mind-body interventions. *Diabetes Spectrum*. 2001;14(4):213–217.
2. Pelletier K. *The best alternative medicine: what works? What does not?* New York: Simon & Schuster; 2000.
3. Jenn. Mind, body intervention [Altmedinstitute]. Available at: http://www.altmedinstitute.com/mind-body-intervention.htm. Accessed January 4, 2011.
4. Mipham S. *Turning the mind into an ally*. New York: Riverhead Books; 2003.
5. Kabat-Zinn J. *Coming to our senses: healing ourselves and the world through mindfulness*. New York: Hyperion; 2005.
6. Rinpoche S. Essential advice on mediation. Available at: http://www.sacred-texts.com/bud/tib/essmed.htm. Accessed January 4, 2011.
7. Wallace A. *Tibetan Buddhism: from the ground up: a practical approach for modern life*. Somerville, MA: Wisdom; 1993.
8. Cianciosi J. *The meditative path: a gentle way to awareness, concentration, and serenity*. Wheaton, IL: Quest; 2001.
9. Somerville R, ed. *The alternative advisor*. Alexandria, VA: Time Life Books; 1997.
10. Vipassana Dhura Meditation Society. What is Vipassana? Available at: http://www.vipassanadhura.com/whatis.htm. Accessed January 7, 2011.
11. Meditation Is Easy. Vipassana: the technique of Gautama Buddha. Available at: http://www.meditationiseasy.com/mCorner/techniques/Vipassana.htm. Accesesd January 7, 2011.
12. Maharishi University of Management. Transcendental meditation technique. Available at: http://www.mum.edu/tm.html. Accessed January 7, 2011.
13. The transcendental meditation program. Available at: http://www.tm.org/meditation-techniques. Accessed
14. Zen Mountain Monastery. Zen Meditation Instructions. Available at: http://www.mro.org/zmm/teachings/meditation.php. Accessed January 7, 2011.
15. A View on Buddhism. What is meditation? Available at: http://viewonbuddhism.org/meditation_theory.html#1. Accessed January 8, 2011.
16. Meditation techniques: Taoist meditation methods. Available at: http://1stholistic.com/meditation/hol_meditation/hol_meditation_taoist_meditation.htm. Accessed January 8, 2011.
17. Story F. *Buddhist meditation*. Sri Lanka: Buddhist Publication Society; 1986. Available at: http://www.freemeditations.com/buddhist_meditation.html. Accessed January 8, 2011.
18. Macinerney C. Yoga stories and essays. Available at: http://www.yogateacher.com/text/essays/spring2005.html. Accessed January 10, 2011.
19. Kiann N. Persian dance and its forgotten history. Iran Chamber Society. Monday, September 5, 2011. Available at: http://www.iranchamber.com/cinema/articles/persian_dance_history02.php Accessed September 5, 2011.
20. Esenko L. Image of Sufi dancing in Cairo. Available at: http://lh5.google.com/luka.esenko/R39r7ZoInjI/AAAAAAAAAoM/iL4sPGI8qMI/s8. Accessed January 10, 2011.
21. McQueen M. What is Sufi dancing? Available at: http://openheartmusic.org/whatis.html. Accessed January 10, 2011.
22. Erzen J. The dervishes dance—the sacred ritual of love. Available at: http://www.contempaesthetics.org/newvolume/pages/article.php?articleID = 514. Accessed January 10, 2011.
23. Gurdjieff Movements. Available at: http://www.danze-di-gurdjieff.it/Templates/English/HomeE.htm. Accessed January 10, 2011.
24. Mehta A. Meditation techniques, types and practice—a comprehensive guide. June 6, 2007. Available at: http://www.anmolmehta.com/blog/2007/06/05/meditation-techniques-types-and-practice-a-comprehensive-guide/. Accessed January 11, 2011.
25. Maharshi R. Ramana Maharshi on "Who am I" meditation. Available at: http://www.messagefrommasters.com/Life_of_Masters/Ramana-Maharshi/Who-am-I.htm. Accessed January 11, 2011.
26. Contemplative meditation. The meditation newsletter. Available at: http://www.themeditationsite.com/7-contemplativemeditation.html. Accessed January 11, 2011.
27. Mehta A. Guided meditation #2: sound awareness meditation technique. Available at: http://www.anmolmehta.com/blog/2007/04/18/free-online-guided-meditation-book-sound-awareness-meditation-technique-ch-2/. Accessed January 11, 2011.
28. Osho. The mystic rose meditation: laughter, tears, and silence. Available at: http://www.osho.com/Topics/TopicsEng/MysticRose.htm. Accessed January 11, 2011.
29. Biography Online. Biography Osho—Bhagwan Shree Rajneesh. Available at: http://www.biographyonline.net/spiritual/osho.html. Accessed January 11, 2011.

30. Hurley T. Mandalas for meditation and coloring. Available at: http://stress.lovetoknow.com/Mandalas_for_Meditation_and_Coloring. Accessed January 12, 2011.
31. Wong C. Coloring mandalas as a meditation technique. Available at: http://altmedicine.about.com/od/mindspiritandself/ss/mandala.htm. Accessed January 12, 2011.
32. Project-Meditation.org. Benefits of meditation. Available at: http://www.project-meditation.org/benefits_of_meditation.html. Accessed January 12, 2011.
33. ABC-of-Yoga.com. Meditation—benefits of meditation. Available at: http://www.abc-of-yoga.com/meditation/benefits.asp. Accessed January 18, 2011.
34. Borysenko J. *The beginner's guide to meditation* [CDs]. Hay House; 2006.
35. National Institutes of Health, National Center for Complementary and Alternative Medicine. Research results by date. Available at: http://nccam.nih.gov/research/results/spotlight/. Accessed January 12, 2011.
36. Lawlis F. *Mosby's complementary and alternative medicine: a research-based approach*. St. Louis: Mosby; 2001.
37. Nidich SI, Rainforth MV, Haaga DAF, et al. A randomized controlled trial on effects of the transcendental meditation program on blood pressure, psychological distress, and coping in young adults. *Am J Hypertens*. 2009;22(12):1326–1331.
38. Davidson J, Kabat-Zinn J, Schumacher J, et al. Alterations in brain and immune function produced by mindfulness meditation. *Psychosomatic Med J*. 2003;65:564–570. Complete article available at:http://www.stat.psu.edu/%7Edhunter/016/fall2006/yogaorig.pdf. Accessed January 20, 2011 and September, 2011.
39. Aubrey A. Meditation a hit for pain management. NPR September 4, 2011. Available at: http://www.npr.org/templates/story/story.php?storyId=7654964 Accessed September 6, 2011.
40. Weil R. Yoga. Available at: http://www.medicinenet.com/yoga/article.htm. Accessed January 22, 2011.
41. Shaynebance. History of yoga—a complete overview of the yoga history. Available at: http://www.abc-of-yoga.com/beginnersguide/yogahistory.asp. Accessed January 22, 2011.
42. Bradford N, ed. *The one spirit encyclopedia of complementary health*. London: Hamlyn; 1996.
43. Ernst E. *The desktop guide to complementary and alternative medicine: an evidence based approach*. New York: Mosby; 2001.
44. Google. Yoga images. Available at: http://www.google.com/images?hl=en&rlz=1G1GGLQ_ENUS368&q=yoga+images&um=1&ie=UTF-8&source=univ&ei=glPoTIffFMT7lweixOmeCQ&sa=X&oi=image_result_group&ct=title&resnum=1&ved=0CCIQsAQwAA&biw=1194&bih=1136. Accessed January 23, 2011.
45. WebMD. The health benefits of yoga. Available at: http://www.webmd.com/balance/the-health-benefits-of-yoga. Accessed January 23, 2011.
46. Saradananda S. *The power of breath: the art of breathing well for harmony, happiness, and health*. London: Duncan Baird; 2009.
47. Kiecolt-Glaser JK, Christian L, Preston H, et al. Stress, inflammation, and yoga practice. *Psychosomatic Med*. 2010;72(2):113–121.
48. Pilkington K, Kirkwood G, Rampes H, Richardson J. Yoga for depression: the research evidence. *J Affect Disord*. 2005;89(1):13–24.
49. Kirkwood G, Rampes H, Tuffrey V, Richardson J, Pilkington K. Yoga for anxiety: a systematic review of the research evidence. *Br J Sports Med*. 2005;39:884–891.
50. Nagarathna R, Nagendra H. Yoga for bronchial asthma: a controlled study. *Br Med J (Clin Res Ed)*. 1985;291:1077.
51. Raub J. Psychophysiologic effects of hatha yoga on musculoskeletal and cardiopulmonary function: a literature review. *J Altern Complement Med*. 2002;8(6):797–812.
52. Mayo Clinic. Hypnosis. Available at: http://www.mayoclinic.com/health/ hypnosis/. Accessed January 28, 2011.
53. American Society of Clinical Hypnosis. General info on hypnosis. Available at: http://asch.net/Public/GeneralInfoonHypnosis/MythsAboutHypnosis/tabid/135/Default.aspx. Accessed January 28, 2011.
54. University of Maryland Medical Center. Hypnotherapy. Available at: http://www.umm.edu/altmed/articles/hypnotherapy-000353.htm. Accessed January 28, 2011.
55. Goudas L, Carr DB, Bloch R, et al. Management of cancer pain. AHRQ Pub No. 02-E002. Rockville, MD: Agency for Healthcare Review.
56. Godot D. Hypno-oncology: hypnosis in the treatment of cancer. 2007. Available at: http://chicagopsychology.org/davidgodot/hypno-oncology/. Accessed January 28, 2011.
57. Peynovska R, Fisher J, Oliver D, Mathew VM. Efficacy of hypnotherapy as a supplement therapy in cancer intervention. *Eur J Clin Hypn*. 2005;6(1):2–7.
58. Patterson DR, Wiechman SA, Jensen M, Sharar SR. Hypnosis delivered through immersive virtual reality for burn pain: A clinical case series. *Int J Clin Exp Hypn*. 2006;54(2):130–142.
59. Askay S, Patterson D, Jensen M, Sharar S. A randomized controlled trial of hypnosis for burn wound care. *Rehab Psychol*. 2007;52(3):247–253.
60. Thieme K, Gracely RH. Are psychological treatments effective for fibromyalgia pain? *Curr Rheumatol Rep*. 2009;11(6):443–450.
61. Wilson S, Maddison T, Roerts L, Greenield S, Singh S. Systematic review: the effectiveness of hypnotherapy in the management of irritable bowel syndrome. *Aliment Pharmacol Ther*. 2006;24(5):769–780.
62. Richardson J, Smith JE, McCall G, Richardson A, Pilkington K, Kirsch I. Hypnosis for nausea and vomiting in cancer chemotherapy: a systematic review of the research evidence. *Eur J Cancer Care*. 2007;16(5):402–412.
63. Shenefelt P. Biofeedback, cognitive-behavioral methods, and hypnosis in dermatology: is it all in your mind? *Dermatol Ther*. 2003;16:114–122.
64. Shenefelt P. Hynosis in dermatology. *Arch Dermatol*. 2000;136:393–399.
65. National Board for Certified Clinical Hypnotherapists. Find a hypnotist. Available at: http://www.natboard.com/index_files/Page548.htm. Accessed January 29, 2011.
66. The Complete Guide to the Alexander Technique. What happens during an Alexander Technique lesson or class? Available at: http://www.alexandertechnique.com/lesson.htm. Accessed January 30, 2011.
67. Goldberg M. The F.M. Alexander Technique. Available at: http://www.alexandercenter.com. Accessed November 3, 2010.
68. Rickover R. The Alexander lesson. In: *Fitness without stress*. Portland, OR: Metamorphous Press; 1988: Chapter Four.
69. Benor DJ. Spiritual healing: a unifying influence in complementary therapies. *Compl Ther Med*. 1995;3(4):234–238.
70. Little P, Lewith G, Webley F, Evans M, Beattle, A, Middleton K, Barnett J, Ballard K, Oford F, Smith P, Yardley L, Hollinghurst S, Sharp D. Randomised controlled trial of Alexander Technique lessons, exercise, and massage (ATEAM) for chronic and recurrent back pain. *BMJ*. 2008;337:a884. Full text available at: http://www.bmj.com/content/337/bmj.a884.full. Accessed January 30, 2011.
71. Austin JH, Ausubel P. Enhanced respiratory muscular function in normal adults after lessons in proprioceptive musculoskeletal education without exercises. *Chest*. 1992;102(2):486–490.
72. Cacciatore T, Horak F, Henry S. Improvement in automatic postural coordination following Alexander Technique lessons in a person with low back pain. *Phys Ther*. 2005;85(6):565–578.
73. Runcke B. What is biofeedback? Available at: http://psychotherapy.com/bio.html. Accessed February 2, 2011.
74. University of Maryland Medical Center. Biofeedback. Available at: http://www.umm.edu/altmed/articles/biofeedback-000349.htm. Accessed February 2, 2011.

75. Hosker G, Cody J, Norton C. Electrical stimulation for fecal incontinence in adults. *Cochrane Database Syst Rev.* 2007;(3):CD001310.
76. Terra MP, Dobben AC, Berghmans B, et al. Electrical stimulation and pelvic floor muscle training with biofeedback in patients with fecal incontinence: a cohort study of 281 patients. *Dis Colon Rectum.* 2006;49(8):1149–1159.
77. Monastra V, Monastra D, George S. The effects of stimulant therapy, EEG biofeedback, and parenting style on the primary symptoms of attention-deficit/hyperactivity disorder. *Appl Psychophysiol Biofeedback.* 2002;27(4):231–249.
78. U.S. Department of Health and Human Services. Find a biofeedback practitioner. Available at: http://www.healthfinder.gov/docs/doc07988.htm. Accessed February 3, 2011.
79. Andromida. Noetic sciences definition & experiments—science of subconscious mind power & thoughts. Available at: http://hubpages.com/hub/noetic-sciences-experiments-definition-science-of-subconscious-mind-power. Accessed February 3, 2011.
80. Sicher F, Targ E, Moore D, Smith HS. A randomized double-blind study of the effect of distant healing in a population with advanced AIDS—report of a small-scale study. *West J Med.* 1998;169:356–363.
81. Krucoff M, Crater S, Green C, Maas A, Seskevich J, Lane J, Loeffler K, Morris K, Bashore T, Koenig H. Integrative noetic therapies as adjuncts to percutaneous intervention during unstable coronary syndromes: Monitoring and actualization of noetic training (MANTRA) feasibility pilot. *Am Heart J.* 2001; 142(5):760–769.
82. Palmer R, Katerndahl D, Morgan-Kidd J. A randomized trial of the effects of remote intercessory prayer: interactions with personal beliefs on problem-specific outcomes and functional status. *J Altern Complement Med.* 2004;10(3):438–448.
83. Hodge D. A systematic review of the empirical literature on intercessory prayer. *Res Soc Work Pract.* 2007;17(2):74–187.
84. Image of Caduceus. Available at: http://www.google.com/images?hl=en&rlz=1G1GGLQ_ENUS368&q=image+of+Caduceus.&um=1&ie=UTF-8&source=univ&ei=OoXoTNaRHoL6lwf-uYjpCw&sa=X&oi=image_result_group&ct=title&resnum=1&ved=0CC0QsAQwAA&biw=1194&bih=1136. Accessed February 5, 2011.
85. Castro J, Blaylock W. Religion: a shrine to faith and healing. *Time.* Available at: http://www.time.com/time/magazine/article/0,9171,949777,00.html. Accessed February 6, 2011.
86. Kime R. *The informed health consumer.* Guilford, CT: Dushkin; 1992.
87. Christian Science. Who is Mary Baker Eddy? Available at: http://christianscience.com/questions/about-mary-baker-eddy/. Accessed February 6, 2011.
88. Way of Life Literature. Agnes Sanford. Available at: http://www.wayoflife.org/files/316792f23d7a7101cb047f0ae4a95b02-148.html. Accessed February 6, 2011.
89. Articlesbase. Do famous spiritual energy healers manifest miracles? October 6, 2008. Available at: http://www.articlesbase.com/alternative-medicine-articles/do-famous-spiritual-energy-healers-manifest-miracles-592422.html. Accessed February 6, 2011.
90. Brennan B. *Hands of light: a guide to healing through the human energy field.* New York: Bantam; 1987.
91. Spiritual Science Research Foundation. Overcoming addiction to alcohol. Available at: http://www.spiritualresearchfoundation.org/articles/id/spiritualresearch/mentalhealth/addiction/addictioncasestudy. Accessed February 6, 2011.

APPENDIX 14.A

Guided Basic Zen Meditation Technique

It is important to meditate in a quiet and still environment. This might be in a bedroom or den in your house. The lighting should be low or, if daytime, sit without the sun directly on you. You can set a timer but it is not necessary.

1. Sit in a comfortable position. You can sit on a zafu in a lotus or cross-legged position.[27] People who use a zafu sit on the forward part of the cushion so that the hips are higher than the knees. Sometimes it may require sitting on more than one zafu to raise the hips higher than the knees. You may also sit on a chair. If so, keep both your feet planted on the floor.
2. Lengthen your spine. It should be upright, but allowing for the spine's natural curve.
3. Rest your hands on your thighs.
4. Try to relax your shoulders and your arms.
5. Tuck in your chin a little.
6. Shut your eyes until they are half open. You may focus your gaze on the floor in front of you or on some other point in the room. You also may close your eyes completely if you wish.
7. Relax your face and jaw. It helps to relax the jaw by placing your tongue on the roof of your mouth. Stillness of the body is important at this time. It is the time to calm the mind as well as the body.
8. Concentrate on your breathing. You may take a few deep, slow breaths through the nose and breathe out through the mouth. Try not to manipulate your breathing after those first few breaths. Just pay attention to it and become aware of when the breath is relaxed.
9. Some people are taught to count their inhalations and exhalations up to a certain number and then to start again. You may try that for the first week of meditating. Inhale deeply and count one. Exhale deeply and count two. Inhale again and count three. Exhale again and count four.[27] The next week, try counting only the inhalations but not the exhalations. The third or fourth week that you meditate, try not counting at all. Just sit in stillness and be aware of the moment, the state of stillness.

APPENDIX 14.B

Guided Sound Awareness Meditation Technique

Guided sound awareness meditation is another variation on meditation. The first steps are the same as guided Zen meditation. The last steps are a little different.

1. Sit in a comfortable position. You can sit on a zafu in a lotus or cross-legged position. People who use a zafu sit on the forward part of the cushion so that the hips are higher than the knees. Sometimes it may require sitting on more than one zafu to raise the hips higher than the knees. You may also sit on

a chair. If so, keep both your feet planted on the floor.

2. Lengthen your spine. It should be upright, but allowing for the spine's natural curve.
3. Rest you hands on your thighs or your lap.
4. Try to relax your shoulders and your arms.
5. Tuck in your chin a little.
6. Close your eyes or shut your eyes until they are half open. You may focus your gaze on the floor in front of you or on some other point in the room.
7. Relax your face and jaw. It helps to relax the jaw by placing your tongue on the roof of your mouth.
8. Take a few deep, slow breaths through the nose and breathe out through the mouth. Don't try to control your breathing, but pay attention to it.[27]
9. When your breathing becomes relaxed, begin to pay attention to sounds in your immediate environment. Then begin to pay attention to sounds that are more distant. Try to just listen and attend to those sounds. Note if the sound is loud or soft, high or low, or it changes beat. Try not to get involved with the sounds, but become a detached observer who is listening to the music of life.[27] You may find yourself thinking about personal issues. If so, observe those thoughts but then return to attending to the sounds in your environment.
10. After a period of time, turn your attention from distant sounds to sounds closer to you.
11. Lastly, turn your attention to only the sounds closest to you and to your breath.
12. Open your eyes and slowly become aware of all your surroundings. Stand and breathe deeply.

Energy Therapies

LEARNING OBJECTIVES

As a result of reading this chapter, students will:

1. Identify typical practices considered to be energy therapies.
2. Characterize chi and its role in energy therapies.
3. Contrast the practices of Reiki and therapeutic touch.
4. Examine the challenges related to "mainstreaming" energy therapies.
5. Identify whether research exists to support the use of energy therapies.

WHAT ARE ENERGY THERAPIES?

Energy therapies are a method of health care characterized by an attempt to harness, manipulate, or direct energy in an effort to improve health. In Eastern cultures and alternative medicine practice, it is believed that energy, often referred to as chi (also spelled qi), is a therapeutic force. The central concept is that life force energy, chi, is embodied in all things, living and nonliving, and as such that energy can play a role in one's well-being. The National Center for Complementary and Alternative Medicine (NCCAM)[1] places energy therapies into two categories called biofield and bioelectrical therapies. Biofield practices are said to affect the energy in and around the body. There is no effective and efficient mode of measuring biofield energy, thus these forms of treatment are quite controversial. Bioelectrical energy is measurable, with energy forms using a specific frequency or wavelength, and is most often a magnetic force, light energy, or a type of radiation.

The NCCAM goes on to state that practitioners of energy therapy believe that the body possesses and emits "subtle energy" (chi), and it is the disruption in the flow of this energy that causes disease and illness. Thus, therapy involves the restoration of a positive and efficient flow of subtle energy. Warber indicates that most practitioners of Western medicine acknowledge the human body emits a low level of energy, but see it as a by-product of cell activity, nothing of significance, and most certainly not something that can be manipulated for personal well-being.[2]

This chapter will introduce readers to putative (yet to be measured successfully) energy therapies, such as qi gong, Reiki, and therapeutic touch, and veritable (measurable) therapies such as bioelectromagnetic, light, and sound therapies.

WHAT IS QI GONG?

Qi gong (also spelled qigong) is an ancient method of Chinese health care utilizing physical forms, focused breathing, and deliberate movement. According to the Qigong Association of America, qi gong comes from the combination of two Chinese words: *qi* (pronounced "chi"), meaning energy, and *gong* (pronounced "kung") referring to action, or more specifically, skill.[3] As mentioned earlier, qi is described as an energy force found in all things, living and nonliving. Therefore, energy is all around us. Practitioners of qi gong believe energy can be manipulated, gathered, utilized, and influenced through meditation and movement designed to increase and focus the flow of that energy. In this sense it has both a physical component and an intellectual one, where the mind is used as much as the body in gathering and directing energy. Qi gong therefore is a reference to the skill or practice of cultivating energy. Not everyone believes this is a legitimate form of healing and explain potential effects and benefits in other ways. See **BOX 15.1** for an example called the placebo effect.

As in all Chinese medical practices, practitioners of qi gong believe disease or illness takes hold when there is a blockage or disruption in the flow of qi. Qi gong, then, is designed to improve or redirect the flow of energy, and as a result, improve well-being.

When used strictly as a form of exercise, proponents of qi gong point to the multidimensional nature of the art form as "better" than traditional exercise. Benefits are expanded because you must integrate mind with body.

History of Qi Gong

Summarizing 3,500 years of history is no easy task, and we can provide only minimal information here. In short, qi gong history falls into four predominant time frames. The first of these starts when the art was introduced, around 1000 BCE, and continues approximately 800 years. It is during this time period that shamans performed traditional animal dances as a form of spiritual cleansing at New Year's.[4] In addition, the *Chinese Book of Changes* introduced the concept of qi and the relationship among man, heaven, and Earth. Qi was first recorded as a source of energy in ancient carvings. In 300 BCE, Zhuang Zi, a Daoist philosopher, described the connection between breathing and personal health.

The second phase occurred during the Han Dynasty (206 BCE–220 AD). Meditation and Buddhism were introduced in China from India, where qi gong had been used for thousands of years. Because of the new Buddhist influence, this time is often referred to as the religious era of qi gong. In this phase, qi gong focused only on health and well-being, and the introduction of faith practice to the art significantly broadened its emphases. Unfortunately, the masses were not allowed to practice, because the religious leaders kept most of the information secret. If the practice had not been secretly passed on through the Buddhist monasteries, we may not have ever seen qi gong in the general population.

The third phase (500 AD–1911) began during the Liang dynasty, when qi gong became used as a martial art, and ran through the end of the Qing dynasty. Many, many martial art forms were created using principles of qi gong. It was deemed to increase physical strength in addition to simply improving general health and well-being. It is also during this phase when the animal forms came to being: the tiger, leopard, dragon, snake, and crane. Each form represents a different style and sequence of movement representing the most cherished and revered animals of the time.

The final phase runs from 1911 to the present time. Qi gong today is a mix of practices from a multitude of countries. The secrecy of the religious elders has been broken, and qi gong has become an activity of the masses. It is during this current phase that research began to take place, a more pronounced emphasis on wellness and qi gong was seen, and its worldwide visibility increased.[5]

> **Box 15.1**
>
> **Placebo Effects**
>
> People get better because they believe they will get better. That is the explanation many physicians and researchers give to explain the "benefit" of most energy therapies (and many other complementary medicine therapies). It's called the placebo effect. A placebo effect is a situation in which people believe a particular medicine or treatment is curing their illness, but they are experiencing a pill or treatment known to have no medicinal benefit (e.g., sugar pill). In short, studies have shown a percentage of people who are told they are taking a real medicine, even though it is a fake medicine (commonly referred to as a sham), will perceive that their health has improved. They get better because they have the *expectation* that they will get better. The more a person believes they will improve, the better they may become.
>
> When it comes to energy medicine, and the practitioners and patients are working with a form of energy that has yet to be accurately measured, like chi (through therapeutic touch or Reiki), physicians tend to believe that the placebo effect is occurring.

Forms of Qi Gong

According to the Qigong Association of America, the art can be categorized as internal or external.[3] Internal qi gong is similar to meditation, using mind, breath, and visualization to guide bodily energy and energy immediately surrounding an individual. These forms of qi gong are designed to increase qi, to circulate qi, or to use qi to cleanse or heal self. External qi gong involves movement.[6] This movement is said to hold many health benefits, from reduction of blood pressure to increased flexibility. External qi gong can also involve projection of qi outside one's body to assist or affect another. In this latter example, qi gong is completed for the benefit of another.

Activities and movements included in qi gong are done either as a singular movement, in combination, or in sequence. These movements or sequences are referred to as forms. Forms are generally designed to address a specific health issue, such as heart health or lung health. Some forms are designed for general well-being or lifelong fitness. They go by names such as Everyday Stretching Qigong and Eight Brocade Exercises.[6,p17] See **BOX 15.2** for an example called Remedy Routines. There are countless forms available to learn and practice, with a growing number of videos and community-based exercise programs available to teach qi gong as well. Most forms involve a significant emphasis on flexibility. All forms incorporate an emphasis on the flow of qi, the opening of the body's meridians, and breathing. Because of the physical nature of the external form, as with any form of activity,

Box 15.2

The Remedy Routine: Qi Gong[7]

Remedy Routine: Discharging Turbid Substances from the Liver

Part 1. Preparation

Stand with your feet as wide apart as your shoulders and pointing straight ahead, knees slightly bent. Let your shoulders relax. Allow your hands to fall at your sides naturally. Place the tip of your tongue on your upper palate, just behind your teeth. Relax the root of your tongue. Smile slightly. Keep your eyes level and open, thinking of nothing.

Use your mind to relax your head, your neck, your shoulders, your elbows, your wrists, your fingers, your chest, your stomach, your back, your waist, your hips, your knees, your ankles, your feet, and your toes. Gather qi into your lower dan tian (belly button level). Concentrate your mind on your lower dan tian for a little while.

Direct qi from your lower dan tian down to hui yin (groin area) and back up and along du mai (channel through the center middle of the body) to da zhui (neck level). At this point split the qi into two streams and direct it through the middle of the shoulders, down through the arms to lao gong (middle of palm). Shift your body weight onto your left leg and place your right foot a half step forward with the heel on the ground and toes up pointing to a tree, some wood, or wooden furniture.

Part 2. Taking Back the Qi

Turn your palms forward and using your shoulders as pivot, raise your arms while holding a ball of outer qi, and then beam it into bai hui (point at top of skull). Open your chest by spreading out your elbows. With palms down and fingertips pointing at each other, let your hands descend in front of your body guiding qi through your middle channel into shan zhong, or heart area. See Forms 1–4 in **FIGURE 15.1**.

Part 3. Discharging Turbid Substance from the Liver

Move your hands parallel to your right chest and then descend along your right side thinking that you are guiding the turbid substance (spent qi) from your liver through the inner side of your right leg. Discharge it out of your body from da dun (the inner side of your right big toe) to the tree, wood, or wooden furniture. When your hands have descended and become straight, turn your palms facing the tree, wood, or wooden furniture thinking the spent qi has been pushed into it. Then allow your arms to fall naturally at your sides. See Forms 5–8 in Figure 15.1.

If you do it continuously, you should separate your two hands instead of allowing them down, and then push your hands out a bit to draw an arc and raise your hands along your hips and then turn your palms forward and start to do it again. You may do it continuously from 9 times to 30 times until you feel your liver area is comfortable. It all depends on the need of the individual, but you cannot do it too many times.

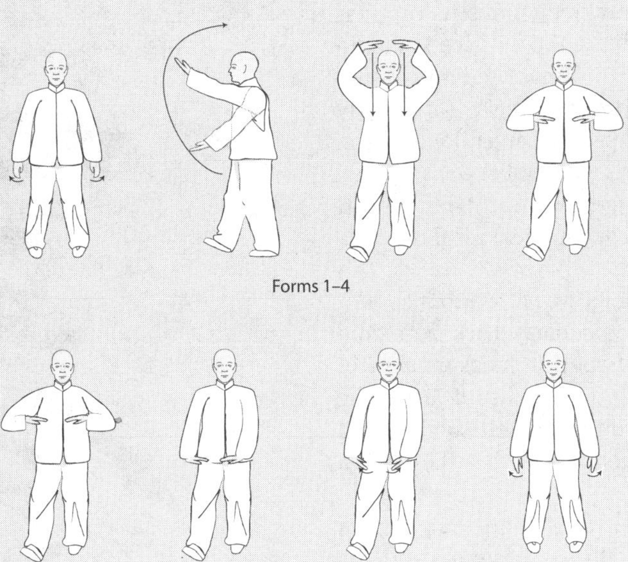

FIGURE 15.1 Remedy routine associated with cleansing of the liver.

Source: Courtesy of Qigong Association of America.

it is recommended you discuss a new program with your physician before initiating practice.

The Science Behind Qi Gong

A challenging component to interpreting the research on qi gong is that most is completed in Chinese culture, where the concept of qi as a universal life force found in all things is a given, not something to be proven. Qi gong is famous in China for curing chronic disease and promoting health. Western practitioners do not appear to have a clear consensus on the effect of practicing qi gong, because there is still the challenge of measuring qi itself.

Yan, Lu, and Kiang, while recognizing the shortcomings of the research such as lack of randomization and control groups, identify a moderate number of studies supporting the notion that the presence and application of external qi (energy delivered from a practitioner to something like cancer cells) reduces the growth rate of cancerous cells, increases blood flow to vital organs, lengthens the time a cancer patient survives, or increases the growth of healthy cells in living animals.[8] The results have been replicated in lab experiments as well.

Clinical research on qi gong is more extensive, with a primary focus on the issue of hypertension and internal qi gong. Mayer conducted a review of 33 studies, the vast majority again published in Chinese literature, to gain a sense of the overall success of qi gong as a method of controlling hypertension.[9] The analysis revealed a results pattern supporting the notion that qi gong can reduce or stabilize blood pressure for those who use the technique. In many of the studies, participants were able to reduce or eliminate their medication. Along with blood pressure adaptations, results included increases in blood flow, reductions in vascular tension, reduced viscosity (thickness) of the blood, and increased volume of blood flow to the limbs. Additional studies show the positive effects on fibromyalgia, particularly in the areas of functioning and pain.[10] Larger, longer-term studies have reported reductions in a number of cardiovascular disease issues such as congestive heart failure, heart attack, and stroke (and in turn, death rates) for those who practice qi gong twice daily.[9,11]

As with lab studies, these results are not without controversy, particularly in research methodology. Lack of random assignment of subjects, lack of specific measurement of treatment effects (was it the qi gong, or was it just being active, or did the ailment just run its natural course), and expectancy bias all were common issues with the studies included in the review.

What does this mean for the practice of qi gong and its health benefit? It depends, actually. By Eastern standards and measures, qi gong is rooted in 7,000 years of historical success, and the documentation of that success is clear and evident. Identifying, measuring, and studying qi are not necessary. It is readily accepted that life force energy exists, and can be accessed at the individual level. Through the eyes of a Western medical practitioner, however, there has not been enough controlled experimentation, accounting for all potential bias, to determine clinical significance of the practice. That being said, there appears to be a positive health effect to the practice of qi gong, and at a time when two out of three U.S. adults are overweight or obese, movement such as qi gong for healthy purposes is a positive alternative.

WHAT IS REIKI?

Combining two Japanese words, *Rei* and *Ki*, gives the word *Reiki*. Literal translation is always challenging when trying to describe something unseen, but Rei has been defined as the wisdom of God, a higher power (in general), or a reference to a cosmic, universal energy. Ki (essentially the same as chi or qi) is the unseen energy that gives or causes life.[12] When placed together, Reiki becomes a reference to an energy force guided by a greater power. Practitioners are quick to point out, however, that the general public should not associate a "greater power" reference to religion or specific dogmatic practice. Reiki is considered to be a universal practice that, once trained, any individual can use to help themselves or others. The symbol for Reiki is two Japanese *kanji*, one over the other: the top representing Rei, the bottom, Ki (see **FIGURE 15.2**).

The International Center for Reiki Training (ICRT) describes the practice of Reiki as a Japanese technique for

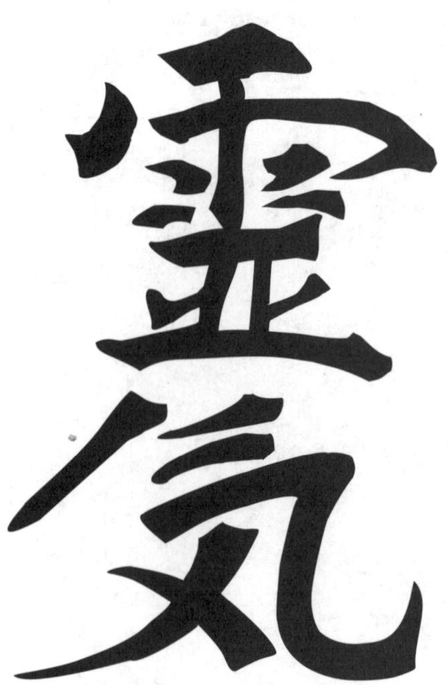

FIGURE 15.2 Japanese Reiki character.

stress reduction and relaxation that also promotes healing.[13] Like other Eastern philosophy techniques, Reiki focuses on chi, the life force energy. It is this energy that causes us to be alive. ICRT summarizes the notion by stating, "If one's life force energy is low, then we are more likely to get sick or feel stress, and if it is high, we are more capable of being happy and healthy."

The exact history of Reiki involves some uncertainty. According to Tanmaya Honervogt, in her book *The Power of Reiki*, the development of Reiki is attributed to a Japanese professor, Dr. Mikao Usui, who left a faculty position to search for the secrets behind the healing and miracles of Jesus Christ.[11] On his journey, which included an extended stay at a Buddhist monastery, Usui was meditating upon a mountain. During that meditation, he was given the power of healing. Although he was able to assist others in their physical healing, he didn't feel as though he was helping people change their lives, and from this notion he created the Reiki rules for life, or the Reiki Principles (see **BOX 15.3**). He also discovered that the desire to be healthy was not by itself enough for healing to occur. A person must *ask* for healing, and one must *give* something in return. The history presents a challenge in that all records of the "lineage" of Reiki were destroyed in World War II, and it has now become more like folklore than fact.

The Principles were written to help people understand that you must make a conscious decision to improve oneself, and accept responsibility for your healing, for the process to have lasting results.

Reiki came to the United States after World War II through a Reiki master named Hawayo Takata. She carried on the practice of Reiki in the United States, and began training new masters in 1975. Before her death in 1980, she had trained 22 new masters. Reiki healers are not trained in a school, but rather have the art passed on to them from another master. Today one can find Reiki practitioners all over the world.

The Reiki practitioner is said to serve as a channel for life force energy. A relatively simple concept, the practitioner uses their hands to transmit life force energy to the ill. The ICRT Web site describes the experience as "a wonderful glowing radiance that flows through and around you ... including body, emotions, mind and spirit, creating many beneficial effects that include relaxation and feelings of peace, security and wellbeing."[13]

Box 15.3

The Original Reiki Principles

Just for today, be free and happy.

Just for today, have joy.

Just for today, you are taken care of.

Live consciously in the moment.

Count your blessings with gratitude.

Honor your parents, teachers, and elders.

Earn your living honestly.

Love your neighbor as yourself.

Show gratitude to all living things.

Source: From B. Muller and H. Gunther, *A Complete Book of Reiki Healing*.[14]

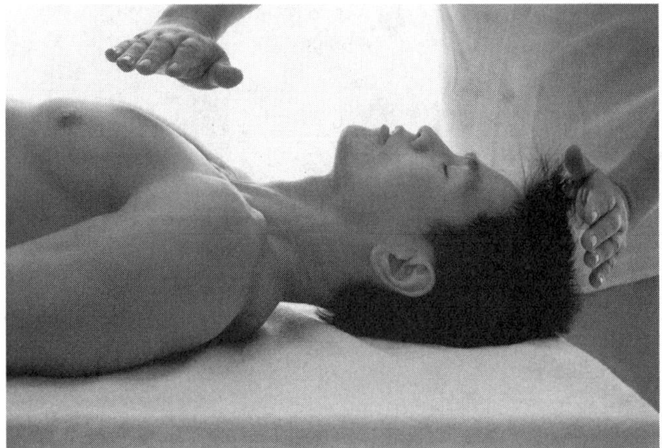

Reiki healing

REIKI SYMBOLS

Reiki symbols (shown in **TABLE 15.1**) are used through movement of the center of the palm or the fingers, through a visualization of the symbol, or by spelling the symbol name three times. Whichever method of activation is used, it is done over an energy center or the ailing component of the recipient of services. Symbols and *mantras* (words spoken internally that represent the symbols) are used during the healing process to create vibration. Vibration creates and accesses energy. The first symbol activates available energy. The second symbol adds peace and harmony, the third is for intuition, the fourth for healing and restoring the flow of energy, and the final symbol, used only by Reiki masters, opens one to a higher energy.[12,p40]

The Concept of Attunement

The process of using Reiki as a healing modality, or of using Reiki on another person, begins with attunement. Attunement is the ceremony of initiation to the force of energy, and is the precursor to an individual becoming a practitioner. The

Table 15.1
The Symbols

SYMBOL NAME	ALIAS	SYMBOL	USE
Cho Ku Ray (choh-koo-ray)	The Power Symbol		Increases power by drawing energy from the surrounding area
Sei Hei Ki (say-hay-key)	The Mental/Emotional Symbol	2 1 3 4	Mental, emotional healing; calming the mind; balance
HonSha Ze Sho Nen (Hanh-shah-zay-show-nen)	The Distance Symbol		Sends Reiki over distance and time (past, present, future), to anyone and anything
Tam-a-Ra-Sha (Tam-ara-sha)	The Balancing Factor		Grounds and balances energy; unblocks chakra centers
Dai Ko Myo (dye-ko-me-o)	The Master Symbol	1 2	Most powerful symbol; used only by Reiki masters; heals the soul

Source: Adapted from reiki-for-holistic-health.com.

student receives this energy, or attunement, from a master, opening up the chakras and channels to allow the energy to flow through the body. Energy is released through the hands, and once "attuned," a student can then use the energy on another person. The energy never leaves you once your channels are opened.[14]

Reiki Degrees

Reiki practitioners can progress through three levels of training, or degrees. The first degree, and most basic, contains the initial attunements, opening up the energy channels for transmission of energy to another person (or animal, see **BOX 15.4**). According to Potter, the energy will go where it is needed, so there need not be any specific placement of the hands.[15] The Reiki practitioner could rest his or her hands on the patient's hands, and the energy flow would make its way from the practitioner, through the patient's hands, and continue through the patient's body until it reaches the area of need. All hand placements for healing physical ailments are trained at level one. A second-degree Reiki practitioner integrates symbolism into the healing process. At this level, the practitioner has been further trained in the placement of hands for the purpose of healing the nonphysical realm, in deep emotional and mental healing, and in sending energy over distance. The third degree, or Reiki master, is studied when one is ready to lead a life of healing. The Reiki master training is much more personalized, with mastery of the Reiki symbols the focus. The Reiki master is expected to then train new practitioners, passing along skills and attunements.

> **Box 15.4**
>
> **It's Not Just for Humans**
>
> One of the fastest growing areas for the use of Reiki is in the animal kingdom. Reiki masters are using their training to heal pets, farm animals, and show animals. A 2004 article in *Farmer's Weekly* discusses a Reiki master who has established a training facility to help horse owners learn to better care for their animals.[16] She states that practicing Reiki on horses can reduce negative habits, like spooking, and other ailments with emotional roots. A doggie spa in Hollywood, California, offers Reiki to injured or hurting animals, with scores of happy pets and pet owners as the end result. A 2008 *New Straits Times* article references the use of Reiki in distant healing in an area of Kuala Lampur.[17] Here, when animals get sick they tend to be abandoned. Distant healing practices help the pet owners keep their animals healthy and in the home. And in New Mexico, a local Reiki healer works with family pets to ease anxiety and fear in the animals, helping them to be more pleasant and cope with being in a home with more success.[18]
>
> Most of the pet owners, and even some of the practitioners, cannot fully describe what is at work. Skeptics will say it is simply the one-on-one attention the pet receives—something the owner should be doing anyway. Believers in Reiki will reinforce the tenets of healing and the ability of energy to be focused for the good of the animal. Most pet owners simply know that their animal is more calm, less noisy in many cases, and, overall, better behaved.

WHAT IS THERAPEUTIC TOUCH?

Therapeutic touch, in practice, is much like Reiki. An individual unfamiliar with either practice would not be able to distinguish them, with the notable exception that therapeutic touch does *not* involve touch (in most instances). Reiki, in most cases, involves actual placement of the hands on the recipient. Other distinctions between the two are found primarily in philosophy, history, and training. The actual art of laying on of hands and healing through touch is almost as old as mankind. It is described in virtually every history or spiritual practice available. Therapeutic touch's specific form, description, and function of healing was designed and introduced in the 1970s by a New York University nursing professor, Deloris Krieger.[19] Krieger took the ancient philosophies and designed a form of healing to be used by nurses in practice, although her vision was that anyone and everyone could be a healer.

Therapeutic touch is performed in four stages. The first of these stages, centering, is a form of meditation that allows the therapeutic touch practitioner to focus on their own

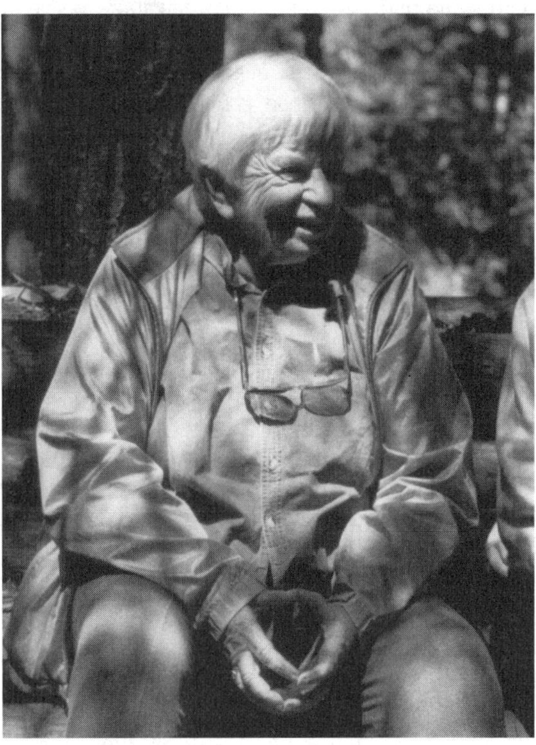

Deloris Krieger, designer of therapeutic touch

energy field in preparation for transmission to the patient. McCormack describes the necessity of the process, stating the importance of the healer working without judging the patient, and that doing so requires a clear mind.[19,p188] Once the practitioner is centered, an assessment of the energy surrounding the patient is performed. This stage is a clear distinction from Reiki practice. Assessment involves the passing of the healer's hands 2 to 6 inches away from the patient's body in an attempt to detect disruptions in energy flow or in the patient's energy field.[2] The practitioner will move their hands in a sweeping motion, palms facing the patient, attempting to sense a distinction in energy in moving from one place to the next.

In the third stage, unruffling, the objective is to "smooth out" the patient's energy field. Hands are moved in long sweeping strokes, much like one would use to smooth out a bed sheet while making a bed. This effort is designed to unruffle the energy field; allow for energy to flow in a positive, undisturbed fashion; and allow the patient to then heal more efficiently. The final stage is the treatment phase, sometimes referred to as modulation. In this final phase the practitioner uses stationary hand positions to direct energy to a specific location. This is said to transfer energy from the practitioner to the patient, correcting any further imbalance in the patient's energy field.[19,p189]

Recipients of therapeutic touch report a variety of outcomes, some positive, some not. In her 2004 article in *Nursing Standard*, Annie Hallett reported on seven cancer patients and their experience with therapeutic touch.[20] Reactions varied with some patients mentioning relaxation, peace, focus, or understanding. Others reported that the "clarity" they found actually brought back negative memories, or regrets, or what one patient described as his "demons."

WHAT RESEARCH EXISTS RELATED TO REIKI AND THERAPEUTIC TOUCH?

As you might imagine, therapy and medicine based on a mystical presence of energy surrounding the human body is likely to be criticized. Significant debate exists over whether there actually exists a field of energy surrounding the body. The manipulation of that energy, then, would seem even more debatable. Although proponents of energy therapies say there is proof of the human energy field, demonstrated for instance with Kirlian photography, others believe such techniques are not measuring a "manipulatable" field of energy. Nonetheless, significant published research exists. Ann Marie McClintock (Reiki) and Guy McCormack (therapeutic touch), in *Complementary Therapies and Wellness* (2003), discuss the myriad of research outcomes related to the use of energy therapies.[19,21] Both note that few rigorous studies (by Western medical standards) have been conducted related to practice, and that the evidence presented demonstrating positive effect ranges from purely anecdotal to research with rigor. Both also note that although criticized for a weak scientific approach, the vast majority of research shows some positive influence of the practice on illness, healing, sense of well-being, stress levels, and/or pain reduction, warranting further research. In summary, the research related to energy therapies indicates a significant reduction in the pain levels of cancer patients, a reduction in state anxiety, a reduction in blood pressure, and increases in immune system hormones and chronic disease improvements; however, there are also articles containing significant criticism of both practices.

Supporting Research

A study with one of the largest samples of recipients of therapeutic touch was published in 2003 in the journal *Holistic Nursing Practice*.[22] As part of a quality improvement process at a New York hospital, more than 600 recipients of therapeutic touch were surveyed and monitored. The results indicated patient satisfaction with the process and improvements in pain reduction, calmness, and overall well-being.

A 2003 Kumar and Kurup study reviewed the impact of Reiki and meditation practices on individuals with seizure disorders proving untreatable by other means.[23] The 15 people in the study participated in Reiki sessions over a 3-month period. In the end, participants showed significant positive changes to the imbalances in magnesium, tryptophan, tyrosine, dopamine, and norepinephrine, all of which were related to an increase in seizure frequency. All participants experienced a reduction in seizure frequency of at least 50 percent, with most experiencing a decrease of 75 percent (as an example, a drop from 12 seizures per month to 2).

A short-term 2006 study of 24 seniors, half of whom received four weekly Reiki treatments and half of whom did not, revealed small but nonstatistically significant improvements in the mental function of those involved in the study.[24] Participants, between 60 and 80 years of age, most commonly reported improvements on scales related to memory and depression. Short-term memory of recent events, recall of location of items, and concentration ability showed improvement. Emotional state improvements in degree of sadness, degree of worry, and measures of self-esteem were seen as well.

Stress reduction is often a desired impact in the practice of energy therapies. A 2004 study measured the influence of Reiki on several mechanisms in the autonomic nervous system, the component of the central nervous system responsible for initiating and disengaging the stress response.[25] The study found significant positive influences for the reduction of mean blood pressure, diastolic blood pressure (a reflection of the relaxation response), heart rate, frequency of respirations, and vagal tone (pre- and post-Reiki measurement). *Vagal tone* is the difference in the pace of the heartbeat when breathing in versus when breathing out. Heart rate normally increases during an inhalation and slows during an exhalation. A small difference in heart rate during inhalation and exhalation would indicate a weak or poor vagal tone, and a reflection of increased stress levels. Participating in an activity that increases the vagal tone would suggest the reduction of stress. It should be noted that differences were also significant when compared to a control group receiving no treatment. Interestingly, a placebo group (subjects believed they were receiving Reiki, but were not) also showed a pre/post-test improvement in several of the measured areas. Environmental stress has also been positively affected by Reiki. Baldwin and Schwartz compared the Reiki practice to a sham practice (people simply sitting next to the subject with their hands up and facing) and a control group, and found Reiki to be an effective tool in reducing the impact of white noise on systematic stress in laboratory animals.[26]

Some Examples Against

One of the more compelling pieces pointing to therapeutic touch as fraudulent is a 1998 article published in the *Journal of the American Medical Association*, featuring a study conducted by a sixth-grade student in Colorado.[27] The study asked 21 practitioners of therapeutic touch to show they could detect a human energy field. Practitioners sat at a table with their hands on the table, palms up. The researcher placed one of her own hands 3 to 4 inches above one of the practitioners' hands. The practitioner, with vision of the hands blocked, was to indicate which hand was covered. The practitioners were only able to correctly identify to researcher's hand placement 42 percent of the time, less than what would be expected by random guessing.

Reiki tenets also have been challenged in the literature. It is believed the Reiki practitioner is independent of the energy transmission process, and functions merely as a "go-between" in the healing process. One 2006 study found the practitioner's own energy field did have an impact on the healing and growth of *E. coli* cultures in a laboratory setting.[28]

A 2002 study again placed doubt on the legitimacy of a Reiki practitioner to accurately identify energy fields, or to have a significant effect on the health process for, in this case, stroke victims.[29] A Reiki master trained several hospital employees in Reiki, with only half going through full initiation, the process giving them the ability to be a healer. Results did not indicate a difference in treatment responses between fully initiated and fake Reiki healers, nor a difference in the new healers' ability to determine whether they had been fully initiated.

WHAT IS BIOELECTROMAGNETIC THERAPY?

As stated at the outset of the chapter, veritable (measurable) energy therapies use a predetermined wavelength and/or frequency to emit energy on a patient as a healing force.

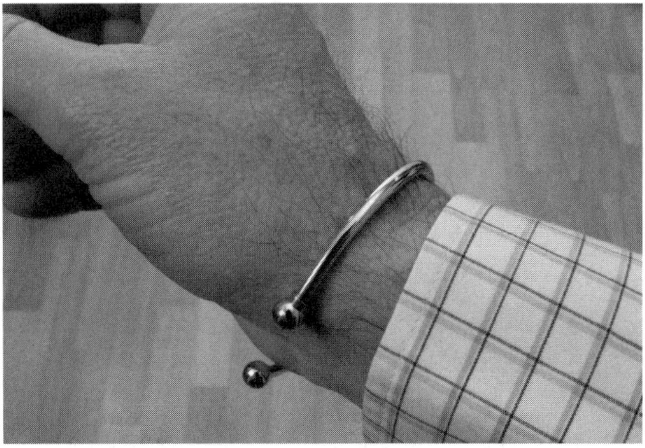

Healing magnet bracelet

Although light and sound therapies are included in this subcategory of energy therapies, magnet or magnetic therapies are the most commonly seen and most controversial of the group. The use of magnets for healing has occurred for centuries. The relationship between human energy and magnets became more popularized in the late 1700s when Franz Mesmer "demonstrated" his ability to use magnets to alter the human energy field.[30]

Magnets, Polarity, and Healing

If one accepts the concept that we each possess a human energy field, or biofield, as has been discussed throughout the chapter, then what is acknowledged is the existence of *universal polarity*. Consider a time in your childhood when you played with magnets. Magnets, you were told, had a north pole and a south pole. One end of the magnet attracted and one end repelled, and most kids figured out how to make one magnet spin by turning another magnet above it. The strength of the magnetic pull is called Gauss rating (see **BOX 15.5**).

The energy found in and around the human body, chi, is said to move because of the tension between polarities.[30,p95] Anderson explains the tension between opposing polarity "pulls" energy through the body, and keeps it in constant motion.[30] If illness is a disruption or blockage in the flow of energy, then the manipulation of polarity can return flow to normal. This is the basis of magnet therapy.

Research Related to Bioelectromagnetic Therapies

The majority of research on the use of magnets for health purposes is in the area of pain control. Ratterman, Secrest, Norwood, and Ch'ien report the literature claims related to magnetic therapy's impact on fibromyalgia, and chronic and soft tissue pain.[31] The group points out that research supporting the claims is sparse, and what exists is predominantly anecdotal. Of the seven pieces of research summarized in

Box 15.5

Gauss Ratings

The claim reads, "We have the most powerful magnets on the market today! 12,500 gauss! There is nothing better for your health, so buy yours now. Supplies are limited on this incredibly powerful magnet!" The key to the advertisement is the term "gauss."

Gauss is used to describe magnetic strength or power. In general, the term is used to answer the question, "How magnetic is it?" A typical consumer often believes that bigger is better. If 300 gauss is a good magnet, then 12,500 gauss must be awesome! When it comes to products for magnetic therapy, however, consumers should know that gauss ratings are only part of the story. You must also consider the size, weight, and material used for the magnet.[33]

An example of this is the Earth's magnetic field, which possesses a gauss rating of 0.5, compared to a refrigerator magnet, which has a gauss rating of about 8–10. Is the refrigerator magnet 50 times more powerful than the Earth? Well, no, of course not. Because it is not *just* about the gauss rating; it has to do with the size and mass of the Earth compared to the size and mass of the refrigerator magnet. A one-quarter-inch round iron magnet has the same gauss rating as a 12- by 12-inch iron plate. The gauss rating is based on the material, iron. The plate would be more powerful overall, because of its greater size, and would have a magnetic pull from a greater distance, as opposed to just right next to the magnet.

If you are interested in utilizing magnet therapy, don't be manipulated by claims like the one above. Most therapy-related magnets range from 300–3,000 gauss. When looking for products, be certain to investigate. Check the company's reputation, any business claims made by consumers, and cost. Use the gauss rating, but also review the size and mass of the magnet, its cost, and return policies if you experience no benefit from the therapy.

the article, six show a positive improvement on pain and/or fatigue, but all show deficiencies in study design.

Like the other energy therapies, some magnet therapy research also shows little to no benefit from the method. A stereotypical article of this nature is a 2002 study on the use of real magnets on individuals with carpal tunnel syndrome compared to sham magnets with no polarity.[32] Both groups showed improvement, but to a degree the authors attribute to no more than chance, or placebo effect. This is a common finding throughout the literature. The authors also mention the general lack of rigor and scientific merit in energy therapy research.

HOW SHOULD I CHOOSE AN ENERGY THERAPY?

A quick search of the Internet will identify thousands of people identifying themselves as therapists using energy-based techniques, and no less than 350,000 hits for a search on "healing magnet dealers." Like all alternative therapy practices, follow the basic guidelines from the NCCAM to protect yourself.[34]

- Keep your primary health care provider informed. Seek their recommendation for a practitioner in the type of healing you seek.
- List CAM practitioners and gather information about each before making your first visit. Read the research for use of a practice for your ailment.
- Ask the practitioner some basic questions: What are your credentials? How long have you been in practice? Where did you receive you training? What licenses or certifications do you have? What is your success rate? Can I talk to other clients of yours?
- Ask how much the treatment will cost. How many sessions of treatment would you need? Check to see whether your insurance will cover the cost.

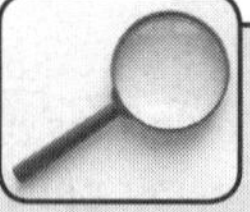

Case Study

Janine is a 47-year-old woman who recently has been struggling with her health. In the last 12 months, Janine has been feeling extremely fatigued. Continuous aching throughout her body compounds this sense of "tired." She has been to see her family practice doctor on several occasions, who first treated her for flu, then arthritis, but has now determined that the symptoms are too random and are therefore untreatable. She feels like she has been on every medication in the book. The pain for Janine has become almost unbearable. She has lost her job because she cannot make it through the day without taking breaks due to her tiredness and her pain. Money is getting tight in her family, and her husband is working extra to try and support Janine and their two children. She is starting to think that no one believes her, and that this is all in her head. She has even contemplated suicide, although she has no real desire to die, she just has had enough of the pain.

Questions:

1. What might Janine's issue be?
2. Which energy therapies discussed in this chapter, if any, have been shown, at some level, to assist with Janine's issue?
3. How might Janine go about determining whether an energy therapy, or a specific energy therapist, is right for her?

- Make a list of questions for the first visit, and come prepared to answer questions about your personal health history. Decide after the first visit if the practitioner is right for you. Did you feel comfortable with the practitioner? Could the practitioner answer your questions? Did he or she respond to you in a way that satisfied you? Does the treatment plan seem reasonable and acceptable to you?

CONCLUSION

Energy therapies are often considered some of the most controversial of alternative medical practices. The emphasis on the mental and spiritual aspects of healing leaves room for much debate over the actual physiological influences and what might be attributed to mere suggestion. Those who claim to have benefitted from these practices, as well as the growing number of practitioners in the realm of energy therapies, will continue to tout the advantages of taking part in mind-body-spirit modalities.

Review Questions

1. What is a veritable energy therapy?
2. What is a putative energy therapy?
3. For what ailments is qi gong potentially an appropriate therapy?
4. How do Reiki and therapeutic touch differ? Explain each difference.
5. Why might the mystic/spiritual component of touch therapies present a problem for researchers?
6. What is the theory behind the use of magnet therapy as an approach to healing?
7. What steps should a person take before committing to an alternative medical practitioner?

Key Terms

assessment A process in Reiki wherein the practitioner determines where and how the energy of the patient is moving.

attunement A Reiki right of passage where the ability to heal is passed on to a new Reiki practitioner from a Reiki master.

biofield The energy emitted from the human body.

channel In Reiki, the role of practitioner. Energy sent to the patient simply flows through the Reiki healer, who is the channel.

degrees, reiki Levels of advancement in the art of Reiki.

external qi gong Bodily movement related to the practice of qi gong.

form A series of predetermined and/or scripted movements designed to increase, unblock, or promote healing through the acquisition of energy (qi).

gauss rating The degree of magnetic strength based solely on materials used to construct the magnet.

internal qi gong A form of qi gong emphasizing breathing, meditation, and visualization.

magnet therapy The use of magnets on or around the human body to restructure the flow of energy in the human body for purposes of healing and well-being.

putative A type of energy that has yet to be effectively measured by science.

qi (chi) Life force energy. The centerpiece of energy therapies.

qi gong A type of energy therapy that uses gentle movement to access and redistribute energy surrounding and within the human body.

Reiki An energy therapy characterized by laying hands on an individual at specific locations, and the transfer of energy from the practitioner to the patient.

subtle energy Generic term used to describe all energy not easily or readily categorized by modern science.

therapeutic touch An energy therapy characterized by holding the hands several inches away from the patient, sending energy to the patient via the hands, in an effort to heal.

universal polarity Concept of all energy being influenced and moved by opposing polar magnetism.

unruffling In Reiki, the process of smoothing out energy fields surrounding the patient.

veritable A form of energy that can be measured scientifically.

References

1. National Center for Complementary and Alternative Medicine. What is CAM? February 2007. Available at: http://nccam.nih.gov. Accessed May 2009.
2. Warber SL, Kile G, Gillespie BW. "Energy" healing research. In: Jonas WB, Crawford CC, eds. *Healing, intention, and energy medicine*. Edinburgh: Churchill Livingstone; 2003: 83–102.
3. Qigong Association of America. February 5, 2008. Available at: http://www.qi.org. Accessed January 11, 2009.
4. Cohen KS. *The way of qigong: The art and science of Chinese energy healing*. New York: Random House; 1997.
5 Wudang Internal. The brief Qigong history. 2009. Available at: http://www.internalstyle.com. Accessed June 2010.
6. Kuei S, Comee S. *Beginning qigong: The ancient Chinese method of healing and strengthening the body, mind, and spirit*. Tokyo: Tuttle; 1993.
7. Johnson D. *Chinese soaring crane qigong*. Corvallis, OR: Qigong Association of America, 1997.
8. Yan X, Lu PY, Kiang JG. Qigong: basic science studies in biology. In: Jonas WB, Crawford CC, eds. *Healing, intention, and energy medicine*. Edinburgh: Churchill Livingstone; 2003:103–119.

9. Mayer M. Qigong clinical studies. In: Jonas WB, Crawford CC, eds. *Healing, intention, and energy medicine*. Edinburgh: Churchill Livingstone; 2003:121–137.
10. Chen KW, Hassett AL, Hou F, Staller J, Lightbroun AS. A pilot study of external qigong therapy for patients with fibromyalgia. *J Altern Complement Med*. 2006;12:851–856.
11. Sancier KM, Holman D. Multifaceted health benefits of medical qigong. *J Altern Complement Med*. 2004;10:163–166.
12. Honervogt T. *The power of Reiki*. London: Gaia; 1998.
13. International Center for Reiki Training. What is Reiki? Available at: http://www.reiki.org. Accessed March 20, 2010.
14. Muller B, Gunther H. *A complete book of Reiki healing*. Mendocino, CA: LifeRhythm USA; 1995.
15. Potter P. What are the distinctions between Reiki and therapeutic touch? *Clin J Oncol Nurs*. 2003;7(1):1–3.
16. Ellis S. Healing for your horse: find out the best therapy yourself. *Farmer's Weekly*. 140:21, 2004.
17. Farida M. Much cheaper way to heal pets. *New Strait Times*. June 21, 2008:7.
18. Swan B. Healing force. *Santa Fe New Mexican*. April 5, 2008:E4.
19. McCormack G. Noncontact therapeutic touch. In Carlson J, ed. *Complimentary therapies and wellness*. Upper Saddle River, NJ: Prentice Hall; 2003:186–213.
20. Hallett A. Narratives in therapeutic touch. *Nurs Stand*. 2004;19(1):33–37.
21. McClintock A. Reiki. In Carlson J, ed. *Complementary therapies and wellness*. Upper Saddle River, NJ: Prentice Hall; 2003: 214–231.
22. Newshan G, Schuller-Civitella D. Large clinical study shows value of therapeutic touch program. *Holist Nurs Pract*. 2003; 17(4):189–192.
23. Kumar R, Kurup PA. Changes in isoprenoid pathway with transcendental meditation and Reiki healing practices in seizure disorder. *Neurol India*. 2003;51:211–214.
24. Crawford SE, Leaver VW, Mahoney SD. Using Reiki to decrease memory and behavior problems in mild cognitive impairment and mild Alzheimer's disease. *J Altern Complement Med*. 2006;12:911–913.
25. Mackay N, Hansen S, McFarlane O. Autonomic nervous system changes during Reiki treatment: a preliminary study. *J Altern Compliment Med*. 2004;10:1077–1081.
26. Baldwin AL, Schwartz GE. Personal interaction with a Reiki practitioner decreases noise-induced microvascular damage in an animal model. *J Altern Complement Med*. 2006;12(1):15–22.
27. Rosa L, Rosa E, Sarner L, Barrett S. A close look at therapeutic touch. *JAMA*. 1998;279:1005–1010.
28. Rubik B, Brooks AJ, Schwartz GE. In vitro effect of Reiki treatment on bacterial cultures: role of experimental context and practitioner well being. *J Altern Complement Med*. 2006;12(1): 7–13.
29. Shiflett S, Nayak S, Bid C, Miles P, Agostinelli S. Effect of Reiki treatments on functional recovery in patients in poststroke rehabilitation: a pilot study. *J Altern Complement Med*. 2002;8:755–763.
30. Anderson E. Introduction to energy therapies. In Carlson J, ed. *Complementary therapies and wellness*. Upper Saddle River, NJ: Prentice Hall; 2003:92–99.
31. Ratterman R, Secrest J, Norwood B, Ch'ien AP. Magnet therapy: what's the attraction? *J Am Acad Nurse Pract*. 2002;14(7): 347–353.
32. Carter R, Hall T, Aspy CB, Mold J. The effectiveness of magnet therapy for treatment of wrist pain attributed to carpal tunnel syndrome. *J Fam Pract*. 2002;51(1):38–40.
33. Magnet Therapy Magnets.com. Measuring magnetic gauss. Available at: http://magnetictherapymagnets.com/gaussmeter Accessed May 1, 2010.
34. National Center for Complementary and Alternative Medicine. Selecting a complementary and alternative medicine practitioner. Available at: http://nccam.nih.gov/health/decisions/practitioner .htm. Accessed June 2009.

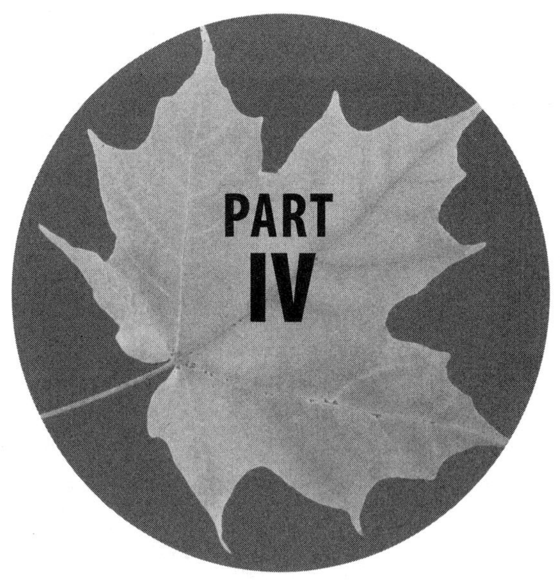

Avoidance of Scams and Costly Treatments That Don't Work

Frauds and Quackery

LEARNING OBJECTIVES

As a result of reading this chapter, students will:

1. Explain what separates conventional medicine from health quackery.
2. Describe the most common forms of consumer health fraud.
3. List guidelines for determining if a health practice is fraudulent.
4. Summarize the quackery of some modern-day scams.
5. Explain the reasons the nutrition market is particularly susceptible to health quackery.

WHAT IS HEALTH QUACKERY?

"Medical or health quackery is not a new problem in the United States. It has always flourished in the areas of disease where no cures had yet been found by legitimate medicine, or where treatment was long and perhaps painful. Quackery, indeed, flourishes because it promises cures, promises which are false, but which a man in pain, unhappy, or afraid would accept without question."[1]

—Congress on Medical Quackery, 1962

Because of the ease of access to health information today, and the skill and design of current advertising, it has become difficult to tell what really has the potential to aid the consumer in addressing personal health issues and what simply is nonsense. Some products have true value in the medical community . . . others do not. The National Council Against Health Fraud (NCAHF) says it is becoming more difficult for consumers to separate quality treatments from quackery, and so has identified five categories for assessing the legitimacy of alternative treatments[2]:

Scientific medicine: Established conventional or mainstream knowledge, based on standard methods of prevention, diagnosis, and treatment, reviewed by medical schools, research centers, professional organizations, professional journals, and governmental offices.

Investigational medicine: Approved for testing on consumers, but not yet fully approved for distribution—under investigation. Treatments are discontinued if they prove to be harmful, outmoded, or not useful.

Unproven treatments: Treatments of unknown value. Not yet proven worthless or effective.

Home or folk remedies: The NCAHF acknowledges that some folk remedies can be effective for very specific things, but are not a panacea for all disorders or illnesses, and should not be considered such. They also note some home remedies are bunk, and absolutely worthless.

Quackery: Treatments proven to have no benefit, or to improperly use conventional medicine. Generally, the claims made are unrealistic or phony.

You see quackery every day, but may not realize what you are looking at. You might be watching television, when an attractive woman appears on the screen and tells you she lost 50 pounds in 3 weeks with this new miracle weight loss drug. Perhaps you are reading a magazine, and somewhere in the final few pages you see an advertisement for a device that can do everything, from relieving arthritis pain, to easing nausea, to curing cancer. If you are a relatively healthy person who is not experiencing any major health issues at the moment, you most likely let those types of claims fade away without much thought. But if you were a consumer who was struggling to overcome the debilitating nature of arthritis, or were recently diagnosed with a terminal form of cancer, your reaction may be very different—and that is exactly what the advertising agency is hoping.

Cure-all's, quick fixes, and miracle drugs are promoted and practiced all the time. In the health arena, these are referred to as quackery. Quackery is defined in many different ways, but the central theme of all definitions is that it is the practice of deceit or trickery specifically confined to the medical field. In the eyes of the government and the law, it is a form of fraud. Most generally, an unskilled or ignorant health care practitioner searching for financial gain promotes the cure-all. In all cases, quackery preys on the unwell, sometimes desperate, individual who has tried and failed to address their health concern, sees no hope, and is now willing to do anything to find a cure.

WHAT IS A HEALTH QUACK?

If "quackery" is the practice of medical fraud or medical deceit, then the person promoting that practice is the "quack." The *Merriam-Webster* dictionary defines a quack as a "charlatan, or pretender of medical skill."[3] The term originated in the 1600s as *quacksalver*:

> A physician of the time by the name of Paracelsus [see **FIGURE 16.1**] seems to be the first physician "lucky" enough to be labeled a *quack*. He made a salve that had a bit of mercury in it. He massaged it into a patient's syphilitic rash, and the rash went away. Other physicians of the time claimed that the rash did not go away but went further and deeper into the patient's body. They called him a quack for using *quacksalber*.[4]

In the health arena, anyone who offers false hope of recovery or elimination of a health care concern through practices, techniques, or use of equipment that has no real chance of resolving the health condition is called a quack. The National Council Against Health Fraud states a quack is "Anyone who promotes health schemes and remedies known to be false, or which are unproven, for a profit."[5]

Financial gain may indeed be a motive for promoting worthless health products. The individuals who do this are deceitful and manipulative, preying on the vulnerabilities of sick people. But not all quacks are outright, or even intentionally, deceitful. Many believe very strongly in their cause (see Box 16.1), and have developed their opinions through time and personal experience, or through their interpretation of existing research. They are educated and many times respected by their peers, and at some point their perspective alters from the mainstream medical community. This is when the great debate begins: Are they crazy, or have they gained insight into something others have missed? Traditional medical practitioners, who want to see practices tested and researched thoroughly before they are promoted to the public, will dismiss these ideas as quackery. Consumers who are willing to experiment, or who have tried all other approaches and failed, may very well become immediate believers. Health professionals committed to protecting the latter group, the susceptible and vulnerable, will fight vehemently to protect the consumer.

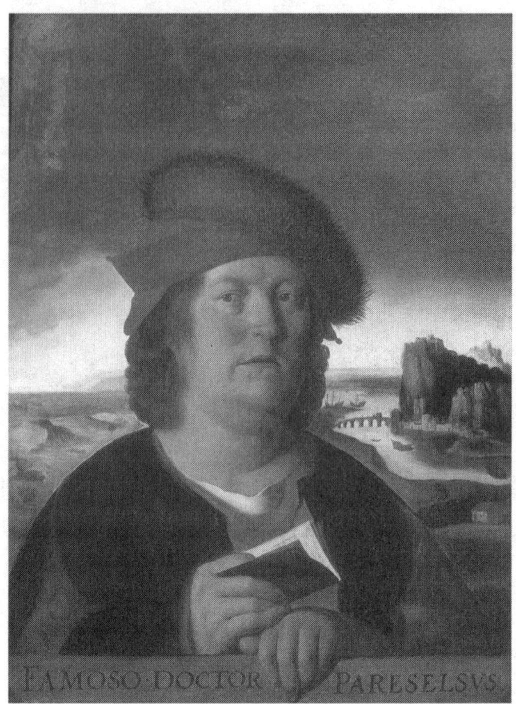

FIGURE 16.1 Paracelsus

WHAT ARE THE MOST COMMON TYPES OF HEALTH FRAUD TODAY?

Clearly, quackery or health fraud is not a new phenomenon. In fact, according to Medical World News, quack products or treatments are a multi-billion-dollar per year industry in the United States.[6] The Food and Drug Administration estimates that 38 million Americans have used a fraudulent health product within the past year, with 1 out of 10 people who try quack remedies harmed by side effects.[7] The Internet explosion of the last 15 years has created a new and simple method for scam artists and quacks to take advantage of the general public.

A review of the May 2009 *Consumer Health Information*[8] from the FDA points to the following as the most common fraudulent health claims:

Cancer fraud: The Hoxsey Cancer Treatment is an herbal procedure that promises to draw cancer out from the skin. The FDA has issued specific warnings against the treatment (see **FIGURE 16.2**). Black salves are marketed as having a similar effect. Neither has been shown to have any benefit and can be corrosive to tissues.

Box 16.1
Immunizations and Autism

In 1998, British researcher Andrew Wakefield published what was then a landmark paper in *The Lancet*, a highly respected medical journal. In essence, the article drew a link between children who received vaccination (specifically the measles, mumps, rubella vaccine) and an increase in the likelihood of developing autism. Since that time, great debate has been held regarding the findings in that study. It was criticized highly for the small number of children actually studied (12) and the associations and conclusions drawn.

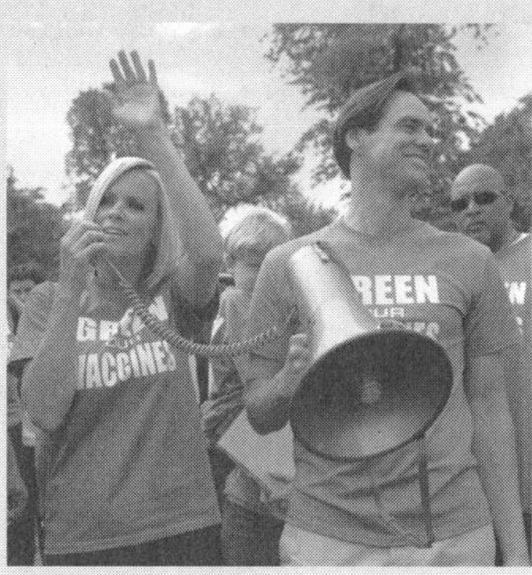

As is the case with many "causes," celebrity support and use of public forums became increasingly visible as performers such as Jenny McCarthy, Jim Carrey, and Holly Robinson Peete called for parents to reconsider vaccinating their children. They claim vaccines are simply promoted for making money (conspiracy theory) and that our children are paying a significant price because of the volume and timing of all the shots. They have been successful, because the number of parents choosing not to vaccinate has been growing over the last decade.

However, there is an issue with this. Since the original Wakefield publication, more than half of the co-authors have distanced themselves from the work, or dismissed it completely. Almost 15 independent studies have been conducted since then, none of which shows any link between vaccination and autism. It appears a conflict of interest may have been at hand, because Wakefield was paid over $600,000 to conduct the study by a lawyer looking to sue the pharmaceutical companies. And then in late 2010, it came to light that Wakefield had actually doctored the research, falsifying information to fit the needs of the study.

The primary damage here is to the children. Although all the anti-vaccine promotion work is done in good faith, in a perceived effort to help children, it may in fact be hurting them. The reality is that parents are delaying or neglecting important vaccinations for serious illnesses, raising the susceptibility of their children to these diseases. And because a growing number of children are going unvaccinated, all other children are at risk of exposure as well.

Public Beware!

WARNING AGAINST THE HOXSEY CANCER TREATMENT

Sufferers from cancer, their families, physicians, and all concerned with the care of cancer patients are hereby advised and warned that the Hoxsey treatment for internal cancer has been found worthless by two Federal courts.

The Hoxsey treatment costs $400, plus $60 in additional fees—expenditures which will yield nothing of value in the care of cancer. It consists essentially of simple drugs which are worthless for treating cancer.

The Food and Drug Administration conducted a thorough investigation of the Hoxsey treatment and the cases which were claimed to be cured. Not a single verified cure of internal cancer by this treatment has been found.

Those afflicted with cancer are warned not to be misled by the false promise that the Hoxsey cancer treatment will cure or alleviate their condition. Cancer can be cured only through surgery or radiation. Death from cancer is inevitable when cancer patients fail to obtain proper medical treatment because of the lure of a painless cure "without the use of surgery, x-ray, or radium" as claimed by Hoxsey.

Anyone planning to try this treatment should get the facts about it.

For further information write to:
U. S. DEPARTMENT OF HEALTH, EDUCATION, AND WELFARE
Food and Drug Administration
Washington 25, D. C.

FIGURE 16.2 Announcement issued by the FDA regarding the Hoxsey treatment.

HIV/AIDS fraud: Although treatments exist that can slow the progression of HIV, there is still no cure for the virus. Early initiation of the drug regimen for HIV is important, and experimentation with other products only delays the onset of using medicines demonstrated to have an effect. The FDA has approved only one at-home test device for HIV, called the Home Access HIV-1 Test System, which tests for HIV-1 (the cause of most cases) (see **FIGURE 16.3**).

Arthritis fraud: There are so many fraudulent arthritis cures marketed today that the U.S. Federal Trade Commission estimates Americans spend nearly $2 billion every year on them. But chronically pained consumers will keep trying to find something to relieve their discomfort. Some of the more common items claimed to cure arthritis are emu oil, colloidal silver, living water, snake venom, bee venom, and gin-soaked raisins. There currently is no proven, or consistently demonstrated, cure for arthritis.

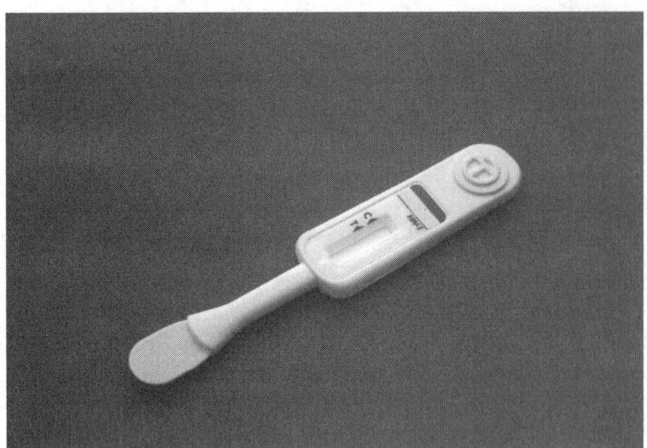

FIGURE 16.3 An at-home HIV test device.

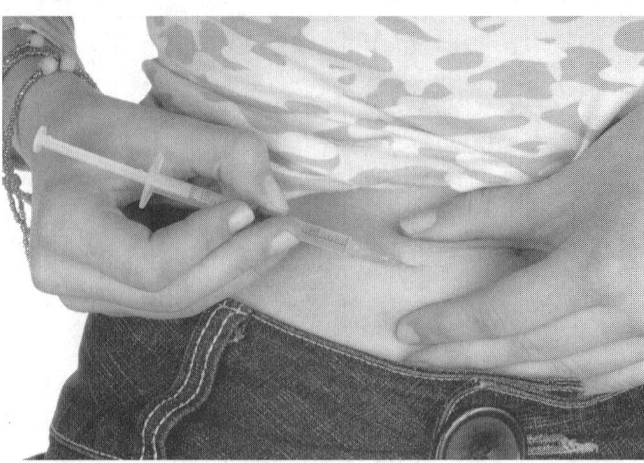

FIGURE 16.4 Questionable practices in weight loss include lipodissolve procedures.

Fraudulent "diagnostic" tests: Blood, saliva, or urine tests that your physician might normally request are used to assist in the detection of many things, such as pregnancy, cholesterol levels, hepatitis, HIV, and blood sugar levels. Unfortunately, there are sources who claim the tests can be used for much more significant purposes. If you are ever curious as to whether a diagnostic test is useful for a particular reason, contact the FDA.

Bogus dietary supplements: There are hundreds of nutritional supplements on the market, and just about as many wild claims regarding what they are good for. We can't even begin to list them all. Here is the best rule of thumb: do your homework. Read everything you can, speak to your physician, and get research and facts, not testimonials.

Weight loss fraud: A Calorie Control Council report indicated that dieting is a "constant concern" for more than 95 million Americans, and that on average dieters make four attempts per year to lose weight.[9] That leaves a lot of room for scam artists to promote their products to the general public. The FDA has worked hard to impose truth in advertising laws and to ensure that claims made by product developers are accurate. Most of what the consumer hears, however, is overblown and not typical of the true effect of the product.

Sexual enhancement product fraud: In 2009[10] the FDA released its latest warning regarding drugs promoted and sold online for treating erectile dysfunction and for enhancing sexual performance. Many of the products are contaminated with drugs that cannot be distributed legally without a prescription and drugs that can cause a significant decrease in blood pressure. One National Institutes of Health (NIH) study found that 77 percent of the sexual enhancement and erectile dysfunction drugs tested were contaminated and posed a serious risk to users.[11]

Diabetes fraud: The FDA has taken numerous compliance actions against sales of fraudulent diabetes "treatments" promoted with bogus claims such as "drop your blood sugar 50 points in 30 days," "eliminate insulin resistance," "prevent the development of type 2 diabetes," and "reduce or eliminate the need for diabetes drugs or insulin."

Influenza (flu) scams: Federal agencies have come across contaminated or counterfeit influenza products. Mostly sold through Internet spam, marketers seized on the 2009 scare when H1N1, or swine flu, hit the headlines. Most of the confiscated products claimed to be generic versions of Tamiflu, which is used to prevent influenza. The drugs, however, were mostly vitamin C and other substances, which have not been shown to treat or prevent influenza.

HOW DO I RECOGNIZE THE POTENTIAL FOR QUACKERY?

The key to success in protecting yourself is to make sure you do your homework on a particular practitioner or treatment modality. The old adage, "If it sounds too good to be true, it probably is," holds very true in this case. Ask questions, seek proof, and don't be convinced by wonderful testimonials. In its Healthy Aging Guide,[12] WebMD suggests you be concerned about an alternative therapy if the product or advertisement you are researching:

- Promises a quick or painless cure
- Claims its formula is secret or special and only available by mail or from one sponsor

- Claims to have the cure the medical community doesn't want you to know about
- Uses testimonials or undocumented case histories from satisfied patients
- Claims to be a cure for everything
- Claims to know how to cure a disease no one else understands (like HIV or cancer)
- Offers an additional "free" gift or a larger amount of the product as a "special promotion"
- Requires advance payment and claims limited availability of the product

It takes only a moment of consideration to see why a product making these claims is most likely untrue. Why would someone have a cure for cancer and not be using it to provide comfort to the millions suffering from the disease? Why would someone have the cure for AIDS and not help people who were HIV positive? Although the medical community may not be perfect, it is unreasonable to think they are evil and would knowingly withhold a potential cure to a major illness.

WHAT CAN I DO IF I FEEL I HAVE BEEN DUPED?

The reality of the situation is that consumers are responsible for their own susceptibility to quackery, which means that you are also responsible for protecting yourself (see *caveat emptor*, discussed in Chapter 2). The Food and Drug Administration lists the following "red flags" regarding health products fraud.[13] You should be concerned if a product or device:

- Claims to be a quick, effective cure-all or a diagnostic tool for a wide variety of ailments
- Suggests that it can treat or cure all diseases
- Promotes itself using words such as "scientific breakthrough," "miraculous cure," "secret ingredient," and "ancient remedy"
- Has descriptive text with impressive-sounding terms such as "hunger stimulation point" and "thermogenesis" for a weight loss product
- Cites undocumented case histories by consumers or doctors claiming amazing results
- Has limited availability and advance payment requirements
- Promises a no-risk, money-back guarantee
- Promises an "easy" fix
- Claims that the product is "natural" or "nontoxic" (which doesn't necessarily mean safe)

Sometimes, it can be challenging to determine if a product or service is legitimate. If you have concerns about a product, device, or service, you can and should file a complaint. If your complaint is about a product that is mislabeled or misrepresented or that you believe might be harmful to those who use it, contact the U.S. Food and Drug Administration or the Federal Trade Commission.

U.S. Food and Drug Administration
Consumer Information
10903 New Hampshire Ave
Silver Spring, MD 20993
1-888-INFO-FDA

Federal Trade Commission
Bureau of Consumer Affairs
600 Pennsylvania Ave NW
Washington, DC 20580
1-877-FTC-HELP

One additional place to begin might be your state's attorney or attorney general's office. That state division will have a mechanism for registering consumer complaints. Check your phone book or search the Internet for your state's governmental Web site. Depending on the product or device you are concerned about, there are a multitude of organizations that might also be able to assist you. Check Chapter 18 for details.

WHAT ARE EXAMPLES OF RECENT QUACKS AND THEIR QUACKERY?

There are many, many examples of entrepreneurial individuals who used quackery to make fortunes, even though their approaches were at some point determined to be completely bogus. Some recent examples include Wilhelm Reich, Mylan Brych, Hulda Clark, and Ruth Drown.

Dr. Wilhem Reich was a psychiatrist in the 1950s who promoted a product called the Orgone Energy Accumulator.[14] Orgone, according to Reich, was a gas undetected by science, yet it permeated all things in life. Orgone was the central life force, also responsible for the creation of the universe and gravity. Reich told people they could harness this energy and, because it was the most prominent source of energy, they could heal any illness known to man. The Accumulator was essentially a box, sat in by the participant, made of celetex and a steel interior. The individual, according to Reich, would soak up the orgone energy and relieve illness or symptoms related to illness. Even though it is unmeasurable, the notion of a "central life force" is believed in by millions in the world, and most likely not a cause for concern with this gadgetry. The Accumulator itself, however, could not be verified to perform as it claimed.

The FDA pursued Reich, and eventually he was arrested for fraud and jailed in 1957, where he died that same year. However, Reich's believers carry on his work still today, promoting products such as discs, pendants, and modules. Each is described as having the power to harness the universal life force, thus balancing the individual and making them healthier.

Mylan Brych was a Czechoslovakian-born immigrant in New Zealand in the 1970s when his claims for curing cancer[15] first surfaced. Brych was injecting patients with a serum (later determined to be some combination of steroids and chemotherapeutic chemicals), and some were showing positive results. It was soon determined, however, that Brych was not a doctor, or even trained as one, and so he fled from New Zealand authorities to practice in the Cook Islands—a location where the president welcomed him. Eventually the president was removed from office and Brych again fled, this time to the United States where he continued his practice. Brych was arrested in California for practicing medicine without a license and offering a phony cure to cancer sufferers. He was sentenced to 6 years in jail.

Hulda Clark ran the Century Nutrition clinic[16] in Tijuana, Mexico until her death in 2009. Dr. Clark (she obtained a PhD in zoology from the University of Minnesota) was the inventor of several devices designed to electrocute pathogens. Her premise was that parasites or pollutants caused all disease. Once parasites were in the system, electrical current could destroy them. Her primary invention[17] was called, appropriately enough, the Zapper. The Zapper provided an electrical current designed to kill parasites, and as such, Clark claimed to be able to cure cancer, HIV,[18] and any other disorder caused by "parasite." She also invented the Syncrometer, which was said to be able to measure the frequency of any disease or organ, much like tuning a radio. If you found the correct frequency, you could adjust the Syncrometer to that wavelength, and send the charge directly to where the impulse was needed. This allowed her to cure anything. The mainstream medical community dismissed much of the treatment practice of Clark. However, her practice remained open until just before her passing in 2009.

In the 1930s, Ruth Drown was a promoter of the notion that radionics[19] was the solution to health problems. Drown's Therapeutic Machine[20] was said to be able to access etheric Life Force energy that, when directed though a photographic plate, could produce photographs of tissue found anywhere in the body. The machine required just a dried drop of the patient's blood on a piece of blotter paper. Her techniques, like a few before her, measured the vibration rate of a patient's illness, because it was believed that each organ and each illness produced its own degree of vibration. In 1935, Drown created Radio-Vision;[21] according to Drown, diagnosis with this device did not even require the patient's presence because radio waves travel over distance.

Again, mainstream medical professionals pronounced her work quackery and her inventions useless. Drown's followers of natural healing, however, still believe quite strongly in her philosophies. Natural healing is based in metaphysics, and Drown's followers view auras and orgone energy as acceptable because in metaphysics all existence has a mathematical foundation. Drown was eventually targeted by authorities in the state of California, and after a 1963 sting operation[22] set up by the State Department of Public Health, was arrested with all her staff and charged with fraud. She died in 1965 awaiting trial.

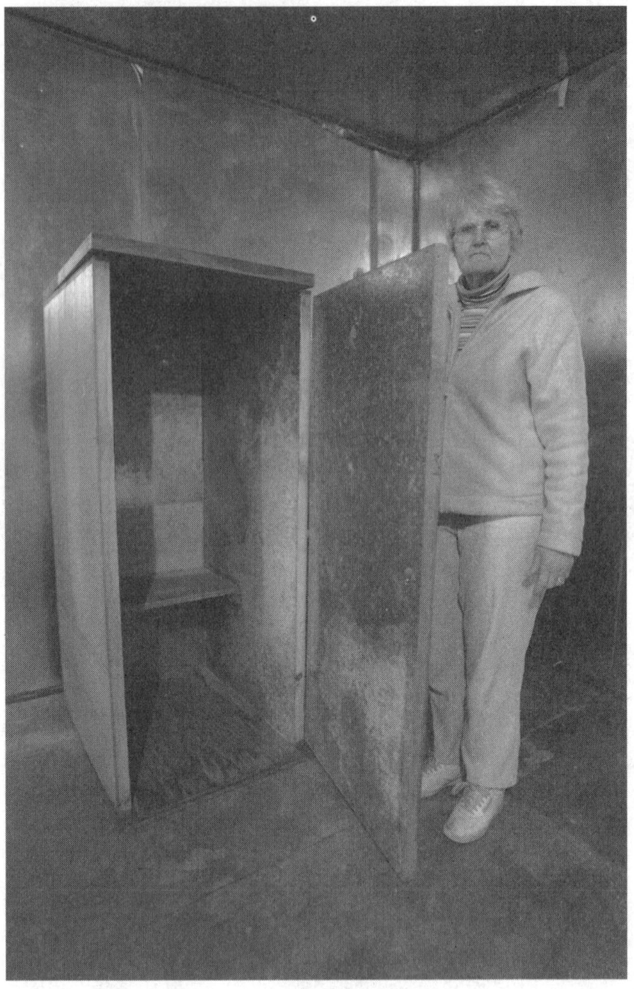

Products found online or over the counter at your local retailer are not immune from quackery. A quick search on the Internet finds a product called a "sport energy band." This product has been growing in popularity as more and more professional athletes are seen wearing them. One Web site tells the consumer that this silicone wristband (which also comes as a pendant or in neoprene!) works with your body's natural energy flow to increase strength, balance, and coordination.[23] The site then list testimonials from dozens of professional athletes supporting the use of the band. The issue here is there is no science presented, and frankly, none exists, that can demonstrate this band has any biological or energy effect on the body. They sell because they are popular.

There also are hundreds of dietary products on the market that are purely gimmicks. Remember, you should always be cautious when a diet claims to have some unique ingredient unknown to science, or has a system and formula the "experts" don't want you to know about. That is usually a clear sign of fraud. One example is the Blood Type Diet. The diet's creator, a naturopathic healer, has posited that one's blood type should dictate one's diet.[24] Again, the diet became popular when promoted by movie stars and athletes who claimed the diet returned their body to its best shape ever. This diet suggests that your blood type is responsible for a specific immunity and digestive function. Because of this, each of the four blood types has a different dietary pattern to follow. However, like all diets and weight loss schemes, if you read far enough into the material, you'll see the indications that not all people respond positively to the diet designed for their blood type. However, you will find substantial opportunities to spend hundreds or thousands of dollars on products designed to help you determine if the diet is best for you.

Many products marketed as dietary supplements are available to consumers. Because dietary supplements are not regulated by the FDA (in fact, all dietary supplement product packaging must contain a disclaimer stating that the FDA has not evaluated the product claims) it is a wide open market for promotion to the consumer. Consumers should be cautious when choosing supplement products, whether buying them over the counter or online. In December 2010, the FDA issued a statement[25] disclosing that many dietary supplements are tainted with ingredients either not listed on the labels or with drugs that require a prescription. In some cases, the products contained ingredients that had been removed from the consumer market due to dangers posed by their consumption. Some of these products were designed for weight loss, others were marketed as supplements for sexual performance or enhancement, and still others were supplements for bodybuilding. The FDA warns consumers to avoid products that claim to work just like prescription drugs, or that claim to contain "legal" alternatives to banned drugs.

IS THERE QUACKERY IN THE NUTRITION INDUSTRY?

Simply stated, people who are overweight make an easy target. According to a report from the Centers for Disease Control and Prevention,[26] 34 percent of Americans are obese and two in every three Americans are classified as overweight. That is approximately 151 million U.S. adults. Essentially, this creates a tremendous market of consumers looking for a quick solution to their weight issues. When you have a society obsessed with weight, and over 150 million people looking for an easy way to accomplish weight loss, it becomes a simple task for quacks and hucksters to promote the "next greatest weight loss product."

It is evident, as well, that Americans are buying. In 2009, there were an estimated 72 million Americans on some type of diet.[27] The estimate for spending by Americans on weight loss products was over $60 million that same year. So what are people doing? Currently, the low-carb diet plans are very popular. This includes diets such as the Atkins Diet, the South Beach Diet, and the Zone. Commercial weight loss companies, such as Weight Watchers and Jenny Craig, are still relatively popular as well, used by almost 7 million consumers in 2008. Marketdata, Inc. estimates that 3–5 million people use meal replacement products. Even with all of these options, the obesity rates in the United States have not changed significantly in nearly a decade.

When reviewing weight loss options, consumers can protect themselves by assessing a diet in five ways.[28] First, does the diet suggest you make significant calorie reductions? Reducing the calories you consume is a common element of diets, but drastic reductions (800- to 1000-calorie diets, or less) are counterproductive. Second, diets that require special pills or powders are usually gimmicks, and will not produce long-term weight loss. In addition, since 2008 the FDA has identified more than 70 weight loss products that have undisclosed components in them, posing serious health risks to the consumer.[14] Third, there is no scientific support for a single food or combinations of foods being the "key" to successful weight loss. If a product makes this claim, you are safe to reject it. Fourth, diets that completely eliminate everything from a single food group have not demonstrated long-term weight loss success. You may see short-term success, but this is more likely due to calorie reductions or reductions in water weight. Once you return to a regular diet, the weight will return. And finally, diets that require you to skip meals will not produce long-term weight loss.

CONCLUSION

This chapter presented some of the more notable quacks and quackery found in the health care arena over the past century. Certainly there are many more. Consumers need to remain active in their investigation of treatment options as to not be fooled into utilizing bogus physicians and products when real health care issues need to be addressed.

Review Questions

1. Why has quackery always been a part of the medical community?
2. What makes quackery hard to distinguish from more readily accepted forms of treatment?
3. What are the five types of treatments, as defined by the National Council Against Health Fraud?
4. Define "quack." Are quacks always liars and cheats?
5. What are the most common forms of health fraud according to the Food and Drug Administration?
6. What is the most common concern regarding sexual enhancement products?

7. What types of claims should the consumer be careful about when looking into a potential treatment option?
8. Identify some of the claims fraudulent products make to the consumer.
9. What should a consumer do if they feel they would like to file a complaint about a product or service?
10. Describe some of the more recent attempts to deceive the public regarding medical treatment.
11. Why is nutrition a popular area for medical quackery?

Suggestions for Class Activities

This chapter contains the list of "red flags" for quack product endorsement provided by the Food and Drug Administration. This activity will give you a chance to critically review advertising found on the Internet.

1. Locate the following four items:
   - A Web page marketing an herbal supplement
   - A Web page marketing a sexual enhancement product
   - A Web page marketing an arthritis drug or technique
   - A Web page marketing a nonstandard cancer treatment
2. Using the red flags, determine how likely the product is to be legitimate. Provide a written explanation for each item you believe may be deceptive in nature, and why you believe this to be true.
3. For *one* of the Web sites you identified, create a mock letter to the U.S. Food and Drug Administration explaining your concerns, and what you believe ought to be done about the issue.

Key Terms

attorney general The principal legal officer who represents a state in legal proceedings and gives legal advice to the government.

autism A mental condition, present from early childhood, characterized by great difficulty in communicating and forming relationships, and in using language and abstract concepts.

deceit Concealment or distortion of the truth for the purpose of misleading.

erectile dysfunction Difficulty in achieving or maintaining an erection; impotence.

Food and Drug Administration A division of the Department of Health and Human Services that protects the public against impure and unsafe foods, drugs, and cosmetics.

fraud Trickery, unethical practice, or breach of confidence, perpetrated for profit or to gain some unfair or dishonest advantage.

naturopathic A system or method of treating disease that employs no surgery or synthetic drugs but uses special diets, herbs, vitamins, massage, and the like to assist the natural healing processes.

orgone A vital, primal, nonmaterial element believed to permeate the universe.

Orgone Energy Accumulator A cabinet-like device constructed of layers of wood and other materials, claimed by its inventor, Wilhelm Reich, to restore orgone energy to persons sitting in it, thereby aiding in the cure of impotence, cancer, the common cold, and other ailments. Also called an orgone box.

quack A person who admits, professionally or publicly, to skill, knowledge, or qualifications he or she does not possess.

quackery The practice of deceit or trickery specifically confined to the medical field.

radionics A dowsing technique using a pendulum to detect energy fields emitted by all forms of matter.

scam A confidence game or other fraudulent scheme, especially for making a quick profit.

Tamiflu An oral antiviral drug that attacks the influenza virus and prevents it spreading inside the body.

traditional medical practitioner A medical doctor practicing under a Western, pharmaceutical-based philosophy.

truth in advertising Laws designed to compel advertisers to give accurate, forthright information regarding products, services, and anticipated outcomes.

Zapper A machine created by Hulda Clark that delivers energy to the body in an effort to cure a myriad of illnesses and diseases.

References

1. Congress on Medical Quackery: Conference Report. *Publ Health Rep*. 1962;77(5):453–455.
2. Doctors Corner Internet Group. Medical quackery. 2004. Available at: http://your-doctor.com/patient_info/alternative_remedies/various_therapy/quackery.html. Accessed December 12, 2010.
3. Merriam-Webster. Quack. Available at: http://www.merriam-webster.com/dictionary/quack. Accessed July 22, 2011.
4. Minnesota Wellness Publications. The history of quackery. 2009. Available at: http://www.mnwelldir.org/docs/history/quackery.htm. Accessed December 11, 2010.
5. National Council Against Health Fraud. Quackery-related definitions. 2001. Available at: http://www.ncahf.org/pp/definitions.html. Accessed December 2, 2010.

6. Hughes EF. Overview of complementary, alternative, and integrative medicine. *Clin Obstet Gynecol.* 2001;44(4):774–779.
7. Food and Drug Administration. Top 10 health frauds. *FDA Consumer*. May 12, 2009.
8. U.S. Food and Drug Administration. FDA101: health fraud awareness. May 2009. Available at: http://www.fda.gov/ForConsumers/ProtectYourself/HealthFraud/default.htm. Accessed December 2, 2010.
9. Calorie Control Council. Majority of Americans think about dieting year-round; number of dieting attempts on the rise—new survey reveals dieting a constant concern. 2007. Available at: http://www.sucralose.org/latest/release_20080201.asp. Accessed December 15, 2010.
10. U.S. Food and Drug Administration. FDA warns consumers on sexual enhancement products: another dietary supplement is found to be contaminated with potentially dangerous ingredient. November 2009. Available at: http://www.fda.gov/NewsEvents/Newsroom/PressAnnouncements/2009/ucm189295.htm. Accessed December 10, 2010.
11. Low MY, Zeng Y, Li L, et al. Safety and quality assessment of 175 illegal sexual enhancement products seized in red-light districts in Singapore. *Drug Saf.* 2009;32(12):1141–1146.
12. National Institute on Aging, U.S. Department of Health and Human Services. Health quackery: spotting health scams. 2005. Available at: http://www.webmd.com/healthy-aging/guide/health-quackery-spotting-health-scams. Accessed December 4, 2010.
13. U.S. Food and Drug Administration. Beware of online cancer fraud. 2008. Available at: http://www.fda.gov/ForConsumers/ConsumerUpdates/ucm048383.htm. Accessed December 12, 2010.
14. The Wilhelm Reich Infant Trust. Biography. 2006. Available at: http://www.wilhelmreichtrust.org/biography.html. Accessed December 1, 2010.
15. Lowenthal R. Snake oil, coffee enemas and other famous nostrums for cancer—a recent history of cancer quackery in Australia. Cancer Forum, v.29, no.3, Nov 2005, p.150-3.
16. Dr. Clark Information Center. In remembrance of Dr. Hulda Clark—1928–2009. 2010. Available at: http://www.drclark.net/en/hulda_clark/about_drclark.php. Accessed December 15, 2010.
17. Dr. Clark Information Center. All you need to know regarding the zapper. Available at: http://www.drclark.net/en/products_devices/devices/zapper.php. Accessed December 17, 2010.
18. Avert. A cure for AIDS. Available at: http://www.avert.org/cure-for-aids.htm. Accessed: December 12, 2010.
19. Kook Science Resistance. Radionics or black box dowsing. August 2010. Available at: http://www.kookscience.com/2010/radionics-or-black-box-dowsing/. Accessed November 29, 2010.
20. Adachi K. Dr. Ruth B. Drown, America's greatest radionics innovator. The untold story, part 1. Available at: http://www.educate-yourself.org/tjc/ruthdrownuntoldstory.shtml. Accessed December 7, 2010.
21. Drown Laboratories. Radio-Vision, scientific milestone. 1960. Available at: http://educate-yourself.org/tjc/radiovisionbookintro30jul03.shtml. Accessed December 14, 2010.
22. Smith RL. The incredible Drown case. *Today's Health.* April, 1968.
23. Wizard Sports. Power Balance wristbands and pendants. Available at: http://www.wizardsports.com/power-balance.html. Accessed January 5, 2011.
24. Eat Right for Your Type. How blood type determines your health. Available at: http://www.dadamo.com/program.htm. Accessed January 5, 2011.
25. U.S. Food and Drug Administration. Tainted products marketed as dietary supplements. Available at: http://www.fda.gov/ForConsumers/ConsumerUpdates/ucm236774.htm. Accessed January 2, 2011.
26. Ogden CL, Carroll MD, McDowell MA, Flegal KM. *Obesity among adults in the United States—no change since 2003–2004.* NCHS data brief no 1. Hyattsville, MD: National Center for Health Statistics; 2007.
27. Marketdata Enterprises. *The U.S. weight loss market*. 10th ed. 2009. Tampa, FL.
28. Gavin M. 5 ways to spot a fad diet [TeensHealth]. May 2010. Available at: http://kidshealth.org/teen/food_fitness/dieting/fad_diet_tips.html. Accessed December 21, 2010.

Traditional Medical Self-Care

LEARNING OBJECTIVES

As a result of reading this chapter, students will:

1. Decide which type of over-the-counter medicine to purchase when not feeling well.
2. Distinguish between medicine for colds and medicine for pain.
3. Understand what self-care items should be kept in the home.
4. Determine when to self-treat and when to see the doctor.

TAKING CARE OF YOURSELF

As the costs of visiting the doctor continue to rise, practicing self-care in the home is often a welcome option. For college students, a lack of disposable income, significant distance between them and their physician, and the generally hectic nature of college life make self-care a necessity! In fact, a 2008 study in the *Journal of American College Health*[1] indicated that 74 percent of college students used some form of over-the-counter medicine in the prior 12 months. With that the case, consumers need to then know what to do, how to do it, and when to act.

HOW CAN I PREVENT ILLNESS IN THE FIRST PLACE?

The best technique to use for self-care is to try not to get sick in the first place. Hundreds of resources exist on preventative approaches to lifestyle and how to make positive choices for a healthy life. The Centers for Disease Control and Prevention (CDC) has summarized much of this information into a short list of general prevention it calls "Tips for a Safe and Healthy Life."[2]

Eat healthy: This includes a diet with a variety of fruits, vegetables, and whole grains daily; limiting calories, sugar, salt, fat, and alcohol; and maintaining a healthy weight.

Be active: You should consider including 2.5 hours of activity that increases your heart rate each week.

Manage your stress: Many American's would say this is the most difficult item on the list. The CDC includes the following suggestions: Balance work, home, and play; maintain a positive attitude; create time for relaxation; and sleep 7–9 hours each night.

Get check-ups: Know what tests, exams, and shots are necessary for someone your age; and know your family health history.

Protect yourself: The CDC has a myriad of suggestions for daily protection that include wearing helmets and seat belts, using sunscreen and insect repellent when outdoors, washing hands, avoiding tobacco smoke, and maintaining healthy relationships. College students in particular should ensure their vaccinations are up to date (see **TABLE 17.1**).

WHERE DO I BEGIN?

To be successful in self-care you must know your own body. When you have taken note of your own physical tendencies, you will more readily know when something odd is occurring. To know your body also means to have an idea of things like your normal blood pressure, cholesterol levels, and family medical history. If there is a dramatic change in your health status, or you begin to exhibit symptoms of an ailment commonly identified in your family, you will have a much better idea of how and when to begin addressing the situation.

Table 17.1
Adult Immunization Chart

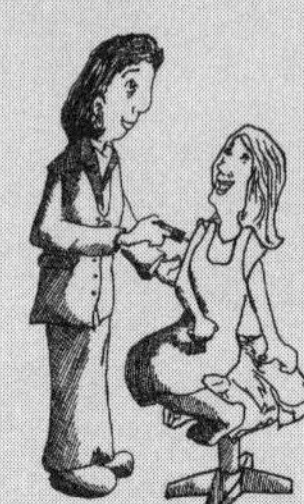

Vaccinations for Adults

You're NEVER too old to get immunized!

Getting immunized is a lifelong, life-protecting job. Don't leave your healthcare provider's office without making sure you've had all the vaccinations you need.

Age ▶ / Vaccine ▼	19–49 years	50–64 years	65 years & older
Influenza	You need a dose every fall (or winter) for your protection and for the protection of others around you.		
Pneumococcal	You need 1–2 doses if you smoke cigarettes or if you have certain chronic medical conditions.*		You need 1 dose at age 65 (or older) if you've never been vaccinated.
Tetanus, diphtheria, pertussis (whooping cough) (Td, Tdap)	Be sure to get a 1-time dose of "Tdap" vaccine (the adult whooping cough vaccine) if you are younger than age 65 years, are 65+ and have contact with an infant, are a healthcare worker, or simply want to be protected from whooping cough. You need a Td booster dose every 10 years. Consult your healthcare provider if you haven't had at least 3 tetanus- and diphtheria-containing shots sometime in your life or have a deep or dirty wound.		
Hepatitis B (HepB)	You need this vaccine if you have a specific risk factor for hepatitis B virus infection* or you simply wish to be protected from this disease. The vaccine is given in 3 doses, usually over 6 months.		
Hepatitis A (HepA)	You need this vaccine if you have a specific risk factor for hepatitis A virus infection* or you simply wish to be protected from this disease. The vaccine is usually given as 2 doses, 6–18 months apart.		
Human papillomavirus (HPV)	You need this vaccine if you are a woman who is age 26 years or younger. One brand, Gardasil, can be given to men age 26 years or younger to prevent genital warts. The vaccine is given in 3 doses over 6 months.		
Measles, mumps, rubella (MMR)	You need at least 1 dose of MMR if you were born in 1957 or later. You may also need a 2nd dose.*		
Varicella (Chickenpox)	If you've never had chickenpox or you were vaccinated but received only 1 dose, talk to your healthcare provider to find out if you need this vaccine.*		
Meningococcal	If you are going to college and plan to live in a dormitory, or have one of several medical conditions*, you need to get vaccinated against meningococcal disease. You may also need additional booster doses.*		
Zoster (shingles)		If you are age 60 years or older, you should get this vaccine now.	

* Consult your healthcare provider to determine your level of risk for infection and your need for this vaccine.

Do you travel outside the United States? If so, you may need additional vaccines. The Centers for Disease Control and Prevention (CDC) provides information to assist travelers and their healthcare providers in deciding the vaccines, medications, and other measures necessary to prevent illness and injury during international travel. Visit CDC's website at www.cdc.gov/travel or call (800) CDC-INFO ([800] 232-4636). You may also consult a travel clinic or your healthcare provider.

Technical content reviewed by the Centers for Disease Control and Prevention, December 2010. www.immunize.org/catg.d/p4030.pdf • Item #P4030 (12/10)

Immunization Action Coalition • 1573 Selby Ave. • St. Paul, MN 55104 • (651) 647-9009 • www.vaccineinformation.org • www.immunize.org

Source: Reprinted from Immunization Action Coalition, www.immunize.org.

You will also need to monitor your symptoms. Symptoms help determine what the cause is, and what approach or medicine could be used to help. Choosing an approach to address your situation will require that you accurately describe your symptoms, including the nature of the symptoms you experienced, when the symptoms started, how long they have lasted, and their severity. Knowing this information will allow you to discuss the situation with a physician if necessary.

WHAT MEDICINES ARE AVAILABLE TO ME OVER THE COUNTER?

One trip to the local drug store or pharmacy and it is clear that the consumer has hundreds of choices of over-the-counter (OTC) medications for virtually every ailment possible. Unfortunately, because anyone can walk up to the counter and buy them, consumers sometimes forget there are potential dangers associated with OTCs, and that they are medications to be used in accordance with accepted guidelines. The Food and Drug Administration is responsible for the monitoring and approval of OTC drugs, and currently states that more than 80 categories of drugs exist.[3] The FDA states that a drug will become available OTC under the following circumstances:

- The drug's benefits outweigh risks.
- The potential for misuse and abuse is low.
- The consumer can use them for self-diagnosed conditions.
- The drug can be adequately labeled.
- Health practitioners are not needed for the safe and effective use of the product.

With 80 categories of drugs available, the actual number of items within those categories can be overwhelming. Of common interest are those drugs related to relieving symptoms of pain, cold, and flu. It is vital the consumer know what they are taking and what each medication is designed to do.

Pain Relievers

Pain relievers, or *analgesics*, come in two forms—acetaminophen and nonsteroidal anti-inflammatory drugs (NSAIDs). Acetaminophen, marketed as Tylenol, for example, is found in over 600 products according to the Food and Drug Administration. Acetaminophen reduces the sensation of pain by blocking pain receptors in the brain and spinal cord.

NSAIDs, in contrast, actually slow the production of a specific enzyme, called prostaglandin.[4] Prostaglandins are responsible for swelling and pain production when the body has suffered an injury. By reducing the amount of this enzyme produced by the body, NSAIDs reduce swelling and pain.

There are many different types of NSAIDs on the market today. Although each acts similarly in the body, it is important to remember that each of these forms of NSAIDs has different dosing requirements. The following are NSAID dosing guidelines approved by the FDA and published by the Agency for Healthcare Research and Quality through the National Institutes of Health.[5]

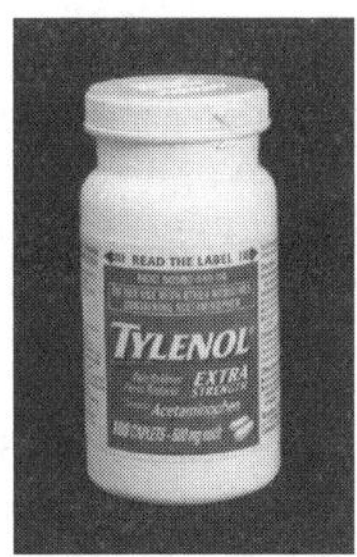

Tylenol contains acetaminophen.

Aspirin: The oldest of the NSAIDs, found in items such as St. Joseph's Aspirin and Bayer. Aspirin also has an added benefit of reducing blood clots, and is often recommended for individuals at risk for their development. Product dosing is unique to the product, so follow the product guidelines for dosing.

Ibuprofen: Found in products such as Motrin and Advil. Can be taken in dosages from 200–800 mg, three or four times each day. The maximum daily dose is 3,200 mg.

Ketoprofen: Found in products like Orudis. Each dose is 25–75 mg, taken three or four times per day. The maximum daily dose is 300 mg.

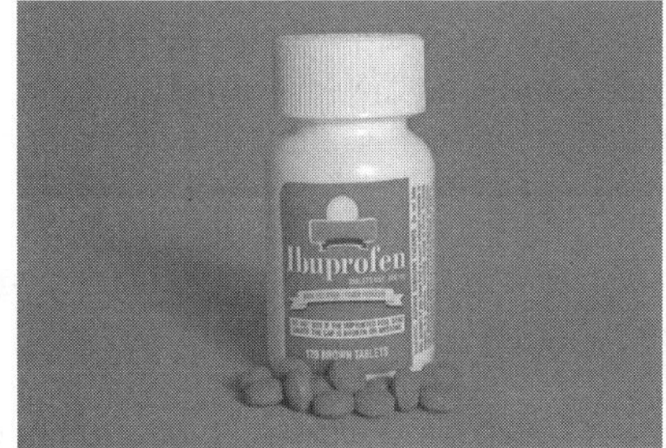

This product contains ibuprofen.

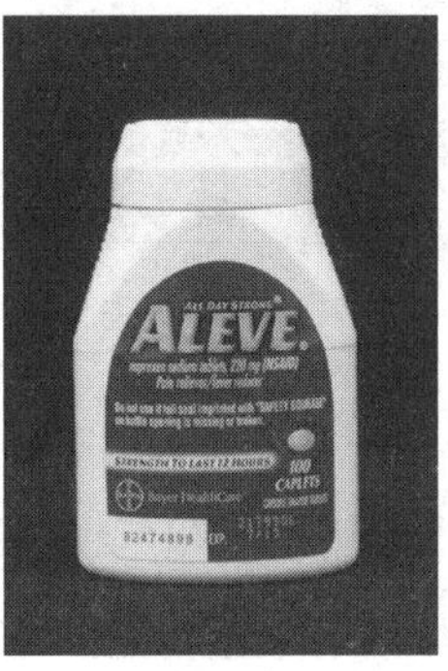

Aleve is the most common OTC drug with naproxen.

Naproxin: Found in products such as Aleve. Although naproxen comes in many varieties, the most common OTC dosage is 200–500 mg, with a maximum of 1250 mg per day.

Allergy Medicine

Antihistamines counteract the symptoms associated with an allergic reaction. When the body responds in a negative fashion to a common item, like grass or a cat, a person is said to have an allergy. When the body senses this foreign agent, it releases a substance called histamine to defend itself. Histamine causes an individual to experience a runny nose, sneezing, and scratchy eyes and throat. There are many antihistamines approved for over-the-counter purchase that can counter the effects of histamine. Brompheniramine (Dimetapp), chlorpheniramine (Actifed, Contac), doxylamine (Alka-Seltzer Plus), and diphenhydramine (Benadryl) are examples of currently available antihistamines.[6]

Medicines for the Common Cold

If symptoms include a stuffy nose and difficulty breathing, a decongestant is the medication needed. Currently there are few decongestants approved by the FDA, primarily pseudoephedrine and phenylephrine. A decongestant works by reducing the blood flow to the nasal capillaries, thereby reducing the swelling of the tissues in the nose. This opens the air passages for easier breathing.[7]

In 2006, President Bush signed a revised version of the Patriot Act, a portion of which directed that products containing pseudoephedrine be pulled from availability as an over-the-counter drug due to the substance's use in the making of methamphetamine. Methamphetamine is a highly addictive, quickly destructive amphetamine that uses pseudoephedrine as its main ingredient. More than half of the individual states in the United States also have laws restricting the availability of pseudoephedrine, most of which limit the amount you can buy, indicate that purchase must come directly from a pharmacist (not OTC), and that a signature documenting receipt of the drug is required.

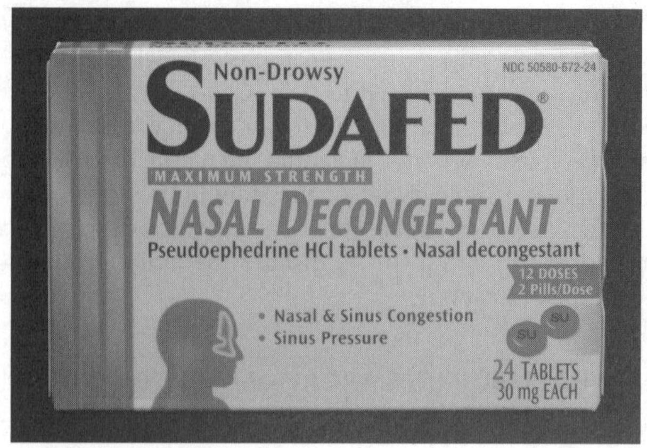

Pseudoephedrine in products like this was removed from the market because of its drug-making capacity.

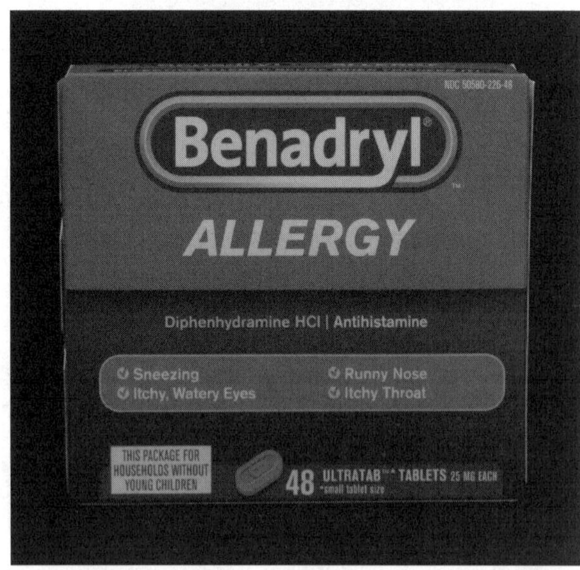

Benadryl is an antihistamine.

Medicines for a Nagging Cough

A common physical symptom of illness is a cough. However, not all coughs are the same, and because of that, medicines to treat cough symptoms also vary. Generally, coughs are caused by excess phlegm (a gooey substance in the throat) or dryness causing a cough reflex. Medicines designed to stop the cough reflex are called antitussives. They work by reducing the sensations in the nerves that tell the brain to cough. Dextromethorphan is by far the most common antitussive on the market today, and is found in virtually all OTC cough suppressants. A cough associated with significant phlegm requires the use of an expectorant. An expectorant

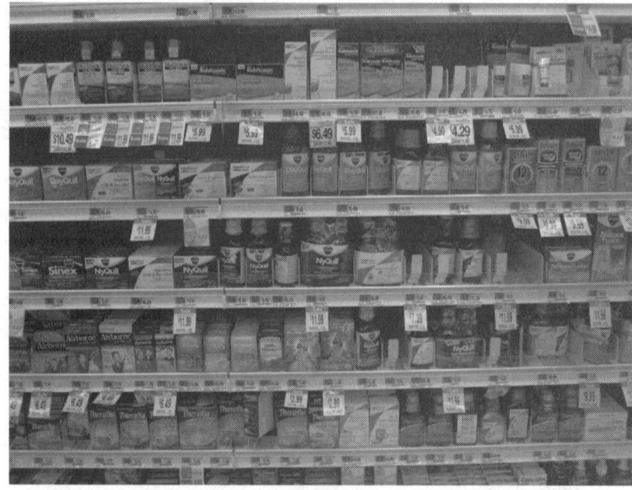

Hundreds of products are available to treat cough and cold.

> ### Box 17.1
> ### OTCs and Children
>
> Parents of young children will tell you: there is nothing worse than a sick child. It can be a helpless feeling for a parent, knowing the child feels miserable and yet being able to do little to ease their suffering. Research indicates children under the age of 6 average between six and eight colds every year. Fever, stuffy nose, aches, sneezing...all are part of the process, and in the meantime, the child (and the parents) just can't function. Parents readily admit administering OTC cough and cold medicine to their children.[8] In fact, a 2007 Kaiser Foundation report revealed that 56 percent of all parents responding had given OTC medicine to their children under 2 years old, and nearly 80 percent had given the same type of medicine to their children under 6 years old.[9]
>
> Nearly $4 billion was spent on cough and cold relief for children, and the Centers for Disease Control and Prevention reports these medicines were connected to more than 1500 emergency department visits.[10] The problem? There is no clinical evidence that OTC medicines for children are effective.
>
> In 2007, manufacturers of infant cough and cold remedies voluntarily removed them from the market. Those medicines were designed for children under the age of 2 years. The current recommendation, supported by research, suggests removal of all products intended for children under age 6. A 2008 study[7] indicates the following:
>
> - Children's cough medicines with dextromethorphan or diphenhydramine were no more effective than a placebo at controlling cough.
> - Sleep was not improved when these medicines were taken.
> - There continues to be little support for the effectiveness of cough medicines for children.
> - Antihistamines do not help kids with cold symptoms breathe better, and can have side effects.
>
> In addition, research has begun to associate the use of acetaminophen with the development of asthma in children and adults.[8] Based on the evidence, decongestants are not recommended for children under the age of 12.
>
> 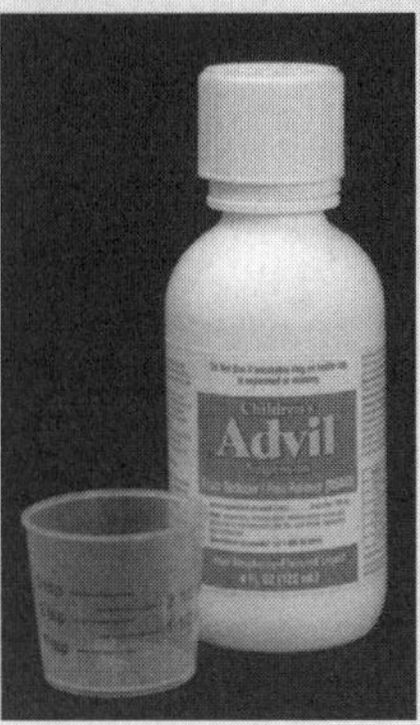
>
>
> The use of OTC medicines for children has been a topic of much debate.

thins and loosens the phlegm so the cough is more "productive," allowing the phlegm's removal. Guaifenesin is the only approved OTC expectorant on the market. Simply stated, the medicine you should choose for your cough, depends on the cough.

WHAT IF I JUST TAKE THEM ALL WHEN I AM ILL?

Products labeled as "cough and cold" or "nighttime flu" medicines will combine many of the products we have mentioned—an analgesic for pain, antihistamine for runny nose, and antitussive for cough, for instance. If you live by the "more is better" mantra, this is one time you may wish to think twice. The rule of thumb is to take only what you need. If you have no cough, then the consumption of a medicine that contains guaifenesin is overkill, and only serves to make your liver work harder. A multitude of combinations of medicines exist on the market today. Finding one that matches your symptoms just takes a little effort. If you get lost in the myriad of products, ask your store pharmacist or your family physician for assistance.

DO OVER-THE-COUNTER MEDICATIONS HAVE SIDE EFFECTS OR DRUG INTERACTIONS?

Like all medications, the potential for side effects and drug interactions does exist with OTCs. Side effects vary depending on the medicine you are taking. Some pain relievers can cause liver damage if used in excess over time. Antihistamines have a history of producing drowsiness in users. Decongestants can cause excitability or make a user feel hyper. Most cough medicines have no consistently noted side effects, but can make some people feel drowsy. Because we are all wired a little differently, the consumer may need to try a couple different brands before finding the one that works best for them.

A drug *interaction* means that taking a medicine may affect a medicine already in your system. A very common drug interaction involves monoamine oxidase inhibitors (MAOIs). MAOIs are used to combat depression and anxiety and are very susceptible to the introduction of other medicines in the user's system. **TABLE 17.2** details some other potential OTC drug interactions.

The most significant side effect for college students appears to be anxiety and distress (a bad type of stress). Students experience these symptoms on a regular basis given the nature of studying, testing, and social situations. However, research suggests that college students self-medicating actually increase their reported level of anxiety.[1] Products containing medicines such as pseudoephedrine (used to keep themselves awake) and valerian (an herbal drug to aid sleep) seem to have the greatest risk of increasing anxiety in students. When medicines are taken in combination, the likelihood of experiencing greater anxiety also increases.

Table 17.2
Potential Drug Interactions for Over-the-Counter Drugs[11]

DRUG	POTENTIAL INTERACTIONS
Pain Relievers	
Acetaminophen (Tylenol)	When taken with the antibiotics rifampin and isoniazid it can affect how the liver processes acetaminophen and increase the risk of liver problems. It also increases the blood-thinning effect of blood thinners.
Aspirin (Bayer, St. Joseph's)	Aspirin increases the blood-sugar-lowering effect of diabetes medicines. Aspirin binds with proteins affecting the work of antiseizure drugs. This can lead to increased antiseizure drug levels in your blood.
NSAIDs, including: Aspirin Ibuprofen (Advil, Motrin) Ketoprofen (Orudis KT) Naproxen (Aleve)	NSAIDs reduce the effectiveness of the kidneys' ability to remove anti-cancer, immune system, and heart drugs, leaving too much in your blood. They also reduce the effectiveness of blood-pressure-lowering drugs and diuretics and increase the blood-thinning effect of blood thinners.
Ibuprofen Naproxen sodium	Ibuprofen and Naproxen reduce how the kidneys clear lithium (a drug for bipolar disorder) out of the body. This can lead to having too much lithium in your blood.
Antihistamines	
Brompheniramine (Dimetapp Cold & Allergy Elixir, Robitussin Allergy & Cough Liquid) Chlorpheniramine (Robitussin Flu Liquid) Dimenhydrinate (Dramamine) Diphenhydramine (Benadryl Allergy, Nytol, Sominex) Doxylamine (Vicks NyQuil, Alka-SeltzerPlus Night-Time Cold Medicine)	Antihistamines increase the depressant effects of anti-anxiety drugs, sleeping pills, or sedatives on the brain.
Decongestants	
Pseudoephedrine (Contac Non-Drowsy, Efidac 24, Sudafed)	Should never be taken with MAOIs. May cause an increase in blood pressure or heart rhythm problems. Increases anxiety when taken with stimulants, and inhibits the positive effects of high blood pressure drugs.
Cough Medicines	
Dextromethorphan (Delsym, Robitussin Maximum Strength, Vicks 44 Cough Relief)	Should never be taken with MAOIs. May cause "serotonin syndrome," increasing the effects of sedatives.

Source: Adapted from the California Department of Alcohol and Drug Programs, http://www.adp.ca.gov.

Table 17.2 provides a summary of some OTC drug interactions to be aware of, but again, the best advice and guidance in this matter comes from your personal physician.

WHAT NONMEDICINE OPTIONS DO I HAVE?

Medicines you buy over the counter are not curing your cold or flu, of course; they are simply easing the symptoms associated with those afflictions. If you would prefer not to take something from the pharmacy, or you have a preference for a more natural approach, research has identified the following items as having some potential to help[12]:

- *Rest:* It seems to be the last thing people do when they get sick, but the fact is, your body only heals while at rest. Thin out your schedule (at a minimum) and allow your body to heal itself.
- *Zinc:* There is some support for the notion that zinc will help lessen the severity of cold and flu symptoms *if taken at the onset of those symptoms*. There

is also some support that zinc can help prevent colds in younger kids.

- *Echinacea:* The research is mixed regarding this product, but those supporting its use indicate that when taken at the first sign of symptoms, there may be some relief in symptom severity.
- *Warm salt water:* Simple and effective. For a stuffy nose, warm salt water can relax nasal passages and allow for better breathing. Warm salt water can also temporarily ease sore throat pain.
- *A hot, steamy shower:* Heat and steam will, again, temporarily help loosen up stuffed nasal passages, and relax sore muscles.

WHAT SHOULD I KEEP AT HOME FOR MY PERSONAL USE?

If you are to take care of yourself from your own home, it is essential to make sure you have items necessary to provide your own care. In addition to items required to manage any special health issues (like diabetes or high blood pressure), the following items are the most commonly used, and are recommended by Carol Lewis of the U.S. Food and Drug Administration (*FDA Consumer Magazine*)[10]:

For Home Medical Care

- Analgesic (relieves pain)
- Antibiotic ointment (reduces risk of infection)
- Antacid (relieves upset stomach)
- Antihistamine (relieves allergy symptoms)
- Syrup of ipecac (induces vomiting)
- Decongestant (relieves stuffy nose and other cold symptoms)
- Fever reducer (adult and child)
- Hydrocortisone (relieves itching and inflammation)
- Antiseptic (helps stop infection)

In the Medicine Cabinet

- Adhesive bandages
- Adhesive tape
- Gauze pads
- Tweezers
- Thermometer
- Calibrated measuring spoon
- Alcohol wipes
- Disinfectant

The FDA also points out two important pieces of information regarding your home health care supplies. First, it is best to keep medicines in a cool, dark, and dry place outside the bathroom. The heat and moisture in the bathroom can cause a medicine to not work properly. Also, the FDA suggests you clean out your home medical supplies, especially medicines with an expiration date, once a year.[13] Outdated medicines should be discarded and restocked.

WHEN IS THE RIGHT TIME TO GO TO THE DOCTOR?

This chapter has focused on how to manage illness yourself. There will be times, however, when you should choose to see your physician. The Yale Medical Group[14] makes the following suggestions when trying to decide whether you should treat yourself or make an appointment with your doctor.

You should treat yourself when:

- The illness is minor, such as a cold, influenza, diarrhea, stomachaches, headaches, and skin rashes or fungal infections. Rest and OTC medications can be effective in these situations.
- You are not on medication for a chronic illness.
- Your symptoms are mild and familiar (you've experienced them before).
- Your symptoms do not last very long, or are not recurring (coming and going over time).
- Your pharmacist has given advice on an OTC medication to take.

You should see a doctor when:

- You have a chronic illness or diagnosed condition.
- Your cold, flu, or stomachache symptoms get worse even though you're resting and taking OTC medicine.
- Your symptoms are unusual, painful, or worrisome.
- You suspect a sinus infection, experience a bad sore throat with a fever, or other symptoms you think may require an antibiotic.
- You experience diarrhea or constipation for longer than a week. You experience bloody diarrhea or diarrhea with mucus.
- You have joint pain that affects your normal activities, or joint pain with redness or swelling.
- You have back pain accompanied by pain that travels down your leg or arm.
- You have feelings of worthlessness or helplessness that last for at least 2 weeks.
- You are injured and can't self-treat.

HOW CAN I PREVENT PERSONAL INJURY?

During the next hour, at least 11 people will die in the United States from unintentional injuries. The causes will be diverse, including automobile crashes, drownings, poisonings, and fires. Unintentional injuries kill more children than all childhood diseases combined. Until recently, the number of fatal unintentional injuries had been steadily declining, reaching a 68-year low of approximately 89,000 in 1994. However, that number has been rising annually since then. The following advice is designed to help minimize your likelihood of unintentional injury.[15,16]

Automobile Safety

Motor vehicle crashes are the greatest cause of preventable death due to injuries, but the number of deaths has been dropping. Approximately 30 percent of automobile fatalities involved alcohol. In addition to deaths, motor vehicle accidents are the leading cause of unintentional injury in the United States. To keep yourself and others safe while riding in automobiles, heed the following recommendations. For general vehicle safety:

- Never drink and drive or take other drugs that impair your ability to drive.
- Always wear your seat belt; this practice reduces by half your chance of injury or death in a motor vehicle crash.
- Slow down and prepare to stop as you approach yellow lights. Many people cause automobile crashes because they try to "beat" the light.
- Yield the right of way at intersections.
- Don't tailgate; allow at least one car length for each 10 mph.
- Know the traffic laws of the state in which you are driving and obey these laws.
- Read and heed traffic signs, especially railroad warning signals and gates. Not all railroad crossings have gates or sound warnings to signal oncoming trains.
- Obey the speed limit.

Pedestrian Safety

Approximately 85,000 pedestrians are injured by vehicles every year, and almost 6,000 are killed. To help prevent pedestrian injuries, practice these safety measures:

- Model safe behavior for children.
- Cross at marked crosswalks and at corners whenever possible. Do not assume that drivers will stop because you are in a crosswalk.
- Stop, look both ways, and listen before deciding that it is safe to cross. Teach children to look left, right, then left again. Continue to look and listen as you cross.
- Cross only on a green light or a "walk" signal.
- Never cross between parked cars.
- Never run into the street.
- Walk on sidewalks whenever possible. If you must walk in the street, walk to the left facing traffic.

Water Safety

Nearly 4,000 people die each year from drowning, not including deaths due to boat-related incidents. Most drowning of children happens in pools, hot tubs, or spas owned by their parents, relatives, or friends. Staying safe involves these tips:

For adults

- Never consume alcohol when operating a boat.
- Always use approved personal flotation devices (life jackets).
- Don't underestimate the power of water. Even rivers and lakes can have undertows.
- Always have a first-aid kit and emergency phone contacts handy.

For children

- Provide barriers to water, such as fences and walls.
- Fence gates should be self-closing and self-latching. The latch should be out of a child's reach.
- Instruct babysitters about pool hazards for young children.
- Do not assume that children will not drown because they know how to swim.
- Never leave a child unsupervised near a pool, and while at the pool, watch small children continuously; do not become preoccupied with something else.
- Children can drown in the bathtub, in a bucket of water, or in the toilet. Never leave children alone when they are in or near any type of water.

For swimmers

Even good swimmers have accidents in the water and drown. For safety in the water, follow these guidelines:

- Never swim alone.
- Don't push or jump on others.
- Check water depth before you dive or jump into the water.
- Never swim in unsupervised areas such as quarries, canals, or ponds.
- Don't swim or use a hot tub or spa while drinking alcoholic beverages or taking other drugs that could impair your judgment, impair your ability to swim, or make you drowsy. (Alcohol is involved in 25 to 50 percent of adolescent and adult deaths associated with water recreation.)

Bicycle Safety

Over 600 people die in traffic-related bicycle crashes each year, and more than 50,000 bicyclists are injured. Many deaths could be prevented if riders wore helmets. By the end of 2009, 21 states, the District of Columbia, and at least 190 local governments had enacted legislation about bicycle helmets, with the majority of laws pertaining to children and adolescents.

For bicycling safety, follow these simple rules:

- Make yourself visible with light-colored clothing and reflective tape.
- Drive on the right-hand side of the road in single file, obeying all traffic signs and signals.
- When cycling in the road, leave a distance of about 3 feet between you and parked cars. You will be more noticeable to drivers and will not be knocked off your bike by the opening doors of parked cars.
- Walk your bike at busy street corners in pedestrian crosswalks.

- When exiting a driveway into a lane of traffic, stop, look both ways, and listen to determine that it is safe to enter.
- Before turning use hand signals and look in all directions.
- Don't ride your bike on rainy nights. Your chances of being involved in a crash are 30 times greater than on a dry night because automobile drivers cannot see bicyclists well in the rain.

Fire Prevention

Eight out of 10 fire deaths occur in the home, the majority caused by careless smoking. Home fires not only cause loss for those in the home, but for firefighters, neighbors, property, and the environment as well. Follow these tips for safety.

Smoke Detectors

- Every home should be equipped with smoke detectors on every level, particularly outside of sleeping areas.
- Ensure that your smoke detectors are tested monthly and batteries are replaced twice a year. Change batteries when you change your clocks.
- Encourage children to help test the smoke detectors. Familiarize them with the sounds of the alarm(s).

Fire Extinguishers

- Keep an all-purpose fire extinguisher in your kitchen (one rated for grease fires and electrical fires.)
- Keep fire extinguishers near the furnace, garage, and anywhere else a fire may start.
- Make sure every able-bodied member of the family is trained and familiar with the proper way to use the fire extinguishers.
- If you must use an extinguisher, make sure you have a clear way out in the event you can't put out the fire.

Flammables

- Keep matches, lighters, and candles out of reach and out of sight of children.
- No one should ever smoke in bed. Make sure that cigarettes/cigars are extinguished properly before dumping ashes.
- Avoid grease build-up in the kitchen and on appliances. Don't leave food cooking on stovetops unattended.
- If a fire should occur, suffocate it with a pot/pan lid or a cookie sheet, or close the oven door.
- Christmas trees are a primary concern. Consider using an artificial tree that is labeled "flame resistant." If you do use an evergreen, water it daily to keep it from drying out. Make sure to inspect stringed lights and window ornaments annually for deterioration.
- Dispose of materials from fireplaces and grills in non-flammable containers.

Electrical Safety and Heat Sources

- Make sure your electrical system is not being overtaxed.
- Inspect wires.
- Make sure space heaters automatically shut off if tipped over. Keep all flammable materials away from heat sources.
- Have your chimney inspected and cleaned annually.
- Keep appliances unplugged when not in use.

CONCLUSION

Managing your own care is a skill that can save you time and money. Having an understanding of the types of medications available to you and how they are safely used can keep you from making frequent and unnecessary trips to your physician.

Case Study

Frank has felt this illness coming on for 2 weeks: a slow drain in his energy level over time, and now the body pain and stuffed up nose. He can barely sleep. He has struggled with depression most of his life, but he is pretty sure this is not related. To complicate things, his 3-year-old son, Jeremy, has the exact same symptoms. Jeremy wakes up crying because he can't breathe and "his head hurts." As things go with children, if Jeremy doesn't sleep, nobody sleeps! Tomorrow Frank is supposed to make a report to the board of directors for his company, and if he doesn't get some rest and start to feel better, he fears the worst.

Questions:

1. Are there over-the-counter products that might help Frank?
2. What should Frank do to help Jeremy?
3. Are there any considerations Frank should make when choosing an OTC medicine?

Review Questions

1. What is an over-the-counter medicine?
2. What is an analgesic?
3. Name three common antihistamines.
4. What is the difference between an antitussive and an expectorant?
5. What is the current status of OTC medicines for children under 12 years old?
6. What are the potential dangers associated with children using OTC cough and cold medicine?
7. What can I try to relieve symptoms if I prefer not to take medicine?

Key Terms

analgesic Any member of a group of drugs used to relieve pain.

antihistamine Drug used to counteract the physiological effects of histamine production in allergic reactions and colds.

antitussive Capable of relieving or suppressing coughing.

decongestant Medication or treatment that breaks up congestion, as of the sinuses, by reducing swelling.

expectorant Promoting or facilitating the secretion or expulsion of phlegm, mucus, or other matter from the respiratory tract.

Food and Drug Administration An agency of the U.S. Department of Health and Human Services responsible for the safety regulation of medicine.

histamine Stimulates gastric secretion and causes dilation of capillaries, constriction of bronchial smooth muscle, and decreased blood pressure.

methamphetamine Used as a stimulant to the nervous system and as an appetite suppressant, and illicitly as a recreational drug.

monoamine oxidase inhibitors (MAOIs) A group of antidepressant drugs that inhibit the action of monoamine oxidase in the brain.

nonsteroidal anti-inflammatory drug Used for reducing inflammation and pain.

over-the-counter medicine Medicine sold without a prescription.

prostaglandin Any member of a group of lipid compounds that sensitize the body to pain.

pseudoephedrine Drug similar in action to ephedrine; used extensively as a decongestant, or illicitly to produce methamphetamine.

self-care Personal health maintenance.

References

1. Stasio MJ, Curry K, Sutton-Skinner KM, Glassman DM. Over-the-counter medication or dietary supplement use in college: dose frequency and relationship of self-reported distress. *J Am Coll Health*. 2008;56:535–547.
2. Centers for Disease Control and Prevention. Tips for a safe and healthy life. Available at: http://www.cdc.gov/family/tips/index.htm. Accessed March 30, 2011.
3. U.S. Food and Drug Administration. Regulation of nonprescription products. Available at: http://www.fda.gov/AboutFDA/CentersOffices/CDER/ucm093452.htm. Accessed August 15, 2009.
4. Griffin RM. How NSAIDs work [WebMD]. 2009. Available at: http://www.webmd.boots.com/osteoarthritis/guide/how-anti-inflammatory-medicines-work. Accessed June 1, 2010.
5. Agency for Healthcare Research and Quality. Comparable NSAID dose levels. Available at: http://www.ncbi.nlm.nih.gov/bookshelf/br.fcgi?book = hscompeff&part = cer4.appendices.app3. Accessed June 9, 2010.
6. Morris N. Over-the-counter allergy medications [Healthology]. 2006. Available at: http://nydailynews.healthology.com/allergies/article41.htm?pg = 3. Accessed December 3, 2008.
7. Stöppler MC. Making sense of OTC cold and cough medications [MedicineNet]. Available at: http://www.medicinenet.com/script/main/art.asp?articlekey = 43412. Accessed December 12, 2008.
8. Etminan M, Sadatsafavi M, Jafari S, Doyle-Waters M, Aminzadeh K, FitzGerald J. Acetaminophen use and the risk of asthma in children and adults: a systematic review and metaanalysis. *CHEST*. 2009;136(5):1316–1323. Available at: Academic Search Premier. Accessed June 9, 2010.
9. National Public Radio/Kaiser Foundation/Harvard School of Public Health. Children's OTC cold medicines: the public, and parents, weigh in. November 2007.
10. Ryan T, Brewer M, Small L. Over-the-counter cough and cold medication use in young children. *Pediatr Nurs*. 2008;34:174–180.
11. California Department of Alcohol and Drug Programs. Drug-drug interactions of common OTC drugs. Available at: http://www.adp.ca.gov. Accessed September 2010.
12. Doheny K. The taming of the flu. *Nat Health*. 2004;34:51–60.
13. Lewis C. Your medicine cabinet needs an annual checkup, too. *FDA Consumer Magazine*. March 2000:34.
14. Yale Medical Group. Self-treat? Or see a doctor? Available at: http://www.yalemedicalgroup.org/stw/Page.asp?PageID = STW001364. Accessed April 1, 2011.
15. National Safety Council. Safety and health fact sheets. Available at: http://www.nsc.org/news_resources/Resources/Pages/SafetyHealthFactSheets.aspx. Accessed May 1, 2011.
16. Alters S, Schiff W. *Essential concepts for healthy living*. 5th ed. Sudbury, MA: Jones and Bartlett; 2011.

Protection and Rights of American Consumers

LEARNING OBJECTIVES

As a result of reading this chapter, students will:

1. Describe the rights consumers have related to use of the healthcare system.
2. Outline their personal responsibility when making choices related to healthcare system use.
3. Explain the purpose of the Patient Care Partnership.
4. Identify the agencies committed to consumer protection.
5. Compare and contrast the roles various agencies play in consumer protection.
6. Explain how a consumer can know a product will be effective.
7. Describe the federal government's role in consumer protection.

CONSUMER RESPONSIBILITIES AND RIGHTS REGARDING HEALTH CARE

Over the last 20 years, consumers have become much more involved in decisions related to health and health care.[1] No longer are we passive receptacles of medical information. We ask questions, we compare costs, we demand quality care, we research illness, we review and experiment with alternative care. The result of this metamorphosis in health care is the substantial demand from consumers that quality care is a right. With that more active role, however, consumers have needed to become more responsible for their care.

The balance of right and responsibility was at the front of the political debate during the presidency of Bill Clinton. In early 1997, in response to the escalating cost of health care and increasing consumer dissatisfaction, then-President Bill Clinton created the Advisory Commission on Consumer Protection and Quality in the Health Care Industry. This 32-member council was charged with keeping the president informed on the status of the healthcare system, and to recommend actions to improve the quality and value of health care, its consumers, and its employees.

WHAT WAS THE RESULT OF THE COMMISSION'S WORK?

The end product of the commission's work was *Consumer Rights and Responsibilities (CRR)*,[2] a document that discusses the rights of consumers related to eight areas of health care: the disclosure of information related to plans, physicians, and facilities, consumer choice of providers and plans, consumer access to emergency services, the participation of the consumer in treatment decisions, respect and nondiscrimination of consumers utilizing the healthcare system, confidentiality of consumer's health information, the right to file complaints and appeals, and the responsibilities of consumers when accessing the healthcare system. These will be discussed in the following sections.

Information Disclosure

The commission indicated that information given to consumers should be accurate and easily understood. Also, when necessary, consumers should receive assistance to make informed health care decisions. The information provided should include (1) cost, licensure, and emergency services under health plans; (2) certifications, experience, and consumer satisfaction related to health care professionals; (3) experience and accreditation of health care facilities; and (4) appropriate consumer assistance programs.

Choice of Providers and Plans

Part two of the CRR referred to consumer choice. This included having sufficient providers and emergency services in the network to meet consumer demand, ensuring access to those providers was available, having sufficient women's health services (i.e., gynecology and midwifery), authorizing an appropriate number of specialist visits, and providing a variety of plan options for consumers.

Access to Emergency Services

Part three of the CRR addresses access to emergency services. Specifically, health plans are encouraged to let consumers know the availability of emergency services and other appropriate options, as well as to convey to the consumer that emergency costs, when appropriate, will be covered by the plan.

Participation in Treatment Decisions

The CRR established the right of consumers to play a role in their treatment decisions. Communication and easily understandable information is the key. This section reinforces the consumer's right to choose no treatment, to be told of all risks and potential side effects of treatment options, and to discuss the use of advanced directives.

Respect and Nondiscrimination

The CRR establishes the consumer right to nondiscrimination. It states, "Consumers who are eligible for coverage under the terms and conditions of a health plan or program

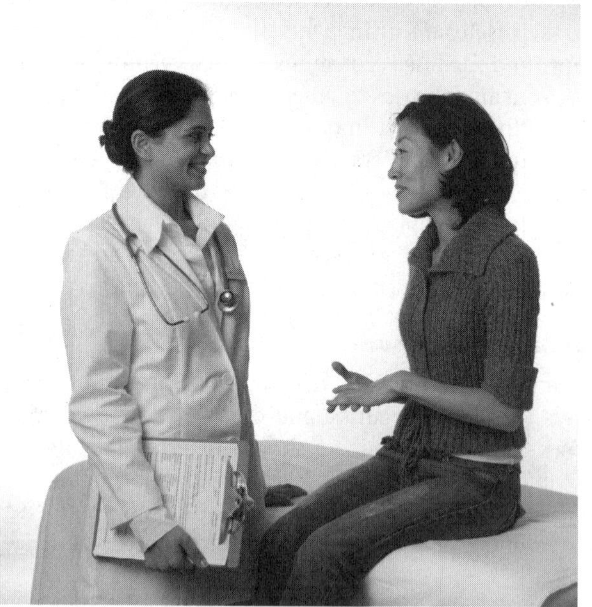

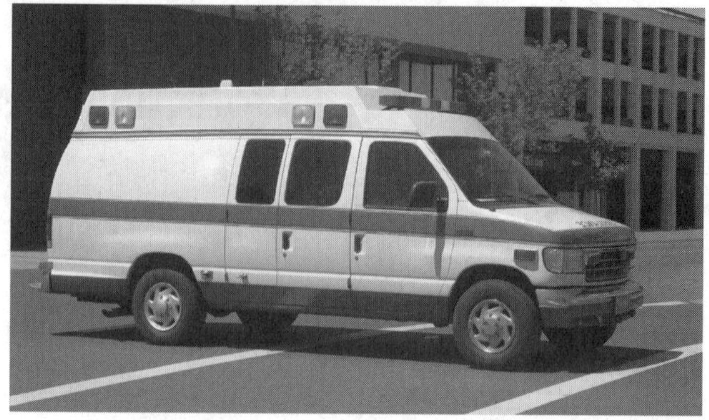

or as required by law must not be discriminated against in marketing and enrollment practices based on race, ethnicity, national origin, religion, sex, age, mental or physical disability, sexual orientation, genetic information, or source of payment."

Confidentiality of Health Information

Consumers have a right to the confidentiality of their information, and the confidence that information will not be disclosed without their specific consent. Health care practitioners and facilities should make every attempt to use nonpersonal identification numbers (like Social Security numbers) to identify patients under their care.

Complaints and Appeals

When consumers believe they have been treated unfairly, they should have the right to make a complaint and express their concerns. The CRR encourages conflicts to be handled internally whenever possible. The procedure for addressing situations such as incorrect billing, mistreatment by a staff member, or timeliness of services should be clearly explained to the consumer. When consumers act inappropriately, the facility also has the right to terminate services, but should do so in writing, with a complete

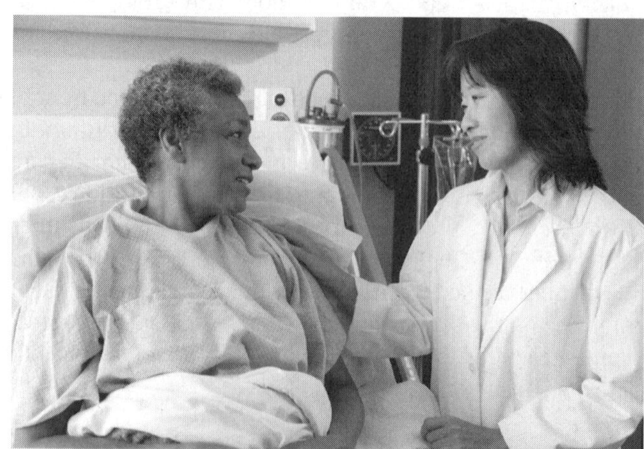

explanation of the circumstances and resolution done in a timely manner.

When internal processes do not meet the satisfaction of the consumer, an external appeal may be necessary. This would happen in cases such as refusal of services, denying payment, or reduction in treatment, and should be conducted by individuals trained for that responsibility and not involved in the original decision. Again, completion of the appeal in a timely fashion is recommended.

Consumer Responsibilities

The final component of the CRR reviews consumer responsibilities. Making the healthcare system functional requires all parties, not just providers, to make an effort for success. The following items are included in consumer responsibilities:

- Take responsibility for maximizing healthy habits, such as exercising, responsible alcohol use, managing stress, not smoking, and eating a healthy diet.
- Become involved in specific health care decisions.
- Work collaboratively with health care providers in developing and carrying out agreed-upon treatment plans.
- Disclose relevant information and clearly communicate wants and needs.
- Use the health plan's internal complaint and appeal processes to address concerns that may arise.
- Avoid knowingly spreading disease.
- Recognize the reality of risks and limits of the science of medical care and the human fallibility of the health care professional.
- Be aware of a health care provider's obligation to be reasonably efficient and equitable in providing care to other patients and the community.
- Become knowledgeable about your health plan coverage and health plan options (when available) including all covered benefits, limitations, and exclusions; rules regarding use of network providers; coverage and referral rules; appropriate processes to secure additional information; and the process to appeal coverage decisions.
- Show respect for other patients and health workers.
- Make a good-faith effort to meet financial obligations.
- Abide by administrative and operational procedures of health plans, health care providers, and government health benefit programs.
- Report wrongdoing and fraud to the appropriate resources or legal authorities.

WHAT DOES CRR MEAN FOR THE CONSUMER?

Primarily, *Consumer Rights and Responsibilities* spells out what is believed to be the optimal functioning capacity of the U.S. healthcare system. Individual consumers have the right to accurate, professional, and understandable systems and treatments, while at the same time hold the responsibility to be honest, forthcoming, and timely regarding health and personal well-being. When patients, doctors, and hospitals begin the process of trying to accomplish the same goals, the system works for everyone.

WHAT IS THE PATIENT CARE PARTNERSHIP?

The American Hospital Association (AHA) first wrote the Patient Bill of Rights in the 1990s. It was an initial attempt to build a bridge between physicians and patients at a time when consumers believed the system was getting too impersonal. Doctors and hospitals believed that the usage patterns established by consumers were often unnecessary and were creating a financial burden on an increasingly expensive system to run. The AHA document was an attempt to get consumers and the medical system to work together to improve care, and at the same time reduce costs.

In 2003, the AHA released a new version, entitled the Patient Care Partnership. The document, like its predecessor, was created to inform consumers of what they should expect during a hospital stay, and what rights and responsibilities the consumer held.

Your Rights Under the PCP

The Patient Care Partnership[3] focuses on areas of care and the consumer's rights associated with them. The consumer should expect high quality hospital care. This includes the right to know the names of your medical staff and their level of expertise, and to receive appropriate care where and when you need it. Consumers should expect a clean and safe environment, and be notified of issues that arise and how they might affect the consumer's care.

The component of the PCP most focused on is the consumer's involvement in their care. The Partnership includes the right to discussions regarding your condition and your care (benefits, risks, long-term outcomes, posthospital care, and financial impact). The Partnership also includes involvement in the discussion of your personal treatment plan. Usually this involves the signing of documents signifying you have been consulted about treatment and your agreement or refusal of that treatment. It also includes the consumer identifying who should be responsible for making decisions about health care if the patient cannot make those decisions for themselves. The Partnership emphasizes the consumer's role in the provision of complete and accurate information regarding past illness, allergies, medications, and health plan. And finally, being involved in the health care decisions means both sides understanding the patient's health care goals.

The PCP believes in the consumer's right to the protection of patient privacy, and the health care facility's commitment to following state and national laws in that regard. Finally, the PCP discusses ensuring the patient understands post-hospitalization guidelines, and can receive assistance in understanding billing and payments when necessary.

WHAT DOES THE PCP MEAN TO THE CONSUMER?

Much like the efforts placed behind the creation of the *Consumer Rights and Responsibilities* document, the PCP sends the message to consumers that the hospital will do all it can to make your hospital visit the best it can be, but needs the consumer to play an active role in that process. When hospital and consumer work together, the quality of care is improved.

CRR, PCP, and Consumer Confidence in Medical Care

In 2005, the Department of Health and Human Services, Centers for Medicare and Medicaid Services (CMS), approved and mandated the Hospital Consumer Assessment of Healthcare Providers and Services.[4] The intent was to receive consumer feedback about their experience in the healthcare system. CMS required hospitals to complete the assessment in order to receive full reimbursement for services provided to consumers. Therefore, the data are comprehensive and extensive, pooling information from 2,700 hospitals nationwide. Data covering the first quarter of 2008[5] indicate consumers are most satisfied with communication with physicians and discharge information. Responsiveness of hospital staff and communication from hospital staff were the greatest areas of concern, with hospitals reporting just over half of their consumers satisfied with these components of the hospital experience.

According to the 2008 Hospital Pulse Report,[6] a survey of almost 3 million consumers from nearly 2,000 hospitals, patient satisfaction with health care is improving, but still has room for more improvement. Overall patient satisfaction with hospitals and physicians has shown modest yet steady increases since 2003 from 83.4 percent to 84.7 percent. The top priorities, according to the report, continue to focus on communication between staff and the consumer and the display of empathy toward consumers. The most significant areas of concern for consumers, starting with the most important, were (1) response to concerns or complaints during the hospital stay, (2) the degree to which the hospital addressed consumer emotional needs, (3) staff effort to include the consumer in decisions about treatment, (4) how well nurses kept consumers informed, and (5) promptness in staff response to "from room" calls (the patient call button). Level of patient satisfaction was good for smaller facilities, but showed steady decline in satisfaction rates as the facility grew in the number of beds available. Also, emergency department satisfaction among consumers was lower than nonemergency department satisfaction.

There seems to be much agreement about the rights consumers have regarding the use of the healthcare system. Protected privacy, open communication, involvement in the decisions regarding treatment and nontreatment options, and communication are central to the process of a successful health care experience. The new tools available for long-term comparison of consumer satisfaction will tell the tale over time as to whether we have been successful in providing a healthcare system that both works and is satisfactory to the consumer.

AM I A "CONSUMER" OF HEALTH CARE?

Health care is not usually something we think of in terms of "consumption," but as you have read, we are all consumers of health care. There are the obvious uses in the healthcare system, such as seeing your family doctor or a specialist, receiving prescription drugs, or visiting an emergency department, but the consumer market for health care is much larger. If you have ever purchased ibuprofen for a headache, an antihistamine for allergies, a treadmill for a workout, a diet book, nutritional supplements, or self-help books or videos you have contributed to the health consumer market. And you are not alone. In 2007, Americans spent about $7,500 each ($2 trillion total) on medical health care, plus $20 billion on over-the-counter health-related products, $40 billion on diet plans, and $3 billion on home fitness equipment. Health care is big business in the United States.

Who do you trust? What do you believe? How do you know that a product will be effective? How do you protect yourself? In many cases, laws exist protecting the consumer from fraudulent advertising or product fraud. The same is true for products in the health arena, including medical malpractice. As the business of health care and the market for health products continue to grow, challenges arise for the consumer.

WHAT ORGANIZATIONS ARE AVAILABLE TO ME IF I HAVE A CONSUMER ISSUE?

Consumers have the right to be treated fairly and appropriately whether they are utilizing the health care system, purchasing a car, or deciding whether a crib is safe for their newly born child. Fortunately, a wide array of governmental and public agencies have formed to protect citizens from fraud and danger. Each agency in the following section has been serving consumers for decades and are well established. While each agency may have a special focus, the central focus is the protection of the consumer. For more information, see Table 18.1 for agency Web site addresses.

Public Citizen

In 1971, Ralph Nader's efforts to protect the consumer came to fruition in an organization titled Public Citizen that was dedicated to protecting the consumer. It was the first of its kind. Its Web site[7] states its mission clearly and succinctly:

> We fight for openness and democratic accountability in government, for the right of consumers to seek redress in the courts; for clean, safe and sustainable energy sources; for social and economic justice in trade policies; for strong health, safety and environmental protections; and for safe, effective and affordable prescription drugs and health care.

The efforts of Public Citizen are varied. Each division (e.g., Auto Safety, Congress Watch, Energy Program, Global Trade) focuses on a specific aspect of consumer safety. One division, Health Research Group, has been a watchdog of the healthcare industry, publicly calling for increased access to health care for all, promoting safe and affordable drugs and medical devices, and improving work standards.

The group also publishes two very popular books: *Worst Pills, Best Pills,* which addresses the types of medicines people access and their effectiveness and potential harm, and *20,125 Questionable Doctors Disciplined by State and Federal Governments*.

U.S. Public Interest Research Group

The U.S. Public Interest Research Group (PIRG) conducts research, provides advocacy, and conducts community organizing to address consumer issues of public concern.[8] Representatives of the Public Interest Research Group at the state level comprise the group, which promotes itself as an agency that "stands up to powerful special interests." In fact, the U.S. PIRG's mission promotes activism designed to protect health and encourage fair treatment of consumers, free of the influence of lobbying from special interest groups.

Historically, the state PIRGs have had an influence on several notable changes in consumer safety and public health.[9] Some of these accomplishments include:

- Passage of generic drug laws in the 1970s
- Conducting studies that led to the ban on asbestos as an insulation material
- Raising awareness for stronger antiflammable children's sleepwear
- Passage of the nation's first lemon laws (laws protecting consumers when a newly purchased vehicle is defective)
- Superfund laws
- Reforms on toxic pollution control and public notification
- Disclosure of credit card financial information
- Fair credit reporting

One of the more visible efforts of the U.S. PIRG each year is the Toy Safety Report. First published in 1986, and now in its twenty-third edition, the report has resulted in the removal from the market more than 100 dangerous toys. In 2007, the group played a significant role in the development of lobby reform and prescription drug safety and review reform, and promoted laws designed to protect consumer identity.

Consumer Federation of America

The Consumer Federation of America (CFA) is an association of non-profit consumer organizations that was established in 1968 to advance the consumer interest through research, advocacy, and education. Today, nearly 300 of these groups participate in the federation and govern it through their representatives on the organization's Board of Directors. CFA is a research, advocacy, education, and service organization.

- As a research organization, CFA investigates consumer issues, behavior, and attitudes through surveys, focus groups, investigative reports, economic analysis, and policy analysis. The findings of such research are published in reports that assist consumer advocates and policymakers as well as individual consumers. They provide an important basis for the policy positions and work of the organization.
- As an advocacy organization, CFA works to advance pro-consumer policies on a variety of issues before Congress, the White House, federal and state regulatory agencies, state legislatures, and the courts. We communicate and work with public officials to promote beneficial policies, oppose harmful ones, and ensure a balance debate on issues important to consumers.
- As an education organization, CFA disseminates information on consumer issues to the public and news media, as well as to policymakers and other public in-

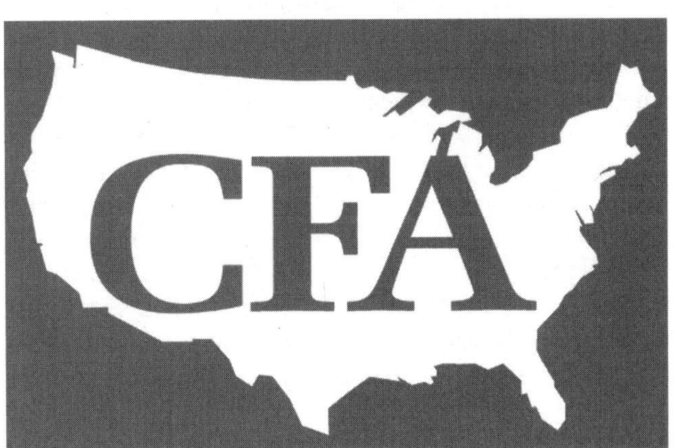

terest advocates. To do so, we utilize reports, books, brochures, news releases, press conferences, a newsletter, conferences, forums, and this Web site. Of special importance are the on-line newsletter CFAnews Update, three annual conferences—Consumer Assembly, financial services conference, and food policy conference.

- As a service organization, CFA assists individuals and organizations. Our principal service to individuals is through the America Saves campaign which we organized in 2000 and have managed since then. Our services to organizations, with a special focus on CFA member groups, includes CFAnews Update, our three annual conferences, our State and Local Resource Center, our Consumer Cooperative Advisory Group, and our annual Awards Dinner that recognizes distinguished public, consumer, and media service.[10]

Consumers Union

Consumers Union (CU) is best known as the organization responsible for the publication of *Consumer Reports* magazine. CU strives to create a safe marketplace for consumers by providing a thorough analysis of the safety, reliability, and quality of commonly used and purchased items.[11] Unique to public magazines and periodicals found on the newsstand, *Consumer Reports* prides itself on not accepting advertising, thereby allowing the organization to be honest, frank, and unbiased in its analyses of consumer products.

Better Business Bureau

The Better Business Bureau's (BBB's) mission is "to be the leader in advancing marketplace trust." By design, the BBB strives to enhance the consumer experience by[12]:

- Creating a community of trustworthy businesses
- Setting standards for marketplace trust
- Encouraging and supporting best practices
- Celebrating marketplace role models
- Denouncing substandard marketplace behavior

The BBB builds its relationship with the public in several ways.[13] First, consumers can access BBB Reliability Reports. Reliability Reports provide an array of information on businesses including consumer experiences. These reports can assist individuals with making an informed choice on whether to support a business or purchase goods from a business. Second, the BBB provides a dispute resolution service. For example, the BBB Auto Line is a dispute resolution program for consumers who believe their automobile warranty is not being honored. The BBB also trains consumers to act as mediators and arbitrators to resolve consumer conflicts. The third method for building a relationship with the public is BBBOnLine, which encourages companies to strive for accuracy and quality on their Web sites. If companies meet the criteria established by the BBB, they can advertise this on their site, increasing consumer confidence in the company's products.

WHAT GOVERNMENTAL AGENCIES ARE INVOLVED IN CONSUMER PROTECTION?

The government has also integrated consumer protection into its structure. As with public agencies, each has a particular area of expertise. In addition, several have the additional responsibility for administering laws applicable to that area of expertise.

Box 18.1

Influences of the FDA[16]

The following information shows the major events, milestones, issues, and accomplishments of the US Food and Drug Administration during the last 150 years. While not nearly all-inclusive, it shows the broad spectrum of influence the FDA has had on the health and well being of people in the United States.

1820–1900

First compendium of standard drugs for the United States, Drug Importation Act; 1862: Bureau of Chemistry formed, predecessor to the Food and Drug Administration

1900–1969

Purity of serums, vaccines, and similar products; prohibition of interstate commerce of adulterated food/drugs; stops use of poisonous preservatives and cure-all claims for worthless and dangerous patent medicines; prohibits false therapeutic claims in labeling; requires food package contents to be clearly identified on the outside of the package; requires prescriptions for certain narcotics; imposes controls on cosmetics and therapeutic devices; requires new drugs to be shown safe before marketing; regulates biologicals and communicable diseases; requires directions and purpose for use on drug labels; imposes safety limits for pesticide residues on vegetables; bans hazardous toys without adequate label warnings

1970–1990

Categorizes drugs based on abuse and addiction potential compared to their therapeutic value; initiated over-the-counter drug review; ensures safety and effectiveness of medical devices; issues tamper-resistant packing regulations; expedites the availability of less costly generic drugs; approves AIDS test for blood

1990–Today

Identifies anabolic steroids as controlled substances; requires packaged food nutrition and health labels; accelerates the review of drugs for life-threatening diseases; requires nutrition labeling for supplements; institutes an over-the-counter drug labeling format; requires labeling foods for trans fat content; bans OTC materials used to make steroids; bans dietary supplements containing ephedrine

The Food and Drug Administration

The Food and Drug Administration (FDA) is the most significant governmental player in the protection of consumer rights. With origins dating back to the 1820s, protecting consumer welfare has long been a priority in U.S. government. The FDA is housed in the federal Department of Health and Human Services and is responsible for regulating a wide range of areas including the nation's vaccines and blood supply; the safety and labeling of cosmetics; over-the-counter and prescription drug approvals (as well as labeling and manufacturing standards); the labeling and safety of all food products (except poultry and beef, which are regulated through the Department of Agriculture); approval, manufacture, performance standards, and malfunction reporting of medical devices; and the standards and assessment of radiation-emitting equipment.[14]

Beginning its work as the Division of Chemistry and later the Bureau of Chemistry, the FDA began to function as a regulatory agency in 1906 with the passage of the Federal Food and Drug Act.[15] Since its original passing, Congress has amended or added to the law more than 40 times. Each amendment added to the FDA's regulatory and oversight responsibility. Examples include the Import Milk Act (1927), Fair Packaging and Labeling Act (1966), Controlled Substances Act (1970), Prescription Drug Marketing Act (1987), Nutrition Labeling and Education Act (1990), Dietary Supplement Health and Education Act (1994), and Pediatric Research Equity Act (2003). A full list of the laws the FDA has regulatory responsibility for are located on the agency's Web site.

Bureau of Consumer Protection (BCP)

The BCP is a division of the Federal Trade Commission designed to protect consumers from businesses that choose to use fraud or deception in the sale of their product. The BCP will investigate claims from consumers in an attempt to stop unfair practices. The bureau also uses its authority to provide education to the public, establish policy related to fair business practices, and when necessary, file suit against companies that break the law. The BCP provides services through seven divisions, summarized in the following list from the BCP Web site[17]:

Division of Advertising Practices

- Enforces:
- Truth-in-advertising laws
- Children's Online Privacy Protection Act
- Fairness to Contact Lens Consumers Act
- Federal Cigarette and Smokeless Tobacco Acts
- Dietary supplement guides, and restriction of transportation of dietary supplements across borders

Division of Consumer and Business Education

- Conducts education with public regarding rights
- Works with industry to explain compliance regulations

Division of Enforcement

- Legal branch that enforces consumer protection laws
- Works with FTC on enforcement of court rulings in civil cases

Division of Financial Practices

- Focuses on enforcement in the financial services industry
- Ensures fair and safe lending practices, loan servicing, debt collection, and credit counseling or other debt assistance practices
- Aids consumers in understanding costs and terms related to credit cards and financial services
- Works to stop unfair mortgage lending practices, including discriminatory credit practices as defined in the Equal Credit Opportunity Act
- Works to ensure mortgage payment collection practices are fair and ethical
- Works to halt deceptive telemarketing practices
- Works to ensure that those who work in the debt collection, debt reduction, and credit counseling industries do so ethically

Division of Marketing Practices

- Works to halt direct-mail, telecommunications, and Internet fraud, including spam, investment, and work-at-home schemes
- Enforces the Do Not Call component of the Telemarketing Sales Rule, which prohibits unwanted or late-night telemarketing calls
- Enforces the CAN-SPAM Rules, for labeling sexually explicit commercial e-mail
- Requires franchise sellers to provide details on business potential to those who might buy into the franchise (Franchise and Business Opportunity Rule)
- Enforces the 900 Number Rule, making charges clear and prohibiting their being marketed to children
- Requires funeral directors to be upfront and complete regarding charges for services
- Enforces the Magnuson-Moss Act, which gives consumers upfront information related to product warranties

Division of Planning and Information

- Provides a consumer response system to collect and handle complaints
- Manages a Web site of millions of FTC consumer fraud complaints

Division of Privacy and Identity Protection

- Enforces the laws that prohibit unfair or deceptive acts or practices
- Protects the use of consumers' personal information
- Enforces the Fair Credit Reporting Act (accuracy of, and access to, credit bureau information)
- Enforces the Gramm-Leach-Bliley Act (confidentiality of customer information)
- Operates the Identity Theft Data Clearinghouse

Consumer Product Safety Commission

The U.S. Consumer Product Safety Commission (CPSC) is what is referred to as a federal regulatory agency. The commission has oversight responsibility on a vast array of products around the home and in sports, recreation, and schools. The CPSC investigates claims of products that may cause a fire; pose an electrical, chemical, or mechanical hazard; or cause injury to children. Specifically, based on the CPSC Web site, the commission is responsible for[18]:

- Developing voluntary standards with industry
- Issuing and enforcing mandatory standards or banning consumer products if no feasible standard would adequately protect the public
- Obtaining the recall of products or arranging for their repair
- Conducting research on potential product hazards
- Informing and educating consumers through the media, state and local governments, and private organizations, and by responding to consumer inquiries

The CPSC provides regular reports and statistical analysis on deaths and injuries related to consumer products, when use results in poisoning, carbon monoxide exposure, electrocution, fire, or sport- and recreation-related injury. All reports are available from the CPSC or on the CPSC Web site. Consumers can request reports, receive injury statistics, or review specific products' injury history. One can access laws and regulations related to consumer-purchased products. Finally, if a consumer has a grievance with a product's safety, they can file a report with the commission.

The CPSC is not a testing or certification group, nor does it recommend products for consumers to use. Instead, when enough reports have come in regarding a product, the commission may order a recall or replacement for safety

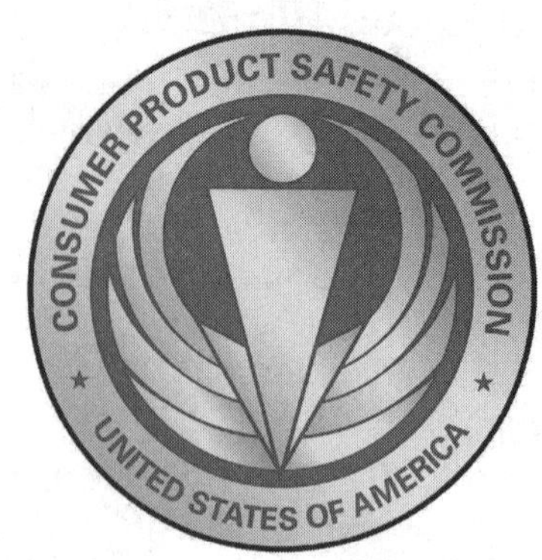

Table 18.1
Web Sites for Consumer Agencies

Agency	Web site
Public Citizen	http://www.citizen.org
U.S. Public Interest Research Group	http://www.uspirg.org
Consumer Federation of America	http://www.consumerfed.org
Consumers Union	http://www.consumersunion.org
Better Business Bureau	http://www.bbb.org
U.S. Food and Drug Administration	http://www.fda.gov
Bureau of Consumer Protection	http://www.ftc.gov/bcp
Consumer Product Safety Commission	http://www.cpsc.gov

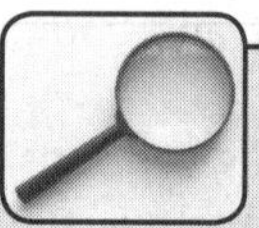

Case Study

Miguel and Maya have just learned that they will be having their first child in 6 months. They are very excited to begin the process of preparing for their new arrival. However, not having had children before, they are unaware of what products are of high quality and what products may present a danger to their new baby.

Question

Where could Miguel and Maya find accurate information on the following products and services:

- Cribs
- Children's clothing
- Infant toys
- A reliable minivan
- Medications for their child
- Child care facilities

reasons. All manufacturers, retailers, and distributors of consumer products are covered under the laws and regulations of the CPSC.

WHAT ROLE DOES THE CONSUMER PLAY?

In 1962, when then-President John F. Kennedy[19] told congress that the American people had the right to safety, information, choice, and voice, he set the parameters clearly for protecting people from consumer misfortune. The primary role the consumer plays comes to life in the "voice" piece. When you believe a company is providing false or misleading information, or when you believe a product is unsafe, consumer agencies need to hear your voice. Let businesses know you expect to buy quality products that are safe for you and your family at fair prices.

CONCLUSION

In most cases, consumers can be confident that they are dealing with ethical, well-intended agencies and health providers. In the event, however, that a consumer believes they are being mistreated, or have been misled, public and governmental agencies are available to assist with their issue. Consumers have the opportunity to learn the laws related to their situation, and access consumer protection agencies to help resolve the situation.

Review Questions

1. What items are covered under information disclosure in Consumer Rights and Responsibilities?
2. In what ways can the consumer participate in their own treatment decisions?
3. According to Consumer Rights and Responsibilities, what categories should be protected from discrimination?
4. Identify 10 consumer responsibilities related to use of the healthcare system.
5. What is the Patient Care Partnership? What is it designed to accomplish?
6. What seem to be the early trends in survey data related to patient satisfaction in the United States?
7. What consumer protection group was founded by Ralph Nader? What is that agency's role in consumer protection?
8. What do Public Interest Research Groups do? Name three examples of PIRG accomplishments.
9. What organization is responsible for the production of *Consumer Reports*?
10. What organization is responsible for informing the public when a company is deemed untrustworthy?
11. How long has the U.S. Food and Drug Administration been helping to protect U.S. consumers?
12. Identify the different divisions active in the Bureau of Consumer Protection.
13. What agency is responsible for establishing industry standards for product safety?

Key Terms

activism A doctrine or practice that emphasizes direct vigorous action, especially in support of or opposition to one side of a controversial issue.

adulterate To corrupt, debase, or make impure by the addition of a foreign or inferior substance or element.

biological Any substance, such as a serum or vaccine, derived from animal products or other biological sources and used to treat or prevent disease.

compendium A brief summary of a larger work or of a field of knowledge.

consumer A person that uses economic goods.

defraud To deprive of something by deception or fraud.

equity Justice according to natural law or right; freedom from bias or favoritism.

franchise The right or license granted to an individual or group to market a company's goods or services in a particular territory; a business granted such a right or license.

fraud Intentional perversion of truth in order to induce another to part with something of value or to surrender a legal right.

globalization Marked especially by free trade, free flow of capital, and the tapping of cheaper foreign labor markets.

lobby To attempt to influence or sway someone (such as a public official) toward a desired action.

malpractice An injurious, negligent, or improper medical practice.

misbranding To brand falsely or in a misleading way; to label in violation of statutory requirements.

redress To set right; to make up for; to remove the cause of (a grievance or complaint).

spam Unsolicited usually commercial e-mail sent to a large number of addresses.

References

1. Lumsdon K. Baby boomers grow up: health active baby boomers begin to flex their muscles as health care consumers. *Hosp Health Network*. 1993;67(18):24–26.

2. Advisory Commission on Consumer Protection and Quality in the Health Care Industry. *Consumer rights and responsibilities*; Washington DC, 1998.
3. American Hospital Association. *Patient care partnership: understanding expectations, rights and responsibilities*; Atlanta, GA, 2003.
4. Centers for Medicare and Medicaid Services. CAHPS hospital survey. January 8, 2009. Available at: http://www.hcahpsonline.org. Accessed January 15, 2009.
5. Centers for Medicare and Medicaid Services. Summary of HCAHPS survey results. Available at: http://www.hcahpsonline.org. Accessed January 4, 2009.
6. Press Ganey Associates. *Hospital pulse report 2008, patient perspectives on American health care*. South Bend, IN: Author.
7. Public Citizen. About us. Available at: http://www.citizen.org/Page.aspx?pid = 2306. Accessed January 14, 2009.
8. U.S. Public Interest Research Group. Available at: http://www.uspirg.org. Accessed January 12, 2009.
9. U.S. Public Interest Research Group. A history of action in the public interest. Available at: http://www.uspirg.org/results/a-history-of-action-in-the-public-interest. Accessed January 12, 2009.
10. Consumer Federation of America. Available at: http://www.consumerfed.org. Accessed January 12, 2009.
11. Consumers Union. About Consumers Union. Available at: http://www.consumersunion.org/about/. Accessed June 12, 2010.
12. U.S. Better Business Bureau. Vision, mission and values. Available at: http://www.bbb.org/us/BBB-Mission. Accessed June 16, 2010.
13. U.S. Better Business Bureau. Programs and services. Available at: http://www.bbb.org/us/Consumer-Programs-Services. Accessed June 16, 2010.
14. U.S. Food and Drug Administration. What FDA regulates. Available at: http://www.fda.gov/comments/regs.html. Accessed January 6, 2009.
15. U.S. Food and Drug Administration. History of the FDA. Available at: http://www.fda.gov/AboutFDA/WhatWeDo/History/origin/default.htm. Accessed January 6, 2009.
16. U.S. Food and Drug Administration. Significant dates in U.S. FDA food and drug law history. Available at: http://www.fda.gov/AboutFDA/WhatWeDo/History/Milestones/ucm128305.htm. Accessed January 6, 2009.
17. Federal Trade Commission. About the Bureau of Consumer Protection. Available at: http://www.ftc.gov/bcp/about.shtm. Accessed June 15, 2010.
18. Frequently Asked Questions. US Consumer Product Safety Commission. Available at: http://www.cpsc.gov/about/faq.html#wha. Accessed June 11, 2010.
19. JRank. Consumer protection history. Available at: http://law.jrank.org/pages/22685/Consumer-Protection-History.html. Accessed January 14, 2009.

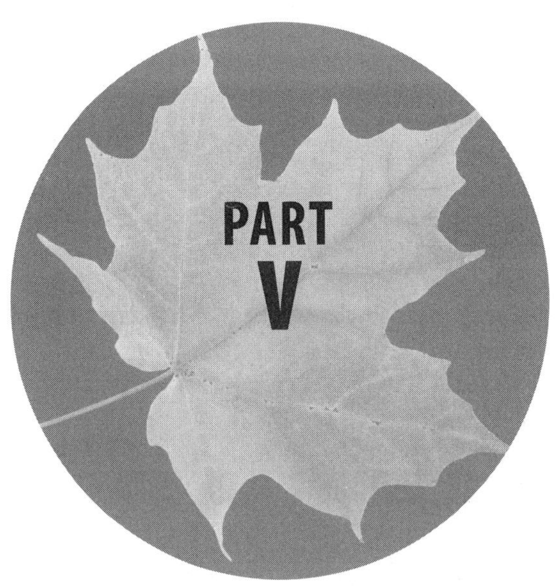

Health Insurance and Health Resources

Health Insurance in the United States

LEARNING OBJECTIVES

As a result of reading this chapter, students will:

1. Explore what the rights of citizens should be regarding health insurance.
2. Differentiate among Medicare, Medicaid, and the Patient Protection and Affordable Care Act and explain how they are funded.
3. Analyze what the impact of the Patient Protection and Affordable Care Act will be on the U.S. economy.
4. Assess the future of Medicare and Medicaid in terms of funding and public support.

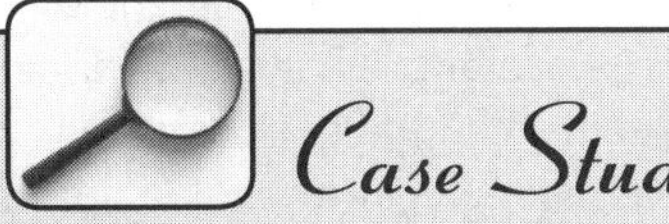

Megan Smith is getting ready to graduate in May. Like many college students, it took her more than 4 years to complete her degree. She will be 23 in April and will not be eligible to remain on her parents' health insurance after graduation. She has a job offer from a school district in her small hometown to teach for $35,000 per year, or about $2,300 a month after taxes. Her hometown is about 45 minutes from a larger town. Megan has grown up in this town and has gone to the same doctor all of her life. When she looked at the insurance options offered through the school district she had no idea how to choose. One of her choices is an HMO at $75 per month, which includes copayments of $25 per doctor's visit and $10 for prescriptions. There is no deductible to meet. This insurance includes vision. However, there are no HMO providers in her hometown; she would have to drive 45 minutes to go to a doctor.

The next option is a PPO plan. Her hometown doctor is in the preferred network of providers, so she would not have to travel to see a doctor. The cost for the PPO plan is $200 per month. The plan has a $500 deductible and then pays 80 percent of the remaining medical costs for the calendar year, including prescriptions. Vision is not included.

The district also offers vision insurance for $10 a month and dental insurance for $50 a month. They have a free life insurance policy for $5,000, if she dies for any reason after the first 6 months of employment. There is also optional life insurance ($100,000 of coverage for $25 per month), disability insurance ($25 per month), and long-term care insurance ($15 per month). Megan is completely confused about what insurances she will need and chooses the PPO and all of the other insurance choices to make sure she is covered just like her parents are covered. The monthly cost for all of her insurance coverage is $325.

Questions:

1. Did Megan make the right choices?
2. What would happen if she did not have health insurance and later got into a car crash and sustained multiple injuries?

WHAT CAN YOU DO TO BECOME AN INFORMED HEALTH INSURANCE CONSUMER?

Many people have high medical bills even if they have health insurance. What can an informed consumer do to prevent themselves from getting stuck with high medical bills?

Ask Questions

If you have insurance:

- Ask your health insurance company whether the procedure is covered, not your doctor!
- Does the procedure require prior approval?
- Has your deductible been paid for the year, or will you need to pay the deductible?
- Will you have to pay other fees such as copayments and coinsurances?[1]

If you don't have insurance:

- Find out the costs upfront; costs are different for those paying cash than for the insured.
- Ask whether the hospital will negotiate and accept less than the requested amount.
- Get any payment arrangements in writing.
- Ask whether there are programs that can help you afford care.
- Be prepared to show proof of financial need to find out if you qualify.[1]

Visit In-Network Providers

You will save money by using doctors and hospitals in your health insurance network.

- Get the names of the physicians and facilities you plan to use and ask your health insurer whether they participate before you receive services.
- Don't assume that a doctor or hospital is in-network just because they accept your insurance.
- Be aware that even though a hospital may participate in your plan, other physicians at the hospital such as anesthesiologists and pathologists may not be part of your plan. Check with your insurer to find out about these costs.
- If you feel that you must use an out-of-network provider, you can request an exception to cover the services at your in-network benefit level.
- Be sure to ask your insurance company before you receive out-of-network services.[1]

Understand Your Rights

- If your managed care insurer denies a claim or doesn't pay as much as you expected, you can contest the decision through the appeal process.
- If your appeal is denied after the first level, you may be able to seek additional reviews.
- You're entitled to a copy of the criteria the health plan uses to decide if the surgery, treatment, test, or device is medically necessary.
- You have the right to get a copy of your medical records unless the physician feels releasing them could endanger you or someone else. You may need copies of your medical record if you're planning to go elsewhere for treatment or want to appeal a denial from your insurer.
- The physician or facility has the right to charge a reasonable fee for preparing and copying records.[1]

Understand Your Responsibilities

- Take the time to understand your health insurance coverage.
- Contact your insurer to get a copy of your benefits. Read them and ask any questions you have about your policy.
- Make sure the physicians, hospitals, and other health care facilities you visit have your complete health insurance and contact information.
- Understand that medical care costs can be a heavy financial burden.
- Keep in mind that you can be sent to collections for medical bills even if you're making minimum monthly payments towards the debt you owe.[1]

HOW MANY AMERICANS DO NOT HAVE HEALTH CARE INSURANCE, AND WHAT ARE THE COSTS?

As shown, health insurance has been one of the top news stories in the United States. The 2010 U.S. census showed that 50.7 million people in the United States are without health insurance; with the price of oil rising, all goods and service prices will rise as well, leaving less available income for people to spend on health insurance.[2] According to a study by Harvard University, 50 percent of people who file for bankruptcy felt that it was the result of high medical expense debt.[3]

National health expenditures grew 4 percent to $2.5 trillion in 2009 and accounted for 17.6 percent of the gross national product (GNP). By the year 2019, that amount is estimated to exceed 19.3 percent of the GNP.[4] In 2010, employer health insurance premiums increased to $13,770 for a family of four and $5,049 for an individual.[5] The costs for medical care are rising due to many factors including poor management practices, lawsuits, inappropriate care, fraud, waste, and abuse. As the cost for medical care increases, the cost of average annual premiums for family coverage increased from 1999 to 2010 (see **FIGURE 19.1**).[6]

Health insurance expenses are the fastest growing cost for employers and are expected to overtake profits in a few years. Forty-five percent of families report that health insurance is their top personal expense concern, ahead of higher taxes and retirement security.[3] During the last 9 years, fewer people have had private insurance or employer-based health insurance and more people are using Medicaid.

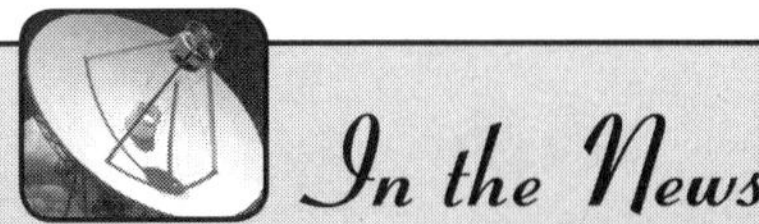

In the News

Much debate has occurred over nationalized health insurance since the Clinton administration tried to develop a plan during his first term in office (1993–1997). Once President Obama was elected, he, leaders in his administration, and members of Congress attempted again to reform the nation's health insurance programs. On the other hand, other members of Congress, the Republican party, and a large percentage of the U.S. population opposed such an act. The following excerpts demonstrate how the news media and the governmental news releases can sway the public.

First, an example of the deep negative emotions surrounding the passage of the Affordable Care Act is exemplified in a news article published on *Business Week's* Web site in June 2008.[7] The article highlighted several appearances by various people on the Fox News channel at differing times and gave their views regarding the Affordable Care Act. The following is a summary:

March 2008: Bill O'Reilly on *The O'Reilly Factor*: "The president must know Obamacare is a huge risk for the country, and at this point, I believe the risk is not worth taking." He further provided a comparison between President Bush, who sincerely believed Saddam Hussein was a threat to the world, and President Obama sincerely believing that health care reform will make America stronger.

Laura Ingraham is a U.S. radio host, author, and conservative political commentator who is a frequent guest host and Fox News contributor. She hosted *The O'Reilly Factor* one evening in March 2008. Previous to her appearance, she placed a message on her Twitter account that said, "Let's kill the bill!"

Fox Business Network senior correspondent Charles Gasparino said that if he were a member of Congress he would vote against the health care bill.

Fox News senior judicial analyst Andrew Napolitano claimed on Fox News that the reform was unconstitutional and was a step on the road to socialism. He urged the Republican party to be the party of no and to stop that train (health care bill).

January 4, 2009: On a Fox broadcast of *America's Newsroom*, substitute anchor Gregg Jarrett agreed with former Republican official Ken Blackwell's criticisms that the health care bill is unconstitutional. At the end of the segment he told Blackwell that all his arguments were good ones and that he agreed with them.

August 31, 2009: A Fox News contributor, Peter Johnson Jr., spent 5 minutes rejecting the reform bill.

November 2, 2009: A senior VP of *Business News* who was a "Your World" host announced that he was opposed to the bill and that the bill was "bad" and "awful."

November 2009: Fox Nation declared "Victory!" over Democratic setbacks. *Fox Nation* has run the following headlines:

"Fox Nation Victory! Senate Removes 'End of Life' Provision"
"Fox Nation Victory! Obama Backs Down From Gov't-Run Health Care!"
"Fox Nation Victory! Congress Delays Health Care Rationing Bill"

Question:

After reading the above commentary, what do you think was the impact on listeners and readers?

In contrast, on the White House blog, one can find a great deal of information promoting the benefits of health insurance reform. The title of this particular blog is, "Putting Americans in Control of Their Health Care." Answers to the following frequently asked questions were offered at the White House blog[8]:

- Can I afford coverage?
- Can I get insurance if I have a pre-existing condition?
- Am I going to be forced into a government plan?
- How will I know which plan is best for me?
- Can I buy insurance in another state?
- Will the government decide what treatment I can get?

Moreover, the White House blog contains headings such as "Investing in a Healthier Nation," "Protecting Patients' Rights," "Answering Your Healthcare Questions," and "The Affordable Care Act: How It Helps You." A link to videos promoting the new health insurance reform act also is offered.

Question:

How do you think the White House blog may have affected listeners and readers?

A White House news release was published on the Internet on June 7, 2010.[9] The title was, "Secretary Sebelius Announces $51 Million in Affordable Care Act Grants to Innovate, Improve, and Enhance Health Insurance Premium Rate Review." The news release discussed the offering of $250 million in Affordable Care Act grants to states over a 5-year period to fund a review of health insurance premium rates. Further, the news release quoted Secretary Sebelius as saying, "This is an important step in putting consumers back in control of their health care," and that the grants would help provide protection to consumers because it would make insurance companies accountable for their rates. Other statements intended to promote the Affordable Care Act grants were offered in the news release (found at http://www.hhs.gov/news/press/2010pres/06/20100607a.html).

Questions:

1. After having read the preceding news reports, do you have a better understanding of the impact of the news (print, Internet, and television) on readers and listeners?
2. How can you discern what statements are truths and which are lies?
3. How can you become a better news consumer?

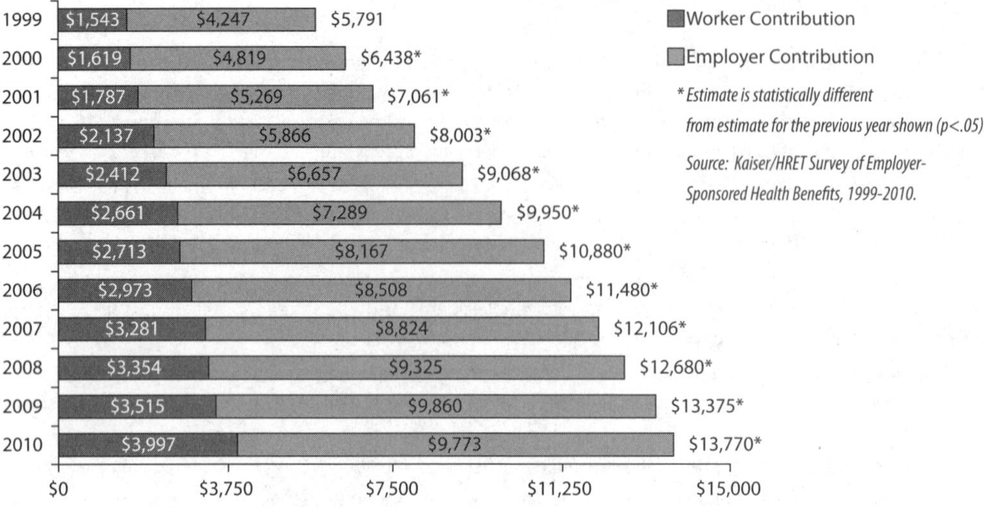

FIGURE 19.1 Average annual premiums for single and family coverage, 1999–2010.
Source: The Henry J. Kaiser Family Foundation. Kaiser/HRET Survey of Employer-Sponsored Health Benefits, 1999-2010. Chart Pack, Slide 2. Available at: http://www.kff.org/insurance/index.cfm. Accessed August 23, 2011

In 2009, U.S. insurance coverage was broken down as follows: 49 percent of Americans had employer-sponsored insurance; 17 percent were uninsured; 5 percent participated in private, nongroup insurance; Medicaid or other public insurance accounted for 17 percent, and Medicare accounted for 12 percent. See **FIGURE 19.2**.[10] The total cost for health insurance was $303.3 million.

Many people with lower incomes do not have health insurance, which results in fewer doctor visits and more visits to emergency rooms for late-stage illnesses when they are more difficult to treat. **FIGURE 19.3** depicts nonelderly uninsured by poverty levels and age, 2009.[11] As you can see, 50 million people were uninsured in 2009.

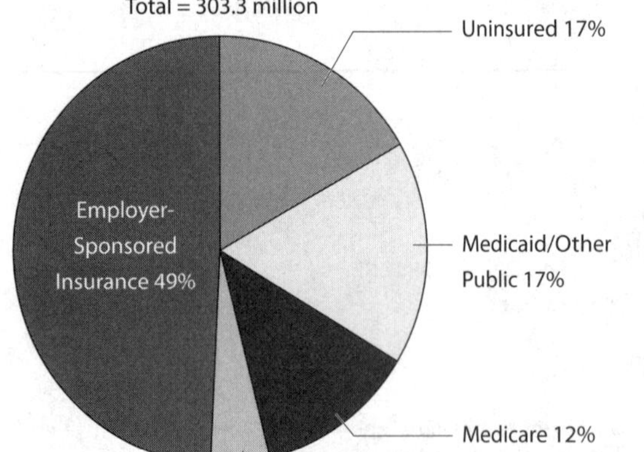

Note: Includes those over age 65. Medicaid/Other Public includes Medicaid, CHIP, other state programs, military-related coverage, and those enrolled in both Medicare and Medicaid (dual eligibles).

FIGURE 19.2 Health insurance coverage in the United States, 2009.
Source: The Henry J. Kaiser Foundation. KCMU/Urban Institute analysis of 2010 ASEC Supplements to the CPS. Available at: http://facts.kff.org/chart.aspx?ch=1476

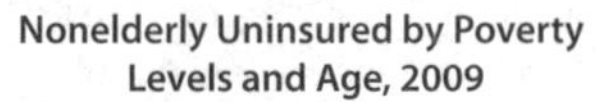

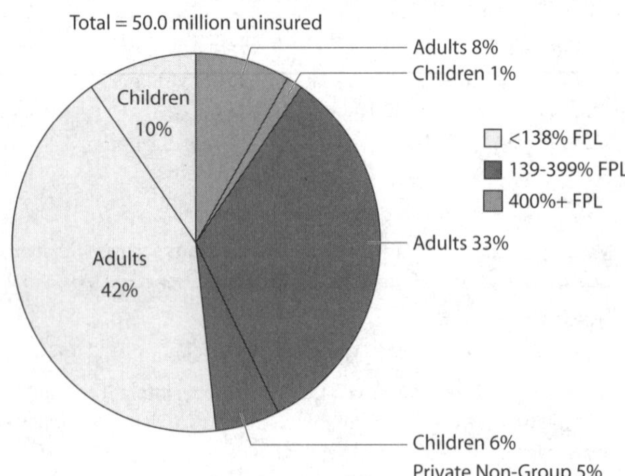

Note: Federal Poverty Level (FPL) for a family of four in 2009 is $22,050/year.

FIGURE 19.3 Nonelderly uninsured by poverty levels and age, 2009.
Source: The Henry J. Kaiser Family Foundation Commission on Medicaid and the Uninsured/Urban Institute analysis of March 2010 CPS. Available at: http://facts.kff.org/chart.aspx?ch=477

WHAT ARE THE FACTS ABOUT HEALTH INSURANCE?

Health insurance helps individuals and families to afford medical expenses. Health insurance was originally designed to cover extraordinary expenses due to a serious injury or illness, not doctors' visits for colds and minor injuries. It was typically the lifeline for many people as depicted in **FIGURE 19.4**.

However, medical costs have risen enough in the last 50 years that most individuals and families cannot afford regular medical expenses without health insurance.[12] There is a link between health and having health insurance. People with health insurance are healthier than those without health insurance.[12]

Private health insurance companies, like other types of insurance companies, determine the insurance premiums based on the risk factors for disease or injury. Some risk factors include being overweight, having high blood pressure, geographical location, age, and family history of disease. The fewer risk factors for disease or injury, the lower the health insurance premiums. People who are in a higher risk category pay a higher premium than those with few risk factors. All premiums are placed in a pool of funds. Insurance companies then withdraw medical costs as people make insurance claims. The insurance company dips into the pool of money created from well clients to pay for people with high medical expenses. This is a very simplified explanation of insurance; the risk calculations are much more complex.

WHAT ARE THE AVAILABLE HEALTH INSURANCE OPTIONS?

Most college students are on the student university health insurance plan or are on their parents' health insurance plan and do not think much about what type of health insurance they use. Whether a student or adult, certain relevant questions must be asked. For instance: Up to what age am I covered on my parents' plan? Can I only go to one doctor? If I need a specialist, do I have to get a referral from my doctor? Is there a copay for each visit? Do I have to pay for x-rays or other diagnostic tests separately? Should I be concerned about meeting the yearly deductible? These are just some of the questions that would give some clues about the type of health insurance you need and can afford. The following offers a more detailed explanation of various options.

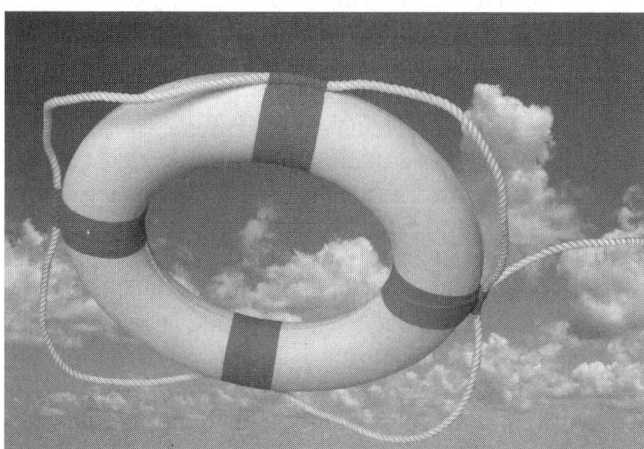

FIGURE 19.4 Health insurance rescues individuals from financial ruin.

Indemnity Insurance

Indemnity insurance allows the individual to choose their health care providers. An individual can go to any doctor or hospital.[6] An indemnity plan reimburses the person or the health care provider for services rendered; however, there is a yearly deductible that needs to be met prior to reimbursement. There is also a yearly maximum out-of-pocket expense; after this is met the plan begins to pay reimbursable expenses in full. Often, the plan requires preapproval for procedures and hospital stays.[13]

Point-of-Service (POS) Plans

Point-of-service plans are similar to indemnity plans because doctors refer patients to doctors within the plan for the lowest copayments. However, with this type of plan, the primary caregivers can refer patients to providers outside of the network and the plan will pay most of the bill. If you choose a specialist outside the plan, you will have to pay a much higher copayment.[13]

Basic Health Plans

Basic health plans offer health insurance at a greatly reduced cost for the consumer. These plans cover a variety of procedures, but the coverage varies from plan to plan. It is extremely important to read the specifics of a basic health plan to make sure of what it covers. The premiums on this type of policy differ by age, gender, health status, and geographic location.[13,14]

Health Maintenance Organizations (HMOs)

HMOs are usually provided through an employer and are less expensive than most kinds of insurance. There are restrictions about what physicians are available and the primary care doctor must refer specialists. The HMO company must pre-approve most tests and procedures. HMOs have an extensive network of physicians and hospitals. Doctors are paid a salary rather than an income from visits and procedures, which is supposed to make the doctors less likely to require extensive medical tests that are unnecessary. The insured chooses a doctor from a list and that doctor becomes the gatekeeper for medical care. All referrals for specialists come from this primary caregiver. The fees are lower than point-of-service or preferred provider organizations.

The patient pays a copayment for all doctors' visits that includes all services provided during that visit, including lab tests and x-rays. The out-of-pocket expenses can be much cheaper for the patient with this kind of health insurance. The caveat for this type of insurance is the patient cannot go out of the network for services, nor can they see a specialist without a referral.[13]

Preferred Provider Organizations (PPOs)

PPOs are networks of physicians that work with an insurance company. A negotiated rate for services has been prearranged for persons insured under the plan for in-plan doctors. Doctors who are not listed as providers are called *out-of-network doctors*, and the copay is higher. With PPOs, there is a prenegotiated rate for each kind of service. The insured pays the prenegotiated fees with the plan's doctors. If the insured decides to go outside the plan's providers for services, he or she must pay the difference between the negotiated rate and the outside provider's fee.[13]

Health Savings Accounts

Health savings accounts were signed into law by President Bush in 2003. They allow the employee to deduct an amount each month on a pretax basis that gets deposited into a savings account specifically for health-related expenses.[12] This means the person does not pay taxes on the amount saved or spent on health care. Only people with high-deductible health insurance can have these types of accounts. These savings accounts can be used for a variety of medical expenses, including over-the-counter drugs, copays for doctor visits, copays for prescriptions, or any out-of-pocket medical expenses. The only caveat is that the money must be spent by the end of the fiscal year, or it is lost.[12–14]

Flexible Spending Arrangements

These are savings accounts set up by employers that allow employees to contribute on a pretax basis to reimburse health care expenses. These accounts can be used with any type of health insurance. Money saved into the account must be used within the year that the contributions are made. However, some companies now allow employees a 2 $^{1}/_{2}$ month window after the end of the year for employees to spend down the account.[12,13]

Archer Medical Savings Accounts

These are individual accounts that may be set up by self-employed individuals and those who work for small businesses (less than 50 employees). Either the employees or the employer can deposit money into the account, but only one or the other can make deposits during a calendar year. People who have high-deductible health plans can enroll in this type of plan.[12,13]

High-Deductible Health Plans

High-deductible health plans have very high deductibles and are usually called catastrophic insurance because the insurance does not start reimbursing for medical services until the deductible is paid. Deductible amounts can be as high as $1,000 for individuals and $2,000 for families. These plans can be a good choice when there is no employer health insurance and money is tight. Although the deductible is high, it is still better than being without insurance and paying the entire amount in an emergency or sudden serious illness.[12,13]

Government Insurance Plans

Medicaid and Medicare are available to people who meet the programs' qualifications. Medicare is available for U.S. citizens who are over the age of 65, persons with disabilities, and those with chronic renal failure.[11] Medicare reimburses medical expenses for hospitalization, doctor bills, home health care, and skilled nursing care. There is a monthly charge for Medicare, which is taken out of the Social Security checks of those over age 65. Medicare does not reimburse 100 percent of medical expenses.

Medicaid is available for some women and children who meet the very low income qualifications and for those disabled who do not meet the Medicare qualifications. Medicaid is a state program that is subsidized by the federal government. Participants must meet the state set income levels to be eligible. Medicaid covers both physicals and illnesses. Not all doctors accept new Medicaid patients.

Patient Protection and Affordable Care Act

The Patient Protection and Affordable Care Act (ACA) is nationalized health insurance for U.S. citizens. The main points of this insurance reform include the following[15,16]:

Overall approach: The ACA would require most U.S. citizens and legal residents to have health insurance.

Cost: Could be $940 billion over 10 years.

Effect on deficit: The Congressional Budget Office (CBO) estimates it would reduce the deficit by $143 billion over the first 10 years, and further reduce it by $1.2 trillion in the second 10 years.

Coverage: The ACA would expand coverage to 32 million Americans who are currently uninsured. It would provide new coverage for those with pre-existing health conditions and extend coverage for young adults until age 26. It will extend coverage for early retirees who no longer will be eligible for employer insurance but who are not yet eligible for Medicare. It also will hold insurance companies accountable for unreasonable rate hikes.

Health insurance exchanges: The uninsured and self-employed would be able to purchase insurance through state-based exchanges with subsidies available to individuals and families with income between 133 percent and 400 percent of poverty level. Effective in 2014, separate exchanges would be created for small businesses to purchase coverage. Funding will be available to states to establish exchanges within 1 year of enactment and until January 1, 2015.

Subsidies: Individuals and families who make between 100 percent and 400 percent of the Federal Poverty Level (FPL) and want to purchase their own health insurance on an exchange are eligible for subsidies. They cannot be eligible for Medicare or Medicaid and cannot be covered by an employer. Eligible buyers receive premium credits, and there is a cap for how much they have to contribute to their premiums on a sliding scale.

Paying for the plan: The Medicare Payroll Tax was expanded in 2012 to include unearned income. This is a 3.8 percent tax on investment income for families making more than $250,000 per year ($200,000 for individuals). Beginning in 2018, insurance companies will pay a 40 percent excise tax on so-called "Cadillac" high-end insurance plans worth over $27,500 for families ($10,200 for individuals). Dental and vision plans are exempt and will not be counted in the total cost of a family's plan. There will be a 10 percent excise tax on indoor tanning services.

Medicare: The ACA closes the Medicare prescription drug "donut hole" by 2020. Seniors who hit the donut hole by 2010 received a $250 tax-free rebate. In 2011, seniors in the gap received a 50 percent discount on brand name drugs. The bill also includes $500 billion in Medicare cuts over the next decade.

Medicaid: The ACA expands Medicaid to include people at 133 percent of the federal poverty level, which is $29,327 for a family of four. The act requires states to expand Medicaid to include childless adults starting in 2014. The federal government pays 100 percent of the costs for covering newly eligible individuals through 2016. Illegal immigrants are not eligible for Medicaid.

Insurance reforms: Six months after enactment, insurance companies could no longer deny children coverage based on a pre-existing condition. Starting in 2014, insurance companies cannot deny coverage to anyone with pre-existing conditions. Insurance companies must allow children to stay on their parents' insurance plans until age 26.

Abortion: The bill segregates private insurance premium funds from taxpayer funds. Individuals would have to pay for abortion coverage by making two separate payments. Private funds would have to be kept in a separate account from federal and taxpayer funds. No health care plan would be required to offer abortion coverage. States could pass legislation choosing to opt out of offering abortion coverage through the exchange.

Individual mandate: In 2014, everyone must purchase health insurance or face a $695 annual fine. There are some exceptions for low-income people.

Employer mandate: Technically, there is no employer mandate. Employers with more than 50 employees must provide health insurance or pay a fine of $2000 per worker each year if any worker receives federal subsidies to purchase health insurance. Fines are applied to the entire number of employees minus some allowances. Employers with 25 or less employees with average wages less than $50,000 who offer insurance to their employees will receive a tax credit.

Immigration: Illegal immigrants will not be allowed to buy health insurance in the exchanges—even if they pay completely with their own money.

Caregivers: The health reform legislation creates a new Medicare pilot program aimed at helping patients and caregivers successfully negotiate the transition from a hospital stay to their homes or other care settings. It also provides new funding for Aging and Disability Resource Centers, which provide information and assistance to caregivers and people with long-term care needs.

Long-term care: The legislation establishes a nationwide system for states to run background check programs for employees of long-term care facilities and providers. This proposal builds on a successful pilot program, which operated in seven states and kept thousands of individuals who had disqualifying records out of the long-term care workforce.

As you can see, it is an amazing task to choose the right type of health care for each person's needs. Beyond what is available for families, there are other governmental programs that provide health care for children and the military, insurance for people who are disabled, and vision insurance. Those are described next.

State Children's Health Insurance Program (SCHIP)

State Children's Health Insurance Programs are offered through the various states. This insurance is offered to children whose parents do not qualify for Medicaid, but have a low enough income level that they cannot afford private insurance.

Military Health Care

There are two types of military health care: one for people who are currently enlisted in the Armed Forces and their families, and one for veterans. Both groups have doctors that are in the military network.[13] There are no co-pays for people in the service for any medical care, including dental and vision.

Disability Insurance

Disability insurance covers loss of income due to illness or injury that keeps a person from working. Disability insurance comes in long-term and short term varieties. Short-term disability insurance covers the individual after missing only a few days of work, usually 1–14 days. Long-term disability insurance covers the individual after several weeks to several months and continues coverage for years to the rest of their life. Most companies are required to have short-term disability insurance for their employees and can cover up to 60 percent of their monthly paycheck. According to the Institute for Insurance Information, 43 percent of people over the age of 40 will have a disability incident before they reach 65 years old.[13]

Social Security can cover unemployment due to disability, but the person has to qualify and not be able to do any form of work. Many people apply for this type of benefit, but few qualify. Another type of loss-of-income insurance is workman's compensation, if you are injured at work. However, it will only pay a small percentage of your monthly check and is only in force for a few months to years.[13]

Employer-paid disability will only cover a percentage of the person's paycheck to encourage the person to come back to work. The money received from employer-based disability insurance is taxable by the federal government. Individually purchased disability insurance is not taxable and can pay up to 100 percent of the person's paycheck[13]

Disability premiums are based on how risky your profession is and how much income you are trying to protect. If you have little risk to your job, than your premium should be fairly low.[13]

Vision Insurance

Vision insurance helps defray the costs of eye exams, eyewear, and other vision services. Typically, vision insurance covers eye exams with a set copayment. Eyewear is also covered with a copayment, which varies with the type of insurance. Insurance companies cover a specific dollar amount for frames, lenses, and contact lenses with a copayment. For instance, one vision insurance company may pay $100 for frames and $100 for lenses with a $25 copayment. If the person would like $150 frames and $200 lenses, they must pay the $25 plus the difference between the actual cost of the frames and lenses and the $200 coverage; therefore, the person would pay $175 for the $350 pair of glasses. The same applies to contact lenses. The same insurance company pays $50 per eye for contact lenses for 6 months. If the contact lenses cost $55 per box per eye and the copayment is $25, then the person must pay $35 for a 6-month supply of contacts costing $110.

Some vision insurance companies will also pay for a portion of the cost of laser surgery to correct vision impairment. Check with the vision insurance company prior to considering this type of vision correction, because coverage varies among insurance companies.

This section discussed various types of health insurance. The following discusses life insurance and long-term care insurance.

WHAT IS LIFE INSURANCE?

Life insurance pays money to the beneficiary when the policy holder dies. The beneficiary is the person who receives the death benefit. You can name from one to any number of people, a charity, your estate, or a trust fund you've set up as the beneficiary. If you do not name a beneficiary, the death benefit will go to your estate. There are two levels of beneficiaries, primary and contingent beneficiaries. Primary beneficiaries receive the death benefit upon the policy holder's death. The contingent beneficiaries receive the death benefit when the policy holder dies and the primary beneficiaries are also deceased or cannot be found. If no contingent beneficiaries are living or cannot be found, the death benefit is paid to the estate.

WHAT FORMS OF LIFE INSURANCE ARE AVAILABLE?

There are basically two types of life insurance, term life and permanent insurance.

Term Life Insurance

Term life insurance comes in two types, level term and decreasing term. Level term life insurance pays the same amount at the death of the policy holder at any time during the life of the policy. Decreasing term life insurance decreases over the life of the policy. As the amount of years go by, decreasing term life insurance plans diminish in value. Term life insurance does not earn interest and pays the face value of the policy to the beneficiary at the death of the policy holder. The cost of term life insurance is dependent upon the person's age and health status at the beginning of the policy. Premiums usually remain the same throughout the life of the policy and end at a specified age or term. Normally, insurance companies do not sell term life insurance that ends past the person's eightieth birthday. Level term policies can be for 5–30 years in 5-year spans. With a 5-year term, it is renewable every 5 years. The premium can change at the end of each fifth year. Ten-, 15-, 20-, 25-, and 30-year term policies end at the end of the term and are not renewable. At the end of the term, a new policy must be purchased with a new premium based on the person's age and health status. For this reason, many people choose 20- or 30-year terms.

Term life insurance can be purchased through an employer, from an insurance agency, from a mortgage lender, or from another lender. Many times mortgage lenders and motor vehicle dealerships offer term life insurance when a purchase is made. The term life insurance pays off the loan upon the death of the borrower. If a person thinks that this is necessary, it may be better to buy a whole life policy or term life insurance for a much larger amount to assist the family in paying other expenses at their death, besides just the car or house.

Permanent Insurance

Permanent insurance includes whole life, universal or adjustable life, variable life, and variable universal life. *Whole life insurance* offers a death benefit and a savings account. Part of the premium goes to a life insurance policy and part goes towards a savings account that grows based on the dividends paid by the insurance company. *Universal or adjustable life insurance* also has a savings account feature called a cash value account, which earns interest at the market rate. If there is enough money in the cash value, either the premiums can be reduced or the cash value can pay the premium until the cash value runs out. If the financial situation changes for an individual, the cash value can help keep the policy in force; however, if the cash value runs out the policy will be cancelled. *Variable life insurance* uses part of the premium to purchase stocks, bonds, and mutual funds. Variable life can increase the earnings of the policy, but can also decrease the value of the cash value and the death benefit depending on the market. Some companies who offer variable life offer a minimum death benefit that cannot change with market fluctuations. *Variable universal life insurance* combines the best features of universal and variable life insurance. The policy has the same risks and benefits of bonds, stocks, and mutual funds and can adjust the premium with the cash value earnings.

If you have no dependents, enough money saved to pay for your burial, and no indebtedness you do not need life insurance of any kind. That description fits very few individuals. If you have dependents, you will want to buy enough life insurance to replace the income that you would have earned if you had lived. You may want to purchase life insurance to create an inheritance or give to a charitable organization. Life insurance should be carefully considered to protect those you love from financial burden, while making sure that having life insurance doesn't become a financial burden.

WHAT IS LONG-TERM CARE INSURANCE?

Long-term care insurance started being offered by employers around 2005. Long-term care insurance covers the individual when someone requires help with many activities of daily living (ADLs). Activities of daily living include getting dressed, bathing, taking medication, doing housework, paying bills, and the like. Long-term care insurance provides care either in-home, in an assisted living center, or in a skilled nursing facility.

Assisted living centers are like apartments that are staffed with people who will help with some ADLs. They provide emergency care 24/7; meals are served three times a day and assistance is provided for getting dressed or taking medication. Assisted living is more expensive than an apartment, but not as expensive as a skilled nursing facility.

Skilled nursing facilities offer nursing care and help with ADLs. Most people in skilled nursing facilities cannot take care of most ADLs, need help with medication and treatments, and are under the supervision of a doctor. They can no longer live independently in either an assisted living center or at home.

In-home care takes place in the person's home, and someone with nursing skills, or other skills depending on the need, comes to help with the ADLs. Sometimes people only require help with ADLs for a short time until they recover from an accident or injury. Sometimes they require care for the duration of their lives.

The premium for long-term care insurance varies depending on the age of the participant—the older the participant the larger the monthly premium. Currently, Medicare pays for only 180 days a year of long-term care and does not pay for in-home care or assisted living centers. If a person needs to stay in a skilled nursing facility, the burden of the cost goes to the family or the individual. The cost of skilled nursing is about $42,000 to $80,000 per year, depending on the state, city, and institution.

WHAT IS COBRA?

The Consolidated Omnibus Budget Reconciliation Act (COBRA) was passed into law in 1986. COBRA is available for terminated employees, those who lose coverage because of reduced work hours, or children who can no longer be on their parents' policy because of age. It provides those people the opportunity to buy group insurance coverage for themselves and their families for limited periods. COBRA allows the person to continue with health insurance, prescription drug coverage, dental insurance, and vision care. COBRA will not cover life insurance.[17]

COBRA covers employees who work for employers with 20 or more employees on more than 50 percent of the calendar workdays. The number includes all part-time and full-time employees. If the employee is covered by the employer's health insurance prior to one of the following events, then the person is qualified for COBRA. Qualifying events for employees include voluntary or involuntary termination (other than gross misconduct) or reduction of work hours. The eligible family members can enroll in COBRA for 18 months after the qualifying event.[17]

Qualifying events for spouses are the same as for employees, plus the employee becoming eligible for Medicare, divorce or legal separation, or death of the employee. Spouses may be insured for 36 months. Children qualify for the events listed for the employee and spouse, plus loss of dependent child status. Children may be covered for 36 months after losing their dependent child status. Qualified persons have a 60-day window to elect to continue coverage through COBRA. The time frame is either the date of qualification or the date the notice to elect COBRA is sent, whichever is later. The premium is paid by the beneficiary of COBRA.[17]

Example 1: Mary has been insured under her mother's health insurance from the university where her mom works. Mary has turned 25 and is no longer allowed to be covered under her mother's insurance. If Mary chooses to pay the premium, she can continue coverage for 36 months.

Example 2: John works but has been under his wife's health insurance plan because it was less expensive. Now John is getting a divorce and he will not be eligible to enroll in his work insurance for another year. If John chooses, he can be covered for 36 months after the date of his divorce.

Example 3: Allen is married with three children. The company that he works for is downsizing and the company has terminated his employment. He is offered COBRA for 18 months, if he chooses to enroll and pay the premium.

HOW DO I CHOOSE A HEALTH INSURANCE PLAN?

The first thing everyone needs to know is that health insurance can be purchased as an individual policy. *Individual insurance* is insurance purchased from an insurance company. *Group insurance* is insurance that is available to groups of individuals, such as employers, unions or professional organizations.

With all of the choices available, someone might ask how to choose a health insurance plan after they are ineligible to participate on their parents' health plan. Most people will get a job after graduation and the employer will offer health insurance. Should you choose to participate in your employer's health insurance plan? The answer is absolutely yes. Employers pay a portion of the premium of the health insurance plan, which will translate into a lower cost for the employee. Plans are cafeteria style and offer different types of health insurance including HMOs, PPOs, dental insurance, vision insurance, and life insurance. However, larger employers will offer a wider variety of plans. How do you choose among the plans?

Many questions need to be answered in order to make an informed choice. If a person has no pre-existing diseases at the time of employment, the questions are going to be how much can you afford now for health insurance and how much money is available if you have an accident or contract a serious illness. Most people want to spend as little as possible on a health insurance plan, because the premium is deducted from gross income. However, the premium is deducted before taxes are deducted from your gross pay, which means that you pay lower taxes. However, if you have a serious accident or you contract a serious disease, will you be able to pay your medical bills? If you have an automobile accident, the costs can be well over $20,000. If the plan has a $1,000 deductible and then pays 80 percent of the remaining bill, the total out-of-pocket expenses will be $4,800. Choosing health insurance should be based on your specific needs and income.

If you do not have a job, high-deductible indemnity health insurance may be the best route to take. Often called catastrophic insurance, you only use it for hospital stays, emergency room visits, and/or repeated doctor's visits that bring your out-of-pocket expenses above the deductible limit. This type of insurance usually pays 80 percent after the deductible is met, which still means that there could be several thousand dollars' worth of debt after the insurance pays. **TABLE 19.1** shows that a $20,000 accident will still cost the insured $4,800. Catastrophic insurance is better than no insurance, because without it, the cost would be $20,000 instead of $4,800. Although $4,800 is not an insignificant amount of money, it would be easier to pay off over time than $20,000.

A healthy person without any serious preconditions might choose an HMO. If your job offers an HMO, choose a doctor who is in the town where you work, because you will be making most of your doctor's visits during normal working hours. If you have children, it would be better to choose a doctor close to home. The premiums are lower for HMOs than for PPO plans and the copays are minimal. One of the most convenient aspects of HMOs is that doctor visits have one copay that includes all diagnostic services. HMOs are also one of the most inexpensive plans.

If you answered that the primary doctor may not have felt a specialist was needed and would not give a referral, you would be accurate. The caveat with HMO plans is that the main provider works as a gatekeeper for diagnostic services and referrals. The main provider may not want to refer a specialist and may want to handle the disease or condition in his or her office. That may or may not be in your best interest. If you have a serious precondition, you may want to choose a PPO. Although the premiums are higher, the plan has more flexibility for specialists. PPOs are also a good choice when there are no HMOs in your area and when you are covering a large family with children going to school outside your area. HMOs cover only emergency care outside of the HMO network.

PPOs have an individual and a family deductible that must be met prior to the insurance plan reimbursing you for medical expenses. The family deductible is to help the

Table 19.1
Automobile Accident Costing $20,000

TYPE OF PLAN	DEDUCTIBLE	COPAY	OUT-OF-POCKET EXPENSES
High-deductible plan: $1,000 per person, pays 80% after deductible	$1,000	$3,800	$4,800
HMO: $50 emergency copay		$50	$50
PPO: $500 per person deductible, pays 80% after deductible	$500	$3,900	$4,400

family if one member has extreme medical costs; however, each person must meet their deductible prior to reimbursement. Most plans have choices for deductible amounts. For instance, there may be a $300 or a $500 deductible amount. The higher the deductible, the lower the premiums are. The best way to choose is to determine how often you use medical services. If you rarely go to the doctor, then the higher deductible may be the right choice. If you are a woman, then you may want to consider the lower deductible because of the yearly visits to the gynecologist and tests that are required with each visit. If you are over the age of 40, it also might be wise to choose the lower deductible because of the increased chances of becoming ill and the greater number of tests that are recommended. After the deductible is met the insured pays for the services and then files a claim with the insurance company for reimbursement of about 80 percent of the medical expenses. The wait for reimbursement depends on the company and the state laws. Most insurance companies reimburse their clients in about 4–6 weeks, which is another consideration.

If you are uninsured and you are pregnant, Medicaid may be able to help you with the cost of medical care. Medicaid is available to people who earn an income that is below poverty level. Medicaid will insure women who are pregnant and children in qualified households. People with disabilities may also qualify for Medicaid. Medicaid pays 100 percent of all qualifying expenses, but does not cover dental or vision services. If you are uninsured and you have a child, the Children's Health Insurance Plan (CHIP) may be able to help you with health insurance. CHIP is subsidized by the federal government but is processed by the state. CHIP has a low premium that is on a sliding scale according to your income, and is available only for children. For instance, in Texas, the yearly premium for insuring a child is $0 or $50 depending on the household income; copays for doctor's visits and prescription drugs are $3–10 depending on the provider. In New York State, the premiums are $0 to $15 a month depending on the household income, and there are no copays for services. Check with your state to determine your eligibility and the costs involved.

If you are over the age of 65, Medicare is available for a monthly premium depending on your income. If your income is below poverty level, you are eligible for Medicaid and Medicare, with Medicaid paying the deductibles and long-term care costs. Medicare reimburses a percentage of certain medical expenses. Like PPOs, people can choose their provider and Medicare reimburses 80 percent of hospital visits through Part B insurance. Part A insurance covers hospital visits, diagnostic costs, and some treatments. People can also enroll in prescription coverage through Part D.

Most health insurance plans cover prescriptions with a set copay or percentage of reimbursement. HMOs generally

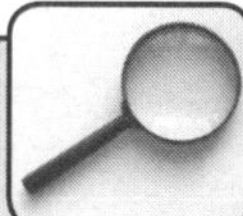

Case Study

Roxanne is a divorced mother of a 6 year old son. Recently the son needed to have reconstructive surgery on his inner ear to restore his hearing. The chain bones in his inner ear were destroyed during his many ear infections when he was younger. Roxanne is covered by a local HMO through her job at a university. Her provider was happy to refer him to an ear, nose, and throat (ENT) specialist. The visit to the doctor had a copay of $25 and the copay for the surgery was $100. This is the second surgery her son had to restore his hearing, and the last time the cost was over $5,000 because Roxanne had a PPO rather than an HMO.

Question

In this instance, what could have been a problem with the son's care because of Roxanne's enrollment in an HMO?

offer prescription benefits with a set copay for formulary drugs and generic drugs. PPOs have a formulary list as well, and only reimburse up to a certain amount for each drug on their formulary list. Formulary drugs are a list of drugs that have been approved by the insurance company. Non-formulary drugs are not on the list and need prior approval to be eligible for the prescription plan. For instance, many people take Allegra D for allergies. Before it became an over-the-counter-drug, an insurance company may have had a new formulary list that had Zyrtec D instead. If the person had switched to Zyrtec D, they would only have had to pay the $25 copay instead of the actual cost of the prescription, which was approximately $156 per month.

HMOs have a lower copay for generic drugs, but not as low as a new service that is being offered across the country. Grocery stores and large retail chains that have pharmacies, along with some pharmacies, are offering $4 to $5 for a one month order of generic prescriptions at commonly prescribed doses and $9 to $10 for 90-day supplies of generic prescriptions. There are no enrollment fees or other costs involved, and anyone is qualified to take advantage of it.

Another choice for insurance from many employers is dental insurance. Each plan will vary in its network of providers. You pay a set fee to plans that reimburse you for a percentage of specific services up to the plan limit. For instance, the network of dentists provides services at a set fee that is well below the regular fee for those services. The plans that reimburse usually pay for cleanings and exams twice a year without a copay and reimburse up to 80 percent for dental services up to a maximum of $1000 per year. Most plans offer a lifetime benefit for braces up to a certain amount, such as $2,500. The premiums for dental insurance are fairly inexpensive, for instance $90 per year for a family.

Vision insurance is also offered through different vision insurance companies. The premiums are very low and the cost of services varies from plan to plan. Some vision insurance is offered through HMOs, with premiums included in the health insurance. The plan offers, for instance, frames up to $50 and plain lenses with either single vision, bifocals, or trifocals for a $10 copay with the eye exam for $25. Other plans outside of HMOs offer lenses that are more expensive and frames for a copay of about $25 for glasses and $25 for the eye exam. Contacts are free with an HMO and have the same copay for glasses on the other plans.

Most employers offer free life insurance to their employees for a small amount of insurance, most of them not large enough to pay for the burial. Additional life insurance is available for a monthly premium. Decisions regarding life insurance are difficult to advise. If there are no children and no large indebtedness, there is little need to purchase additional life insurance.

Another choice to make is for disability insurance. Disability insurance is intended to cover some of your monthly income if you become disabled due to accident or injury while off the job. All employers are required to cover you with insurance in case you are injured on the job, but it is a very small percentage of your monthly income and you are required to visit doctors specializing in job accidents that may not be your doctor. Disability insurance is a personal choice, but most young people should decide if it is worth the premium.

Remember that only about 4 percent of people over the age of 65 are in long-term care, but most people know of at least one person in a long-term care facility. It is a difficult decision to make, but if you are young, you may not want to enroll.

CONCLUSION

The information given in this chapter was intended to raise your awareness about health insurance in the United States. Obtaining employment that offers health insurance benefits will add hundreds of dollars to your total employment package. If you are in-between jobs, COBRA is a choice. Always keep in mind the fact that if you should get a serious disease or disability and you do not have health insurance, you are

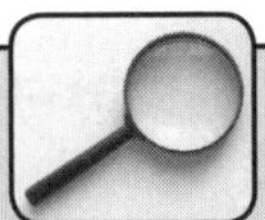

Case Study

Since Megan Smith, referred to in the first case study in this chapter, is only 23, she is less likely to have any serious injury or disease. Because of the high deductible on the PPO insurance she will be paying out of pocket up to $500 per year to see her hometown doctor. It may be in her best interest to buy the HMO coverage for anything serious that might happen and pay out of pocket to see her hometown doctor, because she would be paying out of pocket anyway if she chose the PPO. Also, the HMO covers vision so that she doesn't have to pay the $10 per month extra. The free life insurance is almost enough to cover the cost to bury Megan, so it is probably enough life insurance for now, until she buys a house or gets married and has children. Disability insurance is probably unnecessary because she does not have a high risk job and lives near her home, but it is a personal decision. Long-term care insurance may be an important purchase, but it might be good to take a look at the monthly cost and see if putting that into a savings account would earn enough to pay for long-term care without insurance. What do you think?

at risk of losing everything. Investigate further the Patient Protection and Affordable Care Act to determine if there is aid for you.

Suggestions for Class Activities

1. Form groups in the class. Each group should select one of the following to research: Medicare, Medicaid, traditional health insurance, Affordable Care Act, HMOs, PPOs, and other types of insurance. Each group should write main points about their type of insurance on butcher paper using large markers. Place on a wall and discuss each.
2. Ask people in several age groups to come to the class and form a panel presentation. Before the panel presentation, the members of the panel will be given a list of questions that could be asked. Class members will compose the questions regarding: health insurance, life insurance, views about the ACA, HMOs, PPOs, Medicare, Medicaid and so forth.

Review Questions

1. What is health insurance?
2. What do you feel should be the rights of U.S. citizens regarding health insurance?
3. What percentage of U.S. citizens are covered by employer-sponsored health insurance?
4. What percentage of U.S. citizens are covered by privately purchased insurance?
5. Why is there a difference by ethnicity in the numbers of people who are covered by insurance?
6. Why does health insurance cost so much?
7. What are the main provisions of the Affordable Care Act?
8. What are indemnity plans?
9. What are basic health plans?
10. What are health savings accounts?
11. What are high-deductible health plans?
12. What are managed care options?
13. What are health maintenance organizations (HMOs)?
14. What are point-of-service (POS) plans?
15. What are preferred provider organizations (PPOs)?
16. Who is eligible for government health insurance?
17. What is Medicaid?
18. What is Medicare?
19. Who is eligible for the State Children's Health Insurance Program (SCHIP)?
20. What is military health care?
21. What is disability insurance?
22. What is covered under vision insurance?
23. What kinds of life insurance are available?
24. What is long-term care insurance?
25. What is COBRA?

Key Terms

Archer Medical Savings Accounts Individual accounts that may be set up by self-employed individuals and those who work for small businesses (less than 50 employees).

beneficiary The person who receives a death benefit.

COBRA (Consolidated Omnibus Budget Reconciliation Act) Terminated employees, those who lose coverage because of reduced work hours, or children who can no longer be on their parents' policy because of age may be able to buy group coverage for themselves and their families for limited periods of time.

contingent beneficiaries Receive the death benefit when the policy holder dies and the primary beneficiaries are also deceased or cannot be found.

copayment The amount of money the insured is responsible for paying for each visit or time of service. These amounts are set by the insurance company.

decreasing term life Insurance that decreases in value over the life of the policy.

disability insurance Insurance that covers the loss of income due to illness or injury.

flexible spending arrangements Savings accounts set up by employers that allow employees to contribute on a pretax basis to reimburse health care expenses

group insurance Insurance available to groups of individuals, such as employers, unions, or professional organizations.

health maintenance organizations (HMOs) Insurance plans usually provided through an employer. Plan has a main provider (doctor) who is a gatekeeper for all services.

indemnity insurance Allows the individuals to choose their health care providers.

individual insurance Insurance for one individual purchased from an insurance company.

level term life Life insurance that pays the same amount on the death of the policy holder at any time during the life of the policy.

Medicaid Government insurance for people who meet financial need criteria and for people who are disabled.

medical necessity A procedure that is required for the benefit of a person's physical health. Cosmetic surgery is not considered a medical necessity, for instance.

medical savings account Allows a person to save pretax dollars to use for medical expenditures that are not covered by insurance.

Medicare Government insurance for everyone who has paid Social Security and is over the age of 65 and some disabled people.

pre-existing conditions Medical problems that an insured person already has prior to acquiring health insurance. Some pre-existing conditions are not covered by insurance.

preferred provider organizations (PPOs) Networks of physicians that work with an insurance company with a negotiated rate for services.

primary beneficiaries Receive the death benefit upon the policy holder's death.

State Children's Health Insurance Program Insurance offered to children whose parents do not qualify for Medicaid, but do not have health insurance.

variable life insurance Uses part of the premium to purchase stocks, bonds, and mutual funds.

variable-universal life insurance Provides death benefits and cash values that vary when the investment portfolio changes (money market, government bond accounts, equity accounts).

whole life insurance Offers a death benefit and a savings account.

References

1. Cooper R. How to make the most of your health care coverage. April 30, 2007. Available at: http://www.ncdoj.gov/News-and-Alerts/Consumer-Columns/How-to-make-the-most-of-your-health-care-coverage.aspx Accessed June 30, 2008 and September 5, 2011.
2. U.S. Census Bureau. Income, poverty, and health insurance coverage in the United States: 2009. Available at: http://www.census.gov/prod/2010pubs/p60-238.pdf. Accessed June 6, 2011
3. National Coalition on Health Care. Health insurance cost: facts on the cost of health care. 2008. Available at:http://nchc.org/sites/default/files/resources/Fact%20Sheet%20-%20Cost.pdf. Accessed September 5, 2011.
4. Centers for Medicare and Medicaid Services. NHE fact sheet. Available at: https://www.cms.gov/NationalHealthExpendData/25_NHE_Fact_Sheet.asp#TopOfPage. Accessed April 28, 2011.
5. Kaiser Family Foundation. Employer health benefits 2010 annual survey. Average annual worker and employer contribution to premiums for family coverage, 1999–2010. Available at: http://ehbs.kff.org/?page = charts&id = 1&sn = 6&p = 1. Accessed June 3, 2011.
6. Kaiser Family Foundation website. Average annual worker and employer contributions to premiums for family coverage, 1999–2010. Available at: http://facts.kff.org/chart.aspx?ch = 1545. Accessed June 3, 2011.
7. Business Exchange. News commentary on the Affordable Care Act. Available at: http://bx.businessweek.com. Accessed June 2008.
8. White House. Blog: putting Americans in control of their health care. Available at: http://www.whitehouse.gov/health-care-meeting/questions/no-insurance. Accessed March 6, 2011.
9. U.S. Department of Health and Human Services. News release: Secretary Sebelius announces $51 million in Affordable Care Act grants to innovate, improve, and enhance health insurance premium rate review. Available at: http://www.hhs.gov/news/press/2010pres/06/20100607a.html. Accessed June 4, 2011.
10. Kaiser Family Foundation website. Health Insurance Coverage in the U.S., 2009. Available at: http://facts.kff.org/chart.aspx?ch = 477. Accessed June 3, 2011.
11. Kaiser Family Foundation. Nonelderly uninsured by poverty level and age. Available at: http://facts.kff.org/chart.aspx?ch = 1476. Accessed June 2, 2011.
12. Agency for Healthcare Research and Quality. What is consumer-directed coverage? Available at: http://www.ahrq.gov/consumer/insuranceqa/insuranceqa6.htm. Accessed June 20, 2008.
13. Insurance Information Institute. What are my health insurance choices? Available at: http://www.iii.org/individuals/healthinsurance/ Accessed June 20, 2011.
14. Torpy JM, Burke AE, Glass RM. Health care insurance: the basics. *JAMA*. 2007;297(10):1154.
15. HealthCare.gov. Provisions of the Affordable Care Act, by year. Available at: http://www.healthcare.gov/law/about/order/byyear.html. Accessed June 20, 2011.
16. Kaiser Family Foundation. Focus on health reform. Available at: http://www.kff.org/healthreform/upload/8061.pdf. Accessed June 20, 2011.
17. Pension and Welfare Benefits Administration. COBRA insurance summary. 1994. Available at: http://www.cobrahealthinsurance.com/Cobra_Health_Insurance_Summary.html. Accessed June 25, 2008.

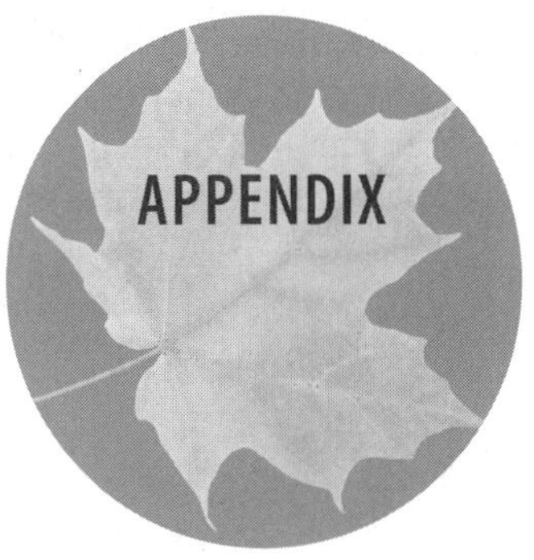

APPENDIX

Available Internet Health Resources

PROTOCOL FOR EVALUATING HEALTH RESOURCES ON THE INTERNET

The following eight criteria are used by the Health on the Net Foundation (HON) to award its approval for quality health information found on the Internet. According to its Web site,

> The Health On the Net Foundation (HON) promotes and guides the deployment of useful and reliable online health information, and its appropriate and efficient use. Created in 1995, HON is a non-profit, non-governmental organization, accredited to the Economic and Social Council of the United Nations. For twelve years, HON has focused on the essential question of the provision of health information to citizens, information that respects ethical standards. To cope with the unprecedented volume of healthcare information available on the Net, the HON code of conduct offers a multi-stakeholder consensus on standards to protect citizens from misleading health information.

HON has reviewed 5,533 sites in 72 countries covering 32 languages, and has accredited over 1.2 million Web pages. More information on the Health on the Net Foundation can be found at http://www.hon.ch/pat.html.

Consumers can look for the HON designation on a Web site, in the criterion search in their search engine, or use the descriptions themselves to determine the legitimacy of the information they retrieve.

According to HON, a Web site should be (or have):

1. *Authoritative:* Indicate the qualifications of the authors.
2. *Complementarity:* Information should support, not replace, the doctor–patient relationship.
3. *Private:* Respect the privacy and confidentiality of personal data submitted to the site by the visitor.
4. *Attribution:* Cite the source(s) of published information, data, and medical and health pages.
5. *Justifiability:* Site must back up claims relating to benefits and performance.
6. *Transparency:* Accessible presentation, identities of editor and Webmaster, and accurate e-mail contact information.
7. *Financial disclosure:* Identify funding sources.
8. *Advertising policy:* Clearly distinguish advertising from editorial content.

WHAT ARE THE BEST WEB SITES FOR DISEASE AND CONDITION INFORMATION?

The Consumer and Patient Health Information Section (CAPHIS) of the Medical Library Association compiles the most complete online listing of credible health information Web sites into what is called the CAPHIS Top 100 List. CAPHIS uses the Criteria for Assessing the Quality of Health Information on the Internet created by the Health Summit Working Group. The criteria used to create the list are quite similar to the HON criteria and include credibility, sponsorship/authorship, content, audience, currency, disclosure, purpose, links, design, interactivity, and caveats. The Web site breaks down the list into categories for easy review by the consumer. You can find the list at http://caphis.mlanet.org/consumer/.

WHERE CAN I FIND INFORMATION REGARDING HEALTH HOTLINES?

The most comprehensive roster of organizations offering "hotline" assistance is managed and updated by the National Library of Medicine (NLM), a component agency of the National Institutes of Health. The database describes more than 14,000 resources, listed by topic area or by group disseminating the information on a particular disease. All numbers contained in the listing are verified by the NLM. The database can be found at http://healthhotlines.nlm.nih.gov/index.html.

IS THERE A SIMPLE WAY TO IDENTIFY A DOCTOR, SPECIALIST, HOSPITAL, OR CLINIC?

The National Library of Medicine also manages a database of physicians, clinicians, hospitals, clinics, dentists, midwives, specialists, and virtually every type of health care professional you might need. This easy to use link-oriented Web site will redirect you to the appropriate agency or organization that hosts the directory. You can find the listing at http://www.nlm.nih.gov/medlineplus/directories.html.

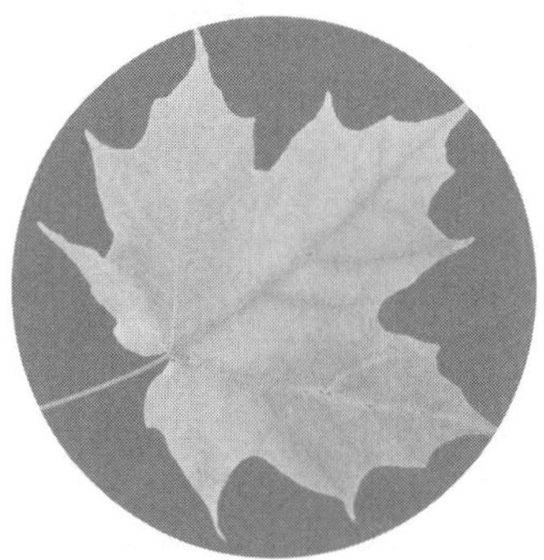

Glossary

A

absolutes Plant extractions that are obtained by using chemical solvents.

activator A small tool used by chiropractors that delivers a light and measured force to correct a misalignment.

active release technique (ART) Technique designed to treat scar tissue adhesions, which can cause symptoms such as pain, weakness, and restricted range of motion. It is also used to treat overused muscles that may have small tears or are not getting enough oxygen.

activism A doctrine or practice that emphasizes direct vigorous action, especially in support of or opposition to one side of a controversial issue.

acupressure The application of pressure or localized massage to specific sites on the body to control symptoms such as pain or nausea.

acupuncture Procedure that increases the flow of qi energy to treat illness or provide local pain relief by the insertion of stainless steel needles at specified sites on the body.

acupuncture point injection Sterile syringes are used to inject vitamins or herbal products into the system via the trigger points.

adjustment A process of manipulating misaligned vertebrae or other joints in the body (e.g., wrist bones and joints) back into place.

adulterate To corrupt, debase, or make impure by the addition of a foreign or inferior substance or element.

advertising The act or practice of calling public attention to a product or service.

Alexander technique A process in which people can learn to release muscular tension and habitually overtightened muscles that cause our bodies to become distorted, unbalanced, and compressed.

alkaloids A group of chemicals alkaloid in nature.

allopathic medicine A system in which medical doctors and other health care professionals (such as nurses, pharmacists, and therapists) treat symptoms and diseases using drugs, radiation, or surgery. Also called biomedicine, conventional medicine, mainstream medicine, orthodox medicine, and Western medicine.

allopathic physician A traditional or orthodox physician who is a medical doctor (MD).

alternative medicine Those medical or health related treatments used as a replacement for traditional medical practices (e.g., use of a special diet to treat cancer rather than surgery or chemotherapy) are known as alternative.

anatripsis The act of rubbing up during massage.

anointing Involves dipping a finger in oil and touching a person either on the forehead or on another body part as part of a religious ceremony.

Archer Medical Savings Accounts Individual accounts that may be set up by self-employed individuals and those who work for small businesses (less than 50 employees).

aromatherapist A person trained in the use of essential oils.

aromatherapy Means "treatment using scents"; the use of concentrated plant oils.

asanas Another name for yoga poses.

Asclepions Sanctuaries of healing. They had their roots in ancient Greece on the island of Kos.

assessment A process in Reiki wherein the practitioner determines where and how the energy of the patient is moving.

astringent A substance or preparation that constricts tissue. It can lessen discharges such as mucus or blood.

attorney general The principal legal officer who represents a state in legal proceedings and gives legal advice to the government.

attunement A Reiki right of passage where the ability to heal is passed on to a new Reiki practitioner from a Reiki master.

auricular acupuncture Uses points in the ears that correspond to areas of the body and bodily symptoms.

autism A mental condition, present from early childhood, characterized by great difficulty in communicating and forming relationships, and in using language and abstract concepts.

Ayurveda Sanskrit word that means science of life or science of lifespan.

Ayurvedic medicine (ayurveda) A form of holistic alternative medicine that is the traditional system of medicine of India. It may have influenced ancient Chinese medicine and the humoral medicine practiced by Hippocrates in Greece.

B

Bach® Original Flower Remedies Tinctures made from flowers to treat emotions rather than disease.

bandwagon Advertising technique in which mass appeal is used to attract customers.

basti Medicated enema or colonic irrigation.

behavioral advertising Tracking a consumer's pattern of Internet use in an effort to display specific types of advertising that might appeal to those use patterns.

beneficiary The person who receives a death benefit.

biased Unknown or unacknowledged error created during the design, measurement, sampling, procedure, or choice of problem studied.

biofeedback A mind–body intervention that helps train people to control their own bodily functions by using their minds. This is done by being connected to electrical sensors that help people visualize information about their bodily functions and thus allow them to learn how to control them.

biofield The energy emitted from the human body.

biological Any substance, such as a serum or vaccine, derived from animal products or other biological sources and used to treat or prevent disease.

biologically based therapies Use of natural techniques to maintain health and/or treat diseases.

biomedical physician A physician trained in the application of the principles of the natural sciences, especially biology and physiology, to clinical medicine.

biomedicine The application of the principles of the natural sciences, especially biology and physiology, to clinical medicine.

bioresonance The practice of using an electronic device to measure the body's electromagnetic radiation and electric currents.

biotypes Body types or body constitution that naturopaths use to aid a diagnosis because they believe that each type has certain characteristics that are related to risk of particular diseases.

blood lactate A chemical associated with stress.

bonesetters People who set the broken bones of people without conducting surgery.

botanical A drug, medicinal preparation, or similar substance obtained from a plant or plants.

Bravewell Collaborative Founded in 2002 by a small group of leading philanthropists dedicated to transforming the culture and delivery of health care and improving the health of the public through integrative medicine.

Buddhism A religion that originated in India by Buddha (Gautama) and later spread to China, Burma, Japan, Tibet, and parts of southeast Asia. It holds life is full of suffering caused by desire, and the way to end this suffering is through enlightenment that enables one to halt the endless sequence of births and deaths to which one is otherwise subject.

Burmese position Sitting on the floor and using a zafu—a small pillow—to raise the hips just a little, so the knees can touch the ground. Sitting on the pillow with two knees touching the ground forms a tripod base that gives 360-degree stability.

C

calibration To adjust instrumentation so that it will be precise.

cardiac glycosides These chemicals have a marked action on the heart, strengthening the force and speed of systolic contractions.

carotenoid pigments Pigments found in yellow to red plants such as carrots, sweet potatoes, red and yellow peppers, squash, and tomatoes.

carrier oils Base or vegetable oils used to dilute CO_2s and absolutes before applying them to skin.

channel In Reiki, the role of practitioner. Energy sent to the patient simply flows through the Reiki healer, who is the channel.

chelation therapy Use of a drug to bind with, and remove, excess or toxic amounts of metal or minerals from the blood.

chiropractic A discipline and profession that focuses on disorders of the musculoskeletal and nervous systems under the belief that the effects of these disorders negatively impact health.

chiropractic medicine A method of treatment based on the belief that the nervous system, skeletal system, and muscular system interact and if that interaction is blocked, disease and/or pain will occur.

chiropractic mixers A group of chiropractors who believe that subluxations can lower resistance to disease or cause a neurological imbalance within the body, thus lowering resistance to disease. They would use adjustments to treat back pain, neck pain, and other musculoskeletal disorders. They would also use other modalities such as heat, ice, water, electricity, vitamins, colonic irrigation, and other physical and mechanical adjuncts.

chiropractic objective straights A group of chiropractors who focus only on the correction of chiropractic vertebral subluxations.

chiropractic reformers Chiropractors who recommend chiropractic care only for musculoskeletal disorders and do not believe that spinal joint dysfunction is the cause of disease; therefore, they do not focus on subluxations only.

chiropractic traditional straights A group of chiropractors who claim that chiropractic adjustments are a plausible treatment for a wide range of diseases.

chlorophyll Pigment found in green plants and dark green leafy vegetables such as spinach, parsley, kale, green beans, and leeks.

cholera An acute infectious disease characterized by profuse diarrhea, vomiting, and cramps.

chondritis Inflammation of a cartilage.

Christian Science A healing methodology that does not use medicine. Mary Baker Eddy founded Christian Science and based it on the healing methods of Phineas Quimby.

CO_2s Plant oils extracted by the carbon dioxide method.

chronic Relating to an illness or medical condition that is characterized by long duration or frequent recurrence.

COBRA (Consolidated Omnibus Budget Reconciliation Act) Terminated employees, those who lose coverage because of reduced work hours, or children who can no longer be on their parents' policy because of age may be able to buy group coverage for themselves and their families for limited periods of time.

cold-pressed extraction Process involving mechanical pressure to force the oils out of citrus fruit, nuts, and seeds.

compendium A brief summary of a larger work or of a field of knowledge.

complementary and alternative medicine A group of diverse medical and health care systems, practices, and products that are not generally considered to be part of conventional medicine.

concentration technique Involves concentrating on an external object as a focus point for the mind.

concrete Waxy mass that remains after solvent extraction. The waxy concrete is then processed to remove the waxy materials.

constitution Pattern of energy that comprises or makes up a person.

consumer One who buys products or services for personal use and not for the purpose of resale.

contemplative meditation techniques Use introspection, self-study, and reflection. Contemplative meditation is supposed to help people gain a deeper understanding of some aspect of reality.

contingent beneficiaries Receive the death benefit when the policy holder dies and the primary beneficiaries are also deceased or cannot be found.

copayment The amount of money the insured is responsible for paying for each visit or time of service. These amounts are set by the insurance company.

cortisol A chemical associated with stress.

D

deceit Concealment or distortion of the truth for the purpose of misleading.

decoction The process of boiling a substance in water to extract its essence.

decreasing term life Insurance that decreases over the life of the policy.

defraud To deprive of something by deception or fraud.

degenerative arthritis Chronic breakdown of cartilage in the joints; the most common form of arthritis, occurring usually after middle age.

degrees, Reiki Levels of advancement in the art of Reiki.

dementias Gradual and progressive decline in cognitive and reasoning skills plus loss of memory. The most common is Alzheimer's disease.

demographic A single vital or social statistic of a human population, such as the number of births or deaths.

deregulation To remove governmental regulations and control.

dervish dancers Turkish dancers who dress in a particular style and seem to dance to the rhythm of the cosmos or the universe.

diagnosis Identification of a diseased condition.

diet therapy Prescribed to increase qi energy; it is grounded in the theories of five elements and eight guiding principles.

direct-to-consumer Advertising sent directly to the consumer, not through a third-party provider.

disability insurance Insurance that covers the loss of income due to illness or injury.

distant healing Involves people praying for and healing others at great distances away (sometimes without the ill person knowing it). Also known as intercessory prayer.

Doppler ultrasound A form of ultrasound that can detect and measure blood flow.

dosha Five elements, space (akasha), air (vayu), fire (agni), water (apu), and earth (prithvi) make up the body's constitution called dosha. There are three doshas: Vata, Pitta, and Kapha.

E

echinacea A genus of herbaceous flowering plants in the daisy family, *Asteraceae*. It is an herb used to fight infections, especially upper respiratory conditions such as the common cold.

ectomorph Body type in which the appearance of the body is thin.

effleurage Massage using contours of the body; uses a smooth stroke.

electro-acupuncture Mild electrical pulses are relayed via acupuncture needles to various trigger points in the skin.

empirical A word derived from the Greek word for experience or observation.

empty mind meditation Involves sitting still, often in a full lotus or cross-legged position, and letting the mind go silent on its own.

endemic Diseases belonging exclusively or confined to a particular place.

endomorph Body type in which the appearance of the body is round and soft. The physique presents the illusion that much of the mass has been concentrated in the abdominal area.

endorphins Natural pain-killing substances produced in the human body and released by stress or trauma.

epidemic Diseases that affect many persons at the same time, and spread from person to person from one locale to another.

equity Justice according to natural law or right; freedom from bias or favoritism.

erectile dysfunction Difficulty in achieving or maintaining an erection; impotence.

essential oils Distilled liquid from the leaves, stems, flowers, bark, roots, or other elements of a plant.

experimental Subjects are randomly selected or assigned into a treatment or control group.

expression A method to extract essential oils from the rinds of citrus fruit without using heat. Requires squeezing by hand and collecting oils with a sponge.

external qi gong The practice of transferring the practitioner's qi to another person for healing purposes. This form of qi gong is similar to other body work modalities in the West, such as therapeutic touch.

F

facet joint A synovial joint that helps support the weight and control movement between individual vertebrae of the spine. Facet joints are at the back on either side of the spinal column, between the discs and the vertebral bodies. The bony prominences of each vertebrae form a joint with the vertebrae above and below. The role of the facet joints is to limit excessive movement and provide stability for the spine.

faith or spiritual energy healing Has occurred since earliest times among all cultures, religions, and medicinal practices. Various healing techniques are used (including chants and prayer, touching, or placing the hands close to the body within the energy fields that surround the body). Popular current methods include Reiki therapy, therapeutic touch, qi gong healing, and crystal healing.

fasting To abstain from all food.

feeling and emotion meditation techniques These may be used independently but also may be combined with other types of meditations.

five elements (or tattwa) Earth, water, fire, air, and ether or space.

fixed oils Referred to as vegetable, carrier; or base oils; they contain nutrients such as minerals, antioxidants, and fat-soluble vitamins.

flavonoids A set of chemicals that include brilliant plant pigments seen in fruits and vegetables.

flaxseed A member of the genus *Linum* in the family *Linaceae*. It is a blue flowering plant that contains rich oily seeds. It is recommended for general well-being and digestive health.

flexible spending arrangements Savings accounts set up by employers that allow employees to contribute on a pretax basis to reimburse health care expenses.

florasols/phytols extraction method A process that uses gaseous solvents to extract essential oils.

Food and Drug Administration A division of the U.S. Department of Health and Human Services that protects the public against impure and unsafe foods, drugs, and cosmetics.

form A series of predetermined and/or scripted movements designed to increase, unblock, or promote healing through the acquisition of energy (qi).

franchise The right or license granted to an individual or group to market a company's goods or services in a particular territory; a business granted such a right or license.

fraud A deceitful, tricky, or willful act committed to gain an unfair or dishonest advantage or to make a profit (make money off someone else).

free radicals Unstable oxygen molecules that can cause tissue damage.

full lotus position A seated position in which each leg is placed on the opposite thigh.

fumigation Burning of plant oils to create a great deal of smoke.

G

galvanic stimulation Uses direct high-voltage pulsed current to create an electric field over the area to be treated. Two pads are used. One slows circulation and decreases swelling and the other pad causes increased circulation to speed up the healing process.

gauss rating The degree of magnetic strength based solely on materials used to construct the magnet.

genomics A recent scientific discipline that strives to define and characterize the complete genetic makeup of an organism.

ghee A mixture also known as sneha made from cow's milk into an edible oil or medicated butter.

globalization Marked especially by free trade, free flow of capital, and the tapping of cheaper foreign labor markets.

glucosamine A natural compound found in healthy cartilage. Glucosamine sulfate is used for arthritic conditions.

group insurance Insurance available to groups of individuals, like employers, unions, or professional organizations.

Gurdjieff Sacred Dances A technique wherein the movements are very defined and different parts of the body seem not to be related to each other.

guru One who is regarded as having great knowledge, wisdom, and authority in a certain area and who uses it to guide others.

H

half lotus position A seated position in which the left foot is placed onto the right thigh and the right leg is tucked under the left thigh.

halitosis Offensive odor of the breath.

health care conglomerates Composed of hospitals, clinics, and research facilities that either include, or are affiliated with, a medical school.

health maintenance organizations (HMOs) Insurance plans usually provided through an employer that have a main provider who is a gatekeeper for services.

hemochromatosis A disorder wherein the body is not able to break down iron; therefore, too much is absorbed from the gastrointestinal tract, causing abdominal pain and fatigue.

herbalist A practitioner of, and contributor to the field of, herbal medicine.

holistic A concept in medical practice upholding that all aspects of people's needs, psychological, physical, mental, emotional and social, should be taken into account and seen as a whole.

homeopathic medicine An alternative approach to medicine based on the belief that natural substances, prepared in a special way and used most often in very small amounts, restore health. According to these beliefs, in order for a remedy to be effective, it must cause in a healthy person the same symptoms being treated in the patient.

homeopathy The use of extremely diluted substances given to cure disease using the law of similars: *like cures like.*

hydrosol Floral water or distillate water that remains after distilling an essential oil.

hydrotherapy The treatment of physical disability, injury, or illness by immersion of all or part of the body in water to facilitate movement, promote wound healing, and relieve pain. It is usually done under the supervision of a trained therapist. May involve the use of hot, moist soaks or dry heat for pain relief and to promote healing.

hypnosis A mind–body technique that focuses on awareness and attention to internal stimuli, much like what is learned while doing meditation. The word "hypnosis" comes from the Greek word *hypnos*, meaning sleep. It was first termed "animal magnetism."

hypnotherapy Therapy using hypnosis to gain access to the deeper levels of the mind so that a change in thinking and behavior will occur.

hypnosis The induction of a person into a state of consciousness in which he or she is responsive to a suggestion/s by a therapist.

hypothesis A proposition, or set of propositions, set forth as an explanation for the occurrence of some specified group of phenomena. There are four types of hypotheses: nondirectional, directional, correlative, and null.

I

immobilization therapies Use of splints, casts, wraps, and traction to immobilize body parts so that the injured part may heal.

incontinence Inability to control excretion of urine and feces.

indemnity insurance Allows the individual to choose their health care providers.

individual insurance Insurance purchased by an individual wherein the policy only applies for that person.

infrastructure The basic, underlying framework or features of a system or organization.

infomercial A product commercial of significant length designed to look like a television show.

information and communications technologies (ICT) An umbrella term that includes any communication device or application, including radio, television, cellular phones, computer and network hardware and software, satellite systems, and so on, as well as the various services and applications associated with them, such as videoconferencing and distance learning.

infused oil Carrier oil that has been mixed with one or more herbs.

integrative medicine Combines treatments from conventional medicine and CAM for which there is evidence of safety and effectiveness.

intercessory prayer Involves people praying for and healing others at great distances away (sometimes without the ill person knowing it). Also known as distant healing.

interferential current (IFC) A kind of TENS therapy in which high-frequency electrical impulses are introduced into the tissue near the pain center.

internal qi gong Uses certain movements and breath work or visualization to gather and circulate qi in the body.

iridology The examination of the iris or colored portion of the eye for markings that supposedly reveal changing conditions of every part and organ of the body.

J

Japanese-style acupuncture Uses fewer and thinner needles with less stimulation than traditional Chinese acupuncture.

K

Kirlian photography Colorful photographs of images surrounding the body and within the body that are made after applying high-frequency electrical currents to a patient's body.

Koan meditation technique Meditations from the Zen School of Buddhism that are designed to break down an ordinary pattern of thinking.

Korean acupuncture Uses points in the hand that correspond to areas of the body and bodily symptoms.

L

laser acupoint stimulation Uses rays or laser beams rather than acupuncture needles to facilitate the trigger point.

level term life Life insurance that pays the same amount on the death of the policy holder at any time during the life of the policy.

lignans Phytoestrogens with weak estrogenic or anti-estrogenic activity.

lobby To attempt to influence or sway someone (such as a public official) toward a desired action.

M

maceration Soaking aromatic plants in animal fats or vegetable oils to prepare for vacuum distillation.

magnet therapy The use of magnets on or around the human body to restructure the flow of energy in the human body for purposes of healing and well-being.

malas Waste products such as urine, feces, or sweat.

malpractice (medical malpractice) An injurious, negligent, or improper medical practice or treatment as by a physician or other health professional.

mandala Means completion or circle; from the classical Indian language of Sanskrit. They may be made from paper, textiles or colored sand in various sizes and colors. They are often used as a point of focus during meditation.

mantra meditation A word or phrase repeated during meditation.

marmas Ayurvedic massage pressure points.

martial arts Encompass understanding the relationship of the power of breath, the life force (qi energy), the mind, and the concept of oneness.

massage May come from the Arabic verb *mass*, meaning to touch, or from the Greek word *massein*, meaning to touch, to handle, to knead, or to squeeze.

medial Pertaining to the middle.

Medicaid Government insurance for people who meet financial need criteria and for people who are disabled.

medical acupuncture Acupuncture performed by a Western medical doctor.

medical necessity A procedure that is required for the benefit of a person's physical health. Cosmetic surgery is not considered a medical necessity, for instance.

medical savings account Allows a person to save pretax dollars to use for medical expenditures that are not covered by insurance.

Medicare Government insurance for everyone who has paid Social Security and is over the age of 65 and some disabled people.

meditation A way of being, a way of seeing, and even a way of loving.

menopause The period of permanent cessation of menstruation, usually occurring between the ages of 45 and 55.

meridians Unseen channels in the body in which qi energy circulates.

mesmerize Term stemming from Dr. Franz Anton Mesmer, who defined the discipline of hypnotism.

mesomorph Body type in which the appearance of the body is a natural, athletic physique.

metabolic rate The amount of energy liberated or expended in a given unit of time.

mindfulness meditation To become aware of your physical, emotional, and mental activities in the here and now.

misbranding To brand falsely or in a misleading way; to label in violation of statutory requirements.

modalities The application of therapeutic agents, usually physical therapeutic agents.

morbidity The proportion of sickness or of a specific disease in a geographic locality.

mortality The relative frequency of deaths in a specific population; death rate.

mother of tincture The homeopathic mixture first made from plants that is diluted in alcohol and left to sit for 2 to 4 weeks.

moxibustion The stimulation of an acupuncture point by burning herbs called moxa, which are placed at or near the point.

muscular dystrophy A genetic disease group that is characterized by progressive weakness and degeneration of the skeletal muscles that control movement. More than 30 genetic groups of muscular dystrophy have been identified. Depending on the genetic group, the disorders differ in terms of the which muscles are affected and the extent of the muscle weakness, the age of onset, and the rate of progression.

muqame makhssos Muslim massage pressure points.

N

nanotechnologies The study of the controlling of matter on an atomic and molecular scale. Generally nanotechnology (or nanotech) deals with structures that are 100 nanometers or smaller in at least one dimension, and involves developing materials or devices within that size.

NARB (National Advertising Review Board) A group of advertising professionals organized to self-regulate the advertising industry.

nasya Nose or sinus irrigation.

naturopath A practitioner trained in the field of naturopathy who uses holistic and natural healing techniques such as spinal mobilization/manipulation, stretching, and massage.

naturopathic A system or method of treating disease that employs no surgery or synthetic drugs but uses special diets, herbs, vitamins, massage, and the like to assist the natural healing processes.

naturopathic medicine A holistic, whole body health care system based on the belief that the body has the potential to heal itself and that the physician's role is to support the body's efforts. A system or method of treating disease that employs no surgery or synthetic drugs but uses special diets, herbs, vitamins, massage, and so on to assist the natural healing processes.

NCCAM (National Center for Complementary and Alternative Medicine) A center in the National Institutes of Health that conducts research to prove the effectiveness of complementary and alternative therapies.

needs assessment Investigation to determine health needs. May investigate at the community, county, state, or national level.

neo-dissociation model A model that suggests hypnosis activates a subsystem of both psychological and physiologic parts.

neti pot Used to give nose or sinus irrigation, usually using a mild salt solution.

noetic science The study of the mind and health healing. Noetic means the power of inner knowing, and is a branch of metaphysics.

nurse practitioner (NP) A registered nurse who has obtained advanced education and clinical training. Most obtain a master's or doctorate degree in nursing practice studies.

nutritional supplements Also called dietary supplements. Nutritional supplements are preparations that provide additional nutrients and may include vitamins, minerals or herbs.

O

objectivity in research Findings must not be biased by a researcher's personal beliefs, perceptions, biases, values, or emotions.

oncology The study of cancer.

organic Agriculture conducted according to certain standards, especially the use of only naturally produced fertilizers and nonchemical means of pest control.

orgone A vital, primal, nonmaterial element believed to permeate the universe.

Orgone Energy Accumulator A cabinet-like device constructed of layers of wood and other materials, claimed by its inventor, Wilhelm Reich, to restore orgone energy to persons sitting in it, thereby aiding in the cure of impotence, cancer, the common cold, and other ailments. Also called an orgone box.

orthodox medicine A system in which medical doctors and other health care professionals (such as nurses, pharmacists, and therapists) treat symptoms and diseases using drugs, radiation, or surgery. Also called allopathic medicine, biomedicine, conventional medicine, mainstream medicine, and Western medicine.

orthomolecular medicine Emphasizes supplementing the diet with mega doses of vitamins, minerals, enzymes, hormones, and amino acids.

osteoarthritis A type of arthritis of the joints that leads to joint pain, stiffness, and swelling.

osteopathic physician (DO) A traditional or orthodox physician who has similar training as a medical doctor but who has advanced studies in the interconnection of the muscles, bones, and nerves.

osteopathy A therapeutic system originally based on the premise that manipulation of the muscles and bones to promote structural integrity could restore or preserve health. Current osteopathic physicians use the diagnostic and therapeutic techniques of conventional medicine as well as manipulative measures.

P

panchakarma treatment Five types of cleansing therapy (vomiting, purging, colonic cleansing, nose and sinus cleansing, and blood detoxification).

parasympathetic nervous system Responsible for causing heart rate and breathing to slow down, blood vessels to dilate, and digestive juices to increase.

pathogen A disease-producing agent such as a virus, bacterium, or other microorganism.

pathology The science or the study of the origin, nature, and course of diseases.

pathya vyavastha treatment Use of diet and activity.

peer review A means to validate the study design, methodology, and results.

periodontitis Gum disease that begins when permeability of the mouth tissue permits pathogenic bacterial components to invade deeper periodontal connective tissues.

petrissage The act of kneading using the whole hand, with fingers together and thumbs outstretched so that the rounder contours of the body are squeezed.

pharmacopoeia A pharmaceutical book that contains a list of drugs, their formulas, methods for making medicinal preparations, requirements and tests for their strength and purity, and other related information.

physician assistant (PA) A professional who can provide many health care services and works under the guidance of a physician.

physiology The functions and activities of the body.

phytoestrogen Estrogen-like chemicals that can act like the hormone estrogen.

phytotherapy Plant therapy. Using botanical medicine to treat disease conditions.

placebo A substance having no pharmacological effect but administered as a control in testing experimentally or clinically the efficacy of a biologically active preparation.

plant coumarins Oral anticoagulants. Coumarin was isolated from the tonka bean (*Dipteryx odorata*), which is in a classification known as coumarou; thus, similar plants were named plant coumarins.

podiatrist A person qualified to diagnose and treat foot disorders.

prakriti Dosha balance.

prana Energy.

predictive science The researcher makes a guess or prediction about the research problem based on the probability that the prediction is accurate. The study tests the prediction using specialized statistical techniques.

pre-existing conditions Medical problems that an insured person already has prior to acquiring health insurance. Some pre-existing conditions are not covered by insurance.

preferred provider organizations (PPOs) Networks of physicians that work with an insurance company with a negotiated rate for services.

prevalence The total number of cases of a disease that is present in a particular population at a specific time.

primary beneficiaries Receive the death benefit upon the policy holder's death.

product claim advertising A form of DTC advertising that reveals the product name and full disclosure of the product uses and side effects.

psychic energy The concept of a principle of activity powering the operation of the mind, soul, or psyche.

pulse taking There are three types of pulses: snake pulse, which denotes vata dosha; frog pulse, which denotes pitta dosha; and swan pulse, which denotes kapha dosha.

purva-karma treatment Precleansing procedures before shodhanam or shamanam treatment. It involves snehan and swedan treatments.

putative A type of energy that has yet to be effectively measured by science.

putrid Having the odor of decaying flesh.

Q

qi In traditional Chinese culture, an active principle forming part of any living thing; frequently translated as "energy flow."

qi (chi) According to TCM, a bodily energy that flows through unseen channels in the body called meridians. Illness is believed to occur when qi is blocked.

qi gong A type of energy therapy that uses gentle movement to access and redistribute energy surrounding and within the human body. Incorporates posture, movement, breathing, meditation, visualization, and conscious intent in order to move qi energy throughout the body.

qi gong therapist Energy therapist who uses posture, exercise, breathing techniques, and meditation. According to Chinese philosophy, qi gong is used to enhance *qi*, the fundamental life energy responsible for health and vitality.

qualitative research Research that seeks to provide an understanding of human experiences, perceptions, motivations, intentions, and behaviors.

quack A person who admits, professionally or publicly, to skill, knowledge, or qualifications he or she does not possess.

quackery The practice of deceit or trickery specifically confined to the medical field.

quasi-experimental Comparison groups in a study are not randomly selected, and many things may cloud (or confound) the findings.

quinine A white, bitter, slightly water-soluble alkaloid, having needlelike crystals, obtained from cinchona bark. Used in medicine chiefly in the treatment of resistant forms of malaria.

R

radio frequency rhizotomy Application of heated radio frequency waves.

radionics A dowsing technique using a pendulum to detect energy fields emitted by all forms of matter.

raktamoksha Detoxifying the blood by bloodletting or using certain herbs.

rancid Having a bad smell or taste. Fats and oils when stale become spoiled or rancid.

randomized controlled study A study in which there are two groups: one is the treatment group and one is a control group who does not get the treatment to be tested. Participants are assigned to each group by a random draw.

redress To set right; to make up for; to remove the cause of (a grievance or complaint).

reflexology A form of massage that involves applying pressure to points on the feet, hands, and ears.

Reiki An energy therapy characterized by laying hands on an individual at specific locations, and the transfer of energy from the practitioner to the patient.

reliability The consistency of a measurement, or the degree to which an instrument measures the same way each time it is used under the same condition with the same subjects. In short, it is the repeatability of your measurement. It is important to remember that reliability is not measured, it is *estimated*.

reminder advertising A form of DTC marketing that only provides the product name, without including details about its use or side effects.

reputable Considered to be good or acceptable usage; standard.

Rescue Remedy Five Bach Remedy flowers that make up a formula to treat a crisis.

research design Divided into two main categories: experimental or quasi-experimental.

research questions Formulated to provide the basis for a research study. As a result of testing the research questions, hard facts will be discovered that help solve a problem, produce new research, add to theory, or improve services.

rheumatoid arthritis A chronic autoimmune disease characterized by inflammation of the joints, frequently accompanied by marked deformities, and ordinarily associated with manifestations of a general, or systemic, affliction.

rhythm and song methods of meditation A combination of rhythm, chanting, music, and breath used during meditation to achieve a desired state of calmness.

S

salicylates and salicins Aspirin-like compounds that have pain-relieving and anti-inflammatory action.

Salvia labandulaefolia Plant known as Spanish sage. Used for healing purposes.

saponins Glycosides or chemicals found in plants such as oats, vegetables, and beans that cause plants placed in water to "soap up," or froth to form a lather.

satvajaya treatment Use of mental hygiene/psychotherapy.

scam A confidence game or other fraudulent scheme, especially for making a quick profit.

seer Master of the healing tradition. A person who knows.

self-correcting research If results of a previous research study are later found to be false, the research should be conducted again so that the conclusions or results may be modified.

sensor technologies Devices such as a photoelectric cell that receives and responds to a signal or stimulus.

serotonin Levels of this chemical influence moods and behavior; low levels are associated with depression, headaches, and insomnia.

seven tissues (dhatu) Plasma, blood, muscle, lipid, bone, nervous system, and reproductive system.

shamanam treatment A balancing treatment.

shamanism An anthropological term referencing a range of beliefs and practices regarding communication with the spiritual world.

Sherley amendment The section of the Pure Food and Drugs Act specifically designed to limit the amount of time commercials can be shown during a television program.

shodhanam treatment A cleansing treatment using five procedures; called panchakarma treatment.

significance level The probability that the test statistic will reject the null hypothesis when the hypothesis is true.

silent mind meditation Technique involving directly perceiving and feeling the world around us by focusing on how we are thinking.

snehan treatment Internally it involves ingesting medicated edible oil or butter; externally it is medicated body massage.

social psychological model A model that suggests during hypnosis, an altered state of consciousness does not occur; instead, hypnosis is explained by suggestibility, positive attitudes, and expectations.

solvent extraction Process of washing blossoms with a solvent such as hexane to dissolve the nonaromatic waxes, pigments, and volatile aromatic molecules.

spam Unsolicited usually commercial e-mail sent to a large number of addresses.

spirituality An ultimate or immaterial reality; an inner path enabling a person to discover the essence of their being; or the "deepest values and meanings by which people live."

stagnate To stop developing, growing, progressing, or advancing.

State Children's Health Insurance Program Insurance offered to children whose parents do not qualify for Medicaid, but do not have health insurance.

subluxation Refers to one or more bones of the spine that have moved out of position and are causing pressure on or irritating spinal nerves.

subtle energy Generic term used to describe all energy not easily or readily categorized by modern science.

succussion Homeopathic mother of tincture solution that is further used to make different potencies by repeatedly diluting with water or alcohol and then vigorously shaking it.

Sufi dancing Said to be the dance of universal peace and is supposed to bring participants to a mystical experience and cultivate inner peace and harmony. The dance involves whirling by oneself or with partners. Dancers whirl with arms in various positions, such as reaching out and reaching to the heavens.

sweat lodge Used for a purification ceremony; a place built as a ceremonial sauna lodge.

swedan treatment Use of dry or wet fomentation or heat therapy to facilitate sweating.

sympathetic nervous system Responsible for the "fight-or-flight" response produced during times of stress.

T

tai chi A Chinese exercise system that uses slow, smooth body movements to achieve a state of relaxation of both body and mind.

Tamiflu An oral antiviral drug that attacks the influenza virus and prevents it spreading inside the body.

tannins Polyphenols obtained from various parts of plants. Found in tree bark, wood, fruit, leaves, and roots.

tapotement Massage that is given by tapping the body or face. It may be done by cupping, hacking, and pinching.

temporomandibular disorder (TMD) A condition characterized by pain and tenderness of the jaw when chewing and opening the mouth.

testimonial An advertising technique in which an individual client is used to share with consumers how a product or service worked for them.

therapeutic touch An energy therapy characterized by holding the hands several inches away from the patient, sending energy to the patient via the hands, in an effort to heal.

thought and laughter methods of meditation Using positive thinking, self-hypnosis, power of intention (strong thought), and even laughter to achieve the meditative state.

tonify Gentle stimulation of an acupuncture point

traditional Chinese herbal medicine (CHM) The study and use of plants for medicinal purposes.

traditional medical practitioner A medical doctor practicing under a Western, pharmaceutical-based philosophy.

transcendental Beyond common thought or experience; mystical or supernatural.

transcendental meditation A technique that is a simple, natural, effortless process practiced 15–20 minutes twice daily while sitting comfortably with eyes closed. The TM technique allows your mind to settle inward, beyond thought, to experience the silent reservoir of energy, creativity, and intelligence found within everyone—a natural state of restful alertness.

transcutaneous electrical nerve stimulation (TENS) Delivery of electrical stimulation through small electrodes placed inside an elastic-type belt.

tri-doshic Having fairly equal characteristics of vata, pitta, and kapha.

truth in advertising Laws designed to compel advertisers to give accurate, forthright information regarding products, services, and anticipated outcomes.

tuberculosis An infectious disease that may affect almost any tissue of the body, but especially the lungs. It is caused by the organism *Mycobacterium tuberculosis*, and is characterized by tubercles.

tuina A type of massage to stimulate or subdue qi energy in the body and bring the patient's body back into balance.

turmeric A plant that contains curcumin. Used for healing purposes.

U

ultrasound Use of deep heat by sound waves to treat muscle pain and spasms and to reduce swelling and inflammation.

universal polarity Concept of all energy being influenced and moved by opposing polar magnetism.

unruffling In Reiki, the process of smoothing out energy fields surrounding the patient.

urinary retention Involuntarily holding urine in the urinary bladder.

V

vacuum distillation A process to remove the alcohol and what is left behind to make a floral absolute.

validity The strength of conclusions, inferences, or propositions. Validity is the extent to which the test predicts the outcome it is supposed to predict.

VALS™ Marketing model used to design advertising to appeal to a particular group of consumers.

vamana Forced vomiting.

variable life insurance Uses part of the premium to purchase stocks, bonds, and mutual funds.

variable-universal life insurance Combines the best features of universal and variable life insurance.

veritable A form of energy that can be measured scientifically.

veterinary acupuncture Acupuncture used on animals to treat a variety of conditions (e.g., arthritis and hip problems, back pain and disc disease, incontinence and urinary retention).

vikruiti Dosha imbalance.

Vipassana Is known as insight meditation. Mindfulness is employed during meditation. Requires being watchful of your breath during inhalation and exhalation.

virechana Forced purging.

visceral organs Internal organs of the body, specifically those within the chest (as the heart or lungs) or abdomen.

visualization techniques Used to achieve a meditative state.

volatile oils Compounds of vegetable origin that evaporate at room temperature and allow us to enjoy the smell.

W

walking meditation Focuses on awareness of self, the process of walking, and the environment.

warranty A warranty is a written guarantee that a product is free of defects and that parts are expected to last and function for a specified period of time or the manufacturer will repair them at manufacturer's cost.

WHO AM I Focuses on negating the false self in order to realize one's true nature or enlightenment.

whole life insurance Offers a death benefit and a savings account.

World Health Organization The directing and coordinating authority for health within the United Nations system.

Y

yin-yang Two energies that control different bodily systems but cannot exist without each other.

yoga Requires full awareness of posture and movements. Attention is focused on the breath during all movements and helps open up the energy channels. Thought to be a powerful meditation technique.

Z

Zapper A machine created by Hulda Clark that delivers energy to the body in an effort to cure a myriad of illnesses and diseases.

zazen The breathing technique of Zen meditation, also known as the meditation of the Buddha. This involves awareness and concentration during the breathing process to help build or shape the mind and to free oneself from dualistic thinking (separation of mind and body).

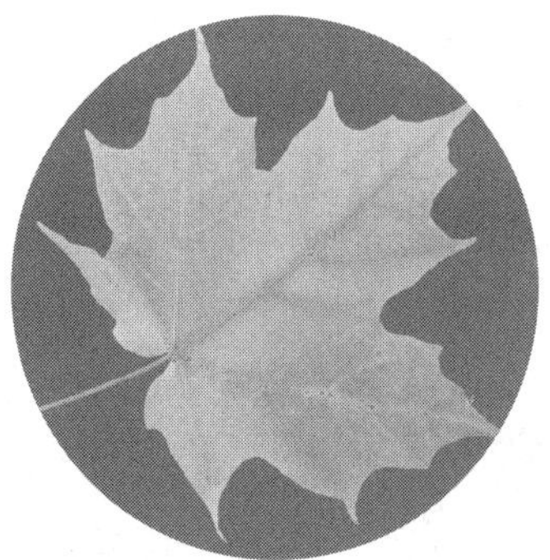

Index

Note: Italicized page locators indicate photos/illustrations; tables are indicated with *t*.

C

H

N

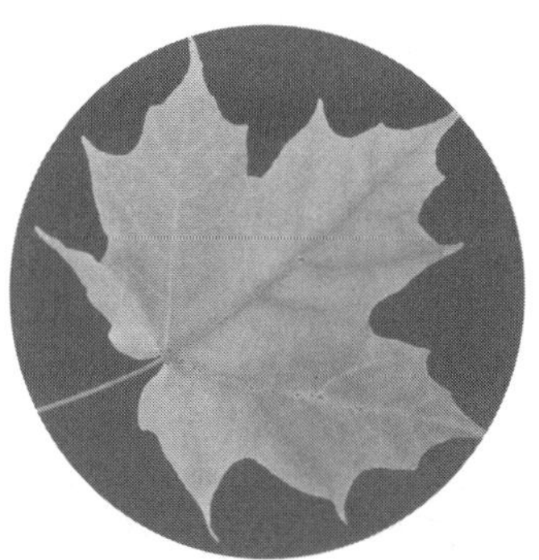

Photo Credits

Openers and features

Maple Leaf © AbleStock; Satellite © Sergei Chumakov/ShutterStock, Inc.; Magnifying glass © Denis Selivanov/ShutterStock, Inc.

Chapter 1

Courtesy of Renee Autrey; 1.2 Courtesy of Southeastern Louisiana University.

Chapter 2

2.1 © Dana Ward/ShutterStock, inc.

Chapter 6

6.1 © Suzanne Kreiter/The Boston Globe/Getty Images; 6.2 With permission from Dr. Bernard Siegel; 6.3 With permission from Dr. Andrew Weil; 6.4 © Diane Bondareff/AP Photos

Chapter 7

7.2 © Eduardo Rivero/ShutterStock, Inc.; 7.3 © Jeffrey T. Kreulen/ShutterStock, Inc.; 7.4 Courtesy or National Library of Medicine; 7.5 Courtesy of Library of Congress, Prints & Photographs Division [reproduction number LC-USZ62-5877].

Chapter 8

8.5 © Logical Images, Inc.; 8.6 © iStockphoto/Thinkstock; 8.7 © Anan Kaewkhammul/ShutterStock, Inc.

Chapter 9

9.2 © Roman Sotola/ShutterStock, Inc.; 9.3 (fire) © Wade H. Massie/ShutterStock, Inc.; (earth) © Ali Ender Birer/ShutterStock, Inc.; (metal) © K. Chelette/ShutterStock, Inc.; (water) © Jo Ann Snover/ShutterStock, Inc.; (wood) © Jonathan Wilson/ShutterStock, Inc.; 9.4 Courtesy of Dr. Steven Orloff, Traditional Healing Acupuncture Clinic; 9.5 © doglikehorse/ShutterStock, Inc. ; 9.6,9.7,9.8 Courtesy of Dr. Kenneth Chow; 9.9 © Chinese School/The Bridgeman Art Library/Getty Images; 9.10 © ARCO/Diez, O/age footstock; 9.11 © mikeledray/ShutterStock, Inc. ; 9.12 © Tyler Olson/Dreamstime.com

Chapter 10

10.1 © Scott Camazine/Alamy Images; 10.2 © Bernard Jensen International;

Chapter 11

11.1 © Andrei Rybachuk/ShutterStock, Inc.; 11.2 Courtesy of John Martin (http://www.geocities.com/herbalogic 2001/index.html); 11.3 © pinkannjoh/age footstock; 11.4 © iStockphoto/Thinkstock; 11.5 © FLPA/Keith Rushforth/age footstock; 11.6 © Siri Stafford/Lifesize/Thinkstock; 11.7 © iStockphoto/Thinkstock; 11.8 © sunsetman/ShutterStock, Inc. ; 11.9 © GFC Collection/age footstock; 11.10, 11.11 © iStockphoto/Thinkstock; 11.12 © TH Foto/age fotostock

Chapter 12

12.1 © James Wibberding/ShutterStock, Inc.; 12.2 © iStockphoto/Thinkstock; 12.3 © Sergey B. Nikolaev/ShutterStock, Inc.; 12.4 © Hemera/Thinkstock; 12.5 © Yehuda Boltshauser/ShutterStock, Inc.; 12.6 © iStockphoto/Thinkstock; 12.7 © Madlen/ShutterStock, Inc.; 12.8 © Tamara Kulikova/ShutterStock, Inc.; 12.9 © Pierre-Yves Babelon/ShutteStock, Inc.; 12.10 Courtesy of Nelsons; 12.11 © Kletr/ShutterStock, Inc.; 12.12 © Mauro Rodrigues/ShutterStock, Inc.; 12.13 © Garden Picture Library/age footstock; 12.14 © Hemera/Thinkstock; 12.15 © iStockphoto/Thinkstock; 12.16 © zuender/ShutterStock, Inc.;12.17 © iStockphoto/Thinkstock; 12.18 © odze/ShutterStock, Inc.; 12.19 © Jiri Sebesta/ShutterStock,

Inc.; 12.20 © iStockphoto/Thinkstock; 12.21 © kosam/ShutterStock, Inc.; 12.22 © Irineos Maliaris/ShutterStock, Inc.;12.23 © iStockphoto/Thinkstock; 12.24 © lafoto/ShutterStock, Inc.; 12.25 © Premaphotos/Alamy Images; 12.26 © Dale Wagler/ShutterStock, Inc. ; 12.27 © iStockphoto/Thinkstock; 12.28 © Henk Verbiesen/age foot-stock; 12.29 © Hemera/Thinkstock

Chapter 13

13.1 © Special Collections and College Archives, Palmer College of Chiropractic; 13.4 © Hemera/Thinkstock; 13.5 Courtesy of International Institute of Reflexology, www.reflexology-usa.net; 13.6 © Peter Gardiner/Photo Researchers, Inc.; 13.7 © Hywit Dimyadi/ShutterStock, Inc.

Chapter 14

14.2 © Motoyuki Kobayashi/Digital Vision/Thinkstock; 14.2 © Lakhesis/ShutterStock, Inc.; 14.3 © Paul Prescott/ShutterStock, Inc.; 14.4 © Hemera/Thinkstock; 14.5 © OSHO International Foundation, www.osho.com; 14.6 © Eliot Elisofon/Time Life Pictures/Getty Images; 14.7 © Matthew Naythons/Liaison/Getty Images; 14.8 © MedusArt/ShutterStock, Inc.; 14.9 © Markovka/ShutterStock, Inc.; 14.10 © grafvision/ShutterStock, Inc.; 14.11 © OtnaYdur/ShutterStock, Inc.; 14.12 © Sally and Richard Greenhill/Alamy Images; 14.13 Courtesy of National Library of Medicine; 14.14 Courtesy of Library of Congress, Prints & Photographs Division [reproduction number LC-USZ62-53514].

Chapter 15

15.2 © Daniela Illing/ShutterStock, Inc.; page 223 © Jupiterimages/Goodshoot/Thinkstock; page 225 Courtesy of Pumpkin Hollow Retreat Center; page 227 © Barry Mason/Alamy Images

Chapter 16

16.1 © Photos.com//Thinkstock; 16.2 FDA. This week in FDA History - Sept. 21, 1960. Available at http://www.fda.gov/AboutFDA/WhatWeDo/History/ThisWeek/ucm117863.htm. Accessed August 23, 2011.; page 235 © Yuri Gripas/Thomson Reuters; 16.4 © ajt/ShutterStock, Inc.; page 238 © Robert F. Bukaty/AP Photos

Chapter 18

Page 254 (left) © iofoto/ShutterStock, Inc.; (top right) © David Scheuber/ShutterStock, Inc.; (bottom right) © Monkey Business Images/Dreamstime.com; page 257 © Consumer Federation of America; page 260 © United States Consumer Product Safety Commission

Chapter 19

19.4 © R. Gino Santa Maria/ShutterStock, Inc.